PHARMACY PRACTICE TODAY
for THE PHARMACY TECHNICIAN

LiAnne C. Webster, PhTR, CPhT
Health Professions Administrator
Richland College
Dallas, Texas

ELSEVIER

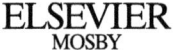

ELSEVIER
MOSBY

3251 Riverport Lane
St. Louis, Missouri 63043

PHARMACY PRACTICE TODAY FOR THE   ISBN: 978-0-323-07903-7
PHARMACY TECHNICIAN

Notices

Knowledge and best practice in this field are constantly changing. As new research and experience broaden our understanding, changes in research methods, professional practices, or medical treatment may become necessary.

Practitioners and researchers must always rely on their own experience and knowledge in evaluating and using any information, methods, compounds, or experiments described herein. In using such information or methods they should be mindful of their own safety and the safety of others, including parties for whom they have a professional responsibility.

With respect to any drug or pharmaceutical products identified, readers are advised to check the most current information provided (i) on procedures featured or (ii) by the manufacturer of each product to be administered, to verify the recommended dose or formula, the method and duration of administration, and contraindications. It is the responsibility of practitioners, relying on their own experience and knowledge of their patients, to make diagnoses, to determine dosages and the best treatment for each individual patient, and to take all appropriate safety precautions.

To the fullest extent of the law, neither the Publisher nor the authors, contributors, or editors, assume any liability for any injury and/or damage to persons or property as a matter of products liability, negligence or otherwise, or from any use or operation of any methods, products, instructions, or ideas contained in the material herein.

International Standard Book Number 978-0-323-07903-7

Vice President and Publisher: Andrew Allen
Executive Content Strategist: Jennifer Janson
Associate Content Development Specialist: Kate Gilliam
Associate Content Development Specialist: Elizabeth Bawden
Publishing Services Manager: Julie Eddy
Senior Project Manager: Rich Barber
Designer: Paula Catalano

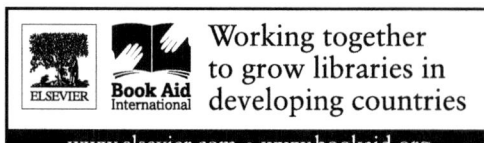

Contributors and Reviewers

Contributors

Mark Floyd, CPhT, CSO
Chief Executive Officer
EDGE Education Group Institute, Inc.
Dallas, Texas

Katrina Harper, PharmD, MBA
Medication Safety Officer
Parkland Health and Hospital System
Dallas, Texas

Rick Leyva
Pharmacy Math Instructor
Richland College
Dallas, Texas

Michelle D. Remmerden, RPT, CPhT, BS
Program Director—Pharmacy Technician
Everest University
Pompano Beach, Florida

Reviewers

Anthony Guerra, PharmD
Chair Pharmacy Technician Program
Des Moines Area Community College
Ankeny, Iowa

Becky Schonscheck, BS, CPhT
Home Office Program Manager – Pharmacy Technician
Anthem Education Group
Phoenix, Arizona

Bobbi Steelman, BS, MA, CPhT
Pharmacy Technician Program Director
Daymar Colleges Group
Bowling Green, Kentucky

Preface

Pharmacy Practice Today for the Pharmacy Technician gives students a road map that clearly outlines their role within practice sites and the rationale for medication therapy. It uses student-centered methodology to educate students in pharmacy technician training programs in all the knowledge, skills, and attitudes necessary to most effectively help pharmacists provide exemplary patient care. It provides the next generation of technicians with thought-provoking resources for how best to advance pharmacy technician practice and the profession of pharmacy as a whole.

ORGANIZATION

Pharmacy Practice Today for the Pharmacy Technician is separated into three units. Unit I, An Introduction to Pharmacy Practice, provides the basic foundation for understanding pharmacy practice. It includes content on pharmacy law, bioethics, professional organizations, and medical terminology. Unit II, Community Pharmacy Practice, discusses practice in the community pharmacy setting. It includes content on community pharmacy structure and workflow, professionalism, pharmacology, dose forms, pharmaceutical calculations, nonsterile compounding, billing and claims processing, infection control, materials management, and medication safety and error prevention. Unit III, Institutional Pharmacy Practice, is preparation for practice in an institutional setting. It includes content on institutional pharmacy structure and workflow, aseptic admixture and compounding sterile preparations, green pharmacy practice, career path overview, leadership and CQI process management, and certification review. Each chapter contains a list of basic terminology, a Chapter Summary, Review Questions, and Critical Thinking exercises.

LEARNING AIDS

A variety of pedagogical features are included in the book to aid in learning:
- **Learning Objectives** listed at the beginning of each chapter clearly outline what students are expected to learn from the chapter materials.
- A list of **Key Terms** follows the Learning Objectives and identifies new terminology and makes it easier for students to learn this new vocabulary; learning this new terminology is vital to success on the job.
- **Tech Alerts** are found in the margins of the text and alert the student to drug look-alike and sound-alike issues.
- Helpful **Tech Notes** are dispersed throughout the chapters and provide critical, need-to-know information regarding dispensing concerns and interesting points about pharmacology.
- A **Chapter Summary** is found at the end of each chapter and summarizes the key concepts in that chapter.
- **Review Questions** further enhance student review and retention of chapter content by testing them on the key content within the chapter.
- The **Technician's Corner** provides critical thinking exercises that help students prepare for on-the-job experiences by challenging them to pull together a collection of facts and information to reach a conclusion.
- The **Bibliography** provides a list of sources that students and instructors can use for additional information on the chapter's topic.

ANCILLARIES

FOR THE INSTRUCTOR

Evolve

Several assets are available on Evolve to aid instructors:
- **Test Bank:** An ExamView Test Bank with multiple-choice questions that feature rationales, cognitive levels, and page references to the text is included. This can be used as review in class or for test development.
- **PowerPoint presentations:** One PowerPoint presentation is included with each chapter; these can be used "as is" or as a template to prepare lectures.
- **Image Collection:** All the images from the book are available as JPGs and can be downloaded into PowerPoint presentations. They can be used during lectures to illustrate important concepts.
- **Text Answer Key:** All the answers to the Review Questions and Technician's Corner questions from the text are included.
- **Workbook Answer Key:** Answers to all Workbook exercises are included.
- **TEACH:** Including lesson plans and PowerPoint slides, all available via Evolve. TEACH provides instructors with customizable lesson plans and PowerPoints based on learning objectives. With these valuable resources, instructors will save valuable preparation time and create a learning environment that fully engages students in classroom preparation. The lesson plans are keyed by chapter and are divided into logical lessons to aid in classroom planning. In addition to the lesson plans, instructors will have unique lecture outlines in PowerPoint with talking points, thought-provoking questions, and unique ideas for lectures.

STUDENT WORKBOOK

FOR THE STUDENT

Several assets are available in the Workbook to aid students:
- Fill-in-the-Blank Exercises, Multiple Choice Questions, Matching Questions, and True/False Questions reinforce the concepts presented in the textbook.
- Internet Research Activities teach students how to keep current with an ever-changing industry.
- Critical Thinking Exercises help students apply the knowledge they learn in class to real-life scenarios, including testing knowledge of pharmacy calculations.

Acknowledgments and Dedication

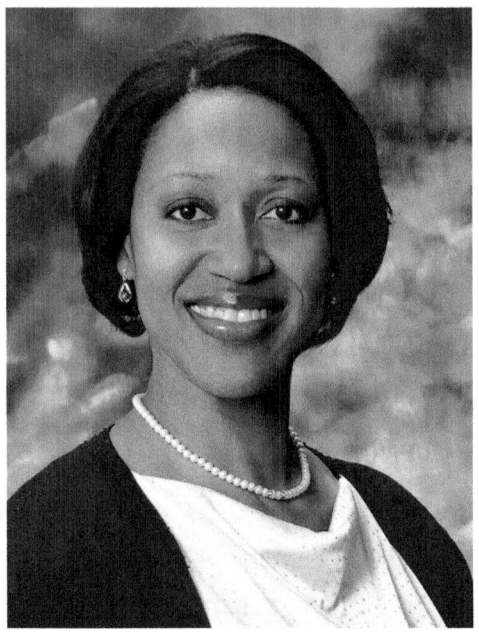

"In large part, we are teachers precisely because we remember what it was like to be a student. Someone inspired us. Someone influenced us. Or someone hurt us. And we've channeled that joy (or pain) into our own unique philosophies on life and learning and we're always looking for an opportunity to share them—with each other, our students, parents, or in our communities."

— Tucker Elliot

To the editors and staff of Elsevier Publishing, whose patience and fortitude guided me through this daunting process. Thank you for believing in this book. I appreciate your expertise and wisdom and for granting me this amazing opportunity to contribute meaningfully to the profession of pharmacy.

To my daughters, Chloe and Cassidy, whose unconditional love and undying sweet spirits carried me through many a sleepless night. I thank God for the gift that you are to me. Mommy loves you so much.

To my colleagues, Shannon Ydoyaga and Jamie Chaney. Without your support and assistance throughout the many challenges that I faced, the writing of this manuscript would not have been possible. My sincerest thanks!

"A good teacher is like a candle: it consumes itself to light the way for others." –Anonymous To my mate, partner, and kindred spirit, Nathan Brown: I am grateful for your inspiration, encouragement, love, and endless support throughout this journey, and in those to come. Thank you for always lighting my way.

To my soul sister, Kia. You have inspired and uplifted me with your grace, savvy, smarts, and loving nature. Love you forever.

To my sisters and dearest friends: Alicia, Danelle, Kathy, Carrie, and Liezel. Our shared laughter along with your encouragement and occasional push kept me going throughout this process.

To my Thunderduck Family at Richland College. Your collective wisdom, passion for teaching and students, and drive toward excellence inspired this project. I am honored and privileged to work with and around so many amazingly talented and genuinely good human beings.

LiAnne C. Webster, PhTR, CPhT

Table of Contents

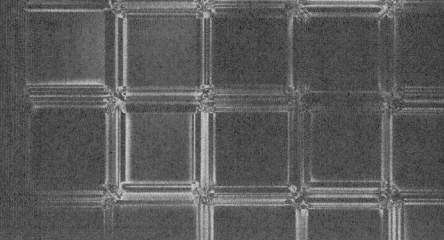

1 Historical Review of Pharmacy Practice

LEARNING OBJECTIVES

By the end of this chapter, students will be able to competently:

1. Discuss the formation of the modern practice of pharmacy, from the early mythos and practice of medicine in ancient cultures, in the following ways:

    a. Identify how each ancient culture contributed to how drugs are used, classified, and prepared.

    b. Examine key historical figures, and describe their contributions to the practice of medicine or pharmacy.

    c. Explain how the role of the pharmacist emerged.

2. Name each of the significant innovations in the twentieth century that revolutionized the use of anti-infective medications.

3. Describe twentieth-century pharmacy practice in the United States, citing how *patent medicines* were developed and their resulting influence on early American culture and the formation of federal drug laws.

4. Describe the pharmacist's role in modern medication therapy management.

5. Relate how pharmacy technician practice has evolved since the 1980s.

6. Define key terminology, and explain its historical relevance to the modern practice of medicine.

KEY TERMINOLOGY

Apothecary: A person who was specifically skilled in the art of preparing and packaging medicinal compounds; a pharmaceutical system of measurement for both solids and liquids. Also, another name for the druggist's shop, now commonly referred to as a pharmacy.

Ars medicina: Translated from Latin as "the art of healing"; the word *medicine* is derived from this expression.

Bodily humors: Elemental fluids of phlegm, yellow and black bile, and blood once thought to contribute to disease in the human body when out of balance.

Efficacy: The capacity or power to produce a desired effect.

Homeostasis: The tendency to maintain, or the maintenance of, normal, internal stability in an organism by coordinated responses of the organ systems that automatically compensate for environmental changes; balance.

Patent medicines: Drug compounds that were marketed and sold as "cure-alls," most which possessed little or no true medicinal value; often contained mostly water, in addition to a highly addictive ingredient such as opium or alcohol.

Pharmacognosy: The study of drugs derived from natural sources.

Pharmacopoeia: An established list of approved drugs and their uses, generally established by various nations.

Pharmakon: Translated from Greek as "drug," "medicine," or "poison," depending on the substance's effect on the human body.

Toxicology: The study of the nature, effects, detection, and treatment of poisons.

Wellness: A balance of health and absence of disease on the mutually equal planes of physical, emotional, and spiritual being.

1

An Introspective Look at History

The word *medicine* is derived from the Latin *ars medicina*, or "art of healing." Indeed, the practice of medicine, and more specifically pharmacy, is an art—one that has been crafted over thousands of years. The notion of healing takes on several interpretations. One's perception of healing is often influenced by culture, whether social, ethnic, or even out of one's personal life experiences. To be a *healer* is to embrace the responsibility of approaching each patient's condition—in light of a number of variables—and evaluate how best to restore and sustain health—physically, emotionally, and spiritually. It is interesting that individuals who choose to pursue some area of medicine often choose to do so out of a calling or desire to touch the life of some living creature and, through that touch, nurture them to a place of health and wellness. In approaching pharmacy practice, it is the responsibility of each practitioner to recognize his or her role in the healing of patients. It may appear that a pharmacy technician is further removed from a patient's wellness or disease management treatment plan than a physician, pharmacist, or other direct patient care provider. It is the hope and expectation of any pharmacy technician educator that students begin to fully recognize that pharmacy technicians provide a great deal of patient care, that significantly affects the health and wellness of the patients they serve.

Wellness is a balance of health and absence (or at least, well-controlled maintenance) of disease, on the mutually equal planes of physical, emotional, and spiritual being. Ancient cultures used medical techniques as a means to create or restore balance in the human body as they understood it. Examining the history of both the *art* and *science* of pharmacy practice is key to gaining a sense of purpose and perspective as a patient care provider. The Greek word *pharmakon* may be translated as both "medicine" and "poison." As history has proved, the practice of medicine and the use of drugs derived from various sources may certainly render both positive and negative effects on the human body. When a patient's treatment plan is devised, several patient-specific factors are considered in light of a variety of clinical treatment options and available drugs. Drug therapy must be carefully considered to render the greatest overall therapeutic benefit, in light of possible risks to the patient's health or other medical conditions. In other words, there must be *balance*.

Throughout the ages, the scientific practice of medicine was shaped by those who were considered the great minds of each period. What was evaluated and accepted as concrete truth was often later disproved, as the practice of medicine as an *evidence-based science* replaced practices that were based on folklore, myth, and mysticism. Interestingly, there are a number of plants and minerals that were widely used by common people—many of which have valid medicinal properties and are still in use today. Let's examine a timeline of historical events along with the error, genius, and accomplishments of several notable individuals. Their contributions helped to develop and shape the delicate balance we now know as modern medicine.

THE SPIRIT WORLD

In the earliest civilizations, including those of Mesopotamia (now Iraq), Egypt, and possibly India before 1500 B.C., illness and disease were attributed to evil spirits, or the supreme judgment or punishment of some god or celestial being. Religious belief, among other things, has been used to explain the unknown or unexplainable—which certainly applied to physical and mental illnesses. Priests, shamans (medicine men), and the like acted as physicians and performed rituals to rid the body of disease. The treatment of a disease was to purify a person's soul and, in so doing, his or her body. Realignment of spiritual well-being was thought to then bring realignment of the body as well. In addition, certain compounds were thought to contain mystical or magical powers that could cure a patient's illness. People from many cultures shared this belief, as reflected in a treatment once given to a European king in the Middle Ages. A concoction of crushed pearls and gemstones was mixed in a goblet of wine and given to the king. Although it likely rendered little more than royal stomach upset, such practices were accepted and quite common. Common people passed along folklore that detailed explanations for the outbreak of illness; shamans and other spiritual healers passed down to their apprentices the formulations for concoctions thought to have magical properties that would cure disease.

As the centuries passed, priests attended more specifically to patients' spiritual needs while physicians addressed physical needs. However, the accessibility of trained physicians, in addition to the

TECH NOTE!
Patient care providers should be knowledgeable concerning the religious belief system that is part of many world cultures and how those beliefs will influence a patient's ability and desire to be compliant—or follow through with—medical treatment or drug therapy.

expense of being under the care of a physician, led most common people to either seek out local healers or rely on natural remedies that had been passed down through generations.

THE GREAT MINDS OF ANCIENT GREECE AND ROME (500 B.C.-A.D. 500)

Hippocrates (500 B.C.)

Hippocrates, long referred to as the "father of modern medicine," was a physician and teacher. He taught other physicians on the Greek island of Cos, and he was among the first to approach medicine as a scientific, rather than mystical, process. Like many others during this period, Hippocrates believed that health was created and sustained when one was able to achieve a perfect homeostasis or balance. He, along with other Greeks and Romans of the time, believed that all things were tied to the forces of nature; all things could be broken down into four substances: earth, air, fire, and water. They further believed that those same forces existed in the body, in the form of four elemental fluids, or *humors*. Blood was the humor of air, associated with heat and moisture. Phlegm was the humor of water (as it was secreted from the nose or lungs), associated with moisture and cold. Black bile was the humor of earth, associated with cold and dryness, and yellow bile was the humor of fire, associated with heat and dryness. Based on a patient's condition, he and other physicians of his time might prescribe a treatment that would render an opposing reaction (e.g., therapeutic bleeding to counterbalance the heat of a fever from a patient's body), creating balance in the body. The Hippocratic method of healing was essentially to apply various medicinal compounds to treat patients, carefully monitor their responses to those medicines, and hypothesize about their benefits or side effects before considering other treatments.

Theophrastus (372-288 B.C.)

The philosopher and teacher Theophrastus was a student of Plato and friend of Aristotle and was an educated man in many subjects—including botany. Often referred to as the "father of botany," Theophrastus' written works concerning plants are the earliest of their kind in literature on the subject. Theophrastus, with the help of his students and explorers like Alexander the Great, gathered a great deal of knowledge concerning plants and their natural properties. Two of his greatest works are *Historia de Plantis* (History of Plants or Inquiring into Plants), and *De Causis Plantarums* (The Causes of Plants). His writings covered up to 550 species and varieties of plants. Many plants were cultivated in his botanic gardens at the Lyceum, which is considered by some to be the first botanic garden. They were acknowledged as the standard in the field of botany until the sixteenth century. The next historical figure was a known follower of the works of Theophrastus—a physician known as Dioscorides.

Pedanios Dioscorides (A.D. 1)

Nearly 600 years after the time of Hippocrates, the works of another Greek physician were making history far beyond the shores of the Roman Empire. Dioscorides was an expert on the use of drugs and had traveled to several lands in search of other medicinal products. During his travels throughout Northern Africa, the Middle East, and the Western European land of Gaul (present-day France), he observed the knowledge of physicians that had not been exposed to the Hippocratic methods of healing. After his travels, Dioscorides recorded all that he had learned in a lengthy essay called *De Materia Medica*, which is Latin for "The Materials of Medicine." In this work, Dioscorides described more than 800 plant, mineral, and animal drug sources. *De Materia Medica* cited information on how each was used, where to find them, and even which type of container was most appropriate for their storage and preservation. The significance of Dioscorides' writings is that they brought more organization to the practice of medicine and provided a more scientific basis for the use of various drugs. For this reason, he is often referred to as the "father of pharmacognosy," which is the study of drugs derived from natural sources.

Claudius Galen (A.D. 100)

The works of another Greek physician emerged nearly 100 years after Dioscorides. Galen lived and worked in Rome. His work helped to further organize the practice of medicine by assigning classifications to various drug compounds based on their effects on the bodily humors. Galen acted as his own pharmacist and was very skilled in the preparation of drug compounds that he found were best suited as remedies for different ailments. One of his greatest works is his book, *De Methodo Medendi,* which translates "On the Therapeutic Method." This work was published without changes or challenges until the sixteenth century, which suggests that his knowledge of both drugs and their preparation was far beyond his time.

THE GREAT FINDS OF AFRICA IN ANCIENT EGYPT (1500 B.C.)

Long before the practice of medicine was formally recorded, ancient physicians and folk healers used the elements of nature to help cure their ailments. On another continent and centuries away from the great minds of Greece, evidence has been uncovered that details the medical era and genius of ancient Egyptian physicians. It is a common notion that Egyptian culture was ahead of its time on a variety of levels, including mathematics, the arts, and architecture. The practice of medicine is no exception, as written documents demonstrate. Our knowledge of the ancient art of medicine in Egypt can be attributed to the finds of several nineteenth-century archeologists.

Although the field of archeology was for centuries tainted by greedy treasure hunters and grave robbers seeking only tangible treasures such as gold and jewels, several ancient texts have been recovered and restored that tell us about the practice of medicine in those times. These texts were written on scrolls of papyrus, and some are several feet in length. They served as both medical handbooks (as was translated in the Papyrus Hearst and the Berlin Papyrus), as well as to detail magical rituals conducted by priest-physicians of that time (as was translated in the London Papyrus). One of the most significant finds was the Ebers Papyrus (acquired by a German law student and ancient Egyptian historian Georg Ebers in the mid-1800s). The papyrus gave a detailed account of patients' histories as well as 877 formulas of remedies. Just as in Greek culture several centuries later, Egyptian culture blended the use of natural remedies with mystical folklore related to the origin of disease. These papyri, named after the archeologists or countries that discovered them, altogether record more than a thousand formulas and contain interesting treatments that are the historical basis for antibiotic therapy. One example was the application of moldy bread to treat an infection of the scalp. Unknown to these Egyptian priest-physicians, moldy bread contains the spores of fungi now known to kill a variety of disease-causing organisms.

THE MEDICINES OF MESOPOTAMIA (980 A.D.)

Babylonia was an ancient empire that existed in the Near East in southern Mesopotamia between the Tigris and the Euphrates Rivers. It was home to the ancient Sumerians, who recorded medical practices of their time. On the northern border of Babylonia was Assyria. Both before and after the fall of the Assyrian empire, there is evidence of advancements in medical training in Babylon. Medicine was expressed in both religious and scientific circles—and it was practiced by both physicians (the Asu) and exorcists (the Dsipu). Both referred to extensive texts that contained diagnostic data in which possible symptoms were listed, along with possible diagnoses, prognoses, and treatments.

Avicenna (circa A.D. 980)

The Persian-born Ibn Sina is a highly celebrated philosopher-physician whose contributions to medicine were esteemed on the same level as those of Hippocrates and Galen. In some texts, he is referred to as the "Persian Galen." His name translated in Latin is "Avicenna." He built up a reputation as a physician while still in his teens, but he pursued several other areas of science over the course of his career and life. The works of Avicenna greatly influenced Western medicine from the twelfth through sixteenth centuries. Avicenna is also credited with noting the relationship between emotions and the physical condition.

The most notable of his 16 medical works are the *Canon of Medicine* and *Book of Healing.* The *De materia medica* of the canon details information on more than 760 drugs, with comments on their application and effectiveness. As with all other great works, the canon also provided a clear and concise classification of all of the subject matter. These works not only collected the wealth of knowledge amassed in the preceding 1500 years, but they also stimulated physicians and teachers in Western Europe to pursue further research and medical discoveries.

SIGNIFICANT ADVANCES IN THE PRACTICE OF CHINESE MEDICINE

The earliest Chinese writings date back to the late Shang dynasty (1200 B.C.) and include records of illnesses, medicines, and treatment methods. The Chinese practice of *pharmacognosy* was demonstrated through the use of plant extracts for the treatment of several diseases, many of which have true medicinal value and are still in use today. There are many similarities in the development of medical knowledge in the East as compared to the West, and notable figures often used themselves as test subjects to measure various plants for medicinal properties. This accumulation of practical experience increased their understanding of what is now known as toxicology, or the study of the nature, effects, detection, and treatment of poisons. These pioneers were able to gain valuable knowledge concerning the toxicity and lethal dosage of herbal medicine. As in the West, disease was also often attributed to the mischief or anger of various gods or spirits, and many believed the appeasing of these spiritual entities might lead to restoration of health. According to a Chinese myth, malaria was caused by three demons that enjoyed plaguing humanity. Additionally, the notion of creating balance among the sources of energy in the body was (and continues to be) a major part of the belief system of Eastern medicine. For example, ancient charts show how the human body may be stimulated to interrupt or guide the body's energy flow, thus restoring balance and promoting wellness.

Emperor Shun Nung (A.D. 100)

Emperor Shun Nung is known as the "father of Chinese agriculture," as well as medicine. It is believed that he tasted hundreds of herbs to test their medicinal value. Although the true authorship is not entirely known, Shun-Nung is credited with writing *Shen-nung pen ts'ao ching* (Divine Husbandman's Materia Medica), which is the earliest Chinese pharmacopoeia. The text notes 365 medicines derived from plant, mineral, and animal sources. The great Chinese scholar T'ao Hung-Ching collected the fragmented records of Shen-Nung's Pen-T'sao, arranged them together, and included an additional 365 herbs that were in use at the time. He further divided the herbs into three classes, according to the duration that one would use them to treat various conditions or cure disease. He also classified herbs according to seven basic sources.

During the Ming Dynasty (1368-644 B.C.), Li Shih-chen wrote his *Pen ts'ao kang mu*, or *The Great Herbal*. It summarized knowledge of herbal medicine up to his time and gives a detailed description of the use and medicinal properties of more than 1800 plants, animal substances, minerals, and metals.

MATERIA MEDICA OVER THE PREVIOUS MILLENNIUM

Although the theory of balancing bodily humors was no more accurate than the notion of expelling disease-causing mystical forces, there was no way for people to recognize microorganisms as the cause of disease. This discovery came much later, with the invention of the microscope in 1590. Up to that point, however, people relied on the wealth of knowledge that had been gathered, as well as those traditional remedies that had been passed through generations. As civilizations rose (and fell), increasing populations within a particular area frequently created opportunities for the spread of infectious disease. The average human life span from prehistoric times through the 1800s was generally around 45. Other contributing factors included limited access to medical treatment, along with additional health risks associated with accepted remedies of the day. For example, people in villages usually relied on someone nearby who knew how to make simple remedies from indigenous (local) plants. But, as was also noted early on, *pharmakon* can be both poison and remedy, depending on the ingredients, their source, and preparation. Even treatments administered by physicians did not guarantee recovery from disease. Often, a patient had to survive the medical treatment itself, in addition to the disease! Therapeutic bleeding is a prime example. If a patient did not die from shock as a result of dramatic blood loss, secondary infections could be deadly (aside from whatever medical condition they were being treated for in the first place). The eras of human development, including ages of darkness as well as enlightenment, gave way to medical discovery as well as periods in which little discovery was made. During the Dark Ages of Western Europe, much of the known medical knowledge was either lost or hidden away. Medical minds in the East, however, kept hold of medical writings of the West, as well as new ideas and medicinal formulations. These concepts did eventually make their way westward, enabling a rejuvenation of the development of more advanced techniques in the practice of medicine.

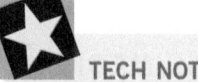 **TECH NOTE!**
Do you have an old family remedy that, although seemingly strange or unscientific, has been an accepted treatment for a particular illness or symptom? Consider some of the ingredients used, and conduct research on the medicinal properties of those components.

In spite of the period of ignorance, the Christian church is credited with keeping alive not only the body of knowledge of Western medicine that had been collected up to that point, but also the pursuit of knowledge and education. Often, priests, monks, and nuns were among the few at that time who could read and write. Much of the printed material related to medical practice was preserved and kept secure in monasteries and convents. Monasteries also served as gardens where medicinal herbs were cultivated—and there were generally a few monks or nuns who were skilled at preparing simple compounds. Examples of the medicinal plants include comfrey, belladonna, foxglove, garlic, and periwinkle. The poor, as well as travelers, could come to convents and monasteries and receive the treatment that they needed, without the expense normally associated with such care.

THE EMERGENCE OF THE APOTHECARY SHOP

As the knowledge of medicines had come to a stand-still until the end of the Dark Ages of Western Europe at the end of the eleventh century, Eastern medicine had made its way to the Western world. One of the greatest social effects of the Crusades was that crusaders brought back the knowledge (and some of the diseases) of the East. Much of the knowledge and drug preparation practices were based on the works of Avicenna, from the twelfth through the sixteenth centuries. The emergence of the druggist or apothecary—one who was specifically skilled in the art of the preparation and packaging of medicinal compounds—came out of the practices of Arab drug makers. Not only were they skilled in the preparation of herbal medicines, but they had also incorporated principles related to maintaining purity and an atmosphere of cleanliness as part of the drug preparation process. Advancements in Arabian medicine also included *alchemy*, an early form of chemistry that involved the process of cooking and combining raw materials into a final preparation. Textbooks in medical schools around Europe widely recognized Avicenna's work as the authority on the practice of medicine, and it became one of the main texts used for teaching medicine and pharmacy until almost the nineteenth century. Drug makers sought to gain power in their communities, and the pharmacists' guilds (formal associations for apothecaries, often in which payment was made in order to gain support and membership) were established in the twelfth century. Pharmacy had become a recognized profession, separate from that performed by physicians, surgeons, and other medical practitioners.

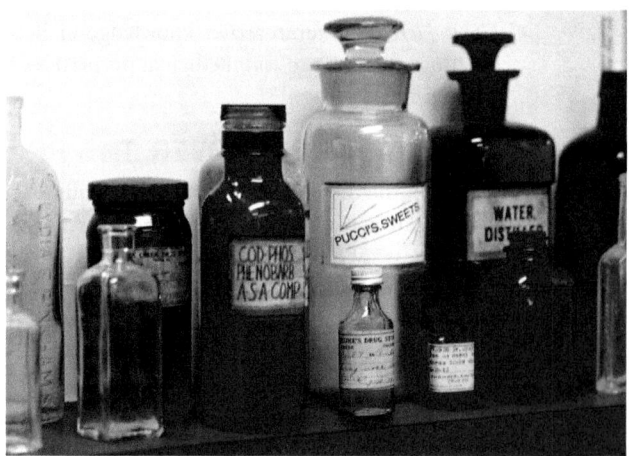

Medications were compounded by hand using a variety of compounds. (From Hopper T: *Mosby's pharmacy technician: principles and practice,* ed 3, Philadelphia, 2011, Saunders.)

The physical structure, content arrangement, weighing equipment, standards of cleanliness, and moral/ethical standards of the apothecary shop were all derived from those shops established by Arabian druggists. Each pharmacy stocked items that included those typically available by regional suppliers, in addition to items the apothecary grew in his own gardens. Apothecary shops also prepared drugs derived from "signed" plants, in which the shape of the plant was believed to be a sign of the body part it was designed to treat. For example, if a plant was kidney shaped, it was believed to have medicinal value in the treatment of kidney disease. Although many of these "signed" plants did possess true medicinal value, many did not—along with hundreds of other useless compounds kept on hand in apothecary shops of the Middle Ages.

As Western Europe moved into the Renaissance period (between the fourteenth and sixteenth centuries), apothecary shops became virtual works of art themselves—with elaborately decorated interiors as well as beautifully crafted drug cabinets and apothecary jars for holding various ingredients. The show globe, which is a beautifully crafted glass vessel filled with brightly colored liquids, became a universal symbol for the apothecary shop. Although it has been rumored that the colors displayed within the show globe were an indicator of disease in an area, the show globe was actually an early marketing tool. Apothecaries could demonstrate their skill with alchemy through the display of brightly colored chemical compounds. That show of skill set apart one apothecary from another in this fiercely competitive marketplace.

Little in the practice of pharmacy changed until the nineteenth century, as it was still unclear to both physicians and pharmacists what the true cause of disease was in the human body. As previously stated, physicians practiced medicine using the knowledge gathered over nearly two millennia, while much of what they considered to be true was not evidence-based nor pointed to microbial activity. Much of the groundbreaking discoveries that would forever change the practice of medicine did not occur until the nineteenth century.

FORMALIZING MODERN SCIENTIFIC PHARMACY PRACTICE

The method by which available drugs were cataloged and evaluated for medicinal efficacy changed as more scientific methods for determining the cause of disease emerged. Existing drugs in various countries were cataloged by name and used on a central compiled listed called a pharmacopoeia (pronounced "faŕ-ma-ka-pē'-a"). Although many pharmacopoeias distinguished drugs used in various international regions, many nations dissolved regional differences by consolidating to a single pharmacopoeia. The first United States Pharmacopoeia (U.S.P.) was published in 1820.

CONVERGENCE OF SCIENCE AND MODERN MEDICINE

Significant scientific discoveries revolutionized the practice of medicine in the nineteenth century. Thanks to the invention of the microscope in 1590, scientists could view organisms unseen by the naked eye, and they began the process of identifying those organisms and their physical characteristics. Most significantly, the discovery that these microorganisms caused human disease allowed the scientific community to make even more important discoveries. It was the French physician Louis Pasteur who confirmed through his "germ theory" that diseases were caused by microorganisms that released toxins in the human body or attacked organs or other anatomical structures. Louis Pasteur is also credited with the later discovery of vaccines for both anthrax and rabies. German bacteriologist Robert Koch expanded on Dr. Pasteur's work by developing an organic substance made of nutrient-rich seaweed gelatin known as agar, which would allow bacteria to survive outside a living body. His assistant, Julius Petri, designed special covered glass dishes that helped speed up the growth of the bacteria being examined and protected the user from unnecessary exposure. This innovation was quite successful, and Petri dishes have been used in laboratories ever since.

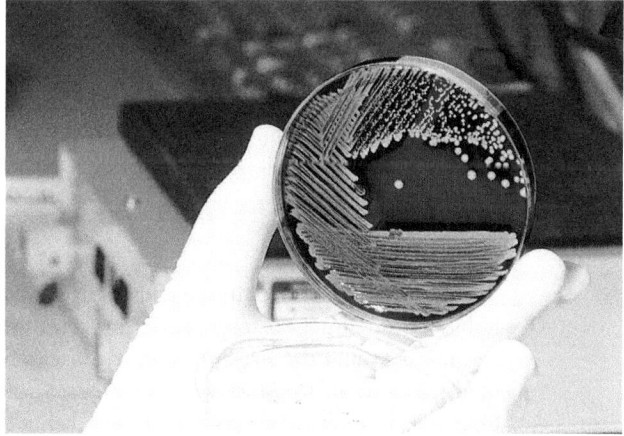

Petri dish growing *Staphylococcus aureus*. (From Gould B: *Pathophysiology for the health professions,* ed 4, Philadelphia, 2010, Saunders. In Stepp CA, Woods M: *Laboratory procedures for medical office personnel,* Philadelphia, 1998, Saunders.)

By the end of the 1890s, medical scientists had discovered a variety of viruses, mold spores, vitamin deficiencies, and other scientific bases for human disease. Though controversial, many of these scientific discoveries were made by identifying diseases infecting livestock, and antibacterial compounds (such as the mold spores from which penicillin is derived) were first successfully applied on animals before they were administered to a human being. Pharmacists now had the unique opportunity to dispense more exact quantities of drug needed to treat various bacterial infections, rather than large quantities of organic compounds with inconsistent therapeutic effects. The U.S. government also began instituting and enforcing laws that regulated the sale of microbes, viruses, and biologically produced medicines such as vaccines. The law required manufacturing plants to be licensed and inspected at will by the Public Health and Marine Hospital Service. The first such law was the Biologics Controls Act of 1902.

The Industrial Revolution gave way to mechanical methods of producing large quantities of drugs, and producing them in multiple dosage forms. Hand-operated machines could form and stamp out pills and even apply a sugar or gelatin coating. Although the concept of the formed pill was several thousand years old, the then-modern machine allowed these pills and capsules to be produced at a rate that far exceeded what a single pharmacist could produce.

ADVANCEMENTS IN PHARMACY EDUCATION

The education required to practice as a druggist or apothecary varied greatly from one country to another in the late eighteenth to the early nineteenth centuries. Whereas those who practiced in large cities typically completed at least 10 years of training, those apothecaries wishing to practice in small towns alternatively served a 6- or 7-year apprenticeship with a master apothecary before attempting to pass an examination given by a local board of physicians. In light of the onslaught of disease epidemics in the nineteenth century—including cholera, smallpox, typhoid, and yellow and scarlet fevers—the need for widespread infectious disease treatment increased. Disease was also spread during time of war; more battlefield casualties resulted from wound infection than from the wounds themselves. Because battlefield medicine was often prepared under hostile and unsanitary conditions, consistent drug purity and potency was a concern. The academic community eventually addressed the need for better-educated pharmacists. By 1820, universities in Europe and the United States were beginning to train pharmacists in the methods of what could be considered modern scientific pharmacy. Curricula focused on drug preparation and dispensing using proper forms. Newer concepts of chemistry, botany, and hygiene were also introduced.

In the United States, one needed only to apprentice with a master apothecary for a period of 6 months before he could be appointed as an apothecary and gather all of the necessary supplies and materials to open a new shop. It was not until 1804 that the state of Louisiana, under the direction of Governor William Claiborne, passed a law requiring a licensing examination for pharmacists wishing to practice their profession. The first pharmacist to pass the examination is said to have been Louis J. Dufilho, Jr. As a result, he is credited as the owner of the first true American apothecary shop.

Formal education in the United States began with the founding of the Philadelphia College of Pharmacy in 1821, followed by the Massachusetts College of Pharmacy in 1823 and the New York College of Pharmacy in 1829. The first organization founded to support the education and practice of pharmacists was the American Pharmaceutical Association in 1852, now known as the American Pharmacists Association. The value and benefit of membership in any number of pharmacy professional organizations will be noted in a later chapter.

TWENTIETH-CENTURY PHARMACY PRACTICE IN THE UNITED STATES

The practice of pharmacy in the United States resembled that of Western Europe, both in form and fashion. Early druggists were physicians, until the distinction between physicians and apothecaries was made around the sixteenth century. Just as in Europe, the artistic interior and exterior design of the American drugstore was consistent with trends that existed. The predecessor to modern drugstores like Walgreens, which was founded in 1901, was the American Soda Fountain. According to historical accounts, the early soda fountain was located inside drugstores. Fountain drinks were pleasantly flavored concoctions containing various drug extracts in carbonated water. The soda fountain provided a social atmosphere in which pharmacists could interact with their customers and build trusting and meaningful relationships. American drugstores also displayed show globes (which were electrified in the early 1900s), and American druggists were often able to market their alchemy skills through "secret" formulas of medicinal fountain drinks.

Many American druggists served fountain drinks that contained both caffeine and cocaine for the treatment of headaches. The use of stimulants was widely accepted at the time, and many were looked upon as safe and effective. However, with the enactment of the Harrison Narcotics Tax Act of 1914, the over-the-counter use of cocaine and opiates was officially banned in the United States. It is interesting that much of the legislation that relates to current pharmacy practice was enacted in large part because of the widespread domestic abuse of narcotics in the United States. This, and many other laws that regulate the practice of pharmacy, will be discussed in a later chapter.

THE EMERGENCE OF PATENT MEDICINES IN THE UNITED STATES

As had been the case in Europe, there was often limited accessibility of medical care, and many citizens relied on traditional remedies to treat their ailments. Because no one at that time really knew the true source of illness, it was difficult to judge whether many medicinal products actually produced the desired therapeutic effect. It was often more cost effective to seek out products that were thought to treat a variety of illnesses.

Many fell prey to the false claims of "miracle cures"—compounds that were sold by local peddlers and scam artists. They took advantage of the public's unawareness of the efficacy, or capacity to produce the stated or desired effect, of their products. These products were known as patent medicines. The name is derived from a practice in England in which manufacturers were, for a large fee to the king, awarded letters of patent that disallowed competing manufacturers from reproducing their products for a period of time. In contrast to many of the products dispensed by physicians, these patent medicines were pleasant tasting and were marketed using clever or misleading names and labels with pictures of attractive women.

Patent medicines made people feel better because many contained opium or alcohol mixed mostly in water. Sadly, consumers would rather quickly develop an addiction to the active ingredients, while whatever illness they were suffering from remained untreated. Patent medicines did not have to be safe or effective—as long as they were considered a new invention, the producer could market the product as a new drug. The first American patent drug was a product called bilious pills; its makers claimed that it cured a range of diseases, such as yellow fever, jaundice, dysentery, dropsy, and worms. Of course, bilious pills cured none of these illnesses, but that did not stop the public from purchasing them. The marketing of these products became quite a booming industry, both for those who made the products as well as those who sold advertisements for these products in local newspapers. Because anyone could advertise just about anything and advertise anywhere that the law permitted, there were no national or ethical guidelines for the content of these ads.

Traveling medicine shows became common practices among the creators of phony drugs, as a way to draw unsuspecting customers. Patent medicine salesmen would travel the countryside, stopping in every local village to set up a stage and "wow" the locals with dramatic stories of romance and adventure associated with the creation of their self-proclaimed *wonder drugs*. Although the art of medicine was rarely practiced, the art of deception was usually in play. Medicine shows hosted by traveling salesmen lasted into the twentieth century, until legislation was passed that either banned or restricted the sale of products without proven efficacy. Patent medicines began to disappear from the market with the enactment of the Pure Food and Drug Act of 1906, which required drug makers to label products with active ingredients as well as inactive ingredients such as coloring or flavors. The intent of the act was to prevent misbranded products from being exported out or imported into the United States. The act also served to prevent the sale of products containing hazardous or habit-forming substances such as alcohol, morphine, opium, chloroform, cannabis, or heroin. Inspectors could also test these products for the presence of dangerous or poisonous substances, such as arsenic.

Into the New Millennia

THE ROLE OF PHARMACISTS IN MEDICATION THERAPY MANAGEMENT

Although pharmacy practice has changed dramatically since the 1800s, the role of the pharmacist has evolved significantly only since the 1960s. Traditionally, physicians had been tasked with the role of diagnosing a patient, determining treatment, and prescribing medication if appropriate. The primary role of pharmacists was to use their skill as chemists to prepare medicinal compounds, dispense them to the patient, and answer any questions that the patient may have had about how to take the medicine. Only since the 1980s have pharmacists been more directly involved in making recommendations on the therapeutic appropriateness of various medicines. This new modern role is known as *medication therapy management.*

Pharmacists may now be found in any of the following pharmacy practice settings:
- Community (retail)
- Compounding
- Long-term care
- Home health
- Managed care
- Hospital
- Correctional facility (i.e., prison)
- Surgical center
- Nuclear medicine
- Oncology

Pharmacists are increasingly sought out as the primary authorities on medication therapy. As students will learn in later chapters, there are a variety of established pharmacy organizations that support the profession of pharmacy and establish standards of practice, regulate pharmacy education, and provide opportunities for pharmacists to further their clinical practice. Pharmacists may even pursue clinical specialties, such as internal medicine or cardiology. These new roles have increased the need for support staff to assist pharmacists, perform nonclinical functions, and increase pharmacists' capacity to engage in medication therapy management. These support staffers are often referred to as *pharmacy technicians.*

THE EMERGENCE OF PHARMACY TECHNICIAN PRACTICE

The pharmacist assistant title was first used in the United States Navy, as the pharmacist mate designation eventually referred to commissioned officers who had completed their education at a college or school of pharmacy. Whereas pharmacists traditionally performed all aspects of medication preparation and dispensing, many of these roles have been assumed by pharmacist assistants, or pharmacy technicians (some states do not recognize the designated title of *pharmacy technician*). Traditionally the role of the pharmacy technician had been limited to administrative roles, such as packaging, cashiering, and general upkeep of pharmacy areas. Pharmacy technician job responsibilities have increased to include cashiering, distributing medications, managing inventory, admixing IVs, and a variety of other nonclinical tasks, under the direction and supervision of a licensed pharmacist. Although pharmacy technicians in the military have been required to complete formal education for a number of years, there is not currently a national requirement for formal training in most U.S. states. As new drug products continue to flood the U.S. market, increasing the potential for medication errors, the need for better-trained pharmacy technicians, who are familiar with drug product names and strengths, becomes increasingly evident. Training for pharmacy technicians is frequently accomplished on the job, under the direction and supervision of a staff pharmacist, using standardized training materials and methods for assessing overall competence. Only since 1995 have pharmacy technicians been subject to a certification examination as a means of determining competence and the attainment of basic subject matter related to their jobs.

The advancement of the pharmacy technician practice has been challenged in part by the availability of training programs, as well as the costs involved. This is particularly true of pharmacy technicians who work in rural areas, where a training program may be many miles away. As the accessibility of formal training increases, the pharmacy profession will benefit from a greater number of better-educated and trained pharmacy technicians. Better-trained pharmacy technicians have a greater capacity to support and assist pharmacists, catch potential errors, provide high-quality customer service, and achieve career advancement within the profession. Just as the roles of pharmacists have evolved, so has the role of pharmacy technicians—who now have more opportunities to gain new skills. Many pharmacy professional organizations, some specifically for pharmacy technicians, also provide opportunities for pharmacy technicians to continue their education. Additionally, some pharmacies offer tuition reimbursement or scholarships to top-performing pharmacy technicians who wish to continue their education to become pharmacists.

In contrast to the evolution of the role of the pharmacist over thousands of years, the pharmacy technician practice has made great strides only since the 1990s. As the pharmacy technician career path continues to change, it is likely that more U.S. state boards of pharmacy will continue to evaluate the need for increased training requirements. A few other countries, such as the United Kingdom and Canada, have instituted a formal training and career path for pharmacy technicians, with favorable outcomes.

Chapter Summary

- In the earliest civilizations, illness and disease were attributed to the actions of spiritual or supreme beings.
- Eleventh century treatments by physicians were aggressive, painful, and often resulted in death.
- Crusaders returned with the medical knowledge of the East, much of which included the works of Avicenna.
- The practice of medicine included the emergence of the druggist or apothecary derived from the practice of Arab drug makers.
- Medicine also incorporated principles of maintaining product purity and an atmosphere of cleanliness as part of the drug preparation process.
- Works of Avicenna became the unchallenged basis for both medical practice manuals and textbooks at universities that educated pharmacists, until nearly the nineteenth century.
- Pharmacy became a recognized profession, separate from that of physicians, surgeons, and other medical practitioners.
- During the Renaissance period, the social focus on the arts transformed apothecary shops into elaborately decorated works of art.
- Physical structure, content arrangement, weighing equipment, standards of cleanliness, and moral/ethical standards derived from shops established by twelfth-century Arabian druggists.
- The art and beauty of the Renaissance period were expressed through the show globe, a universal symbol of pharmacy practice.
- In the eighteenth through early nineteenth centuries, physicians still practiced medicine based on the body of knowledge gathered over two millennia, as little was yet known of the true cause of disease in the human body.
- Germ theory: French physician Louis Pasteur confirmed that diseases were caused by microorganisms.
- German bacteriologist Robert Koch developed a laboratory growth medium, agar, that would allow bacteria to survive outside a living body.
- Prior to the eighteenth century, pharmacists living in large cities were educated in universities for at least 10 years prior to entering the profession.
- Disease epidemics evidenced the need for widespread infectious disease treatment, and concerns with battlefield medicine during time of war further evidenced the need for better education on the importance of a sanitary environment and the need to reduce the contamination of compounded medicines.
- By 1820, universities in Europe and the United States trained pharmacists in the methods of modern scientific pharmacy.
- Pharmacy practice in the United States, in form and fashion, resembled that in Western Europe.
- Distinctions between physicians and apothecaries were made around the sixteenth century.
- Louisiana passed first U.S. state law requiring a licensing examination for pharmacists in 1804.
- Formal education of pharmacists in the United States began with the founding of the Philadelphia College of Pharmacy in 1821.
- Soda fountains were a common service feature inside American drugstores, where many American druggists served fountain drinks that contained both caffeine and cocaine for the treatment of headaches.
- The use of stimulants was widely accepted until the later enactment of the Harrison Narcotics Tax Act of 1914.
- Patent medicines in the United States were often compounds formulated to contrast the unpleasant or unattainable medicinals prescribed by physicians.

- Medicine shows hosted by traveling salesmen lasted into the twentieth century, until the enactment of the Pure Food and Drug Act of 1906, which required drug makers to label their products with all ingredients, including the quantities of chemicals contained.
- Until the 1960s, physicians were considered the authority on medication therapy, whereas pharmacists were responsible for medication preparation and dispensing.
- Pharmacists now are increasingly sought out as the primary authorities on medication therapy and may also pursue clinical specialties, such as internal medicine or cardiology.
- Pharmacists are now found in a variety of pharmacy practice settings. These new roles for pharmacists have increased the need for support staff to perform nonclinical functions and increased pharmacists' capacity to engage medication therapy management.
- The job title and duties of the *pharmacist assistant* first emerged in the United States Navy.
- The pharmacy technician's job responsibilities have increased to include cashiering, distributing medications, managing inventory, admixing IVs, and a variety of other nonclinical tasks.
- In lieu of a formal training requirement, training for pharmacy technicians is frequently accomplished on the job, under the direction and supervision of a staff pharmacist.
- Since 1995, pharmacy technicians have been able to seek certification examination as a means of determining competence and the attainment of basic subject matter related to their jobs.
- More employers recognize the value of well-trained pharmacy technicians, in terms of greater capacity to support and assist pharmacists, catch potential errors, provide high-quality customer service, and achieve career advancement within the profession.

REVIEW QUESTIONS

Multiple Choice

1. Wellness is defined as:
   a. The study of drugs derived from natural sources
   b. The capacity of a drug to render a desired effect
   c. A balance of health and absence or maintenance of disease
   d. The tendency to maintain internal balance

2. These drug compounds had little or no medicinal value:
   a. Patent medicines
   b. Simples
   c. Compounds
   d. *Ars medicina*

3. A list of approved drugs and their uses is known as a:
   a. Pharmacognosy
   b. Pharmacopoeia
   c. Toxicology
   d. Materia medica

4. A pharmaceutical system of measurement of both solids and liquids is:
   a. Homeostasis
   b. Pharmacopoeia
   c. Materia medica
   d. Apothecary

5. The word *medicine* is derived from the Latin:
   a. Materia medica
   b. Apothecary
   c. *Ars medicina*
   d. Pharmacognosy

6. This is the study of the effects and treatment of poisons:
   a. Toxicology
   b. Pharmacognosy
   c. Pharmacology
   d. Apothecary

7. Historical finds that included various drugs derived from nature—along with their uses or how they were compounded—would be described as that culture's:
   a. Pharmacognosy
   b. Materia medica
   c. Efficacy
   d. Pharmakon

8. This historical figure is known as the "father of botany" because of his extensive travels and collection of various plant sources around the world:
   a. Hippocrates
   b. Galen
   c. Theophrastus
   d. Dioscorides

9. The first American College of Pharmacy was founded in:
   a. Philadelphia
   b. New York
   c. Chicago
   d. Dallas

10. This physician, known as the "father of Chinese medicine," is said to have personally tasted hundreds of organic substances to test their medicinal properties:
    a. Pen tsao
    b. Emperor Shen-nung
    c. Li Shih-chen
    d. Ibn Sina

TECHNICIAN'S CORNER

1. Describe at least one common thread in the development of the pharmacy practice among various cultures.
2. Although it was later disproved by scientific evidence, what was the value of Hippocrates' theory of homeostasis?
3. Explain one reason why laws were created in the United States concerning the labeling and sale of pharmaceuticals.

Bibliography

Ahmed, D.M. (1990). *Ibn Sina (Avicenna)—Doctor of Doctors*. Retrieved 3/29/2010, from www.ummah.com/history/scholars/ibn_sina Article originally appears in "Muslim Technologists" in November 1990, and was reproduced with permission on cited website.

Bottcher, H.M. (1964). *Wonder Drugs: A History of Antibiotics*. Philadelphia: Lippincott. Pages 36-43.

Encyclopaedia Iranica Online, volume 3. (1989). *Avicenna xiii. The Influence of Avicenna on Medical Studies in the West*. Retrieved 3/29/2010, from www.iranica.com/articles/avicenna-xiii

Facklam, M.A. (2004). *Modern Medicine: The Discovery and Development of Healing Drugs*. New York: Facts on File.

Helmuth, M., Boettcher, T.F. (1964). *Wonder Drugs: A History of Antibiotics*. Philadelphia: Lippincott.

Feng, M., Doherty, Y., Young, R. (2009). (Website updated in 2009 by Amanda Smith and Roxanne Beatty.) *Classics of Traditional Chinese Medicine*. Retrieved 4/1/2010, from History of Medicine Division–National Library of Medicine: http://www.nlm.nih.gov/exhibition/chinesemedicine Information on website derived from an exhibit of the National Library of Medicine.

Facklam, M.A., Facklam, H., Grady, S.M. (2004). *Modern Medicine: The Discovery and Development of Healing Drugs*. New York: Facts on File. Pages 6, 8, 9 (diagram), 10, 36.

Ohio State University. (2002). *History of Horticulture*. Retrieved 4/1/2010, from www.hcs.ohio-state.edu/hort/history/009.html

Ohio State University. (2002). *History of Horticulture.* Retrieved 4/1/2010, from http://www.hcs.ohio-state.edu/hort/history/023.html

Pure Food and Drug Act. (1906). United States Statutes at Large (59th Cong., Sess. I, Chp. 3915, p. 768-772; cited as 34 U.S. Stats. 768). Medicine in the Americas: Historical Works [Internet]. History of Medicine Division. Bethesda, Maryland: National Library of Medicine (U.S.) 2004. Retrieved 12/20/2012, from http://www.ncbi.nlm.nih.gov/books/NBK22116/

Wiedhopf, R.M. (2010). *Show Globes are Making a Comeback—But Where Did They Come From?* Retrieved 4/2/2010, from University of Arizona College of Pharmacy: http://www.pharmacy.arizona.edu/globes/php

Russell, R. (published date unknown). *Ancient Babylonia.* Retrieved 3/29/2010, from www.bible-history.com/babylonia/BabyloniaMedicine.htm

"Show Globes." Accessed 4/2/10. http://www.pharmacy.arizona.edu/visitors/pharmacy-museum/show-globes

Site Founded and directed by Subhuti Dharmanda, Ph.D. (n.d.). *Famous Doctors: Tao Hung-Ching (Tao Hongjing).* Retrieved 04/01/2010, from Institute for Traditional Medicine: http://www.itmonline.org/doc.taohung/htm

"Soda Fountains" derived from Drug Store Museum, sponsored by Soderlund Village Drug, 2004. http://www.drugstoremuseum.com/sections/level_info2.php?level_id=5&level=1. Accessed 4/28/2010.

Stroud, E.B., Higby, G. (1997). *The Inside Story of Medicines: A Symposium.* American Institute of the History of Pharmacy. Page 31.

Soderlund Village Drug. (2004). *Soda Fountains.* Retrieved 4/28/2010, from www.drugstoremuseum.com/sections/level_info2.php?level_id=5&level=1

Website sponsored by Soderlund Village Drug.

2

Pharmacy Law and State Boards of Pharmacy: Examining Regulatory Standards That Govern Pharmacy Practice

By the end of this chapter, students will be able to competently:
1. Define "law" and how laws impact pharmacy practice.
2. Explain the sources of United States law.
3. Describe, in detail, laws that impact the pharmacy practice.
4. Outline the drug approval process.
5. Discuss the trial process.

Administrative (or regulatory) law: Rules and regulations established by federal agencies with authority from Congress.

Civil liability: Involves conflicts between individuals or entities.

Common (or case) law: Law created based on previous court decisions.

Criminal liability: Results when "an individual commits an act that is considered to be an offense against society as a whole."

Defendant: A person or institution against whom an action is brought in a court of law; the person being sued or accused.

International law: Based on treaties and agreements between two or more countries.

Law: A binding custom or practice of a community; a rule of conduct or action prescribed or formally recognized as binding or enforced by a controlling authority. Another term for a law enacted by a legislature is a statute.

Legislature: An elected body of persons who enact laws.

Malfeasance: An instance in which a person commits an unlawful act.

MSDS: Material safety data sheets—contain information concerning the classification, safe handling, storage, and spill cleanup recommended by the manufacturer of a hazardous chemical substance.

Plaintiff: A person who brings an action (i.e., lawsuit) to a court of law; the person making the complaint.

Statute: An alternate term used to define law.

Statutory law: A body of laws enacted by a legislative body (Congress).

Tort: A civil wrong committed against a person or property.

Verdict: The findings of a jury on issues of fact submitted to it for decision; can be used in formulating a judgment.

Introduction

Law, as defined by the Merriam-Webster dictionary, is "a binding custom or practice of a community: a rule of conduct or action prescribed or formally recognized as binding or enforced by a controlling authority" (Merriam-Webster Online, 2010). Before there were laws established by governments, there were codes, pacts, and agreements among groups of people. These agreements established and defined the behaviors of that group that needed to be followed in order to sustain order within that community. They also served to establish and preserve justice and peace among the people. In the absence of law (or the truthful and fair governance of law), villages, cities, and nations suffer and sometimes fall. Human beings, from infancy, seek boundaries: a set of behaviors that will create a safe environment in which to learn, grow, and develop. History has shown that some laws are static—absolute, irrefutable—whereas others must evolve as the world and the people in it experience change. As human beings, we possess an inherent desire to examine law, to challenge its solidarity, to choose to adhere to it, or to reject it. Therein lies the human right of *choice*. Every choice that is made will render a result, whether positive or negative. Human choices may affect one, or many. All humans must choose, as part of their local and global community, their response to the established *binding customs* that have been instituted and enforced by the controlling authority over them. We, as citizens of a nation, may often disagree with established laws; those who live in a democratic society have the opportunity to express their viewpoints concerning the establishment of, or changes to, the laws of the land through formal or informal discussion forums and through the public vote. Ultimately, one of the roles of government is to pursue the welfare of its citizens and to seek their best interests, often when that is unclear.

As the history of the profession has shown, many principles or *laws* established concerning the practice of medicine have changed based on the traditions, beliefs, and practices of the societies that built them. Many ancient works concerning the medicinal qualities of organic substances have stood the test of time, whereas others have been disproved and replaced by scientific, evidence-based practices. When medicines or medical procedures were found to be a greater harm, rather than benefit, to the patient, those practices were banned or changed for the sake of the patient. Such is true concerning the use of various organic substances that were found to be poisonous or render long-term detrimental effects to the human body. To protect patients, laws have been established concerning the practice of medicine and the dispensing of pharmaceutical products. Because of the free market that exists in the United States, government must intervene in some key instances to regulate the market for the greater good of society—to the extent that failure to intervene would result in harm of the general public or availability of products and services that will protect and sustain public health. The U.S. government will generally intervene and regulate the free market for the following reasons:

- To create access to public goods that a private market might otherwise not provide to the entire population because of inherent risks or limited profit margins (example: requirements for the administration of vaccines for public health and the prevention of disease epidemics)
- To regulate the production or consumption of a product that inadvertently affects others in a fashion that they may not consent to (example: overuse of antibiotics by individuals without a prescription would result in higher resistance to antibiotics in the general population, so antibiotics are only available by prescription)
- To provide incentives to industries that produce a product that costs a great deal more to produce than to supply (such as public utilities like electricity or drugs that are needed by a relatively small population, which are very expensive to develop and produce)
- To require the distribution of information by experts concerning a product for which consumers typically would not possess the knowledge to assess the value and benefit on their own (example: required distribution of patient package inserts as well as drug information to health care providers); such a requirement increases the capacity of both the consumer and the industry experts to make more informed decisions

Standardized curricula have been created for use in colleges and schools of pharmacy and continues to evolve as patient care and biotechnology continue to advance. Pharmacy professional organizations were established, in part, to educate pharmacists using standardized models of practice. This ensured that every provider was empowered with the same basic body of knowledge, skills, and attitudes to best serve and protect the health and welfare of patients. A large part of that knowledge includes established laws that govern the profession. Upon completion of their education, pharmacists begin a process, established by federal law, through which they may obtain a license to practice.

The Bureau of Labor Statistics has noted the stringent requirements for a pharmacist to become licensed. First, pharmacy licensure requires obtaining a PharmD degree from an accredited college of pharmacy. In addition, all states, U.S. territories, and the District of Columbia require successful completion of the North American Pharmacist Licensure Exam (NAPLEX), which tests pharmacy skills and knowledge. Forty-four states and the District of Columbia also require successful completion of the Multistate Pharmacy Jurisprudence Exam (MPJE), which tests pharmacy law. The eight states and territories that don't require the MPJE require a pharmacy law exam specific to the laws of their jurisdiction. All jurisdictions also require a specific number of hours of experience in a practice setting for licensure. Some states also have age minimums, and many others require a criminal background check.

As you might have gathered, pharmacy law is strongly emphasized, and a pharmacy law exam must be passed, in addition to the general licensing exam, in order for a pharmacist to practice in the United States. Pharmacy law is also included on the certification exam for pharmacy technicians—because of its importance and how law defines pharmacy technician practice.

There are forums through which members of the pharmacy profession may discuss current practice standards and make suggestions for change. Pharmacists generally participate at both the state and national level (like a state pharmacy congress), whereas pharmacy technicians may typically voice their viewpoints at the state and local level. Pharmacy technicians should take advantage of every opportunity to voice their opinions, as a means to better educate pharmacists nationally concerning pharmacy technicians' abilities, needs, and concerns. Additionally, many pharmacy technicians entering practice today have transitioned from careers in other professions and may contribute positively and significantly to the profession through their past experiences.

Pharmacy laws were first enacted in the United States for a variety of reasons, but primarily for the safety and welfare of U.S. citizens. These laws were initially established to prevent the manufacture, sales, and distribution of products that were found to be unsafe or that did not yield the therapeutic benefit they claimed. Over the past century, several pharmacy laws have been enacted, and amended, to sustain the protection and welfare of U.S. citizens and their private health information. These laws cover a variety of areas concerning pharmaceutical products, including the following:

- Development, production, and marketing
- Dispensing and distribution processes
- Dispensing and distribution of controlled substances

Pharmacy practice law has been established in accordance with federal and state laws, so those who practice in the profession must adhere to all applicable laws. In addition to established law, there are also government-sanctioned or approved regulatory authorities, such as the *United States Pharmacopoeia* (USP) and *The Joint Commission* (TJC), whose established standards of practice are recognized *as though law* and must be adhered to accordingly.

It is important to both *know* the law and *understand how* it must be applied, given a variety of situations and often-complicated variables. This chapter discusses how and why each of these pharmacy laws was enacted, as well as how pharmacy technicians may apply each of these laws daily in their practice and support of their pharmacists. Students will review case studies to gain perspective on how many of these laws have been applied previously to various patient scenarios. Then comes *choice*. Every pharmacy technician should carefully examine every situation he or she encounters, in light of applicable laws, and *choose* the most appropriate response in order to maintain compliance with legal and regulatory standards. This choice is critical, even when the person involved may not understand or agree with the law or standard that applies. Just remember: the integrity and advancement of the profession of pharmacy technicians depends on it, as well as the health of patients. In the absence of adherence to law, our profession fails, and patient care suffers.

TECH NOTE!
Pharmacy technicians must ensure that they have a working knowledge of the laws and regulations that govern the practice of pharmacy so that they are able to avoid any behaviors or actions that would place them at risk for professional, civil, or criminal disciplinary action.

General Law Review

Author's Disclaimer:
The following information is intended to be a very general law review. The author of this textbook is neither a lawyer nor an expert on government affairs. There can be any number of exceptions to the information provided, particularly as pharmacy practice law varies by state—so this information is intended for educational purposes

only, rather than to serve as the final word on this subject. Students should seek professional legal advice concerning matters of law and legal liability. An excellent resource would include the website of the student's applicable state board of pharmacy, which details all state board rules and statutes that apply to pharmacy practice within that state. Many state boards of pharmacy have on staff code enforcement officers, or staff with a similar title, who are adept at explaining and interpreting that state's laws as it pertains to pharmacy technician and technician trainee practice.

SOURCES OF U.S. LAW

The United States Constitution is the supreme law, so any law that is in conflict with the Constitution is invalid. It was ratified (formally approved) by the Federal Convention in 1787, and the Bill of Rights was added in 1791. Since first enacted, only 16 amendments have been made to the U.S. Constitution. Specifically, the 10th Amendment gives individual states the power to legislate in all areas that do not come into conflict with the U.S. Constitution. A legislature is an elected body of persons who enact laws (also commonly referred to as statutes).

The types of laws that have been enacted for the governance of pharmacy practice would include the following:
- Statutory law: a body of laws enacted by a legislative body (Congress)
- Administrative (or regulatory) law: rules and regulations established by federal agencies with authority from Congress
- Common (or case) law: a law created based on previous court decisions
  - Most common type of case law involves a tort; a tort is a civil wrong committed against a person or property
  - A tort is the most common civil claim in medical law
- International law: based on treaties and agreements between two or more countries.
  - Defines the rules and principles that govern relations between those countries or nations, particularly related to the rights of their citizens

Federal Statutory and Administrative Law

Legislatures may create administrative agencies to implement desired changes in policies or to administer a body of substantive law when the legislature itself cannot perform these functions. Administrative agencies are given the authority to implement laws in which the legislature does not have the ability or the technical expertise to perform these functions. Administrative agencies that regulate the practice of pharmacy include the following:
- The Centers for Medicare and Medicaid Services (CMS), part of the Department of Health and Human Services (DHHS)
- The Food and Drug Administration (FDA), part of DHHS
- The Federal Trade Commission (FTC)
- The Drug Enforcement Administration (DEA), under the jurisdiction of the U.S. Justice Department

The role of each of these agencies in administering and enforcing federal law will be discussed later in this chapter.

State Statutory and Administrative Law

TECH NOTE!
Many state boards of pharmacy have also enacted rules for the regulation of pharmacy technician practice, although the education and practice standards of pharmacy technicians vary greatly from state to state.

On the state level, legislatures form individual state boards of pharmacy in order to monitor the activities of pharmacies and pharmacists on a routine basis. Additionally, many state boards of pharmacy have enacted rules for the regulation of pharmacy technician practice. Appendix A lists states that regulate pharmacy technician practice, along with details concerning requirements for certification, licensure, registration, and education requirements. Some state boards of pharmacy include a list of the roles and responsibilities legally performed by technicians within that state. Although there are well-established standards of education and definitions for pharmacists and pharmacy technicians, education and practice standards for pharmacy technicians vary greatly from state to state. In light of the advancement of the health, welfare, and safety of patients, the need for the proper education and training of pharmacy technicians has been a topic of great interest among state boards across the United States in recent years. A national education standard that clearly defines pharmacy technician practice, such as the American Society of Health-Systems Pharmacists

(ASHP) Model Curriculum, may create more uniformity in the training and skill development of pharmacy technicians in the United States.

Pharmacy laws were designed to shape the day-to-day activities of pharmacists and pharmacy technicians. The intent of pharmacy laws is to protect the health, welfare, and safety of the patient. Therefore, any behavior that would compromise the health, welfare, or safety of a patient is most likely not legal. Although various laws have been enacted, it is equally important that pharmacists and pharmacy technicians exercise sound professional judgment when making decisions and applying the law. As indicated earlier, pharmacy law has been enacted in accordance with both state and federal laws and must not conflict with either, thereby creating a law dilemma and applicable penalties for violation.

Social trends, manufacturing practices, disease epidemics, and several other factors that threatened or compromised the health, welfare, and safety of patients have been addressed at both the national and state level. Most pharmacy laws in place today were enacted during the early twentieth century. Let's examine a timeline of the enactment of pharmacy laws from the standpoint of these four key questions:

- What is the law?
- Why was it enacted?
- Whom did/does it affect?
- How does this law impact the pharmacy technician practice?

Pharmacy Law Timeline

THE PURE FOOD AND DRUG ACT OF 1906

What Is the Law?

This law prohibited the adulteration and misbranding of foods and drugs in interstate commerce. It was amended in 1912 to further prohibit false and fraudulent efficacy claims.

Why Was It Enacted?

This law was enacted to address rising concerns at the time over public health and safety because of unsanitary drug manufacturing practices, as well as poor or misleading labeling and branding of drug products. Adulteration could be defined as contamination by means of unsanitary manufacturing conditions or because of a dispensing container that was composed of or dyed with a poisonous or otherwise unsafe substance. Misbranding was, at that time, defined as labeling a drug with a treatment claim that was false or grossly overstated.

Whom Did It Affect?

The law was intended largely to discourage peddlers of *patent medicines* from marketing and selling drugs under false pretenses, as well as those that contained potentially harmful and habit-forming ingredients such as alcohol, cocaine, morphine, and opium. This law also served to advance the practices of legitimate apothecaries who used good manufacturing practices and appropriately labeled their products. The law did not render its full intended effect because manufacturers did not yet have to test products for toxicity or label medicines with all the ingredients. So although these laws may have led to the removal of false or misleading claims from the bottle label, the medicine itself might still contain poisonous or otherwise unsafe ingredients.

How Does This Law Impact Pharmacy Technician Practice?

This is one of the first federal drug laws and should remind pharmacy technicians of the dangers of unethical pharmacy practice. Because some supplements are labeled with claims that can often be confusing to patients, pharmacy technicians should always encourage patients to consult with pharmacists when making decisions concerning over-the-counter (OTC) supplement and OTC drug selections—particularly in consideration of prescription drugs they may be already taking.

THE FOOD, DRUG, AND COSMETIC ACT OF 1938

What Is the Law?

This law expanded the definition of the Pure Food and Drug Act (PFDA) to provide that no drug could be marketed until it had been proved to be both safe and efficacious. Interestingly, the act exempted drugs marketed prior to 1938. Drug labels were required to contain all ingredients, directions for use, and adequate warnings concerning ingredients that could be habit-forming. Later amendments of the Food, Drug, and Cosmetic Act (FDCA) allowed the FDA to require quality assurance certification testing on products that were batched (mass produced), specifically insulin and penicillin and other antibiotics (later overturned by the Food and Drug Administration Modernization Act of 1997). The FDCA also included the regulation of cosmetic products and medical devices for safety, purity, and good manufacturing practices.

Why Was It Enacted?

The FDCA was primarily enacted to correct the inadequacies of the PFDA and allow the FDA to inspect the warehouses of product manufacturers. The FDCA also gave the FDA the authority to inspect pharmacies, with or without advance notice or declared reason for inspection.

Whom Did It Affect?

The law primarily affected drug manufacturers and better protected the health and safety of consumers—who could make more informed decisions about what medications they wished to purchase from retailers, based on additional information provided on the product label.

How Does This Law Impact Pharmacy Technician Practice?

The FDCA is a current law that is still applicable to practice today. Pharmacy technicians may prepare medications in a community or institutional environment. They are required to complete documentation of all ingredients used in a compound and adhere to all applicable labeling requirements. Those who prepare patient labels must ensure that all necessary prescribing information has been accurately transcribed to the patient's dispensing label. Products that have been batch-prepared must contain all the necessary information as well.

THE DURHAM-HUMPHREY AMENDMENT OF 1951

What Is the Law?

The Durham-Humphrey Act was an amendment to the FDCA and required that all drugs be labeled with "adequate directions for use." The amendment established two classes of drugs: prescription and over the counter. The label of any prescription medicine was required to bear the legend "Caution: Federal law prohibits dispensing without a prescription." Transcribing the prescriber's directions for use by the patient satisfied the "adequate directions for use" provision. The expansive potential for the marketing and sale of over-the-counter brand and generic medications was not realized until years later.

This amendment also provided for the dispensing of medication via verbal order, as well as verbal or written authorization for drug refills. Refills might be authorized either in writing or per verbal order to the pharmacist if the physician found that (1) the drug dosing was appropriate for managing the patient's condition long-term and (2) the drug was safe enough for the patient to continue taking for an extended period of time without the need for monthly consultation.

Why Was It Enacted?

Prior to Durham-Humphrey, drug manufacturers generally determined whether their product was safe for self-administration by the patient, or if it should only be taken under the supervision of a physician. If the FDA disagreed with the manufacturer, the manufacturer could be cited for misbranding. In light of inconsistency among various manufacturers concerning the safety of various drugs for prescription or over-the-counter use, Durham-Humphrey helped to establish criteria for making that determination. Based on a drug's potential for toxicity or method of use, or if it was subject to the FDA's new drug application process, it would be classified as either prescription or OTC.

Whom Does It Affect?

This amendment provided for safer dispensing of drugs, particularly those that needed to be taken under the advice and supervision of a physician. It allowed patients to be dispensed refills on their prescriptions without having to return to their physician once their medication ran out.

How Does This Law Impact Pharmacy Technician Practice?

One of the most frequent tasks that technicians perform in retail practice is processing and filling prescription refills. During this process, there are opportunities for technicians to identify possible problems, such as multiple prescriptions for the same drug or same class of drug in the patient's file or multiple strengths of the same drug. Additionally, pharmacy technicians should be wary of the signs of possible prescription drug overuse/abuse by patients who routinely request refills on their controlled medications earlier than their prescribed days' supply would allow.

THE KEFAUVER-HARRIS AMENDMENT OF 1962

What Is the Law?

This amendment to the FDCA expanded the requirement that a drug must be proved to be not only safe but effective as well. The amendment, also referred to as the Drug Efficacy Amendment, reinforced the FDA's new drug approval process. Other provisions of Kefauver-Harris included the following:

- Transition of jurisdiction for prescription drug advertising from the Federal Trade Commission to the FDA
- Establishment of good manufacturing practices
- Addition of more extensive controls for clinical investigations by requiring the informed consent of research subjects and reporting of adverse reactions

Why Was It Enacted?

This amendment was enacted in response to an epidemic of birth defects involving thousands of newborns across Western Europe. The widely used sedative thalidomide was distributed in the United Kingdom and was pending FDA approval. Thanks to efforts of FDA medical officer Dr. Frances Kelsey, who was concerned about claims of serious birth defects resulting from mothers who had used this sleep aid during pregnancy, the drug was not allowed to be marketed in the United States, so the incidents of resulting birth defects were very low. The drug never gained FDA approval, and this amendment was enacted to ensure that appropriate research and clinical trials provided adequate documentation of every new drug's safety and efficacy.

Whom Did It Affect?

The FDA's response to the premature marketing of this popular but clinically untested product saved thousands of newborns in the United States from suffering horribly disfiguring and debilitating birth defects. This law also alerted drug manufacturers of the necessity of a broad scope of clinical trials prior to drug approval.

How Does This Law Impact Pharmacy Technician Practice?

Although pharmacy technicians may not legally counsel patients on the safe use of their prescription medication, they may certainly encourage patients to review the provided drug monographs, patient package inserts, and to inform their physician and pharmacist right away if they experience any adverse reactions to their medication. Although clinical trials are conducted for several years to identify as many adverse reactions to various drugs as possible, patients should always be informed and aware of their bodies' responses to medication.

THE POISON PREVENTION PACKAGING ACT OF 1970

What Is the Law?

The Poison Prevention Packaging Act (PPPA) defines hazardous household substances as "any substance that is customarily produced for or used in the household," specifically the following:

- A hazardous substance defined in the federal Hazardous Substances Act
- An economic poison under the federal Insecticide, Fungicide, and Rodenticide Act
- A food, drug or cosmetic under the FDCA
- A household fuel when stored in a portable container

The act requires the use of child-resistant containers for packaging most OTC drugs and nearly all prescription drugs. Containers must be manufactured such that at least 80% of children under the age of 5 cannot open them, whereas 90% of adults can. Patients, such as the elderly, may specifically request or have their prescriber request to have their medications dispensed in non-child-resistant containers. Generally patients must sign a statement attesting to that request and cannot make a blanket request for all non-child-resistant caps on their dispensing containers.

Why Was It Enacted?

This law was enacted primarily to educate consumers about the hazards of what were considered common "household" substances, which were often accidentally ingested by children. Clearly defining these substances, and providing information on how each should be labeled and stored, resulted in a significant decrease in the number of cases of accidental ingestion of poisons reported to the FDA. Regulation of the PPPA resided with the FDA until 1973, after which this responsibility was transferred to the Consumer Product Safety Commission (CPSC).

Whom Does It Affect?

To protect children and prevent the accidental ingestion of medication, pharmacies must dispense medication in containers that are child-resistant. Recognizing that elderly patients may have difficulty with child-resistant caps and containers, non-child-resistant packaging is available. Pharmacists must ensure that patients are aware of the risks of non-child-resistant containers and discourage their use in households in which small children reside.

How Does This Law Impact Pharmacy Technician Practice?

If a patient requests non-child-resistant caps and containers, pharmacy technicians who cashier and dispense these prescriptions must ensure that they educate patients on the risks. Pharmacy technicians must have patients sign any required documentation indicating that they have consented to non-child-resistant packaging.

THE OCCUPATIONAL SAFETY AND HEALTH ACT OF 1970

What Is the Law?

The Occupational Safety and Health Administration (OSHA) is a branch of the United States Department of Labor. OSHA is responsible for protecting workers against hazardous working conditions and issuing regulations to ensure safe work environments.

The Occupational Safety and Health Act of 1970 holds employers responsible for the following key tasks:

1. Ensure working conditions are appropriate for workers
2. Comply with standards related to their facility
3. Provide personal protective equipment when necessary for the safety of workers
4. Report employee work-related deaths properly (including heart attacks) within 8 hours, as well as work-related hospitalizations involving three or more workers
5. Communicate hazards on the job, including keeping a record of all non-consumer chemical products in the workplace
6. Post Material Data Safety Sheets (MSDS) in a place accessible to all employees

Why Was It Enacted?

This law was enacted to ensure safe working conditions by implementing regulations that protect the best interest of employees.

Whom Does It Affect?

The law affects every employee and employer that falls under OSHA's authority.

BOX 2-1   Required Information on a Material Safety Data Sheet (MSDS)

- Chemical and common names
- If a mixture, chemical and common names of ingredients
- Physical and chemical characteristics (flash point, vapor pressure)
- Physical hazards
- Health hazards, including signs and symptoms of exposure
- Routes of entry into the body
- OSHA permissible exposure limit (PEL)
- Precautions for safe handling and use
- Procedures for cleanup of spills and leaks
- Emergency and first aid procedures
- Date of preparation of MSDS or date of latest revision
- Name, address, and telephone number of manufacturer, importer, or distributor

How Does This Law Impact Pharmacy Technician Practice?

All pharmacists and pharmacy technicians must be aware of any workplace hazards that exist, how hazardous products must be stored, and any personal protective equipment that must be worn (e.g., gloves, gowns, head covers, face masks, shoe covers). Pharmacy technicians must be trained on how to protect themselves, other employees, and patients from exposure to hazardous substances found in their workplace. Every pharmacy employee should know the location of department MSDSs, as well as hazardous spill kits, eye wash stations, and where to locate all personal protective equipment. See Figure 2-1, a sample MSDS, that notes the type of required information about a hazardous substance, its properties, and instructions for safe handling. It is vital that pharmacy technicians pay close attention during the federally mandated safety training sessions, so that they will know their rights and responsibilities as they relate to workplace safety and the reporting of personal injury while on the job.

THE COMPREHENSIVE DRUG ABUSE PREVENTION AND CONTROL ACT OF 1970 (THE CONTROLLED SUBSTANCES ACT)

What Is the Law?

Prior to the Controlled Substances Act (CSA), several laws had been enacted to regulate the production, labeling, use, and distribution of habit-forming substances. The Harrison Narcotic Act of 1914 required controlled substances above a certain amount to be dispensed only with a prescription, and the pharmacy had to retain records of narcotics dispensed. In 1965, *Drug Abuse Control amendments* were enacted to deal with problems caused by the abuse of depressants, stimulants, and hallucinogens. The *Comprehensive Drug Abuse Prevention and Control Act* replaced previous laws and categorized drugs based on abuse and addiction potential compared to their therapeutic value. The CSA sets forth regulation of the manufacture, distribution, transfer, and dispensing of prescription narcotics and other substances that have been deemed controlled because of their abuse potential or high risk of diversion (theft) from the pharmacy. Drugs that have been controlled have been placed into five primary classifications, per the Drug Enforcement Agency. Table 2-1 details each of the DEA schedules, as well as examples of the types of drugs that fall into each category.

The CSA requires that any entity or person involved in the manufacture, distribution, dispensing, research/chemical analyses of controlled substances; a narcotic treatment program; or the import or export of controlled substances must apply for registration with the DEA. Any pharmacist who wishes to purchase, dispense, or transfer controlled substances via the DEA form 222 (Figure 2-2) must complete DEA form 224 and obtain a DEA number.

Why Was It Enacted?

The CSA was enacted to control the illicit sale, distribution, and use of controlled prescription drugs; to gather and maintain reliable data concerning the dispensing of controlled substances; and to allow for the inspection of controlled substance manufactures, distributors, and dispensers (pharmacies).

MATERIAL SAFETY DATA SHEET (MSDS)		
Date of Issue: 4/28/04		Date of Revision: 8/8/09

SECTION 1   IDENTIFICATION

GENERIC NAME: Glutaraldehyde	INFORMATION TELEPHONE NUMBER: 1 (800) 733-8690
BRAND NAME: Aldecide	EMERGENCY TELEPHONE NUMBER:
MANUFACTURER'S NAME: Brennan Corporation	1 (800) 331-0766
MFG. ADDRESS: P.O. Box 93	
CITY: Camden STATE: NJ ZIP: 08106	

SECTION 2   COMPOSITION OF INGREDIENTS

CAS NUMBER	CHEMICAL NAME OF INGREDIENTS	PERCENT	PEL	TLV
111-30-8	Glutaraldehyde	2.5	0.2 ppm	0.2 ppm
7732-18-5	Water	97.4	None	None
7632-00-0	Sodium Nitrite	<1	None	None

SECTION 3   PHYSICAL AND CHEMICAL PROPERTIES

BOILING POINT: 212° F	SPECIFIC GRAVITY (H_2O = 1): 1.004
VAPOR PRESSURE (mm Hg): 0.20 at 20° C	VAPOR DENSITY (AIR = 1): 1.1
ODOR: Sharp odor	pH: 7.5-8.5
SOLUBILITY IN WATER: Complete (100%)	MELTING POINT: n/a
APPEARANCE: Bluish-green liquid	FREEZING POINT: 32° F
EVAPORATION RATE: 0.98 (Water = 1)	ODOR THRESHOLD: 0.04 ppm

SECTION 4   FIRE AND EXPLOSION HAZARD DATA

FLASH POINT: Not flammable (aqueous solution)	NFPA Rating:
FLAMMABILITY LIMITS: LEL: n/a	Health: 2
EXTINGUISHING MEDIA: n/a (aqueous solution)	Flammability: 0
SPECIAL FIRE FIGHTING PROCEDURES: n/a	Reactivity: 0
UNUSUAL FIRE/EXPL HAZARDS: None	

SECTION 5   REACTIVITY DATA

STABILITY: Stable under recommended storage conditions.
CONDITIONS TO AVOID: Avoid direct sunlight and temperatures above 104° F (40° C).
INCOMPATIBILITY (MATERIAL TO AVOID): Strong acids and alkalines will neutralize active ingredient.
HAZARDOUS DECOMPOSITION BYPRODUCTS: None
HAZARDOUS POLYMERIZATION: Will not occur

FIGURE 2-1 Material safety data sheet. (From Bonewit-West K: *Clinical procedures for medical assistants*, ed 7, St. Louis, 2008, Saunders.)

Both the DEA and each individual state board of pharmacy may exercise the authority to inspect any pharmacy, with or without notice or cause. Inspections are typically conducted to randomly check compliance or to follow up on a formal complaint or suspicion of criminal activity.

Whom Does It Affect?

The CSA affects patients, as well as any person or entity that manufactures, distributes, or dispenses narcotics or other controlled substances. The DEA schedules provide prescribers with the

MATERIAL SAFETY DATA SHEET			
			PAGE 2

SECTION 6   HEALTH HAZARD DATA

ROUTE OF ENTRY: SKIN: yes	EYES: yes	INHALATION: yes	INGESTION: yes

SIGNS AND SYMPTOMS OF OVEREXPOSURE:

SKIN: Moderate irritation. May aggravate existing dermatitis.

EYES: Serious eye irritant. May cause irreversible damage which could permanently impair vision.

INHALATION: Vapors may be severely irritating and cause stinging sensations in the eyes, nose, throat, and lungs. May aggravate pre-existing asthma.

INGESTION: May cause irritation or chemical burns of the mouth, throat, esophagus, and stomach. May cause vomiting, diarrhea, epigastric distress, headache, dizziness, faintness, mental confusion, and general systemic illness.

CARCINOGENICITY DATA: NTP: No	AIRC: No	OSHA: No

SECTION 7   EMERGENCY FIRST AID PROCEDURES

SKIN: Wash skin with soap and water for 15 minutes. If skin redness or irritation persists, seek medical attention. Remove contaminated clothing and wash before reuse.

EYES: Immediately flush with water for 15 minutes. Seek medical attention.

INHALATION: Remove to fresh air. If irritation persists, seek medical attention.

INGESTION: Do not induce vomiting. Seek medical attention immediately. Call a physician or Poison Control Center.

SECTION 8   PRECAUTIONS FOR SAFE HANDLING AND USE

SPILL PROCEDURES: Ventilate area, wear protective gloves and eye gear. Wipe with sponge, mop, or towel. Flush with large quantities of water. Collect liquid and discard it.

WASTE DISPOSAL METHOD: Container must be triple rinsed and disposed of in accordance with federal, state, and/or local regulations. Used solution should be flushed thoroughly with water into sewage disposal system in accordance with federal, state, and/or local regulations.

PRECAUTIONS IN HANDLING AND STORAGE: Store in a cool, dry place (59-86° F) away from direct sunlight or sources of intense heat. Keep container tightly closed when not in use.

SECTION 9   CONTROL MEASURES

VENTILATION: Ensure adequate ventilation to maintain recommended exposed limit.

RESPIRATORY PROTECTION: None normally required for routine use.

SKIN PROTECTION: Wear chemical resistant protective gloves. Butyl rubber, nitrile rubber, polyethylene, or double-gloved latex.

EYE PROTECTION: Safety goggles or safety glasses

WORK/HYGIENE PRACTICES: Prompt rinsing of hands after contact. Handle in accordance with good personal hygiene and safety practices. These practices include avoiding unnecessary exposure.

FIGURE 2-1, cont'd

information they need to protect patients' health and welfare and make informed decisions related to the prescribing of controlled substances, in light of the abuse potential. The provisions of the CSA allow the DEA to better track prescription narcotic use, monitor the activity of controlled substance manufacturers, and ensure compliance by prescribers and dispensing pharmacists.

How Does This Law Impact Pharmacy Technician Practice?

Depending on the state, a pharmacy technician may serve as a narcotics technician under the supervision of a licensed pharmacist, in either community or institutional practice settings. Duties may include the preparation of controlled drugs for dispensing, perpetual inventory of controlled substances in stock, ordering of controlled substances, and daily record keeping. Pharmacy technicians

TABLE 2-1   **DEA Controlled Substance Schedules**

Schedule	Manufacturer's Label	Abuse Potential	Accepted Medical Use	Examples
Schedule I	C-I	Highest potential for abuse	For research only; must have a license to obtain; no accepted medical use in the United States	Heroin, lysergic acid, diethylamide (LSD), cocaine
Schedule II	C-II	Highest possibility of abuse, which can lead to severe psychological or physical dependence	Dispensing severely restricted; cannot be prescribed by telephone except in an emergency; no refills on prescription	Morphine, oxycodone, meperidine, hydromorphone, fentanyl, methylphenidate
Schedule III	C-III	Less potential for abuse and addiction than C-II	Prescription can be refilled up to five times within 6 months if authorized by a physician	Codeine with aspirin, codeine with acetaminophen, anabolic steroids
Schedule IV	C-IV	Lower abuse potential than C-II and C-III; associated with limited physical or psychological dependence	Same as Schedule III	Benzodiazepines, meprobamate, phenobarbital, carisoprodol
Schedule V	C-V	Lowest abuse potential, primarily antitussives	Some sold without a prescription depending on state law; purchaser must be over 18 and is required to sign log and show driver's license	Liquid codeine combination preparations

must maintain the highest level of moral and ethical conduct, carefully considering the consequences of violating federal law. To protect the profession of pharmacy, in consideration of prescription narcotics and drugs with a high risk of diversion, individuals who have a misdemeanor or felony conviction involving theft, drug use, or drug trafficking are generally disallowed from practicing by their state board of pharmacy.

THE DRUG LISTING ACT OF 1972
What Is the Law?

This amendment to the FDCA requires registered pharmacies to provide the FDA with a list of all drugs prepared for commercial distribution. The FDA compiles the data and publishes the drug information in the National Drug Code (NDC) Directory. Each drug listed in the directory is assigned a 10-digit number, called the NDC number, which identifies each product's labeler, product, and package size. See Figure 2-3 for a drug label showing an NDC number.

Why Was It Enacted?

This law enables the FDA to not only effectively track individuals engaging in the manufacture, preparation, propagation, compounding, or processing of drugs, but also to maintain an accurate database of current FDA products that have been assigned an NDC number.

Whom Does It Affect?

The law primarily impacts pharmaceutical manufacturers, distributors, wholesalers, and pharmacies.

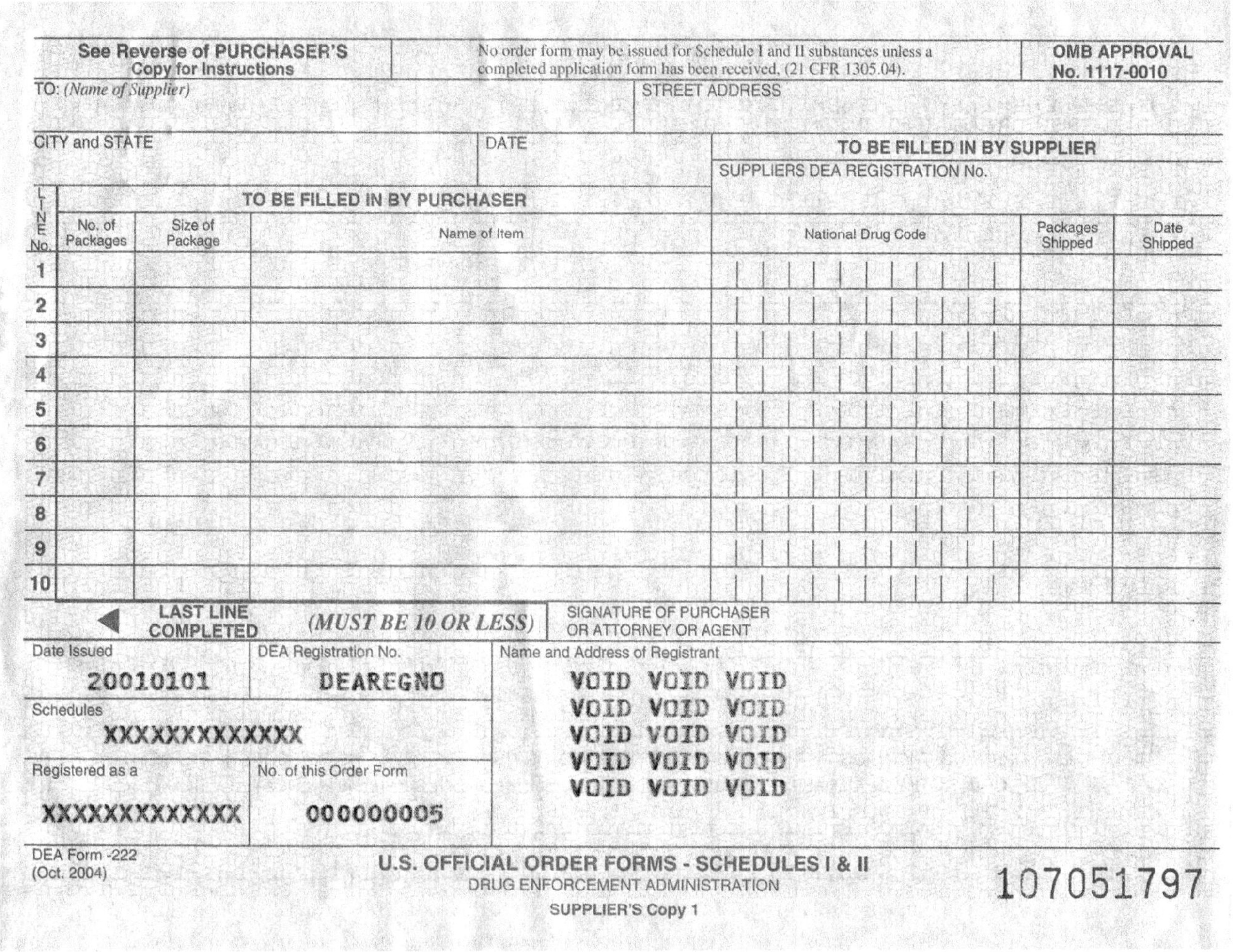

See Reverse of PURCHASER'S Copy for Instructions

No order form may be issued for Schedule I and II substances unless a completed application form has been received, (21 CFR 1305.04).

OMB APPROVAL No. 1117-0010

TO: *(Name of Supplier)*

STREET ADDRESS

CITY and STATE

DATE

TO BE FILLED IN BY SUPPLIER

SUPPLIERS DEA REGISTRATION No.

TO BE FILLED IN BY PURCHASER

LINE No.	No. of Packages	Size of Package	Name of Item	National Drug Code	Packages Shipped	Date Shipped
1						
2						
3						
4						
5						
6						
7						
8						
9						
10						

LAST LINE COMPLETED *(MUST BE 10 OR LESS)*

SIGNATURE OF PURCHASER OR ATTORNEY OR AGENT

Date Issued: 20010101

DEA Registration No.: DEAREGNO

Name and Address of Registrant: VOID VOID VOID VOID VOID VOID VOID VOID VOID VOID VOID VOID VOID VOID VOID

Schedules: XXXXXXXXXXXX

Registered as a: XXXXXXXXXXXX

No. of this Order Form: 000000005

DEA Form -222 (Oct. 2004)

U.S. OFFICIAL ORDER FORMS - SCHEDULES I & II

DRUG ENFORCEMENT ADMINISTRATION

SUPPLIER'S Copy 1

107051797

FIGURE 2-2 Drug Enforcement Administration Form 222. (From Hopper T: *Mosby's pharmacy technician: principles and practice,* ed 3, Philadelphia, 2011, Saunders.)

How Does This Law Impact Pharmacy Technician Practice?

Pharmacy technicians should familiarize themselves with the structure of the NDC number, particularly as technicians are commonly involved in the inventory management processes in both community and institutional pharmacy practice. Gaining familiarity with the labeler identification codes, as well as the package size identifiers, can be very useful when taking inventory and ordering drug supplies. Although every NDC number is unique to each product, and various package sizes between products, it is vital that pharmacy technicians check their prescription order entry and drug fills using multiple product identifiers, in addition to verifying the NDC.

THE ORPHAN DRUG ACT OF 1983

What Is The Law?

The Orphan Drug Act was enacted to encourage manufacturers to develop, research, and produce drugs that treat rare diseases (those that affect fewer than 200,000 people within the U.S. population). The act allows manufacturers a 7-year patent on drugs that receive FDA approval, during which time they may not be produced as generic products by other manufacturers. The law awards manufacturers of these products tax credits against the cost of clinical testing, and research grants.

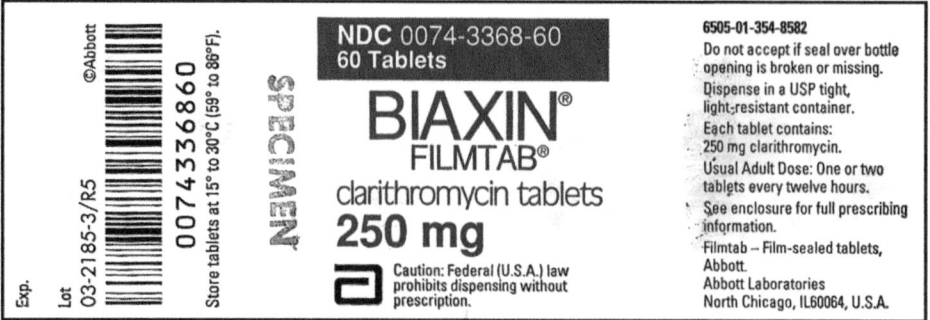

FIGURE 2-3 Drug label with NDC number. All NDCs are divided into three segments. (From Ogden SJ: *Calculation of drug dosages*, ed 8, St Louis, 2007, Mosby. In Hopper T: *Mosby's pharmacy technician: principles and practice,* ed 3, Philadelphia, 2011, Saunders.)

Why Was It Enacted?

The chapter introduction cited situations in which the U.S. government intervenes in a particular industry in order to better serve the health, welfare, and safety of its citizens, and offers incentives to companies that develop products that are more expensive to produce than to provide. The Orphan Drug Act is a great example of such an intervention. Because of the extremely high cost of research and development of drugs, treatment for a relatively small patient population would render such drugs unprofitable. The incentives offered to manufacturers to develop orphan drugs have stimulated ongoing research and subsequent production of such drugs for FDA approval.

Whom Does It Affect?

The Orphan Drug Act has positively served both patients with rare diseases and the pharmaceutical companies that produce the drugs used to treat them. In 2001, the U.S. Department of Health and Human Services Office of the Inspector General conducted an inspection and survey of the implementation of the Orphan Drug Act. According to the findings, the FDA has awarded more than 1000 Orphan Drug designations and has approved more than 200 new drugs. Additionally, the survey found that insurance companies generally pay for these treatments and many companies offer patient assistance programs to increase their accessibility.

How Does This Law Impact Pharmacy Technician Practice?

It is important for pharmacy technicians to recognize the positive impact that this law has had on the lives of patients who suffer from rare conditions. Because of the cost involved, it is important that care be taken during the handling of such products to avoid contamination or waste of such products, particularly as they would be ordered in limited supply.

THE DRUG PRICE COMPETITION AND PATENT-TERM RESTORATION ACT OF 1984

What Is The Law?

Also referred to as the Hatch-Waxman Amendment (U.S. Food and Drug Administration, 2009) to the FDCA, this law allows generic drug manufacturers to submit an abbreviated application for new drug approval (ANDA), without having to duplicate all of the clinical research, data, and trials that had been conducted initially by the manufacturer of the original "parent" drug during the full New Drug Approval (NDA). In the event that the parent drug company submitted a supplemental NDA for a new clinical indication (new therapeutic use for the drug), the company would be granted 3 years of market exclusivity on that new indication if it received FDA approval. This created controversy when generic drug makers could only label their generic products with the indications for which the parent drug did not have exclusive patent rights to—whereas the generic product could still be used for that clinical indication, as it was therapeutically equivalent to the drug that had gained FDA approval for that new use. In the same way, generic drug manufacturers could submit an NDA for a new clinical indication of a previously approved drug. If approved, the generic manufacturer would be granted the same 3-year term of market exclusivity.

Why Was It Enacted?

This law was enacted to allow for the expediting of ANDAs for generic drugs for which there were already clinical data on record providing their safety and efficacy. As many parent drug manufacturers did not wish to compromise the confidentiality of their clinical data, the FDA will accept clinical data that substantiated the approval of the parent drug, so long as the generic drug manufacturer can provide data that prove that the generic drug is bioavailable (renders the same mechanism of action physiologically), is bioequivalent (chemically identical) to the parent drug, and has a proven equivalent rate of absorption and effective drug concentrations in the body as the parent drug. The law also allowed drug companies, which had invested in great expense for clinical data to support an NDA for a new clinical indication, 3 years of market exclusivity to recoup their costs.

Whom Does It Affect?

This law primarily benefits the patient, who may take advantage of lower drug costs once drug patents expire and less expensive generic products become available. This law also benefits parent drug companies by allowing them market exclusivity whenever gaining approval for new clinical uses of existing drugs. Lastly, generic drug manufacturers benefit from the ANDA, as well as the possibility of their products being used to treat new clinical indications (even though their labeling cannot display those indications until after the expiration of the patent extension).

How Does This Law Impact Pharmacy Technician Practice?

This law may affect pharmacy technician practice from the standpoint of insurance claims billing. One of the most frequently performed tasks that the community pharmacy technician performs is the processing of third-party claims electronically to insurance companies. Although a drug may be legally substituted for another that is therapeutically equivalent, *insurance companies* may elect to pay benefits on a particular drug for specified clinical uses. Any other use not specifically named in their criteria (also referred to as an off-label use) may be rejected for payment. Pharmacy technicians must have an understanding of this process so that they may explain claim rejections to patients as well as refer these matters to a pharmacist when appropriate. The pharmacist may need to contact the patient's provider to make recommendations on alternative therapy or perhaps explain to the patient that only the brand name product (at the brand name price) may be filled, in order for their insurance to pay for the claim.

THE PRESCRIPTION DRUG MARKETING ACT OF 1987

What Is the Law?

This amendment to the FDCA provides the following:
- Restricts the import of U.S.–produced drugs that had been previously exported, except by the entity that had originally exported the drug
- Disallows the sale of drug samples or mass distribution of samples directly to patients, which are provided to health care providers for the sole purpose of marketing that product
- Requires wholesale drug distributors to reveal the manufacturer source information for the drugs they intend to distribute to pharmacies or sell to other drug distributors; drug manufacturers must retain, at their corporate headquarters, a list of authorized drug distributors with whom that manufacturer has established an ongoing relationship
- Disallows the sale of wholesale-priced pharmaceuticals by any entity other than those who have been identified by manufacturers as authorized distributors of their products

Why Was It Enacted?

This law was enacted due to the following problems identified by the Food and Drug Administration:

- Reimported drugs could not consistently be verified for the same level of purity and potency as when they had been exported and could be expired or have possibly been adulterated, which presented health risks to the U.S. population.
- Drug samples that were single-dose packaged for provision to patients by providers who wished to determine their efficacy versus other products were being resold to the public and presented health risks involving product expiration or contamination.
- "Submarket" distributors of pharmaceuticals often sought less-than-reputable sources for their products, and it was difficult to trace the sources of compromised products.
- Many pharmacies were investigated for reselling their wholesale-priced drugs to other pharmacies with a price markup, creating unfair competition with authorized drug distributors.

Whom Does It Affect?

This law primarily protects patients from receiving dispensed drugs that came from disreputable sources and could be unsafe for use/consumption. This law also protects manufacturers from being implicated in a lawsuit involving one of their products that may have been compromised by disreputable source, in or outside the United States, by ensuring that they only sell their products to distributors with a proven history of legal and ethical sales and marketing practices. This law also helps to prevent or subvert disreputable distributors from selling their products to pharmacies, as pharmacy entities may verify authorized distributors with drug manufacturers.

How Does This Law Impact Pharmacy Technician Practice?

In the state of Texas in particular, one of the main reasons why technicians lose their registration and ability to legally practice pharmacy is due to the illegal diversion of drugs. Make no mistake, if technicians steal drugs from the pharmacy, they will be caught, will be subject to disciplinary hearings by their state boards of pharmacy, and may be further subject to criminal prosecution. This is one more reason why it is so important that all those in the pharmacy profession exercise sound professional judgment.

THE OMNIBUS BUDGET RECONCILIATION ACT OF 1990 (OBRA '90)

What Is the Law?

This law was the first of its kind to regulate *how* the practice of pharmacy was best applied in terms of patient care—in contrast to the laws up to this point that primarily regulated drug manufacture, sales, and dispensing. OBRA '90 established a set of criteria that individual states were required to meet in order to participate in Medicaid. These criteria addressed three specific areas:

1. Rebates
   a. Pharmaceutical companies provide pharmaceuticals to Medicaid beneficiaries at their "best price."
   b. Manufacturers must pay Medicaid the difference between their lowest price that wholesalers pay, and the average manufacturer's price. So, if their lowest price for drug A was $15 per 100 tablets, and their average wholesale price was $25, the manufacturer would owe Medicaid a rebate amount of $10—thus ensuring that Medicaid always paid the lowest price for pharmaceuticals.
2. Demonstration projects
   a. OBRA '90 funds scientific studies to assess the degree to which patient care improves and health care costs decrease when pharmacists provide drug use review consultive services to patients.
   b. The demonstrative projects also analyze the overall effectiveness of online drug use review, in comparison to face-to-face consultation.
   c. The goal of such ongoing projects is to show that pharmacists can provide cost-effective services to patients, further positioning them within health care as the leading experts on medication therapy and possibly increasing the compensation that pharmacists may receive from government agencies for providing those consultive services.

3. Drug use review—process consists of three key components:
   a. Retrospective review
      i. A drug use review (DUR) board, composed of both physicians and pharmacists, reviews data concerning the long-term use of various medications—to evaluate if a drug's best therapeutic benefit is really gained by patients' overextended use (how does the ideal compare with the actual?).
      ii. Based on treatment plan variables, such as the dosage forms used, duration of therapy, and the effects of drugs being administered at the same time, the board determines if any adjustments could be made that would improve patients' benefit to that prescribed drug treatment.
      iii. Based on the recommended improvements, the DUR board may recommend educational programs be conducted.
   b. Educational programs
      i. These programs may be recommended for delivery to physicians or pharmacists.
      ii. Programs may be delivered via face-to-face consultations, live symposia (lectures), or printed materials delivered to the appropriate professionals.
      iii. Programs present the findings of the DUR board, along with targeted solutions and recommendations on how best to maximize the effectiveness of a specific or range of medication therapy regimen (scheduled treatment plan).
   c. Prospective review—consists of three key requirements:
      i. Screening prescriptions before dispensing: to determine therapeutic appropriateness, in light of known patient-specific variables (i.e., age, gender, ethnicity, health conditions, other medications being taken) for the prevention of possible problems or to make recommendations to the prescriber for a different course of medication therapy.
      ii. Patient counseling (Box 2-2): pharmacists must offer to discuss with each patient or caregiver topics that are pertinent, according to the pharmacist's professional judgment (2-2, which lists common topics that a pharmacist may, in his or her professional judgment, deem necessary to address with the patient or caregiver).
         1. While patients have the right to waive counseling, every effort should be made to offer such counseling, regardless of workload or other factors that would otherwise lead the patient or caregiver to feel that the pharmacist is too busy or unavailable to provide the required counseling.
      iii. Documenting information: OBRA '90 provides that pharmacists must make *a reasonable effort* to retain the following records regarding individuals receiving benefits, including the following:
         1. Name, address, contact phone number, date of birth, and gender
         2. Individual patient history, such as disease history, known allergies, drug reactions, and a comprehensive list of medications (including prescription, over-the-counter, and nutritional supplements) and medical devices being used
         3. Pharmacist comments relevant to the individual's drug therapy

Compliance with each of these measures should create a continuous cycle of medication therapy data collection, which may be reviewed by DUR boards, and recommendations on how best to

---

BOX 2-2   **Patient Counseling Topics per OBRA '90**

- Examples of patient counseling discussion topics for OBRA '90 compliance
- Name and description of the medication
- Dosage form, dosage, route of administration, and duration of drug therapy
- Special directions and precautions for preparation, administration, and use by the patient
- Common severe side effects, adverse effects, interactions, and therapeutic contraindications, including ways to prevent them and the action required if they do occur
- Techniques for self-monitoring drug therapy
- Proper storage
- Prescription refill information
- Action to be taken in the event of a missed dose

maximize treatment outcomes may be provided to the community of health care providers via educational programming.

Why Was It Enacted?

The primary goal of OBRA '90 was to reduce government Medicaid spending. In an effort to optimize government spending on health care, the U.S. government charged the profession with ensuring that physicians and pharmacists made the most appropriate decisions related to prescribing medication therapy, with the intended results of improving patients' therapy outcomes and reducing the costs of patients' health care resulting from inappropriate therapy.

Whom Does It Affect?

This law affects patients, physicians, and pharmacists and the states in which these professionals practice medicine. Each state must provide documentation of adherence to OBRA '90 in order to continue to participate in Medicaid. Patients gain the greatest benefit, as these measures increase the overall quality of medical care as well as provide increased safety and assurance that the medication therapy they have been prescribed is the most cost-effective and appropriate for managing their health issues.

How Does This Law Impact Pharmacy Technician Practice?

It was important to elaborate on the details of this comprehensive bill because of the number of factors that directly impact pharmacy technician practice. There is great value to a pharmacy technician's gaining a working knowledge of the drug use review process. Much of the information recorded by pharmacists for prospective order review is initially collected by pharmacy technicians! Part of the prescription intake process (which will be discussed in greater detail in a following chapter) is the patient interview. During this brief interview, the pharmacy technician should collect pertinent information, including the patient's name, date of birth, current contact information, known drug allergies or significant nonallergic reactions, and any medications or supplements that the patient is taking/using. This critical information allows the pharmacist to better assess the clinical appropriateness of the medications the patient has been prescribed, in light of those data. Further, pharmacy technicians *must* ensure that *every* patient is offered counseling—particularly if the patient is receiving a medication that she or he has never taken before or if a dose or dosing frequency has changed. Whereas pharmacists 50 years ago were the individuals who greeted patients initially and established professional rapport and trust with them, it is now the pharmacy technician who initiates that first contact. It is the *duty* of *every* pharmacy technician to guide and encourage patients to consult with their local medication therapy expert, to receive the information they need in order to safely administer their medication, to identify and prevent possible problems, and to gain the greatest benefit possible from their drug therapy.

THE DIETARY SUPPLEMENT HEALTH AND EDUCATION ACT OF 1994

What Is the Law?

This law requires the manufacturers of nutritional supplements to determine the safety of their products prior to marketing them to the public. Manufacturers of supplements are not required to register their products, although they must register under regulation requirements for manufacturers of food products for good manufacturing practices. The FDA will take action if a manufacturer is found to be unsafe, after it reaches the market, and monitors the safety of postmarket products as well, in terms of product information, voluntary self-reporting of adverse events, claims, and product literature. The Federal Trade Commission regulates dietary supplement advertising.

Why Was It Enacted?

Following the enactment of the Nutrition Labeling and Education Act of 1990, which mandated nutrition labeling on food products and authorized health claims on product labeling (the labeling had to be consistent with FDA guidelines), this law allowed for nutritional supplements to be regulated differently than foods. This allowed the manufacturers of nutritional supplements the freedom to test the safety of their products prior to marketing, without having to register their products with the FDA.

Whom Does It Affect?

This law primarily affected the manufacturers of nutritional supplements.

How Does This Law Impact Pharmacy Technician Practice?

Pharmacy technicians must recognize that the active ingredients of nutritional supplements may, and often do, produce medicinal-type effects in the human body. These products are not regulated by the FDA during the manufacturing process, and their potency can be inconsistent or varying (which is generally stated on the product packaging). Additionally, human clinical trials are not required to prove the safety and efficacy of these products. The medicinal properties of supplements may produce potentially harmful adverse effects when taken in combination with prescription or over-the-counter medication. For the health and safety of consumers, pharmacy technicians must encourage patients to disclose, during the patient interview, all products they may currently be using—including nutritional supplements.

THE HEALTH INSURANCE PORTABILITY AND ACCOUNTABILITY ACT OF 1996 (HIPAA)

What Is the Law?

HIPAA (not to be incorrectly abbreviated HIPPA!) regulation serves to "increase the portability and continuity of health insurance coverage and to prohibit discrimination in health coverage…[and] also regulates the privacy and security of health information." Portability, in terms of health care, may be defined as a "requirement that health plans guarantee continuous coverage without waiting periods for persons moving between plans. The ability for an individual to transfer from one health insurer to another health insurer with regard to pre-existing conditions or other risk factors" (Pohly, 2007). HIPAA defines those entities that must comply with these standards and generally applies to "health plans, health care clearinghouses, and health care providers that conduct financial or administrative transactions electronically."

HIPAA law regulates four major areas of health information:

1. Transaction and code sets

    Those who are required to comply with HIPAA must use a standardized set of codes, whether manual or electronic, for the transmission of health insurance claims and data processing. These standardized codes establish a more efficient means for the identification of patient conditions being treated, as well as standardized codes that identify the types of treatment received each date of service (DOS).

2. National provider entities

    All providers covered by HIPAA must apply to the U.S. Department of Health and Human Services (DHHS) for a National Provider Identifier (NPI), which must be consistently used during the compilation and transmission of claims and data processing.

3. Security

    a. In light of the modern use of electronic medical records, this provision requires the implementation of security safeguards that will protect the confidentiality, integrity, and availability of electronic health information.

    b. These security measures must effectively provide physical and technical safeguards that will protect the information from "unauthorized access, alteration, deletion, and transmission."

    c. Covered entities may establish their own security policies and measures, so long as they adhere to the regulations set forth in HIPAA.

4. Privacy

    a. Those defined as "covered entities" must ensure that they safeguard any information that may be defined as *protected health information* (PHI). Generally, PHI is any information related to the patient's past, present, or future mental or physical health, as well as financial information that is used for billing patients for services rendered. In a broad sense, any information that, if used alone or in combination with other patient identifiers, could positively identify the patient must be safeguarded. Box 2-3 lists each of the 18 items that are considered key patient identifiers that must be safeguarded. A pharmacy may provide only the minimum necessary information that is needed to accomplish the required objective.

BOX 2-3   **Key Patient Identifiers**

Names	Account numbers
Address	Certificate/license numbers
All dates, including date of birth, admission, discharge, deal, ages	Vehicle identifiers and serial numbers, license plate numbers
Phone numbers	Device identifiers and serial numbers
Fax numbers	Web universal resource locators (URLs)
E-mail addresses	Internet Protocol (IP) address numbers
Social Security numbers	Biometric identifiers (finger and voice prints)
Medical or financial record numbers	Full-face photographic images and comparable images
Health plan beneficiary numbers	Any other unique identifying number, characteristics, or codes

    b. The privacy rule allows pharmacies to disclose PHI for three purposes:
      i. Treatment
        1. Allows pharmacies to discuss a patient's PHI with other covered entities, including the patient's health care providers that are directly involved in the patient's care
      ii. Payment
        1. Allows pharmacies to use patients' PHI for the purposes of billing, determining patient eligibility for benefits, and extent of coverage
      iii. Operations
        1. Allows pharmacists to use patients' PHI for administrative functions, such as quality assessment, fraud detection, audits, certifications, and business management
        2. An example would be inclusion of patients' PHI related to their long-term medication therapy outcomes, for the purpose of data submission to a DUR board for review
      iv. Covered entities may also release PHI for government-related purposes, such as the following:
        1. Public health activities
        2. Judicial and administrative proceedings, pursuant to a court order or subpoena
        3. Law enforcement purposes
        4. Suspicion of serious threats to health or safety
        5. As required by law

Pharmacies must provide patients with a "Notice of Privacy Practices" upon initiation of any pharmacy services or retain documentation that the patient refused the notice. So although the privacy notice does not need to be distributed with every prescription, there must be documentation that the patient received the notice upon his or her initial setup and establishment as a customer of that entity. The notice must contain several items, including the following:

• How the pharmacy intends to use and disclose the information
• Summary description of how the pharmacy must legally protect the PHI
• A statement of the patient's rights and how a patient may exercise those rights
• A statement informing patients of their right to complain to the pharmacy or DHHS, and how that complaint may be filed
• A point of contact to which a patient may address any privacy concerns, including that person's name or title and telephone number

Patients must be aware of their rights to obtain, question, or dispute their health information. Pharmacists must fully disclose all PHI to patients during counseling and whenever the patient or designated agent requests. Some pharmacies may charge a small fee for the provision of copies of the patient's medical record, although a patient does not have the right to request to retain their original records. A patient's agent may also receive the full disclosure, whereas a pharmacist should certainly exercise sound professional judgment when determining what would be appropriate and in the best interests of the patient to share with the designated agent.

Pharmacies must ensure that they establish policies and procedures related to the implementation of HIPAA provisions, including actions to be taken against those who violate the policy. Pharmacies must additionally provide training to all new employees concerning their HIPAA policies and must retain documentation that this training was completed. Pharmacy students and pharmacy technician trainee students must also receive this training.

Why Was It Enacted?

This law was enacted as a result of serious abuses involving inappropriate disclosure of PHI for the purposes of target drug/device marketing, fraud, identity theft, inappropriate use by employers in making hiring/firing decisions, and other instances of criminal mischief.

Whom Does It Affect?

As a result, HIPAA ensures that the health information is secure and accessed only when appropriate. This law greatly affects patients and the safe and secure disclosure and transfer of their PHI. This act also impacts physician practices, hospitals, or any other entity that retains medical records, as it stipulates how those entities may handle the PHI contained therein and how and where they may be stored.

How Does This Law Impact Pharmacy Technician Practice?

Pharmacy technicians must ensure that they are aware of their legal responsibilities for adherence to HIPAA laws. They must use professional judgment and common sense when speaking to patients to ensure that PHI is not inadvertently disclosed to surrounding patients or customers. PHI should never be discussed by individuals not involved in a patient's treatment/services and should *never* be discussed in public areas, such as sitting rooms, break rooms, or public elevators. PHI should not be left exposed, whether in print or on a computer screen.

During dispensing, pharmacy technicians *must* ensure that they gain the signature of the patient or the patient's designated agent so that the pharmacy may retain documentation that this individual declared himself or herself as authorized to obtain the patient's medication and received disclosure of the patient's PHI. Pharmacists as well as technicians should exercise sound professional judgment in this instance and may deem it appropriate and in the patient's best interest (particularly if the information or medication is of a serious or sensitive nature) for the patient to pick up the medication in person or call the pharmacy to receive consultation.

THE ANABOLIC STEROIDS CONTROL ACT OF 2004

What Is the Law?

This act classified anabolic steroids as dangerous drugs and amended the CSA to name 59 substances as schedule III narcotics. To control the manufacture, distribution, and dispensing of these products, enforcement of this law is administered primarily by the DEA.

Why Was It Enacted?

This law is an amendment to the original Anabolic Steroids Control Act of 1990, which was enacted to formally identify this drug category and differentiate these products from less harmful over-the-counter nutritional supplements. Congress additionally hoped that this law would discourage these use of these potentially dangerous drugs by college, high school, and even middle school students. A report released by the National Institute of Drug Abuse (NIDA) in 1999 alarmingly reported that more than 500,000 8th and 10th grade students were using anabolic steroids. According to the DEA, "a Youth Risk Behavior Surveillance Survey conducted by The Centers for Disease Control and Prevention (CDC) indicated that in 2001, five percent of all high school students reported use of steroids pills/injections without a physician prescription during their lifetimes" (U.S. Drug Enforcement Administration, U.S. Department of Justice, 2004). Although safe use under the supervision of a physician does promote tissue regrowth and muscle growth for patients with degenerative diseases, prolonged use may render several life-threatening adverse effects. Reported health risks include "heart disease, liver cancer, depression, stunted growth, and eating disorders, not to mention increased episodes of hostility and aggression." Prolonged use of these products can also cause damage to sexual organs. Additionally, the growing concern over the abuse of anabolic steroids and other performance-enhancing drugs by professional athletics has led to a dangerous misconception by youth populations that use of these products does not pose any serious risks. Another concern is that, as many of these products are injected, sharing of needles may also present heightened risks of the transmission of blood-borne infectious diseases, such as hepatitis and HIV.

Whom Does It Affect?

Only practitioners are permitted to dispense substances considered to be anabolic steroids. Any person or agency that manufactures, distributes, dispenses, imports, exports, or researches these substances must have a schedule III registration. Manufacturers and importers must register with the DEA and can only distribute to other DEA registrants.

An intended outcome of this law is to educate and warn young people concerning the dangers and risks involved with the use of these products. Although some performance-enhancing drugs are still classified as over the counter and are widely available, the DEA continues to investigate these products and may expand the definition of these drugs to include any other products that are found to be unsafe.

How Does This Law Impact Pharmacy Technician Practice?

Pharmacy technicians need to be aware of the dangers of these drugs, both as consumers as well as part of the health care community. Use of these products outside of the careful supervision of a pharmacist or other DEA-registered provider presents serious health risks and should be avoided. Technicians in community and institutional practice should be further aware that diversion of these products for distribution or personal use may result in professional discipline, inability to practice pharmacy, and possibly subject offending persons to criminal prosecution (which may result in a felony drug conviction, which may carry penalties up to and including incarceration in a state or federal prison).

THE COMBAT METHAMPHETAMINE EPIDEMIC ACT OF 2005
What Is the Law?

Pseudoephedrine had been sold over the counter in unlimited quantities as a common decongestant until 2004. This drug has a high rate of diversion and use as a main ingredient in the preparation of methamphetamines, which are then illegally sold and used by drug abusers.

Congress passed the Combat Methamphetamine Epidemic Act (CMEA) in 2005 that implemented regulations on the manufacturing, law enforcement, and sale of pseudoephedrine. Each state follows its own regulations on how the drug is distributed, but most states now require a prescription or identification that is used for record keeping in order to obtain the drug.

Why Was It Enacted?

The production of methamphetamine had become a public health epidemic, leading to the need for government regulation of the substance.

Whom Does It Affect?

The CMEA impacts everyone from the consumer to the drug companies. Pseudoephedrine is a very popular and effective decongestant that has historically been sold OTC without restrictions. Patients are now required to seek out guidelines on how to obtain the drug if they have the symptoms that warrant its use. Drug companies that produce pseudoephedrine can experience negative financial impacts if the drug is not as accessible to consumers. Pharmacy staff must also be aware of the regulations of this substance in their state and how to handle dispensing in accordance with local and federal law.

How Does This Law Impact Pharmacy Technician Practice?

The pharmacy technician must know the specifics on how to handle the storage and distribution of pseudoephedrine. A few of the guidelines are as follows:

- Must be stored behind the counter in a locked cabinet
- A log book must document the customer and the amount of the drug being dispensed
- The maximum amount sold may not exceed 3.6 g in a calendar day or 7.5 g per 30 days
- Customers must provide photo identification in order to obtain drug

Each state has its own set of guidelines, and the pharmacy technician must be familiar with their state's regulations.

The New Drug Approval Process: A Closer Look

This chapter has addressed several laws that pertain to the drug approval process, as outlined in the FDCA. In the United States, no drug may be marketed unless an application has been approved. The FDA has established a process whereby drug manufacturers may seek to gain FDA approval of a new drug for which they have gathered clinical data to show its safety and efficacy for use in humans. Manufacturers may submit NDAs for newly developed drugs or for previously approved drugs that contain a new ingredient, are a new combination of previously approved drugs, have been tested for a new intended use, or for a drug in which the dosage, method, or duration of administration has been changed. When a drug has been proved safe in clinical trials on animals, human subject testing may begin. To obtain approval from the FDA, a drug manufacturer must apply for an investigational exemption for a new drug, which is also referred to as an investigational new drug application, or IND. If approved, the manufacturer may proceed with gathering clinical test subjects. The IND application must include the following data:

- Drug name
- Chemical composition
- Methods of manufacture and quality controls
- Data from laboratory and animal investigations regarding the pharmacological (how the drug's chemical composition and properties are applied to various diseases of the body), pharmacokinetics (how the drug is absorbed, distributed, metabolized, and eliminated from the body), and toxicological (potential for toxic or poisonous effects) evaluations

The NDA data collection is conducted as a four-phase process. The FDCA requires that manufacturers secure informed consent for each human subject who has volunteered to participate in the study. The informed consent document must cite all known possible risks, benefits, and alternative courses of treatment. The study must take place in a controlled institutional (hospital) setting. The local institutional review board (IRB) must approve the study, and the IRB committee must review any of the research projects that are conducted on the human subjects. Informed consent must be in writing for all human subjects during phases 1 and 2, whereas consent may be verbal for phase 3 if the attending physician determines medical necessity. Patient consent may not be required if consent cannot be feasibly gained from the patient or a representative or if the attending physician determines that informed consent may not be in the best interest of the patient.

Phase 1: The primary purpose is to determine any possible adverse effects of the drug being tested. The drug is tested on a small group of healthy, disease-free human subjects, and investigators document the drug's effects on the test subjects in terms of the drug's toxicity, metabolism, bioavailability, elimination, and other pharmacological actions. The dosing is administered at a low level then gradually increased. If the drug passes phase 1, then phase 2 begins.

Phase 2: The primary purpose is to test the drug for efficacy with test subjects who have the disease or clinical symptoms as the drug's intended use. Clinical data are collected to measure the drug's safety and efficacy at the manufacturer's recommended dose level for the intended use. If the drug passes phase 2, then phase 3 begins.

Phase 3: This phase allows for mass testing of the drug with hundreds or thousands of patients in a variety of clinical settings. The studies are double-blinded (neither the patient nor the physician knows if the patient is receiving the actual drug or a nondrug placebo, like a sugar pill) and compared with a control group that receives a placebo.

Phase 4: Final Approval: The FDA officially has 180 days to begin review of an NDA. If the NDA is not approved, the manufacturer may request a hearing, although none has been successful in overturning such a decision to date. Additionally, an IND may be terminated at any time if the risks outweigh the clinical benefits of a drug. If a drug receives approval, it will be given its appropriate FDA classification. Thereafter, manufacturers are required to submit postapproval reports (phase 4) concerning ongoing monitoring of the drug's efficacy and safety—including the reporting of any new adverse reactions.

Legal and Administrative Liability for Pharmacy Technicians

Once a pharmacist becomes licensed, he or she becomes obligated, bound by law, and legally liable for his or her actions as a pharmacist, as well as the actions of the pharmacy technicians for whom he or she is responsible. Legal liability extends to both statutory law and administrative regulations and may be either civil or criminal, depending on the circumstances and nature of the offense. The legal term malfeasance defines an instance in which a person commits an unlawful act. Criminal liability is less common and results when "an individual commits an act that is considered to be an offense against society as a whole." In contrast, civil liability involves conflicts between individuals or entities. The most common type of civil offense is a tort, which is a wrongful act committed by one person against another person or personal property for which the filing plaintiff may be entitled to some form of remedy (generally monetary). Lawsuits involving torts are the most common types of civil disputes; both pharmacists and pharmacy technicians may be named in a tort lawsuit and may be held financially responsible for any monetary remedies awarded. Malpractice insurance is commonly offered to pharmacists; pharmacy technicians may also purchase malpractice insurance to protect them against assuming financial responsibility in the event of a lawsuit claim.

FACING A CIVIL OR CRIMINAL OFFENSE

If a pharmacist or pharmacy technician is accused of a civil or criminal offense, he or she may be subject to both legal as well as professional discipline. A pharmacist's license may be suspended or revoked, pursuant to a hearing process conducted by the individual's state board of pharmacy. Depending on the state, a pharmacy technician's license or registration may be suspended or revoked—pursuant to the state board hearing process—and fines may be issued.

In the instance of a civil case, the plaintiffs may bring their case before a judge or jury and must prove their case based on the strength of the evidence presented. The case may go to trial, be dismissed because of technical error, or be settled out of court.

In the instance of *malfeasance*, a police investigation is generally conducted to gather evidence that a criminal act has been committed. The plaintiff (the state) may bring its case before a judge or jury in light of the evidence gathered. The prosecution must prove, beyond reasonable doubt, that the defendant committed a criminal act. If the prosecution proves its case, the court arraigns (calls the accused to answer to the charge[s] being brought against him or her) the defendant. The person may plead either *guilty* or *not guilty*. If the person pleads *not guilty*, a trial will be set. Many cases are settled during the less formal pretrial proceedings and often do not go to trial. If the case goes to trial, the facts of the case will be considered, principles of law related to those facts will be applied, and a conclusion of guilt or innocence will be reached. Depending on the judge's ruling (or the jury's decision), the individual may be issued a verdict of innocent, meaning they are acquitted of the charges, and released. Or the judge may issue a verdict of guilty of a misdemeanor or felony offense, and the defendant will face sentencing. Sentencing may consist of a fine, possibly in combination with probation or imprisonment. A misdemeanor conviction may require a less severe sentence, whereas a felony conviction may be more severe in nature.

Pharmacists and pharmacy technicians must make every effort to avoid situations that could place them in jeopardy of administrative, civil, or criminal liability. Pharmacists must be cognizant of not only their own behavior but that of the pharmacy technicians practicing under the authority of their licenses. A pharmacy technician must never engage in any behavior that would jeopardize not only their ability to practice pharmacy but also the licenses of the pharmacist that they support and assist. It is the responsibility of every pharmacist and pharmacy technician to *know* the law and *how* it must be applied and adhered to.

TECH ALERT!
Ignorance of the law does not preclude an individual from liability, or the resulting consequences.

A Closer Look at Drug Labeling

The Food, Drug and Cosmetic Act, in an effort to prevent misbranding and mislabeling, set forth clear expectations related to drug labeling. Considering that nonprescription medication will be self-administered without the advice of a physician or other health care provider, manufacturers must provide adequate information on the label to allow consumers to use the product safely. Box 2-4 details all the information that must be contained on the prescription drug label. Some medications may be available with both over-the-counter as well as prescription-strength formulations; the approved uses may be different for over-the-counter formulations, as the FDA has determined, through the new drug application process, which clinical indications are safe for the patient to self-treat without consulting a physician or other authorized prescriber. Box 2-5 details all the information that must be contained on the commercial label of a prescription medication. The information contained on the commercial label of a prescription drug is intended for professional use, rather than for viewing by the patient. Additionally, the drug package insert must accompany the drug. The package insert must contain the most essential pharmacological information needed for the safe and effective use by health care professionals.

BOX 2-4   Required Information for Over-the-Counter (OTC) Product Label/Packaging

The drug name, brand or generic, as well as general therapeutic class (i.e., antacid)	"Drug Facts" panel should include the following: Active ingredients, including dosage unit and quantity per dosage unit General therapeutic class Uses (indications) Warnings, such as "Stop using if...," "For external use only," or "Keep out of reach of children" Directions Other information as required Inactive ingredients in alphabetical order "Questions or comments" and a phone number
Name and address of manufacturer, packer, or distributor	Normal dose for each intended use by individuals for different uses and individuals of different ages
Net quantity/volume of the contents within the package	Frequency or duration of administration of the application
Cautions and warnings needed to protect the consumer	Administration or application in relation to meals, onset of symptoms, or other time-related factors
Adequate directions for use	Route or method of administration or application
Any required preparation for use	
National Drug Code (NDC) number and linear bar code	

BOX 2-5   Required Information on the Commercial Label of a Prescription Drug

- Name, address of manufacturer, packer, or distributor
- Established name of the drug product
- Ingredient information, including quantity and proportion of each active ingredient
- Name of inactive ingredients if not for oral use
- Statement of identity (generic and proprietary names)
- Quantity, in terms of weight or measure
- Net quantity or volume of the container

Chapter Summary

- Pharmacy laws were first enacted in the United States for the health, safety, and welfare of citizens. To protect patients, laws have been established concerning the practice of medicine and the dispensing of pharmaceutical products. Pharmacy practice law has been established in accordance with federal and state laws or according to those established standards created by government-approved regulatory authorities.
- Federal legislators may create administrative agencies to implement desired changes in policies or to administer a body of substantive law.
- State legislatures formed individual state boards of pharmacy to monitor the activities of pharmacies and pharmacists on a routine basis.
- The pharmacy-related laws cited in this chapter were enacted for the following key purposes:
  - To prevent the adulteration and misbranding of drugs (The Pure Food and Drug Act of 1906)
  - To require that drug manufacturers prove both the safety and efficacy of drugs (The Food, Drug, and Cosmetic Act of 1938)
  - To define drugs that could be safely administered over the counter with adequate directions for use versus those that must be administered with a prescription and under the supervision of a physician (The Durham-Humphrey Amendment of 1951).
  - To define substances and drugs that should be handled as hazardous substances (The Kefauver-Harris Amendment of 1962).
  - To require the use of child-resistant drug containers (The Poison Prevention Packaging Act of 1970).
  - To define safe conditions in the workplace and the personal protective equipment that may be necessary in the preparation and handling of drugs (The Occupational Safety and Health Act of 1970).
  - To regulate the production, labeling, use, and distribution of habit-forming substances (The Comprehensive Drug Abuse Prevention and Control Act of 1970 [The Controlled Substances Act]).
  - To create a means to maintain an accurate database of current FDA products that have been assigned an NDC number (The Drug Listing Act of 1972).
  - To offer drug manufacturers incentives to offset the extremely high cost of research and development of drugs used to treat a relatively small patient population (The Orphan Drug Act of 1983).
  - To allow for the expediting of ANDAs for generic drugs, for which there were already clinical data on record providing its safety and efficacy; also allows for 3 years of market exclusivity to recoup development and manufacturing costs (The Drug Price Competition and Patent-Term Restoration Act of 1984).
  - To regulate the import and export of drugs in and out of the United States; also prevents the sale of drug samples (The Prescription Drug Marketing Act of 1987).
  - To provide funding for scientific studies to assess the degree to which patient care improves and health care costs decrease when pharmacists provide drug use review consultative services to patients, as well as enact drug use reviews, and optimize government spending on health care (The Omnibus Budget Reconciliation Act of 1990 [OBRA '90]).
  - To monitor the manufacturers of nutritional supplements to determine the safety of their products prior to marketing them to the public (The Dietary Supplement Health and Education Act of 1994).
  - To increase the portability and continuity of health insurance coverage, prohibit discrimination in health coverage, and regulate the privacy and security of health information (The Health Insurance Portability And Accountability Act of 1996 [HIPAA]).
  - To formally identify the anabolic steroid drug category, differentiate these products from less harmful over-the-counter nutritional supplements, and discourage their use and abuse by young adults and athletes (The Anabolic Steroids Control Act of 2004).
  - To regulate the manufacturing and distribution of pseduoephedrine (Combat Methamphetamine Epidemic Act of 2005).
- Pharmacy technicians who have not been formally educated may gain information from their employers and state board of pharmacy concerning the laws that govern their practice.

REVIEW QUESTIONS

Multiple Choice

1. This type of law is established by federal agencies with authority from Congress:
   a. Statutory
   b. Administrative
   c. Case
   d. Tort

2. Individual state boards of pharmacy were created by:
   a. The president of the United States
   b. The federal government
   c. State legislatures
   d. Congress

3. This law prohibited the adulteration and misbranding of food and drugs in interstate commerce, but it did not address their safety or efficacy:
   a. The Pure Food and Drug Act of 1906
   b. The Poison Prevention Packaging Act of 1970
   c. The Food, Drug and Cosmetic Act of 1938
   d. The Drug Listing Act of 1972

4. This law established two classes of drugs: prescription and over the counter:
   a. The Durham-Humphrey Amendment of 1951
   b. The Kefauver-Harris Amendment of 1962
   c. The Food, Drug and Cosmetic Act of 1938
   d. The Controlled Substance Act of 1970

5. This law provides for the dispensing of prescription refills:
   a. The Food, Drug and Cosmetic Act of 1938
   b. The Drug Listing Act of 1972
   c. The Omnibus Budget Reconciliation Act of 1990
   d. The Durham-Humphrey Amendment of 1951

6. This law prohibits the sale of drug samples:
   a. The Prescription Drug Marketing Act of 1987
   b. The Drug Listing Act of 1972
   c. The Orphan Drug Act of 1983
   d. The Controlled Substance Act of 1970

7. A prescription drug with the highest abuse potential would be assigned DEA class:
   a. I
   b. II
   c. III
   d. IV

8. This law requires the pharmacist to offer counseling to every patient:
   a. The Occupational Safety and Health Act of 1970
   b. OBRA '90
   c. The Health Insurance Portability and Accountability Act of 1996
   d. The Poison Prevention Act of 1970

9. This law was enacted in response to alarming trends in the use of performance-enhancing drugs among professional athletes:
   a. The Orphan Drug Act of 1983
   b. The Anabolic Steroids Act of 2004
   c. The Dietary Supplement Health and Education Act of 1994
   d. The Health Insurance Portability and Accountability Act of 1996

10. Phase 3 drug studies must be conducted in the following clinical setting(s):
    a. Physician's office
    b. Hospital
    c. Clinic
    d. All of the above

TECHNICIAN'S
CORNER

1. What is the difference between a retrospective and prospective order review? How does this affect a pharmacist's role in medication therapy management?
2. What is the threefold intent of pharmacy law?
3. Why should a pharmacy technician ask patients about nutritional supplements they may be taking?

Bibliography

Abood, R. (2005). *Pharmacy Practice and the Law*, 4th Edition. Sudbury, Massachusetts: Jones and Bartlett.

Bureau of Labor Statistics, U.S. Department of Labor. (2010). *Occupational Outlook Handbook, 2010-11 Edition, Pharmacists*. Retrieved 5/14/2010, from United States Department of Labor—Bureau of Labor Statistics: http://www.bls.gov/oco/ocos079.htm#training

California State Board of Pharmacy. (2010). *Enforcement Actions: Board of Pharmacy Disciplinary Actions between April 1, 2010, and June 30, 2010*. Retrieved 7/5/2010, from California State Board of Pharmacy: http://www.pharmacy.ca.gov/enforcement/fy0809/ac083232.pdf

U.S. Drug Enforcement Administration, U.S. Department of Justice. (2005). *Drug Scheduling Actions—2005*. Retrieved 6/28/2010, from Office of Diversion Control: http://www.deadiversion.usdoj.gov/fed_regs/rules/2005/fr1216.htm

Food and Drug Administration, United States Department of Health and Human Services (1987). *Prescription Drug Marketing Act of 1987*. Retrieved 6/27/2010, from fda.gov at url: http://www.fda.gov/Regulatory Information/Legislation/FederalFoodDrugandCosmeticActFDCAct/SignificantAmendmentstothe FDCAct/PrescriptionDrugMarketingActof1987/ucm201702.htm

Merriam-Webster Online. (2010). *Merriam-Webster's Online Dictionary*. Retrieved 5/14/2010, from Merriam-Webster Online: http://www.merriam-webster.com/dictionary/law

Occupational Safety and Health Administration. (2010). *Occupational Safety and Health Administration*. Retrieved 6/26/2010, from http://www.osha.gov/pls/oshaweb/owadisp.show_document?p_table=OSHA &p_id=3

Pohly, P. (2007). *Glossary of Terms in Managed Care*. Retrieved 6/28/2010, from Pam Pohly's Net Guide: http://www.pohly.com/terms_p.html

Tamparo, M.A. (2002). *Medical Law, Ethics and Bioethics*, 6th Edition. Philadelphia: F.A. Davis.

The Food and Drug Administration. (2010). *Significant Dates in Food and Drug Law History*. Retrieved 6/26/2010, from fda.gov: http://www.fda.gov/AboutFDA/WhatWeDo/History/Milestones/ucm128305.htm

U.S. Drug Enforcement Administration, U.S. Department of Justice. (2004). *DEA Congressional Testimony— Statement of Joseph T. Rannazzisi–Deputy Director, Office of Diversion Control, Drug Enforcement Agency– Before the House Committee on the Judiciary Subcommittee on Crime, Terrorism, and Homeland Security*. Retrieved 6/28/2010, from U.S. Drug Enforcement Administration website: http://www.justice.gov/dea/pubs/cngrtest/ct031604.html

U.S. Food and Drug Administration. (2009). *Congressional Testimony of August 1, 2003*. Retrieved 6/28/2010, from fda.gov: http://www.fda.gov/newsevents/testimony/ucm115033.htm

U.S. Food and Drug Administration. (2009). *Dietary Supplements*. Retrieved 6/28/2010, from fda.gov: http://www.fda.gov/food/dietarysupplements/default.htm

U.S. Food and Drug Administration. (2010). *National Drug Code Directory*. Retrieved 6/26/2010, from Drug Approvals and Databases: http://www.fda.gov/Drugs/InformationOnDrugs/ucm142438.htm

United States Department of Labor. (2010). *Frequently Asked Questions*. Retrieved 6/26/2010, from dol.gov: http://webapps.dol.gov/dolfaq/go-dol-faq.asp?faqid=258

Word Net Search 3.0. Retrieved 7/5/2010, from www.wordnetweb.princeton.edu

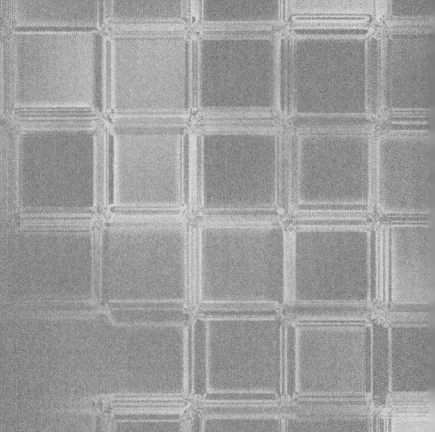

3

The Study of Bioethics in Pharmacy Technician Practice

LEARNING OBJECTIVES

By the end of this chapter, students will be able to competently:

1. Recognize the historical basis and importance of ethics in healthcare.
2. Explain the purpose for informed consent in the delivery of medical treatment.
3. Define core values and explain their importance to the delivery of patient care in pharmacy technicians.
4. Conduct a personal inventory to determine individual core values and how they complement or contrast the Code of Ethics for Pharmacy Technicians.
5. Examine the Code of Ethics for Pharmacy Technicians and 10 core values of professionalism that each represents.
6. Define three key ethical principles that may be applied to pharmacy technician practice.
7. Describe professional situations that may create ethical dilemmas, and apply strategies for resolution using the five steps of the ethical decision-making process.

KEY TERMINOLOGY

Advocacy: Provision of support for a particular group, profession, or cause.

Autonomy: One's right to make decisions about his or her health care independent of the influence of one's health care provider.

Code: A set of rules, principles, or laws.

Core values: The fundamental beliefs, morals, and standards that define one as a person and guide one's behavior.

Ethical dilemma: A situation in which factors to be considered create conflict with one's moral/ethical values or one's interpersonal or work relationships.

Ethics: Principles or conduct governing an individual or a group; the discipline dealing with what is good and bad and with moral duty and obligation.

Integrity: Firm adherence to a code of moral values; the quality or state of being complete or undivided.

Patient autonomy: A patients' right to make decisions about his or her health care independent of the influence of one's health care provider.

Introduction

Ethics, as defined by the Merriam-Webster dictionary, are "principle[s] or conduct governing an individual or a group" and "the discipline dealing with what is good and bad and with moral duty and obligation" (Merriam-Webster Online, 2010). The previous chapter discussed the laws and regulatory authorities that govern the practice of pharmacy. It was further noted that, in addition to adherence to the law, pharmacists and pharmacy technicians must also exercise professional judgment when applying the law. Exercising good judgment and ethical behavior requires the application of ethical or moral principles to various controversial or seemingly controversial situations. Moral principles are often driven by culture, ethnicity, and religious convictions, and they may be further influenced by one's upbringing or life experience. One person's perspective concerning ethics may be different than another's. Yet, the ability to appropriately apply personal or professional ethical principles is of great importance in the practice of patient care. Unlike the concrete definition provided earlier, the line between what is "good" and "bad" is not always easily detected, given a number of variables. However, when one can refer to an established code—that is, a set of rules, principles, or laws (WordNet Search 3.0, 2010)—of model behavior, an individual may more competently determine the "right" decision.

Over the centuries, codes have been established that define and express the primary goals and values of a particular group. Individuals who choose to join that group (or profession, in this context) make a moral commitment to uphold those expressed values and obligations. The following are four historical codes that define and describe moral and ethical obligations concerning the delivery of health care, both in and out of the clinical setting.

HISTORICAL DEVELOPMENT OF MEDICAL CODES OF ETHICS

Hippocratic Oath (5 B.C.)

Written by the Academic Dean of Tufts University School of Medicine, this oath, which is taken by new physicians upon graduation from medical school, is noted in Box 3-1. This oath speaks to the physician's commitment to the well-being of patients and to the honest and true pursuit of all reasonable measures to prevent or treat disease.

Geneva Convention of Medical Ethics (Part of the Fourth Geneva Convention of 1949)

The fourth Geneva Convention, among many other things, set forth universal standards concerning the treatment of those who were—during time of war—wounded, sick, or shipwrecked.

The responsibility of all medical personnel involved in their care was to ensure that such persons were "respected and protected," and the Geneva Convention detailed specific patient rights and the need to obtain consent prior to certain medical procedures.

BOX 3-1   **Modern Hippocratic Oath**

Swear to fulfill, to the best of my ability and judgment, this covenant:
- I will respect the hard-won scientific gains of those physicians in whose steps I walk, and gladly share such knowledge as is mine with those who are to follow.
- I will apply, for the benefit of the sick, all measures [that] are required, avoiding those twin traps of overtreatment and therapeutic nihilism.
- I will remember that there is art to medicine as well as science, and that warmth, sympathy, and understanding may outweigh the surgeon's knife or the chemist's drug.
- I will not be ashamed to say "I know not," nor will I fail to call in my colleagues when the skills of another are needed for a patient's recovery.
- I will respect the privacy of my patients, for their problems are not disclosed to me that the world may know. Most especially must I tread with care in matters of life and death. If it is given me to save a life, all thanks. But it may also be within my power to take a life; this awesome responsibility must be faced with great humbleness and awareness of my own frailty. Above all, I must not play at God.
- I will remember that I do not treat a fever chart, a cancerous growth, but a sick human being, whose illness may affect the person's family and economic stability. My responsibility includes these related problems, if I am to care adequately for the sick.
- I will prevent disease whenever I can, for prevention is preferable to cure.
- I will remember that I remain a member of society, with special obligations to all my fellow human beings, those sound of mind and body as well as the infirm.
- If I do not violate this oath, may I enjoy life and art, respected while I live and remembered with affection thereafter. May I always act so as to preserve the finest traditions of my calling and may I long experience the joy of healing those who seek my help.

Nuremberg Code (1947)

Following the trials of World War II war criminals, this code set forth 10 standards related to the treatment of human subjects during medical experimentation:

- The code required *voluntary informed consent* of the human subject.
- The code recognized that intentional injury or the unnecessary infliction of pain should be avoided.

INFORMED CONSENT

One significant medical practice that has emerged in modern patient care from the Nuremberg Code is the process of properly informing patients of their right to make voluntary and informed clinical decisions concerning their own health. This is also referred to as patient autonomy. Patients must be provided information concerning their health, along with any possible treatment options available and any risks associated with them. The patient may then evaluate the information provided and have any questions answered prior to consenting to treatment.

Figure 3-1 is a sample informed consent form that would be completed by a patient. Figure 3-2 describes the process whereby a patient may exercise his or her autonomy and either consent to or decline recommended treatment options.

Declaration of Helsinki (First Adopted in 1964)

The declaration set forth standards of medical practice for both clinical and nonclinical research conducted on human subjects. In addition, it set forth the expectation that physicians and those involved in the care of human subjects must establish that the medical benefit outweighs any risks involved.

It also indicates that "Special caution must be exercised in the conduct of research which may affect the environment, and the welfare of animals used for research must be respected" (World Medical Organization, December 7, 1996: 313[7070]).

These and many other codes of professional conduct set forth expectations designed to protect the health, safety, and welfare of patients. Regardless of one's background, it is important to recognize that those who voluntarily join a profession should do so with the understanding that they must uphold the values and obligations of that profession in their daily lives, both personally and professionally. Failure to do so may compromise patient safety, and the person who failed to keep this obligation may be subject to professional or legal disciplinary action.

International media coverage does not lack stories that relate to a breakdown in moral or ethical judgment on the part of a pharmacist or pharmacy technician. Students are encouraged to visit the websites of any of the U.S. state boards of pharmacy and conduct a search of code compliance disciplinary actions that are documented as public record. Most of the cases cited are examples of the consequences that result from the exercise of poor professional judgment as well as failed adherence to established laws and rules. It would prove a valuable lesson to learn from the mistakes of others in order to avoid making those same errors. It is often true that those who do not learn from the mistakes of the past are destined to repeat them—which may be one of many reasons why state board disciplinary actions are publicly posted. Pharmacy technicians: Heed the warnings!

The expression of *choice* has been mentioned on several occasions. The lasting value of good decision making, when exercised for the right reasons, is the development of strong moral and ethical character. One must carefully consider a difficult situation, determine the best course of action to take, and then make the most appropriate choices. Believe it or not, good decision making is not always intrinsic—it must be taught and demonstrated. This chapter will approach codes of ethics that set forth definitions of what ideal behavior looks like. Ethical decision-making steps will be detailed along with how each step may be practically applied to pharmacy technician practice.

It is important to carefully examine and discuss how one would respond to an unethical or immoral order or directive. Evaluating options that will allow one to consistently act on moral principles, particularly in the face of opposition, will increase the likelihood of an individual carrying out moral decision making in real-life situations.

A colleague made the following comment concerning the development of a value system: "We don't start out our lives with core values; we learn and develop them. Then, as we grow, mature, and become more emotionally intelligent, we may add to and refine those values" (J. Chaney, 2010).

Tingsboro Hospital Procedure Consent Form	Patient Label Name Medical Record # DOB

Procedure: _____

I,_____, consent to the above treatment procedure as deemed medically necessary by my medical provider. My care provider,_____, has explained to me the nature of my condition, the procedure, the risks and the expected benefits of the above procedure compared with alternative approaches.

My provider has also explained to me the likelihood, and some possible complications of this procedure including, but not limited to, bleeding, infection, loss of limb or organ function, drug reactions or possibly death. I also understand that I may need a blood transfusion during or after this procedure.

I understand that Tingsboro Hospital is a teaching hospital and that students and other trainees may participate in this procedure as permitted by law and hospital policy. I also understand that tissues, blood, body parts or fluid may be removed from the body during the procedure. These materials may be used for diagnostic, therapeutic or research reasons.

Any additional comments:

_____

_____

_____

_____

_____   _____
Signature of Patient   Printed Name

_____   _____
Signature of Provider   Printed Name

Date:_____

FIGURE 3-1 Informed consent document. (From Purtilo R, Doherty R: *Ethical dimensions in the health professions,* ed 5, St. Louis, 2010, Saunders.)

It is up to each pharmacy technician to make the choice and commitment to uphold the values of the profession he or she has chosen. When one demonstrates both moral and ethical behavior on a consistent basis, he or she may set a positive example for others in the profession to follow. But then again, a strong show of character itself is making the decision to *do the right thing*, whether in the face of opposition or if no one else around you chooses to do the same. Choose wisely!

Determining Moral and Ethical Value Systems

DEFINING CORE VALUES

As stated in the chapter introduction, external factors such as one's ethnicity or religious convictions may influence the development of one's personal definition of ethical or moral behavior. Individuals who choose health care as a career path need to be aware of any aspects of their chosen profession that may come into conflict with their cultural or religious beliefs. Given that information, one must decide how he or she will approach those value conflicts; there may be difficult decisions to

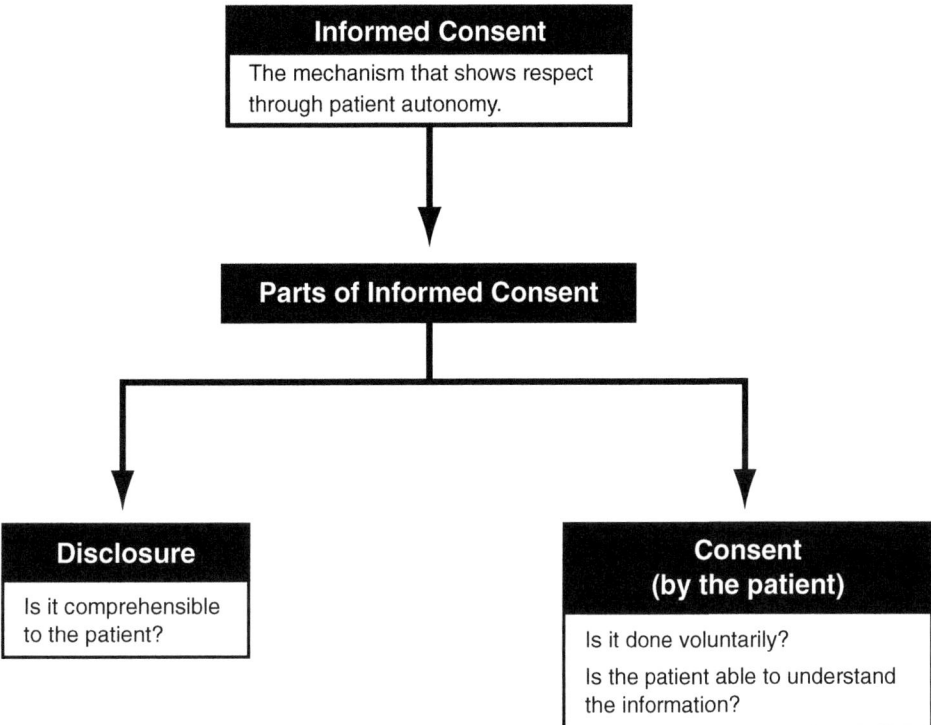

FIGURE 3-2 The two dimensions of informed consent. Relevant facts regarding the process of obtaining consent. (From Purtilo R, Doherty R: *Ethical dimensions in the health professions,* ed 5, St. Louis, 2010, Saunders.)

make as to whether one should continue to pursue pharmacy as a career. The commitment to demonstrate established values, ideals, and obligations is critical to providing the highest level of patient care, achieving career success, and avoiding professional disciplinary action.

One who was indoctrinated with a core value system as a child is far less likely to stray from that value system later on in life. Children who lack parental indoctrination of a *core value system*—or consistent demonstration of those values—may be unduly challenged with adopting core values as adults. Core values, as defined by Tristan Loo, are "the fundamental beliefs, morals, and standards that define you as a person and which guide your behavior. Although other aspects of your life change, your core set of values does not change. Core values are what you tell a person who asks you, 'What do you stand for in your life?'" (Loo, 2006).

Throughout this chapter, it is hoped that each student will reflect inwardly upon the topics discussed and, at the conclusion of the chapter, will have discovered opportunities for personal and professional growth. Students are encouraged to obtain a composition notebook, in which they may record their personal reflections concerning topics discussed. Instructors may choose to use these reflections for classroom discussion and to allow students to share, or the reflections may remain private. Either way, there is great value to journaling personal reflection—one may look back on those reflections and see what changes have taken place since the journaling began.

All individuals must take the opportunity to discover—or reaffirm—where they stand in terms of principles. It will be nearly impossible to demonstrate certain virtues in the workplace that one infrequently models in his or her personal life. Particularly for those who are new to health care, it is challenging early on to demonstrate values that have not been clearly defined or that one has not seen applied in real-life situations. This chapter presents several ethical and moral principles that are common to health care along with examples of how those principles may be applied in given sample case scenarios.

KEY ETHICAL PRINCIPLES TO CONSIDER

Although there are many schools of thought on the subject of ethical principles, there are common key attributes that exist among several sources. Several key themes are most relevant to the practice health care, including the following common principles:

- Respect for persons
- Beneficence
- Justice

Respect for Persons

Each patient has the right to autonomy, or the right to make decisions about one's health care independent of the influence of one's health care provider. Each patient should additionally be respected as an individual who is entitled to dignity and protection. Pharmacy technicians must always treat patients with respect, in both verbal and nonverbal communication. In other words, technicians should extend to patients the same respect *that they or their loved ones would expect to receive* as patients or consumers. Technicians may demonstrate respectful behavior by doing the following:

- Addressing patients professionally
- Demonstrating genuine focus
- Communicating a commitment to meeting patients' needs

Patients generally come to the pharmacy because they are ill and may not be at their best for a variety of reasons. Although their demeanor may not always be pleasant, pharmacists and pharmacy technicians should focus on serving the patient, rather than taking less-than-pleasant treatment as a personal offense. Be assured that patients, regardless of how they are feeling at the time, will generally respond positively to fair and respectful treatment! One of the greatest joys of patient care is the formation of positive relationships with patients, which may be sustained over a number of years. Among the first steps to establishing that relationship are treating patients with dignity and respect and empowering them to make good, informed decisions concerning their medical care.

Consider the following scenario:

John Peterson is a pharmacy technician at a local retail chain store pharmacy. During a busy lunch hour rush, an elderly patient takes several minutes searching through her purse trying to locate her prescriptions. Visibly annoyed, John snidely inquires of the patient, "Can't you just step aside until you find your prescription? It's busy, and you're holding up the line!"

How would you feel if that was the treatment you had received? What if that patient were your mother, grandmother, or close friend? Pharmacy technicians must be sensitive to patient-specific factors, such as age, gender, ethnicity, and any physical or mental incapacity.

Beneficence

All health care professionals must be committed to protecting the well-being of patients by first *doing no harm* and maximizing possible benefits while minimizing possible harm. Pharmacy technicians must ensure that they consistently collect all of the appropriate information from a patient. This will ensure that a pharmacist has all of the necessary data that he or she needs to optimize each patient's medication therapy management. Pharmacy technicians should seek the best interest of patients at all times. A reality of pharmacy practice is that pharmacists and technicians may encounter patients with mental illness or those suffering from chemical dependence issues (i.e., illicit or prescription drug abuse). If patients happen to demonstrate behavior that suggests they may be a danger to themselves or others, pharmacy technicians should immediately alert a pharmacist, store manager, or law enforcement officer as necessary. A pharmacy technician should never engage in any behavior that would harm a patient, physically or emotionally, or inflict harm through the wrongful use of his or her *protected health information* (PHI). In an effort to maximize the possible benefits of medication, patients should seek the expertise and professional advice of pharmacists. Pharmacy technicians must always ensure that patients are offered counseling, regardless of their workload or the patient's perceived demeanor.

Consider the following scenario:

Anila Sharif is the only pharmacy technician working with the pharmacist at a local compounding pharmacy. A new patient comes to the window with a prescription for a product that will require several minutes of careful preparation. As a new patient to this establishment, he will have several forms to complete before Anila may enter his information into the pharmacy computer system. The pharmacy is scheduled to close in 5 minutes. Sighing,

Anila tells the patient, "I'm sorry sir, but we're about to close. Please come back tomorrow morning when we open at 8 a.m."

Is the action that Anila took looking after the best interest of the patient? This is not ethical behavior, for a variety of reasons. A delay in the start of the patient's treatment may present possible health risks, depending on the nature of the drug therapy. Considering that pharmacy compounding is a specialized form of pharmacy, the patient may not have the option of seeking another source in order to have his prescription filled that day. Pharmacy technicians must seek to maximize a patient's medication therapy outcome, which includes the timely preparation and dispensing of prescribed medication. A pharmacy technician should never refuse service to a patient, even if it is close to quitting time!

Justice

Patients should be treated with fairness and equality, regardless of race, creed, gender, sexual orientation, disease state, demeanor, and the like. A homeless patient deserves the same quality of care as a patient with private health insurance. Although pharmacy staff may build relationships with patients, one must be careful not to show preferential treatment or extend greater effort to please or serve a selected patient over others. Every patient should be given the same degree of attention and quality of care.

Consider the following scenario:

Benjamin Okeke has worked at the regional hospital for 7 years. In that time, he has established professional relationships with several regular patients who visit the outpatient pharmacy to pick up prescriptions after visits to one of the hospital's outpatient clinics or physician practices. While Benjamin is engaged in casual conversation with a regular patient at the outpatient prescription window, another patient steps into line behind the first patient. Even though Benjamin notices the other patient, he continues his conversation with the first patient for several minutes before concluding and moving on to the next patient.

Every patient deserves the same level of treatment—failure to assist a patient in favor of another patient is a great injustice, is inconsiderate, and is unethical behavior. Although it is valuable to establish positive professional relationships with patients, that relationship should not compromise the care delivered to other patients (with whom a technician may not have established a rapport or may have a negative rapport).

Application of the principles of, respect for persons beneficence and justice by every pharmacy technician will ensure that every patient receives exemplary customer care. In addition to these core health care principles, there is a core value, or a code of ethics, that has been established specifically for pharmacy technicians. This code will be discussed in the following section.

Code of Ethics for Pharmacy Technicians

When daily workplace situations create conflict with one's moral/ethical values or with one's interpersonal or work relationships, this is considered an ethical dilemma. It may be quite challenging for pharmacy technicians to approach difficult workplace scenarios without a helpful set of tools to guide them through the decision-making process. The Code of Ethics for Pharmacy Technicians, as shown in Table 3-1, is one such tool. Adopted in 1996 by the American Association of Pharmacy Technicians, each of the 10 principles of this code may serve as a guidepost that can help define ideal ethical behavior. When these principles are examined, common values of professionalism emerge. Demonstrating these principles and discovering how they align with each individual's core values will help a pharmacy technician to act professionally and decide the best course of action to take in a difficult situation. It is important to note that the Code of Ethics for Pharmacy Technicians is derived from the Code of Ethics for Pharmacists, ensuring that there is a uniform standard across the profession related to ethical standards of practice.

Oftentimes, personalizing each principle is one of the best ways to discover how to apply it. Students may wish to approach each principle from the standpoint of what their expectation would be if they were on the receiving end of that behavior. Let's take a look at each of the 10 principles, along with the core value of health care professionalism that each describes.

TABLE 3-1 **Code of Ethics for Pharmacy Technicians, Adopted by American Association of Pharmacy Technicians (AAPT) in 2004**

Principle 1	A pharmacy technician's first consideration is to ensure the health and safety of the patient and to use knowledge and skills to the best of his or her ability in serving others.
Principle 2	A pharmacy technician supports and promotes honesty and integrity in the profession, which includes a duty to observe the law, maintain the highest moral and ethical conduct at all times, and uphold the ethical principles of the profession.
Principle 3	A pharmacy technician assists and supports the pharmacist in the safe, efficacious, and cost-effective distribution of health services and health care resources.
Principle 4	A pharmacy technician respects and values the abilities of pharmacists, colleagues, and other health care professionals.
Principle 5	A pharmacy technician maintains competency in his or her practice and continually enhances his or her knowledge and expertise.
Principle 6	A pharmacy technician respects and supports the patient's individuality, dignity, and confidentiality.
Principle 7	A pharmacy technician respects the confidentiality of patients' records and discloses pertinent information only with proper authorization.
Principle 8	A pharmacy technician never assists in the dispensing, promoting, or distribution of medications or medical devices that are not of good quality or do not meet the standards required by law.
Principle 9	A pharmacy technician does not engage in any activity that will discredit the profession and will expose, without fear or favor, illegal or unethical conduct in the profession.
Principle 10	A pharmacy technician associates with and engages in the support of organizations that promote the profession of pharmacy through the utilization and enhancement of pharmacy technicians.

PRINCIPLE 1

A pharmacy technician's first consideration is to ensure the health and safety of the patient and to use knowledge and skills to the best of his or her ability when serving others.

Core Value: Patient/Customer Focus

Above all things, the health and safety of patients must be a pharmacy technician's first priority. Pharmacy technicians must approach each situation with the mindset and intention of utilizing all available resources to ensure that the patient's needs are met. They must make ethical decisions based on what is in the best interest of the patient rather than themselves.

One clear advantage to completing a formal training program is that students gain much knowledge and many skills necessary to best serve patients before approaching the live workplace environment. Individuals who have not sought out formal training may not have as clear an understanding of how patient-focused the pharmacy technician's role must be or of the key ethical behaviors that pharmacy technicians are expected to demonstrate on a daily basis. It is valuable to have the opportunity to consider the principles of ethical behavior so that one may make more informed decisions when approaching patients' issues.

PRINCIPLE 2

A pharmacy technician supports and promotes honesty and integrity in the profession, which includes a duty to observe the law, maintain the highest moral and ethical conduct at all times, and uphold the ethical principles of the profession.

Core Values: Honesty and Integrity

Integrity has two key definitions that one should carefully consider: "firm adherence to a code of moral values" and "the quality or state of being complete or undivided" (Merriam-Webster Online, 2010). Pharmacy technicians may act with integrity not only by modeling moral and ethical behavior but also by coming to terms with any issues in their own lives that might cause them to be divided—or conflicted—with moral or ethical issues. Just as having a core value system helps to establish where you stand on various principles in life, acting with integrity is standing firm in that resolve. Double-mindedness may result in both internal and external instability; in other words, those who are undecided or unsure of where they stand morally or ethically may experience difficulty when faced with making moral or ethical decisions. Pharmacy technicians need to know where they stand, then they must stand firm when it really counts.

PRINCIPLE 3

A pharmacy technician assists and supports the pharmacist in the safe, efficacious, and cost-effective distribution of health services and health care resources.

Core Values: Partnership and Service Orientation

Pharmacy technicians must recognize that they are working under the authority of the staff pharmacists who are responsible for their oversight. Therefore, pharmacists are held accountable for the actions and behaviors of the pharmacy technicians they work with. This relationship is twofold: partnership and service.

Shared Accountability

Quality patient care is based on the competence of both clinical and nonclinical pharmacy staff. Pharmacists must ensure that medication therapy is clinically appropriate; pharmacy technicians must ensure that medications are entered properly into the pharmacy's medication management system, as well as ensure that medications have been accurately counted, measured, or prepared before awaiting a pharmacist's check.

Managerial Accountability

Pharmacists are in a position of direct authority over pharmacy technicians, primarily because of additional educational requirements earned. They are considered the industry experts, and technicians are their support personnel. Pharmacy technicians will certainly increase their knowledge base over years of practice and may hone their skills to the degree that pharmacists may feel comfortable entrusting them with additional responsibilities that do not require professional or clinical judgment. Pharmacy technicians must ensure that they demonstrate service or a genuine desire to attend to the needs of the pharmacist before attending to their own needs. Although pharmacy technicians may possess some clinical knowledge, they may not legally provide that information to a patient, nor may they contradict the professional opinions or perspectives of the pharmacists whom they have been charged to serve.

The Essence of Ethical Service

The word *serve* may take on a negative connotation, as though serving others means taking a lesser role. In terms of pharmacy law, pharmacists and pharmacy technicians are not professionally *equal*. Each is not held to the same level of accountability in many cases; whereas a pharmacist may be professionally disciplined as the result of the actions of a pharmacy technician, it is rare that a pharmacy technician will be held accountable for the actions of a pharmacist. Because a pharmacist's knowledge and expertise far exceed that of a pharmacy technician, technicians must ensure that they ethically perform within the scope, or legal range of duties, of their practice.

Pharmacy technicians should recognize the authority of the pharmacist and follow directions given by the pharmacist. Does this mean that a technician may not question a pharmacist? Certainly not. In fact, most pharmacists welcome questions and challenges, particularly if they help to avoid a medication error. Should a pharmacy technician follow an order that is unethical or illegal? Certainly not. Rather, pharmacy technicians should serve in this partnership with pharmacists to ensure that patients receive the highest level of care and that pharmacy resources are utilized appropriately and responsibly. Pharmacists greatly appreciate pharmacy technicians who can follow and take direction, actively listen, and ask appropriate questions. Truly, pharmacy technicians who make service a priority are much more likely to position themselves for career success and greater opportunities for advancement within the pharmacy technician career path.

PRINCIPLE 4

A pharmacy technician respects and values the abilities of pharmacists, colleagues, and other health care professionals.

Core Value: Respect for Professional Roles

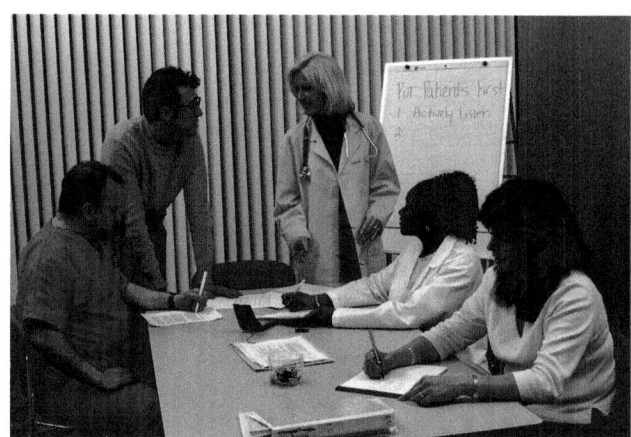

Teamwork and collaboration. (From Bonewit-West K: *Today's medical assistant: clinical & administrative procedures,* St. Louis, 2009, Saunders.)

The culture of today's health care environment fosters more of a team approach. Several health care providers must collaborate to serve the patient. It is important to recognize the role that each member of the health care team brings to patient care. As was so candidly expressed in the modern Hippocratic oath, health care providers must "not be ashamed to say 'I know not,' nor...fail to call in my colleagues when the skills of another are needed for a patient's recovery." The relationship that exists between the various contributors to the health care team must be nurtured with open and honest communication, sharing of information, and demonstration of mutual respect for one another's roles and abilities. The pharmacy technician who wishes to be considered for a supervisory position at any point in his or her career will discover that one of the most valuable management traits is the ability to identify the individual strengths of members of your team. In addition, it is equally useful to identify those areas that are not strengths. Part of acting ethically is to avoid capitalizing on another person's weakness or areas that need further development. Rather, one should seek ways to bridge the gap and work with those individuals to help them to be more successful. After all, the overall success of any team is the sum of the successes of each of its members. As students embark on their careers, they are encouraged to find ways to value, respect, and celebrate the successes and contributions of their co-workers and pharmacists.

PRINCIPLE 5

A pharmacy technician maintains competency in his or her practice and continually enhances his or her knowledge and expertise.

Core Value: Continuous Learning

A pharmacy technician's education does not stop upon graduation from a training program. Pharmacy is an ever-changing industry on many levels. The following is just a brief list of the many things that frequently change in pharmacy practice, for which one will need to stay current and knowledgeable:

- Pharmacy law at both the national and state levels
- Hospital and corporate pharmacy policies
- Pharmacy software and other forms of technology
- Drug products' names, strengths, uses, dosage forms, and so on
- Job titles and responsibilities
- Licensing/registration requirements

Those who have been in the industry for a while may joke that "the only thing that stays the same is that *everything* changes!" Pharmacy technicians must position themselves to adapt to that change and seek out resources for staying current with national, state, and local standards of practice. New roles for pharmacy technicians will continue to emerge; pharmacy technicians should take advantage of every opportunity to learn new things, question pharmacists about clinical processes, read about the drugs they are preparing, and find meaningful sources for continuing their education. For those technicians who must be certified in order to practice in their state, the continuing education (CE) requirement is generally between 10 and 20 CE hours, which must be completed either annually or biennially. Continuous learning is best retained and put to productive use when it is gained on a *continuous* basis. Ethically speaking, one should not wait until a month or two before one's certification expires to begin seeking out sources for CE credit. There are a variety of professional pharmacy organizations that provide opportunities for pharmacy technicians to continue their education.

PRINCIPLE 6

A pharmacy technician respects and supports the patient's individuality, dignity, and confidentiality.

Core Value: Respecting the Patient's Autonomy

This principle speaks to a few of the core ethical principles discussed earlier in the chapter. Patients have the right to make decisions about their own health care: pharmacy technicians should take every opportunity to empower patients with the information they need in order to make informed decisions. Patients should be encouraged to consult with pharmacists concerning their medication therapy or other medication-related concerns. Every patient has the right to be treated with individuality, dignity, and respect. Pharmacy technicians should treat sensitive information delicately and should avoid behaviors that would embarrass or shame a patient.

PRINCIPLE 7

A pharmacy technician respects the confidentiality of patients' records and discloses pertinent information only with proper authorization.

Core Value: Protecting Patient Confidentiality

Protecting patient confidentiality is the law, and pharmacy technicians must strictly adhere to this law at all times concerning patients' PHI. This means never discussing patients' health information outside of that which is necessary to assist them—and this includes maintaining that confidentiality off the job as well. Pharmacy technicians should never access a patient's profile unless they are directly involved in the assistance of that patient. This would include the profile of a friend, family member, or neighbor—even if that person asks you to do so. If a patient's representative comes to pick up the patient's prescription, care should be taken not to disclose any of the patient's PHI without proper authorization. If a technician suspects that a patient's so-called representative is not legitimate, he or she should immediately bring those concerns to a pharmacist.

PRINCIPLE 8

A pharmacy technician never assists in the dispensing, promoting, or distribution of medications or medical devices that are not of good quality or do not meet the standards required by law.

Core Value: Quality Assurance

A patient's degree of confidence in the work that we do is driven by the quality of the final product. Unlike other types of consumer products, the compounding and preparation of pharmaceutical products requires a much higher degree of accuracy and quality. A product that is not prepared according to those quality standards could present serious health risks to the patient. Again, personalization is a great way for pharmacy technicians to measure their behavior in order to ensure that they act ethically. As consumers or patients, technicians would not wish to receive a product that had been contaminated or prepared with incorrect ingredients or with the wrong proportion of ingredients; nor would a technician want to receive a medical device that was not in sound working condition. Pharmacy technicians should prepare every product as though they or one of their family members were the end receiver.

Patients should *not* be dispensed chipped or broken tablets, medication in packaging that was compromised in any way, or a product that was prepared improperly. Pharmacy staff must be further vigilant to ensure that any products that have been subject to a manufacturer's *voluntary recall* are immediately removed from stock and that patients who may have received the product (or a product containing the recalled ingredient) are notified so that they may return that product to the pharmacy.

PRINCIPLE 9

A pharmacy technician does not engage in any activity that will discredit the profession, and the technician will expose, without fear or favor, illegal or unethical conduct in the profession.

Core Value: Accountability to the Profession

Thousands of pharmacy technicians have been cited for various infractions since state boards began regulating and monitoring their activity. Drug diversion is among the top illegal or unethical activity. Pharmacy technicians must realize that the actions of one impact the whole. In other words, the demonstration of unethical—or illegal—behavior by a pharmacy technician most certainly has a negative impact on the health care community and the general public's perception of pharmacy technician practice and the pharmacy profession at large. Consumers may not be able to readily distinguish pharmacy technicians from pharmacists in the community practice setting. When poor customer service is demonstrated or when an error is committed, patients generally do not blame just the individual: blame is assigned to an entire organization or the entire profession. Just as a professional athlete's behavior off the field affects the public's perception about the overall integrity of a sports team, unethical behavior unfairly brands the pharmacy practice.

In addition to accountability for individual behavior, pharmacy technicians are bound to protect the integrity of the profession from unethical or illegal acts committed by another pharmacy technician or pharmacist. Often, individuals who know of illegal activity—whether or not they are acting participants—may be held partially responsible. Just as the driver of a getaway car in a theft may be arrested for acting as an accessory to a crime, a pharmacy technician could be considered an accessory to the criminal or unethical behavior of a colleague. Unfortunately, there is a prevalence of drug diversion from pharmacies, in addition to illegal crime rings involving corrupt medication prescribers writing illegal prescriptions for controlled medications. Any pharmacy staff member who learns of such activity must report it to his or her manager/director, state board of pharmacy, the Food and Drug Administration, the Drug Enforcement Administration, or any other appropriate regulatory authority. Once notified, the most appropriate regulatory authorities, who may then initiate an investigation into the matter. True enough, it may be difficult to report a colleague or staff pharmacist with whom you have built a rapport or share a positive professional or personal relationship. Nevertheless, it is the right thing to do and is considered a professional obligation.

PRINCIPLE 10

A pharmacy technician associates with and supports organizations that promote the profession of pharmacy through the utilization and enhancement of pharmacy technicians.

Core Values: Engagement and Advocacy

Students may be initially overwhelmed by the scope of responsibilities they have to patients, other pharmacy technicians, pharmacists, and the profession at large. It is true—a great deal of responsibility is involved, as well as accountability. However, there are a variety of benefits that those who belong to the profession may take advantage of. Pharmacy technicians should not view their role simply as "something that pays the bills." Although employment does supply the income needed to meet one's living expenses, the pharmacy technician's role is not *just a job*. It is an established career path that requires a body of knowledge, skills, and attitudes that must be appropriately utilized to protect the health, welfare, and safety of patients. Pharmacy technicians must continually seek opportunities to expand their knowledge base, even after they have completed their initial training. One of the best ways to continue one's professional development, while giving back to one's profession, is through membership to one or more professional pharmacy organizations. As mentioned in Chapter 1, professional pharmacy organizations were created to provide support, or advocacy, to pharmacists as well as guidance in terms of educational resources and best practices. Additionally, a variety of professional pharmacy organizations provide resources to their members, including the following:

- Educational programming
- Drug information resources, both print and web-based
- Medication error prevention alerts and studies
- Career and other employment opportunities
- Leadership and management opportunities

Most of these organizations have a branch for pharmacy technician membership and embrace opportunities for pharmacy technicians to become involved at the local, state, and national levels. One of the primary ethical principles approached early in the Code of Ethics for Pharmacy Technicians was *service orientation*. One way for pharmacy technicians to create greater opportunities for themselves is to give back to the organizations that advocates for them. Annual membership dues are generally required, but try to consider it an investment into future career opportunities.

Overcoming Ethical Dilemmas through Ethical Decision Making

Now that the core ethical principles have been outlined and students have had the opportunity to reflect on the development of their own core value systems, it is time to approach how to put those ideals into practice. When entering into a situation that may conflict with one's moral/ethical value system, it is important to employ a process whereby one may determine the most appropriate decision. The *Framework for Ethical Decision Making* details five primary steps:

1. Recognize an ethical issue
2. Get the facts
3. Evaluate alternative actions
4. Make a decision and test it
5. Act and reflect on the outcome

Let's apply each of the decision-making steps to the following scenario:

> *Janet Curry is a pharmacy technician working in a local mail-order pharmacy. One of Janet's co-workers, Rita Jensen, with whom she is friendly, has expressed concern about one of her small children who has been ill with an ear infection for several days. Rita had previously confided that she recently separated from her spouse and has suffered financial difficulty for the past few months as a result. One afternoon, Janet notices that Rita has removed a bottle of Suprax pediatric antibiotic suspension from line stock and set the bottle aside. At the end of her shift, Janet witnesses Rita slipping the bottle into her bag before leaving the staff locker room.*

RECOGNIZE AN ETHICAL ISSUE

It is important to consider whether any applicable laws or regulatory statutes apply to the situation. One should additionally consider any applicable company policies or rules. Generally speaking, if taking action, or *not* taking action, would cause a person to break the law, then the decision is clear-cut. However, if taking action involves choosing the lesser of two or more undesirable outcomes, then that may create an ethical dilemma. Sometimes, when trying to arrive at a personal decision, it may be useful to conduct a brief mental "ethics check." According to Blanchard and Peale in *The Power of Ethical Management*, there are three questions that one may pose when trying to determine the ethical issue at hand:

> *a. Is it legal or in accordance with institutional or company policy?*
> *b. Does it promote a win-win situation for anyone possibly affected by the situation?*
> *c. How would I feel about myself if I were to read about my decision or action in the daily newspaper? How would my family feel? Can I look myself in the mirror?*
>
> **(Lewis M, 2002)**

The reality is that not every ethical decision will leave a person feeling good or satisfied that he or she made the right decision, particularly if that action renders a negative outcome for that person or another person he or she cares about or respects. Although one may seek a win-win solution, it is important to recognize that it may not always be possible. A person who is engaged in illegal or unethical behavior will likely be subject to professional or legal disciplinary action. If one has to self-report (that is, report or face one's own illegal or unethical behavior), one must do so with the recognition of any and all consequences he or she may face as a result.

Referring to the sample scenario, theft of a prescription drug from a pharmacy is a clear violation of federal law, which would make Janet's co-worker subject to potential disciplinary action. The issue that Janet may struggle with involves the personal details she knows about Rita. The actions that Janet witnessed may well be a violation of both legal and company policy; in addition, Rita's actions come into conflict with the core values of the second principle in the Code of Ethics for Pharmacy Technicians: honesty and integrity. Additionally, Janet has the professional obligation to uphold the ninth core value of the code, accountability to the profession, which dictates that she *must* report any observed illegal or unethical conduct "without fear or favor." Janet recognizes which ethical principles may have been compromised, or may be compromised if she does not take action, and then can proceed to the next decision-making step.

GET THE FACTS

It is important to gather all of the facts as well as to identify any stakeholders, or individuals who may be affected, before arriving at any decision, particularly one that involves an ethical dilemma. In the event that there is an investigation, it will be important to disclose any facts or details that may be relevant to the situation. External factors, particularly those that may contribute to the ethical dilemma, should also be taken into consideration.

In the scenario, Janet is aware of certain facts about the person possibly committing a criminal offense. Rita has recently experienced a major life change (divorce and subsequent single parenthood), is suffering financially, and has a sick child for whom she may not have the financial means to gain medical treatment. Although it is normal to feel sympathy or even empathize with the person's situation, the fact remains that stealing—even for the noblest of reasons—will always be considered wrong in the eyes of those who govern the practice of pharmacy.

Rita's actions place her co-workers and supervising pharmacists in professional and legal jeopardy. For example, the inventory technician may have to account for the missing bottle of antibiotic. Perhaps the pharmacist in charge might be held responsible for the missing product during a state board inspection. Perhaps there is a camera that recorded the entire event, and the recording captured not only the theft but any witness who observed the theft. If the witness does not come forward, he or she could be implicated for not protecting the integrity of the profession by immediately reporting unethical/illegal activity. As a result, the person could be dismissed from his or her position.

One must further consider the possibility that there is no true wrongdoing and must consider the person involved to be "innocent until proven guilty." So in fairness, Janet must also consider the possibility that Rita may have spoken with the pharmacist in charge and obtained permission to take the medicine, after producing a written prescription—so her actions might be legal after all. Once Janet has gathered as much information as possible, she may proceed to the next decision-making step.

EVALUATE ALTERNATIVE ACTIONS

One must evaluate each of the possible outcomes of any actions he or she may choose to take and how it will impact anyone else involved. It is important to carefully consider each possible action in terms of cause and effect. If Rita's actions are exposed and she did indeed steal the drug, she will likely lose her job, and she may face professional or criminal disciplinary action. Janet may consider any of the following approaches to taking action in this situation:

- Seek a solution that may result in the least harm. For instance, Janet might confront Rita about what she observed, express her concern and ethical obligation, and allow Rita the opportunity to either explain how her action is appropriate or take the appropriate steps to make it right.
- Take no action. In this situation, Janet may certainly consider doing nothing at all, deciding to mind her own business and "let the chips fall where they may," or ignore what she observed out of sympathy for Rita's personal situation. After all, she's not stealing to sell the drug: she's stealing a drug to take home to give to her sick child.
- Seek a solution that results in all parties' rights being protected or considered. Janet might elect to call the company's fraud, waste, and abuse line to issue an anonymous report of her

observations. This action will not immediately implicate Rita or Janet, and it allows Janet to fulfill her ethical obligation while leaving the pharmacy to take over from there to investigate without her direct involvement.

- Seek a solution that serves the greater good regardless of the outcome, such as bringing the matter directly to a manager or supervisor. This option would allow Janet to state the facts as she witnessed them, releasing her from possible liability, and would allow her supervisor to take the appropriate action from there. This act of self-preservation may keep Janet from possibly facing negative consequences that may impact her employment.
- Seek a solution that leaves the person feeling as though he or she has been true to him or herself from the standpoint of virtue. Perhaps Janet may choose to inform her supervisor of the hardships that Rita has suffered, as an explanation of her unethical behavior. That may make it easier for Janet to rest following that decision, knowing that she shared relevant details that may be taken into consideration and possibly render a less severe outcome for Rita. After all, although a pharmacy may dismiss a technician for stealing, it may or may not choose to pursue criminal charges.

Once Janet has carefully evaluated all possible alternative actions, she may proceed to the next decision-making step.

TECH NOTE!
This applies not only to ethical decision making but to customer service and patient care at large. Pharmacy technicians should be willing to provide every customer the same level of attention, support, and courtesy that they would provide to a family member or close friend.

MAKE A DECISION AND TEST IT

Once an individual arrives at the decision, it may be useful to evaluate that decision again based on the "ethics check" questions. In Janet's situation, she may ask herself, if someone she respected learned of her decision, how would that person feel about it? If the decision were going to affect someone closer to her, like a close friend or family member, would she have arrived at the same decision? As a rule, personalizing behavior or decision making is often quite useful and may quickly change a person's approach to a situation. Pharmacy technicians must take the most appropriate actions, given the facts, possible alternative actions, and possible outcomes—regardless of the outside factors or an individual's closeness to the person involved. That may be extremely difficult, but it is indeed the *right* thing to do.

ACT AND REFLECT ON THE OUTCOME

Janet decides that she does not feel comfortable confronting her co-worker and instead speaks to her supervisor about Rita's situation and the actions she witnessed. Following the meeting, Rita is called in to the pharmacy director's office. She is immediately terminated and is escorted out of the pharmacy. On her way out, Rita approaches Janet tearfully and bitterly remarks, "How could you betray me like that? You know what I've been going through, and now I have no means to support my family!" This type of scenario, as expected, will not end well for the person involved. Janet, upon reflection, feels terrible that Rita lost her job, but she does feel that she made the right decision under the circumstances. It is later determined that the pharmacy's security camera did indeed capture Rita's actions. Had she not come forward, Janet may have faced disciplinary action herself.

Pharmacy technicians will face many ethical dilemmas similar to the scenario just discussed. Although one may not feel good about the outcome in terms of consequences, it is important to make those feelings secondary to acting ethically. One should further assess, during reflection, whether actions taken were implemented with the greatest possible care and attention to the concerns of the persons involved. It is fair to say that the decision Janet came to accomplished that goal. Given the outcome of the situation, Janet should evaluate if she would make the same decision if she had to do it all over again. She should further consider what she has learned from the situation. This scenario will have certainly served as a reminder to Janet and her co-workers of the imminent consequences of stealing: loss of one's ability to earn a living and loss of one's technician license/registration along with one's ability to practice as a pharmacy technician.

Chapter Summary

- Ethics is defined as the "principles or conduct governing an individual or a group" and "the discipline dealing with what is good and bad and with moral duty and obligation."
- Core values were defined as "the fundamental beliefs, morals, and standards that define you as a person and which guide your behavior."

- Every individual must take the opportunity to discover—or reaffirm—where he or she stands in terms of principles.
- Exercising the ability to appropriately apply personal or professional ethical principles is of great importance in the practice of health care.
- Members of a given profession can refer to an established *code* of model behavior, which may effectively lead an individual to practice ethical decision making.
- Pharmacy technicians may have to face their capacity to act on individual conscience when given an order that conflicts with their personal values.
- The three suggested ethical principles on which one may model one's behavior include respect for persons, beneficence, and justice.
- The Code of Ethics for Pharmacy Technicians may be practically applied to workplace scenarios that may present moral or ethical dilemmas, through the application of two decision-making processes including the ethics check and the five key ethical decision-making steps.

REVIEW QUESTIONS

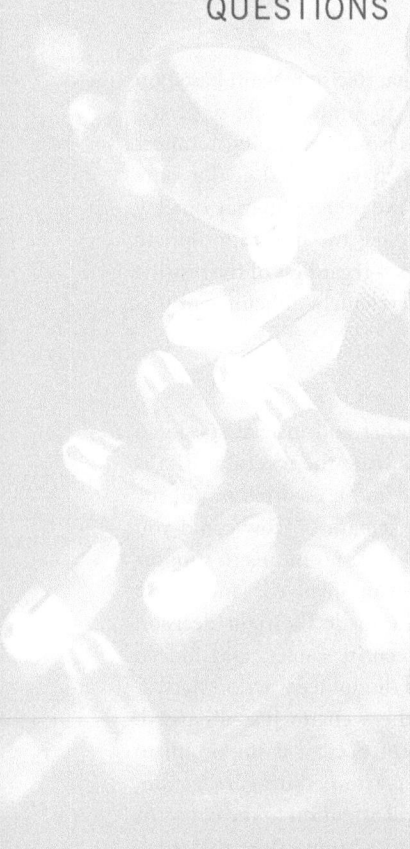

Multiple Choice

1. Advocacy may be defined as:
   a. Support of a particular group or cause
   b. A set of rules, principles, or laws
   c. Firm adherence to a code of moral/ethical values
   d. Patients' rights to make their own decisions about their health care

2. A situation that conflicts with one's moral or ethical values would be considered a(n):
   a. Ethics issue
   b. Ethical dilemma
   c. Compromise of integrity
   d. Exercise of patient autonomy

3. A logical motivation toward thought or action based on moral or ethical principles is the expression of:
   a. Conscience
   b. Ethics
   c. Integrity
   d. Core values

4. The principle or conduct governing an individual or a group is known as the study of:
   a. Ethics
   b. Ethical decision making
   c. Core values
   d. Patient advocacy

5. One who possesses the quality or state of being complete or undivided may act with:
   a. Integrity
   b. Core values
   c. Uncertainty
   d. A code of values

6. The Hippocratic oath's charge to new physicians to ensure that they "call upon colleagues when the skills of another are needed for a patient's recovery" corresponds with which of the Code of Ethics for Pharmacy Technicians' core values?
   a. Patient focus
   b. Respect for professional roles
   c. Advocacy
   d. Continuous learning

7. The Code of Ethics for Pharmacy Technicians' core value of respecting patients' autonomy aligns with the framework ethical principle of:
   a. Beneficence
   b. Justice
   c. Respect for professional roles
   d. Respect for persons

8. A pharmacy technician's commitment to ethical behavior while not at work demonstrates which of the Code of Ethics for Pharmacy Technicians' core values?
   a. Advocacy
   b. Accountability to the profession
   c. Continuous learning
   d. Respect for professional roles

9. Which historical code of ethical practice spoke to the humane treatment of animals during medical experimentation?
   a. Nuremberg Code of 1947
   b. Declaration of Helsinki
   c. Geneva Convention of Medical Ethics
   d. Hippocratic oath

10. The fundamental beliefs, morals, and standards that define a person may be referred to as:
    a. A core value system
    b. Principles
    c. Integrity
    d. Ethics

TECHNICIAN'S CORNER

1. Explain what it means to demonstrate the principle of *respect for persons*.
2. State two specific factors related to the pharmacy practice that may frequently change and necessitate the demonstration of the core value of *continuous learning*.
3. Explain what it means to *personalize* a situation when encountering ethical decision making.

Bibliography

International Committee of the Red Cross. (2005). *International Humanitarian Law—Treaties & Documents*. Retrieved 7/14/2010, from International Committee of the Red Cross: http://www.icrc.org/ihl.nsf/full/470?opendocument#top

Lasagna, L. (2010). *The Hippocratic Oath: Modern Version (written in 1964)*. Retrieved 7/14/2010, from NOVA: http://www.pbs.org/wgbh/nova/doctors/oath_modern.html

Levine, C. (1993). *Building a New Consensus: Ethical Principles and Policies for Clinical Research on HIV/AIDS*. In T. A. Shannon, *Bioethics: Basic Writings on the Key Ethical Questions that Surround the Major, Modern Biological Possibilities and Problems* (p. 303). Mahwah, New Jersey: Paulist Press.

Lewis, M.A. (2002). *Medical Law, Ethics & Bioethics for the Health Professions*, 6th Edition. Philadelphia: F. A. Davis.

Loo, T. (2006). *How to Define Your Life Purpose*. Retrieved 7/11/2010, from Ezine Articles: http://ezinearticles.com/?How-to-Define-Your-Life-Purpose&id=331527

Merriam-Webster Online. (2010). *Merriam-Webster's Online Dictionary*. Retrieved 5/14/2010, from Merriam-Webster Online: http://www.merriam-webster.com/dictionary/law

The Nuremberg Code. (1947). In M. F. Mitscherlich: *Doctors of Infamy: the Story of the Nazi Medical Crimes*. New York: Schuman. Pages 23-25.

Santa Clara University. (2009). *A Framework for Thinking Ethically*. Retrieved 7/14/2010, from Markkula Center for Applied Ethics: http://www.scu.edu/ethics/practicing/decision/framework.html

Vasquez, A.S. (1988). *Conscience and Authority*. Retrieved 7/14/2010, from Santa Clara University: http://www.scu.edu/ethics/practicing/decision/conscience.html

WordNet Search 3.0. (2010). *WordNet Search 3.0*. Retrieved 7/10/2010, from WordNet Search 3.0: http://wordnetweb.princeton.edu/perl/webwn?s=code

World Medical Organization. (1996). *Declaration of Helsinki*. British Medical Journal, 313(7070):1448-1449.

Pharmacy Professional Organizations

By the end of this chapter, students will be able to do the following concerning 10 major national pharmacy organizations:

1. Explain the rationale for the existence of professional pharmacy organizations.
2. Describe pharmacy organizations that are relevant to technician practice and their importance to the profession.
3. Discuss the importance of attending professional conferences and how to prepare.

Health literacy: A consumer or patient's overall knowledge concerning medical treatment, medical terms that pertain to health and medicine, and how to take medication safety and correctly.

White papers: Research studies, reports, and professional commentaries composed by research teams and concerning topics of vital interest to the pharmacy community as well as to the medical community at large.

Introduction

Pharmacy organizations were originally created to provide professional resources that would help pharmacists—then known as apothecaries or druggists—to best protect the health, welfare, and safety of their patients. The early organizations provided resources to colleges and schools of pharmacy to standardize the education and training of new pharmacists in the United States. Many of the current clinical organizations in existence today were formed by members of the first pharmacy organization in the United States. Today, the expansive variety of industry or clinically oriented associations and societies has significantly increased the scope of resources available to the global profession of pharmacy, the health care community, and patients at large.

Although many of these organizations were originally structured to support the education and careers of pharmacist members exclusively (the technician practice was not yet in existence), many that will be noted in this chapter have expanded their educational and career advancement resources to include pharmacy technicians. Most extend membership opportunities as well. Additionally, there are organizations that were founded *specifically* for pharmacy technicians and offer educational and career advancement opportunities that target the pharmacy technician practice. Just as new pharmacy technician students may learn many new things about the profession of pharmacy, students are strongly encouraged to further research these and other professional pharmacy organizations to find out what resources they offer. Professional pharmacy organizations may offer the following:

- Educational programming
- Drug information resources, both print and web based
- Medication error prevention alerts and studies
- Career and other employment opportunities
- Leadership and management opportunities

To stay current with today's technology-driven population, every organization offers electronic resources that may be accessed over the Internet, and most have pages or links to many of the existing web-based social networking media sites. It is important to recognize that these organizations are in place primarily to advance patient care, so one does not have to gain membership to take advantage of many of the professional resources. There is a great deal of information available on the websites of each of these organizations that may be useful to *any* member of the health care team, including physicians, nurses, pharmacists, pharmacy technicians, pharmacy school students, and pharmacy practice residents. Because members of the pharmacy profession play key roles on today's multidisciplinary patient care team, the sharing of information across professional disciplines increases the team's overall ability to best serve patients and optimize the benefits of prescribed medication and other treatment plans.

Professional pharmacy organizations also help to advance the profession of pharmacy by further enlightening the medical community on the education and expertise of pharmacists and by encouraging health care providers to seek out pharmacists as the primary experts on medication therapy. Because members of the pharmacy profession are ethically obligated to adhere to the patient's right to autonomy, many pharmacy organizations also offer resources that are specifically designed to provide information to patients and consumers across the globe. These consumer-based publications are offered not only by pharmacy organizations but by many health care organizations, such as the American Medical Association (AMA). Government agencies, such as the Food and Drug Administration (FDA), also offer consumer safety and product information bulletins and journals that assist patients and increase their ability to make *informed decisions* about their own health care. It is important that all members of the health care team provide resources that will help patients increase their health literacy, or knowledge concerning medical treatment and how to take medication safely and correctly.

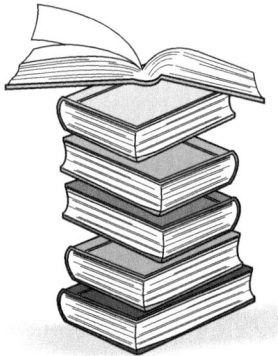

Working together with your colleagues can lead to new ideas while building lasting professional relationships.

Many organizations have sponsored or published research studies, reports, and professional commentaries, sometimes known as white papers. These white papers were composed by research teams and concern topics of vital interest to the pharmacy community as well as to the medical community at large. These research data are often published in professional journals; many of the major pharmacy organizations produce a professional journal that is released biweekly, monthly, or quarterly. The pursuit of knowledge is progressive: each educational resource will direct one to additional resources—there is no end to the knowledge that one may gain, as research and development in the area of medication therapy is ongoing. The fifth principle of the Code of Ethics for Pharmacy Technicians is *continuous learning*. Pharmacy technicians should continually seek opportunities to increase their knowledge base and understanding of how medication is used as well as of the technology that helps increase the efficiency and safety of workflow processes. Pharmacy technicians who seek to continually increase their knowledge base will also gain a great many more marketable skills, which will increase opportunities for career advancement.

Since the late 1990s, the profession of pharmacy has begun to acknowledge the evolving role of the pharmacy technician, thanks in part to studies and information disseminated by professional organizations. The need for better-trained technicians has been increasingly recognized as a patient safety issue that must be addressed across the nation. This chapter examines several organizations and identifies those that have strongly advocated for the pharmacy technician practice. As the 10th principle of the Code of Ethics for Pharmacy Technicians is *advocacy*, pharmacy technicians should seek out organizations that advocate for technicians and offer opportunities for them to contribute productively to the profession and in a manner that protects the health, safety, and welfare of patients.

A Closer Look at Professional Pharmacy Organizations

This chapter covers 10 major national pharmacy organizations, although several other highly respected and recognized organizations exist. For a complete list of pharmacy organizations in existence worldwide, students are encouraged to visit www.pharmacychoice.com/resources/pharmacy_associations.cfm.

Many national organizations also have state-level chapters as well as local chapters within each state. Students are encouraged to seek out additional information concerning the state and local chapters to learn the benefits of gaining membership as pharmacy technician trainees and later as a practicing pharmacy technician (with or without certification).

The subsequent subsections provide the following information about each organization:
- Brief history and description of its membership base
- Primary mission and goals
- Significant accomplishments and contributions to health care and the profession of pharmacy
- Technician advocacy
- Membership information

American Pharmacists Association

HISTORY OF THE ORGANIZATION

The American Pharmacists Association (APhA) was founded on October 6, 1852, in Philadelphia, and it was originally known as the American Pharmaceutical Association. Its headquarters are located in Washington, D.C. APhA was the first professional organization established in the United States and continues to be the largest in existence, with more than 60,000 members. Additionally, many of the national pharmacy organizations currently in existence were originally branches of APhA.

APhA has state- and local-level chapters to which pharmacists, pharmacy technicians, pharmacy residents, and students may gain membership.

PRIMARY MISSION AND GOALS

APhA has five primary mission statements:
- Provide timely information to members
- Increase society's awareness and recognition of pharmacists as the experts in medication therapy and management
- Provide resources to members for continuous professional development
- Educate and influence lawmakers and the public concerning APhA's mission and goals
- Create networking opportunities for members to collaborate across multiple medical disciplines

SIGNIFICANT CONTRIBUTIONS TO THE PROFESSION

The most significant means by which APhA has contributed to the profession has been its long-standing advocacy of the profession of pharmacy through educational programming, as well as its provision of information resources to the health care community and consumers. As the mission statements note, APhA has been very involved in state and federal legislative processes and has exercised influence on lawmakers concerning legislation that impacts the profession of pharmacy. In consideration of today's health care reform issues under debate as new legislation is passed, APhA as an organization has taken strides to stress to lawmakers the degree to which pharmacists make a positive impact when actively involved in medication therapy management. The 2010 executive director and CEO designate of APhA emphasized this point in a statement in which he described the value of pharmacists to patients' safe medication use:

Our Pharmacist members encounter patients every day with medication problems that have real life consequences. Often patients, especially those managing complex medication regimens, don't completely understand how to use their medications correctly and that knowledge gap impacts everyone. Overwhelmingly, data indicate the need for enhanced medication therapy management, and Pharmacists have demonstrated their value in providing it. Health Care Reformers who include Pharmacists' services will one day be seen as visionary.

In the March 2010 issue of the *Medication Therapy Management Digest*, a publication developed by APhA, it was noted that "in the health care reform debate, we educate policy makers about the benefits to consumers when pharmacists are members of the health care team" (Menighan, 2010).

APhA has a variety of other professional publications that are available to members by subscription, including the following:

- *Pharmacy Today*
- *Journal of the American Pharmacists Association*
- APhA Drug Info online
- *Journal of Pharmaceutical Sciences*
- *Student Pharmacist Magazine*
- *Transitions* Newsletter

APhA also publishes a variety of textbooks on the pharmacy practice—and the technician practice.

TECHNICIAN ADVOCACY

APhA provides a variety of resources for pharmacy technicians, including membership. APhA as an organization has generally supported the pharmacy technician practice and has recently made strides in the support of pharmacy technician education and credentialing. At the March 2010 APhA annual meeting, programming included results from a survey that was conducted by the Pharmacy Technician Certification Board (PTCB) concerning the connection between pharmacy technician certification and a reduction in the incidence of medication errors. APhA is also one of the governing organizations that helped form and regulate the Pharmacy Technician Certification Board.

MEMBERSHIP INFORMATION

The APhA membership webpage cites a variety of benefits of membership to its organization. Some of the valuable benefits include the following:

- Pharmacy news/current events
- Educational and drug information resources
- Continuing education programming
- Professional and consumer products and services
- APhA annual meeting and exposition, hosted at various national venues during the month of March
- Educational programming and annual meetings planned and hosted by state or local chapters of APhA

Pharmacy technicians may use the student pharmacists membership application, which includes information related to current annual membership dues. For further information on membership, visit the APhA website at www.pharmacist.com.

American Society of Health-System Pharmacists

HISTORY OF THE ORGANIZATION

The American Society of Health-System Pharmacists (ASHP) began as a part of APhA. ASHP originated as a hospital pharmacist committee that was part of the Section on Practical Pharmacy and Dispensing. Hospital pharmacists later formed the independent organization, then known as the American Society of Hospital Pharmacists, in 1942. As the organization extended its development of pharmacy practice models beyond hospital pharmacy into other areas, such as home care and ambulatory care (community practice), the name was changed to the American Society of Health-System Pharmacists in 1995. ASHP headquarters are in Baltimore, Maryland. ASHP has membership across all areas of the pharmacy profession, although its primary focus (and core membership) is health-system—primarily hospital—pharmacy practice. As of 2010, ASHP had 31,000 members, composed of pharmacists, pharmacy students, interns, residents, and pharmacy technicians.

ASHP has state- and local-level chapters, to which pharmacists, pharmacy technicians, pharmacy residents, and students may gain membership.

PRIMARY MISSION AND GOALS

Since its formation, ASHP was founded on the primary goals of (1) establishing minimal standards for the hospital pharmacy practice, (2) providing a forum for encouraging the development of new pharmaceutical techniques, and (3) aiding the medical profession in extending the economical and rational use of medication. That mission continues, as the organization strives to empower pharmacists with the tools needed to ensure that patients optimize the use of prescribed medication. ASHP advocates for pharmacists and pharmacy technicians concerning the establishment of professional policies and uses its professional rapport and influence to collectively voice issues from across health-system practice that relate to medication use and public health. The primary focus of ASHP's vision statements (which are set forth in great detail as the collective *2015 ASHP Health-System Pharmacy Initiative*) is the establishment of pharmacists as "caring, compassionate medication-use experts" (American Society of Health-System Pharmacists, 2010) who will be sought out by patients and other members of the health-care team in order to maximize the benefits of medication therapy based on proven clinical evidence.

SIGNIFICANT CONTRIBUTIONS TO THE PROFESSION

In the spirit of its founding goals, ASHP has provided the profession with uniform standards for best practice. The *Minimum Standards for Hospital Pharmacists* was originally written in 1943; revisions over the years to the more contemporary *Best Practices for Health-System Pharmacy* have continued to detail standards for those in health-system practice. ASHP further established the *Minimum Standards for Ambulatory Care*, which sets forth practice standards for outpatient or community pharmacy practice. Minimum standards have also been established for pharmacy internships in hospitals.

In the education realm, ASHP has contributed universal educational goals and standards for both pharmacy residency and pharmacy technician training programs. The first *Accreditation Standard for Pharmacy Technician Training Program* was approved by the board of directors in 1982, and ASHP accredited its first pharmacy technician training program at Thomas Jefferson University Hospital in Philadelphia, Pennsylvania. ASHP published the *Model Curriculum for Pharmacy Technician Training Programs* in 1996, developed through the collaborated efforts of the American Association of Colleges of Pharmacy (AACP), APhA, the American Association of Pharmacy Technicians (AAPT), and the Pharmacy Technician Educators Council (PTEC). ASHP is currently the only accrediting body for pharmacy technician training programs, although training programs may also seek accreditation as pharmacy continuing education providers from the Accreditation Council for Pharmacy Education (ACPE).

ASHP has various other professional publications that are available by subscription to members, including the following:
* *American Journal of Health-System Pharmacy (AJHP)*
* AHFS Drug Information and other print and electronic drug references
* *Handbook on Injectable Drugs*
* Special publications
 ASHP also publishes a variety of textbooks and hospital in-house training materials.

TECHNICIAN ADVOCACY

ASHP has a long-standing history of advocacy for the pharmacy technician practice. A detailed historical timeline may be viewed online at www.ashp.org.

ASHP as an organization has concentrated efforts to define the role of pharmacy technicians in hospital practice since the 1950s, as well as to establish educational standards for pharmacy technician training programs. ASHP supported and encouraged the formation of a voluntary pharmacy technician certification exam for a number of years, and the organization has collaborated with APhA, the Illinois Council of Health-System Pharmacists (ICHP), and the Michigan Pharmacists Association (MPA) on the creation of the Pharmacy Technician Certification Board in 1995. The organization has collaborated with several national professional pharmacy organizations to examine pharmacy technician practice, and several related articles have been published in the *American Journal of Hospital Pharmacy (AJHP)* over the years. ASHP has formally endorsed white papers related to the pharmacy technician practice and the need for better-educated pharmacy technicians. The most notable of these white papers was published in 2003 in *AJHP* and was titled "White Paper on Pharmacy Technicians 2002: Needed Changes Can No Longer Wait." The paper was endorsed by nearly every clinical and hospital-related pharmacy professional organization and was a landmark document that alerted the entire profession to the need for quality pharmacy technician education and training as a means to advance patient safety and the clinical roles of hospital pharmacists. ASHP continues to be a strong supporter of pharmacy technician education and has encouraged state boards of pharmacy to consider requiring completion of an ASHP-accredited training program prior to beginning a pharmacy technician practice.

ASHP has involved pharmacy technicians or technician educators on various task forces, councils, and committees concerning technician practice. A pharmacy technician educator has been appointed to the Council on Credentialing, and there is a technician liaison member on the ASHP board of directors.

MEMBERSHIP INFORMATION

Pharmacy technicians may contribute positively to their profession through membership with ASHP. The ASHP membership web pages cites a variety of valuable benefits to members, including the following:

- A free subscription to *Tech Topics* magazine, which contains continuing education lessons
- Member discounts on registration to the annual midyear clinical meeting, held each December in venues across the United States
- Opportunities to retain dual membership to selected state- and local-level societies
- Member discounts on ASHP publications
- Discounted subscription to *AJHP*
- Members-only access to online news and current legislative events

Pharmacy technicians may use the pharmacy technician membership application, which includes information related to current annual membership dues. For further information on membership, visit the ASHP website at www.ashp.org.

American Association of Pharmacy Technicians

HISTORY OF THE ORGANIZATION

The American Association of Pharmacy Technicians (AAPT) was the first established pharmacy technician association in the United States and was founded in 1979 by volunteer pharmacy technicians. This nonprofit international organization is composed of pharmacy technicians from across the United States, Canada, and the United Kingdom. Its membership represents a broad cross section of pharmacy practice settings.

AAPT currently has five state- and local-level chapters, to which pharmacists, pharmacy technicians, and students may gain membership:

- Metro Protech Association of Pharmacy Technicians—New York
- North Carolina Association of Pharmacy Technicians (NCAPT)—North Carolina
- Northland Association of Pharmacy Technicians—North Dakota/Minnesota
- White Rose Association of Pharmacy Technicians—Pennsylvania
- Alamo of San Antonio Association of Pharmacy Technicians—Texas

The national headquarters are in Greensboro, North Carolina.

PRIMARY MISSION AND GOALS

The primary mission of AAPT is to empower student technicians and certified/registered pharmacy technicians with education and resources to increase their capacity to provide exemplary pharmaceutical services that safeguard the health, welfare, and safety of patients. The AAPT also established the Continuing Education Service (CES), which is an official provider of pharmacy technician continuing education credit and programming.

SIGNIFICANT CONTRIBUTIONS TO THE PROFESSION

One of the most significant contributions that AAPT has made to the profession of pharmacy, as discussed in the previous chapter, is the Code of Ethics for Pharmacy Technicians, adopted by the board of directors in 2003. This code, which has been adapted by other pharmacy technician organizations, set the standard and basis for ethical behavior and professional practice. As cited in the previous chapter, the first of the code principles positions the health and welfare of the patient as a pharmacy technician's first concern and focus. The Code of Ethics sets a standard for pharmacy technicians to meet and exceed as they proceed through their careers and challenges them to set a higher standard of practice for those to follow.

For years, AAPT had been the lone voice for practicing pharmacy technicians, aside from other efforts concerted by larger, more established organizations such as ASHP and APhA. These pharmacist-founded organizations have invited AAPT's involvement on their councils and activities (i.e., the development of the Model Curriculum for Pharmacy Technician Training Programs). The groundbreaking efforts of AAPT's volunteer members over the years have created landmark opportunities for pharmacy technicians to be invited to discussions concerning policy making, scope of practice, and possible future roles for pharmacy technicians.

TECHNICIAN ADVOCACY

AAPT provides a variety of resources that pharmacy technicians may take advantage of. Its website features a Career Center where job seekers may search current listings, post résumés, and sign up to receive new posting alerts. Employers may enlist AAPT to post current job openings within their businesses or organizations. The AAPT website provides links to a variety of pharmacy technician resources, including certifying boards, international pharmacy technician associations, various pharmacy publications, a PTCB online study group, and various technician educator resources.

MEMBERSHIP INFORMATION

AAPT offers membership to pharmacy technicians as well as other members of the pharmacy profession who wish to partner with this organization in the support and advancement of the pharmacy technician career path. Membership benefits include the following:

- Resources for free continuing education programming
- Professional enrichment and opportunities for leadership training
- Subscription to a quarterly newsletter
- Discount member rates to AAPT-sponsored events, including the annual convention, which is held during the month of August
- Updates on current industry trends and news/press releases that affect the pharmacy technician practice
- Opportunities for professional networking and community building with pharmacy technicians in the United States and other countries

Pharmacy technicians may use the online membership application, which includes information related to current annual membership dues based on the type of membership. For further information, visit the AAPT website at www.pharmacytechnician.com.

Institute for the Certification of Pharmacy Technicians

HISTORY OF THE ORGANIZATION

The Institute for the Certification of Pharmacy Technicians (ICPT) was founded as the second source through which pharmacy technicians could gain the CPhT credential through competence demonstrated by successfully passing its certification examination, the ExCPT. Once a stand-alone organization, ICPT is now part of the National Healthcare Career Association (NHCA), which partners with various proprietary allied health training programs as a source of credentialing for students of their programs. In 2008, ICPT was granted accreditation through the National Commission for Certifying Agencies (NCCA), which is the accrediting body of the National Organization for Competency Assurance (NOCA).

PRIMARY MISSION AND GOALS

ICPT offers a credentialing exam to individuals seeking pharmacy technician certification, which has gained national visibility as a competitor or alternative to the established examination offered by the Pharmacy Technician Certification Board.

SIGNIFICANT CONTRIBUTIONS TO THE PROFESSION

Like the PTCB exam, the ExCPT examination is computer based and is offered in all 50 states and Washington D.C. The examination is administered by LaserGrade, which is whom applicants contact to secure a testing appointment. Upon completion of the exam, test takers are provided an automatic pass/fail result. Testing is offered more than 300 days a year at various testing locations.

TECHNICIAN ADVOCACY

ICPT seeks to gain more notoriety for its exam across the profession as a viable alternative to the PTCB examination. Although information provided on the organization's website references job tasks typically performed by community pharmacy technicians, the site notes that the exam is offered to applicants from all areas of pharmacy practice. Those who wish to gain certification should check with individual state boards of pharmacy to verify whether their state accepts the CPhT credential awarded by successfully passing the ExCPT examination.

National Association of Chain Drug Stores

HISTORY OF THE ORGANIZATION

The National Association of Chain Drug Stores (NACDS) was founded by the executives of six national drugstore chains in 1933. At this time, chain drugstore practice was very different than it is today and these companies needed a unified voice and strategic plan to remain viable and competitive. Today, the NACDS represents what is now the largest component of the pharmacy practice: membership includes more than 200 chain pharmacy companies (which represent more than 36,000 retail community pharmacies), accounting for over 72% of the 3.2 billion prescriptions dispensed in the United States! NACDS membership also includes more than 900 retail suppliers of goods and services to chain community pharmacies, which includes more than 70 international members from 24 countries (NACDS, 2010). The organization's headquarters are in Alexandria, Virginia. The NACDS has state-level organizations as well, in which pharmacists, pharmacy technicians, pharmacy residents, and students may also seek involvement.

PRIMARY MISSION AND GOALS

The NACDS is the chain pharmacy counterpart to the National Community Pharmacists Association (NCPA). It conversely represents the political and proprietary interests of its member chain companies and suppliers. According to data cited on the NACDS website, chain pharmacy sales equal 26% of the nation's gross domestic product (GDP). The primary mission of this highly influential organization is to "advance the interests of the chain community pharmacy industry, by fostering its growth and promoting its role as a provider of health care services and consumer products." To that end, the NACDS seeks to promote the profession of pharmacy by providing resources to its stakeholders, offering a platform for communication among its members, and assuring members a return on their investment in the organization through strong representation on the political front and continued economical viability.

SIGNIFICANT CONTRIBUTIONS TO THE PROFESSION

The NACDS has had its greatest impact on the pharmacy profession through its involvement in grassroots activities, government, and legislative affairs. NACDS and its stakeholders have been able to effectively influence legislators concerning major health care issues such as increased funding to state Medicaid programs, safe drug disposal policies, and the advancement of health information technology as a means to promote the pharmacy industry's "ability to help patients take their medications correctly, to save and improve lives and reduce health care costs. NACDS highlighted the importance to this effort of technology-based strategies such as electronic prescribing and electronic medication records" (NACDS, 2010). The NACDS has supported and advocated for high-profile pharmacist issues such as keynoting their roles and expertise in such areas as diabetes counseling and education, medication therapy management, and their support of legislation that will target community-specific drug abuse trends. For a comprehensive list of press releases that detail the political activity and advocacy efforts of the NACDS, visit the press release web page at www.nacds.org.

The NACDS was part of a joint effort with APhA and the National Community Pharmacists Association (NCPA) to form the Project Destiny initiative. This partnership was forged to create a future model for pharmacy practice that would create a more central role for pharmacists in community practice, increasing their visibility and ability to lend their expertise to patients and creating an infrastructure for economic profitability for pharmacists concerning clinical consultative services.

In terms of education advocacy for tomorrow's pharmacy leaders, the NACDS Foundation has, since 2010, endowed $280,000 in scholarship money to colleges and schools of pharmacy. The NACDS also offers internships to pharmacy student interns and residents, particularly those who plan to pursue the retail community practice or share an interest in government/political affairs.

TECHNICIAN ADVOCACY

The NACDS has traditionally represented the interests of its primary stakeholders, which are retail chain drugstores and their suppliers. Whereas various retail chains have sought means to standardize or create more quality on-the-job training opportunities for their staff pharmacy technicians, NACDS as an organization has not, to date, specifically advocated for the pharmacy technician practice. The organization has, however, invited and encouraged pharmacy technicians, along with pharmacists, CEOs, patients, pharmacy residents, and students, to take part in its grassroots efforts—which certainly may impact the pharmacy technician practice in the future. Students and technicians may wish to find out more information about the NACDS political action grassroots campaign, RXImpact. Further information may be found at www.capwiz.com/nacds/home/index.

MEMBERSHIP INFORMATION

Because of the nature of the organization, membership is generally established at the corporate—rather than individual—level and is generally extended to entities that comprise four or more chain store pharmacies. It is important to note that certified pharmacy technicians may certainly serve as retail chain store managers in many states; it would be advantageous for individuals who have interest in this area of practice to stay informed of the activities of the NACDS and its members. For more information, visit the NACDS website at www.nacds.org.

National Community Pharmacists Association

HISTORY OF THE ORGANIZATION

The National Community Pharmacists Association (NCPA) was founded in 1898 and was then known as the National Association of Retail Druggists (NARD). NCDA represents the owners of 23,000 community pharmacies. According to information cited on the association's website, the nation's independent pharmacies, independent pharmacy franchises, and independent chains dispense nearly half of the nation's retail prescription medicines (National Community Pharmacists Association, 2009).

PRIMARY MISSION AND GOALS

The primary mission of NCPA is to accomplish the following:
- Expand the growth and prosperity of the nation's independent community pharmacies and ensure that they may compete in a free and fair marketplace
- Use ethically and socially responsible measures to represent and defend the professional and proprietary interests of independent community pharmacists
- Petition the appropriate legislative and regulatory bodies to serve the needs of those they represent

NCPA strives to better educate the public, health care community, and legislators concerning the value of seeking out pharmacists as medication experts, as they are among the most accessible and trusted sources of health care information. A press release from 2009 cited research that indicated only 50% of patients nationally properly adhere to their prescribed medication therapy.

Community pharmacists help the patients that they serve and counsel by ensuring that patients use their medications safely and appropriately, which decreases overall medication therapy costs. According to NCPA, independent pharmacies dispense 1.4 billion prescriptions annually—accounting for $82 billion in sales (NCPA, 2010). Independent pharmacists better serve the public health and reduce health care spending by counseling patients on various treatment options, including the availability of generic products whenever clinically appropriate. NCPA also works to better educate communities concerning the variety of services offered by independent pharmacies, such as charge accounts, hospice and home care medication support, pharmaceutical compounding, and nutrition consultation.

NCPA has a variety of committees on which members may participate. These committees address key issues that affect independent community pharmacists, such as compounding, home health care, long-term care, patient care, legislative/government affairs, and even innovation and technology. NCPA has a news blog titled *The Dose* and has pages or links for the latest online social networking media sites.

SIGNIFICANT CONTRIBUTIONS TO THE PROFESSION

Many of the most impactful contributions that NCPA has made to the profession of pharmacy have been related to its involvement and visibility in government and legislative affairs in support and defense of issues that impact independent pharmacies and pharmacists. NCPA has posted several professional commentaries to government agencies, such as the U.S. Department of Health and Human Services, the Drug Enforcement Agency, the United States Postal Service, and many others. Because of the relatively limited financial capabilities of community pharmacies—in contrast to their corporate chain store counterparts—there are legislative issues that more significantly impact the ability of independently owned pharmacies and independent pharmacists to offer products and services to their patients while remaining competitive in the marketplace. For example, NCPA issued a commentary in July of 2010 to the United States Postal Service in support of the proposed reduction in mail delivery, particularly on weekends. Although larger corporate mail-order pharmacies and pharmacy benefit management corporations might be more visibly affected by this change, NCPA argued that this proposal created an opportunity for patients to reconnect with pharmacists face to face and engage the services provided by their local independent pharmacy. Many local pharmacies offer delivery services to patients' homes, reducing patients' dependence on mail-order sources exclusively (many independent pharmacies have offered this service at no additional charge for many years). The implication is that patients who stay connected to their community pharmacies are more likely to seek out their local pharmacist for consultation and professional advice concerning their medications. The intended result would be greater compliance, fewer compliance-driven adverse drug events, and a long-term reduction in health care costs. NCPA has several resources through which both community pharmacists and consumers may seek out their local and state legislators and have a voice concerning legislation that affects their lives and livelihood. For a list of the letters, commentaries, and other legislative activities of the NCPA, please visit the Legislative and Government Affairs page of the NCPA website at www.ncpanet.org.

To support the advancement of the independent community pharmacy, NCPA worked collaboratively with APhA and the National Association of Chain Drug Stores (NACDS) on a community pharmacy practice model known as Project Destiny. According to the 2008 executive summary, the primary objective of Project Destiny is to expand consumers' knowledge and active use of services provided by their local community pharmacist, who may become the primary source of consultive and dispensing services. Project Destiny developed a proposed vision for the future of community pharmacy, in which community pharmacists would serve as *primary care pharmacists* who would "serve as a trusted and effective resource that is valued by consumers, prescribers, health care funders and payers for their clinical and medical management expertise." Primary care pharmacists would additionally "focus on managing medications, positively impacting health outcomes, reducing overall health care system costs and empowering consumers to actively manage their health" (NCPA, 2008).

In support of education, NCPA offers internships and residencies to students of colleges and schools of pharmacy across the nation. Various student resources are available, particularly for those whose interests lie in grassroots political action or future independent pharmacy management or ownership. NCPA has a variety of other professional publications that are available by subscription to members, including the following:

- The *NCPA Digest*
- *NCPA eNews Weekly*
- *America's Pharmacist Magazine*

TECHNICIAN ADVOCACY

NCPA primarily focuses on the advancement of the independent community pharmacy practice for the benefit of patients within local communities; it also advocates for the legislative and proprietary interests of independently owned pharmacies and the pharmacists who own them. Part of that commitment to advancing the health and safety of community pharmacy consumers includes making educational resources available to the pharmacy technicians who faithfully serve in community pharmacies across the nation.

MEMBERSHIP INFORMATION

NCPA offers membership to pharmacy technicians, as well as pharmacists, pharmacy residents, and student interns. Membership benefits include the following:

- Community pharmacy practice business resources, products, and services
- Professional development opportunities and continuing education programming
- Member rates at the annual NCPA Exposition and Trade Show
- Access to the National Legislation and Government Affairs Conference
- Pharmacy ownership workshop
- Community aging, assisted living, and long-term care certificate programs
- Fight4Rx grassroots campaign forum
- Patient and caregiver resources

Pharmacy technicians may use the pharmacy technician membership application, which includes information related to current annual membership dues. For further information on membership, visit the NCPA website at www.ncpanet.org.

National Pharmacy Technician Association

HISTORY OF THE ORGANIZATION

The National Pharmacy Technician Association (NPTA) was founded by CEO Mike Johnston in 1999 in Houston, Texas. NPTA has grown to be the largest technician-based national association, with more than 30,000 members nationwide. The organization began hosting conferences and seminars targeted at providing opportunities for pharmacy technicians nationally to gather for professional networking opportunities and to take advantage of continuing education programming. Over the years, the role of NPTA has expanded to include political advocacy of the pharmacy technician career path. In 2004 and 2006, NPTA was invited to send a delegate to the United States Pharmacopeial (USP) convention. The USP convention convenes every 5 years and is a consortium of international expert representatives from medical, pharmaceutical, scientific, government, trade, and consumer-based organizations who come together to discuss policy and conduct strategic planning for the organization. NPTA became a not-for-profit organization in 2007 and continues to expand its role and influence in the pharmacy profession.

PRIMARY MISSION AND GOALS

The NPTA has three primary core values that detail the organization's mission:

- Help pharmacy technicians "realize their potential" within the profession
- Provide members with a networking community as well as resources to inspire personal and professional growth
- Provide members with a satisfaction guarantee on all offerings and services

SIGNIFICANT CONTRIBUTIONS TO THE PROFESSION AND TECHNICIAN ADVOCACY

The NPTA was one of the first organizations to offer pharmacy technician–specific continuing education programming during its annual seminar. Many of these sessions were facilitated by pharmacy technicians, which was uncommon in the early 2000s. This organization has done much to inspire pharmacy technicians to aspire to higher levels of practice as well as to contribute in more positive ways to their profession. Among the topics highlighted at the NPTA annual conventions are professionalism, drug information, and considering leadership roles.

Since beginning the process of engaging political involvement in the profession of pharmacy, NPTA has made a positive impact by influencing legislators concerning pharmacy-related issues. Mike Johnston and the NPTA provided support and lobbying assistance to Ohio legislators and the family of Emily Jerry—the toddler who lost her life following an unfortunate fatal chemotherapy compounding error by a pharmacy technician. Mike Johnston and others within the organization have encouraged pharmacy technicians to seek opportunities to voice their concerns regarding the future of their roles within the profession of pharmacy, and NPTA has encouraged members to write their state and local legislators to encourage them to support legislation that impacts the pharmacy profession and practice.

The NPTA has expanded its role as a provider of pharmacy technician continuing education in recent years. The organization offers web-based programming for gaining specialty certifications, such as aseptic intravenous admixture and nonsterile compounding. NPTA's affiliate, Meducation, offers a variety of educational products and training materials for providers of pharmacy technician education, and NPTA has been an active participant in the activities of technician educational resources, such as the Pharmacy Technician Educators Council.

TECHNICIAN ADVOCACY

NPTA engages political advocacy for pharmacy technicians through its nonprofit 503(c) branch Technician Advocacy Group (TAG), which lobbies for the interests of NPTA and its membership. The NPTA also developed a public advocacy campaign aimed at educating consumers, the health care community, and politicians on the significant contributions that pharmacy technicians make to health care at large. NPTA seeks to have a global voice as the only non-European member of the Committee of European Pharmacy Technicians.

MEMBERSHIP INFORMATION

NPTA offers membership to pharmacy technicians as well as other members of the pharmacy profession who wish to partner with this organization in the support and advancement of the pharmacy technician career path. Membership benefits include the following:

- Subscription to the *Today's Technician* bimonthly journal
- *Tech Trends,* a monthly e-newsletter
- Resource and Support Network access
- ACPE-accredited continuing education programming
- Member rates to the RxPO, NPTAs annual convention, held at various times throughout the year
- Regional live continuing education programming

Pharmacy technicians may use the online membership application, which includes information related to current annual membership dues based on type of membership. For further information, visit the NPTA website at www.pharmacytechnician.org.

Pharmacy Compounding Centers of America (PCCA)

HISTORY OF THE ORGANIZATION

PCCA was founded and incorporated in Houston, Texas, in 1981. After a pharmacist was asked to compound a medication that was no longer commercially available, the need for specialty pharmaceutical preparation emerged; a network of pharmacists who faced similar challenges united to form the organization. PCCA has become the nation's comprehensive resource for pharmaceutical compounding, including raw materials, equipment, technology, education, and professional resources.

PRIMARY MISSION AND GOALS

PCCA's primary mission is to strengthen the "role, position, and skill of member pharmacists" who may better serve patients seeking out their unique products and services (PCCA, 2010). The organization primarily focuses on quality, education, and pharmacy consulting. PCCA achieves that mission by providing educational programming, quality assurance testing of the compounding chemicals that the organization repackages and sells to members, and consultive support for pharmacy compounding professionals who are seeking technical support concerning the preparation of a variety of products.

SIGNIFICANT CONTRIBUTIONS TO THE PROFESSION

The primary contribution that PCCA has made to the profession of pharmacy is to establish rapport as a trusted source for unformulated compounding chemicals and ingredients. PCCA is registered and inspected by both the FDA and the Drug Enforcement Agency (DEA) as a manufacturing/repackaging source. The organization's quality control team completes extensive quality assurance testing on all the chemicals that it repackages and distributes, assuring the stability and contaminant-free integrity of pharmaceuticals.

The organization's second significant contribution is pharmaceutical compounding education and training. PCCA provides pharmaceutical compounding training programs at its in-house training facilities in Houston, Texas. This training has been accredited by the American Council for Pharmacy Education (ACPE), and the training facility in Houston serves as a rotation site for students of the University of Houston College of Pharmacy. The PCCA website events page provides an expansive list of educational symposia, seminars, training courses, and workshops available throughout the year.

TECHNICIAN ADVOCACY

PCCA is an excellent educational resource for pharmacy technicians who wish to pursue careers in the specialty practice area of pharmaceutical compounding. Compounding pharmacies often send their staff technicians to PCCA training workshops to gain the knowledge and skills necessary to perform pharmaceutical compounding and to gain proficiency with using pharmaceutical compounding software and equipment.

MEMBERSHIP INFORMATION

Membership is generally extended to compounding pharmacies and pharmacists working within that clinical specialty; membership gives compounding pharmacists access to both educational resources and consulting services. Pharmacy technicians practicing in compounding pharmacies may take advantage of those member resources to support the pharmacists they serve. For a detailed listing of the various educational resources offered by PCCA, visit the organization's website at www.pccarx.com.

Pharmacy Technician Certification Board

HISTORY OF THE ORGANIZATION

The Pharmacy Technician Certification Board (PTCB) was the first national organization in the United States to offer voluntary pharmacy technician certification. It was founded in 1995 by five organizations (the American Pharmacists Association, the American Society of Health-System Pharmacists, the Illinois Council of Health-System Pharmacists, the Michigan Pharmacists Association, and the National Association of Boards of Pharmacy), each of which exercises governing authority over its activities. Its headquarters are in Washington, D.C.

PTCB focuses on quality assurance, and the organization was nationally recognized in December of 2006 when it was granted accreditation through the National Commission for Certifying Agencies (NCCA). NCCA is the accrediting body of the National Organization for Competency Assurance (NOCA), which is responsible for accrediting certification programs. The accreditation process requires that programs adhere to the certification industry's high standards of practice.

PRIMARY MISSION AND GOALS

The primary mission of PTCB is to develop, maintain, promote, and administer a nationally accredited certification and recertification program for pharmacy technicians to enable the most effective support of pharmacists to advance patient safety. The focus of the future vision of PTCB is to promote patient health and safety, as well as to assume the position as the national standard for pharmacy technician credentialing. As cited on the PTCB website, the organization's core vision statements focus on the following aspects of technician practice:

- Providing high standards for the certification of pharmacy technicians
- Supporting the pharmacist–certified pharmacy technician team concept to advance patient care
- Conducting research and documenting the value of the CPhT credential
- Facilitating consensus within the profession on pharmacy technician issues
- Planning and leading public relations strategies on pharmacy technician certification that reflect PTCB's role as a nationally recognized certifying body
- Providing timely information resources related to the PTCB certification program and the role of the pharmacy technician

As of June 2010, 45 states have been identified as state associates with PTCB. These states market the PTCB examination to technicians, provide information about the certification process, and provide pharmacist and technician nominations for PTCB volunteer council participation. Several states have approved the PTCE as the only state-board approved examination. Additionally, as of June 2010, the U.S. Department of Veterans Affairs required all pharmacy technicians employed at the job skill rating of GS-6 and above to gain certification through PTCB. This is a great example of how PTCB's examination credentials have increased the visibility of the pharmacy technician career path and created a means through which a standard of quality may be upheld.

SIGNIFICANT CONTRIBUTIONS TO THE PROFESSION

The most notable contribution that PTCB has made to the profession of pharmacy is the creation of a credentialing examination that validates the base knowledge of pharmacy technicians prior to entering practice. This credential gives greater credibility to the pharmacy technician designation and, in some states, increases the entry-level earning capacity of technicians. Since 1995 when testing began, PTCB has certified 383,457 pharmacy technicians (PTCB, 2010).

PTCB has also been highly instrumental in providing much-needed visibility to the pharmacy technician career path by conducting comprehensive analyses of pharmacy technicians' scope of practice across the profession. From the beginning, PTCB has promoted the examination to all 50 boards of pharmacy. PTCB has conducted surveys of consumers as well as pharmacists and technicians currently in practice (recall the survey results that were presented at a recent annual APhA seminar). The data collected reflect the public's perception of the education and role of the pharmacy technician. PTCB posts statistical data concerning the pass rates of technicians each testing year and what professional demographics are being represented.

Additionally, in 2009 PTCB began providing resources to pharmacy technician educators. The *Educator Bulletin* provides technician educators with a variety of resources that will help them to prepare their students to perform successfully on the PTCE; the resources also give educators the opportunity to expose students to continuing education programming prior to starting their careers.

TECHNICIAN ADVOCACY

PTCB has advocated for technicians primarily by offering them a means through which they can validate their competence. For individuals who are seeking certification, PTCB offers a variety of educational resources. PTCB also offers resources through which PTCB-certified pharmacy technicians may gain information about the activities of their state associations and state boards of pharmacy. PTCB provides its quarterly newsletter, *CPhT Connection*, to all of its certified pharmacy technicians. PTCB also provides opportunities for experienced pharmacy technicians and technician educators to gain involvement in their organization through volunteer committees and other areas such as the following:

- Item writers
  - Each year, PTCB seeks out qualified individuals to write and review questions for inclusion on the PTCE. Pharmacy technicians who have practical industry experience and meet other vital criteria may be selected to participate.
  - Participation is voluntary.
- PTCB Stakeholder Policy Council
  - The council is composed of 16 individuals who provide feedback and recommendations to the PTCB board of governors concerning the direction of the organization.

- The council meets to discuss strategic planning priorities related to pharmacy technician scope of practice, industry trends, and future certification opportunities for pharmacy technicians.

PTCB also provides opportunities for certified technicians to fulfill their continuing education requirements. Free online continuing education is offered periodically through the PTCB website, which also cites several links to organizations that provide online continuing education opportunities.

CERTIFICATION INFORMATION

PTCB awards certification to students who have successfully passed its computer-based examination. In August 2010, the exam application became paperless: all candidates apply online via the PTCB website. In 2007, PTCB moved from print to computer-based testing, which is administered year round, instead of the previous system of designated quarterly testing windows. PTCB partnered with the Pearson Vue professional testing centers, which have several testing locations within each state and offer test takers the flexibility to schedule testing at their convenience.

In addition to the environmental benefit of eliminating the generation of printed testing materials, the computer-based exam allows PTCB to further protect the integrity of exam content within a highly controlled environment at the Pearson Vue testing locations. Those who test will obtain an immediate pass/fail result upon completion of the examination, and the paperless process allows for timelier reporting of detailed exam performance information and mail delivery of the certificate. Applicants may retake the exam no fewer than 60 days following a fail result and are allowed up to two retakes. PTCB also provides information to pharmacy technician educators concerning the certification status of program graduates, which allows them to complete required state and regional exam result reporting. For more information concerning the PTCB certification examination, visit the website at www.ptcb.org.

Pharmacy Technician Educators Council

HISTORY OF THE ORGANIZATION

The Pharmacy Technician Educators Council (PTEC) was founded in 1991 by renowned author and pharmacy technician educator Don A. Ballington. The organization began as a networking resource for pharmacy technician educators and has grown into a network of educators from across the United States and Canada. Its membership comes from a variety of educational settings, including vocational/technical schools, institution-based training programs, community colleges, and 4-year colleges and universities. Its membership includes directors and faculty of certificate, diploma, and associate degree pharmacy technician training programs; PTEC membership is represented by several members of the health care education workforce, including pharmacists, pharmacy technicians, educators of other allied health professions, nurses, and industry consultants.

PTEC is one of the few professional pharmacy organizations in which pharmacists and technicians work side by side as colleagues. Its founding members' input in the well-known 2002 ASHP white paper on pharmacy technician practice earned the organization much-needed credibility within the pharmacy professional community. Since then, PTEC has been invited to contribute to key initiatives involving pharmacy technician education and practice across the profession.

PRIMARY MISSION AND GOALS

The primary mission of PTEC is to promote collaboration among professional pharmacy organizations for the formation and establishment of uniform pharmacy technician education, training, and credentialing standards. To that end, PTEC seeks to advocate for technicians through support of and participation in the activities of other pharmacy organizations. PTEC's long-term vision is that pharmacy technicians will complete formal training program and participate in accredited continuing education programming (throughout their careers).

SIGNIFICANT CONTRIBUTIONS TO THE PROFESSION

PTEC's role in the profession of pharmacy has been to create opportunities for pharmacy technician educators to share ideas and educational resources and to receive training to develop their skills as educators in today's technology-driven educational setting. This role has become more critical in recent years as the pharmacy technician practice continues to evolve and the needs of the industry continue to expand. In the event of the institution of state or national practice standards requiring formal education as a prerequisite for sitting for the credentialing examination, pharmacy technician educators will be tasked with providing a significantly greater volume of students with all of the knowledge, skills, and attitudes critical to technician practice.

Members of PTEC have been consulted on and are actively involved with Pharmacy Technician Program Accreditation, the Scope of Pharmacy Practice Project, and the National Voluntary Pharmacy Technician Certification Exam. PTEC is one of the member organizations of the Council on Credentialing in Pharmacy (CCP) and worked with the other member organizations on the formation of the Pharmacy Technician Credentialing Framework (to be discussed in greater detail in a future chapter), in August of 2009. In summary, this document details the following:

- Key definitions of a *pharmacy technician*
- Uniform definitions for credentialing terms, such as *certification, registration,* and *licensure,* to avoid confusion within the profession and the public regarding the requirements for pharmacy technician practice
- A set of criteria, based on existing educational standards (such as the ASHP Model Curriculum), that state boards of pharmacy may adopt when considering requiring formal education as a prerequisite to sitting for a pharmacy technician credentialing examination

The framework crafted by PTEC and other CCP member organizations was designed to align with the 2015 Future Vision of Pharmacy Practice, which is that "Pharmacists will be the health care professionals responsible for providing patient care that ensures optimal medication therapy outcomes" (Joint Commission of Pharmacy Practitioners, 2007, Revised January 31, 2008). The role that PTEC played in the drafting of this document helped ensure the inclusion of content related to future opportunities for the pharmacy technician career path to broaden and evolve in a way that will support and complement the expanding clinical role of pharmacists. In fact, the framework suggested that the 2015 Vision is not entirely possible without expansion of the roles and practice standards of pharmacy technicians in support of their pharmacists. The collaborative team dynamic that currently exists, along with the future roles of pharmacists and technicians, will be discussed in greater detail in a following chapter.

As noted earlier in the chapter, PTEC was a key contributor to the ASHP Model Curriculum for Pharmacy Technician Training Programs in 1996, in addition to the American Association of Colleges of Pharmacy (AACP), APhA, and the American Association of Pharmacy Technicians (AAPT). This is one of the documents that the CCP reviewed as a basis for creating uniform pharmacy technician education standards.

TECHNICIAN ADVOCACY

Aside from the other significant contributions that PTEC has made to the profession of pharmacy, PTEC advocates for the pharmacy technician practice by providing support specifically for those who educate and train new technicians entering the profession. The organization seeks to educate pharmacy technicians concerning career opportunities that exist in the educational arena and provides technician educator members with significant opportunities to give back to the profession of pharmacy through the provision of quality education to new pharmacy technicians in training.

MEMBERSHIP INFORMATION

PTEC offers membership to pharmacy technicians as well as other health care educators who wish to partner with this organization to promote and advance pharmacy technician education. Membership benefits include the following:

- Opportunities for professional networking
- Leadership opportunities through selection to the executive committee (by vote)
- Continuing education programming
- Member rates at the annual meeting, held in July at interesting venues across the United States
- Subscription to the *Journal of Pharmacy Technology,* the official publication of the PTEC
- Monthly e-newsletter

Pharmacy technicians may use the online membership application, which includes information related to current annual membership dues based on type of membership. For further information, visit the PTEC website at www.rxptec.org.

Annual Meetings: Gaining Involvement in a Fun and Meaningful Way

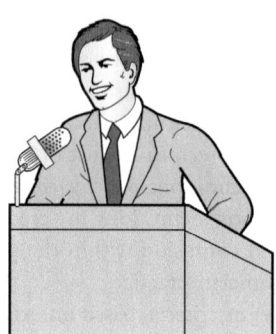

TECH NOTE!

Membership in professional pharmacy organizations does indeed have its privileges and is well worth the investment of time and expense.

Several of the organizations covered in this chapter host annual meetings, which both members and nonmembers across the profession of pharmacy may attend. These meetings are generally hosted at fun and exciting venues across the United States, which provide a pleasant balance of business amenities and entertainment for attendees and their families. Students are encouraged to visit the websites of each of the organizations noted in Box 4-1 to obtain membership and annual meeting information.

WHAT'S THE *POINT*?

The purpose for these meetings is to bring the professional and membership base together for continuing education sessions on a variety of clinical and nonclinical topics, as well as to create opportunities for professional networking. Over a period of 2 to 5 days (usually Thursday through Sunday) live programs cover a variety of topics, such as drug information, clinical procedures, pharmacy law (many states require a designated number of hours of continuing education credit to be in pharmacy law), leadership development, prevention of medication errors, and more. Many programs may be structured as discussion forums or town hall meetings, in which participants are encouraged to join in and provide feedback. Representatives from pharmaceutical companies and other industry venders, whose sponsorship largely funds these events, gather during a 1- to 2-day trade show to display information related to a variety of pharmaceutical products and services. These trade shows, often referred to as expos, also feature educational resources for students, faculty, and administrators of the colleges and schools of pharmacy across the United States. Prospective students may gain information related to entrance requirements; pharmacy school graduates may learn of clinical residency opportunities within various practice settings as well as find out about career opportunities at community pharmacies and hospital systems across the nation.

BOX 4-1   **Professional Pharmacy Organizations**

Association	Website
American Pharmacists Association	www.pharmacist.com
American Society of Health-System Pharmacists	www.ashp.org
National Community Pharmacists Association	www.ncpanet.org
Pharmacy Compounding Centers of America	www.pcca.org
Pharmacy Technician Certification Board	www.ptcb.org
American Association of Pharmacy Technicians	www.pharmacytechnician.com
National Association of Chain Drug Stores	www.nacds.org
National Pharmacy Technician Association	www.pharmacytechnician.org
Pharmacy Technician Educators Council	www.rxptec.org
Institute for the Certification of Pharmacy Technicians	www.nationaltechexam.org

HOW CAN *YOU* GET INVOLVED?

Both pharmacists and pharmacy technicians may have the opportunity to work on research case studies and present their data in the form of a display poster. These posters are entered into a competition and are judged based on technical/clinical merit. Winners receive various prizes, including scholarships, electronics, or other desirable items that are typically donated each year for those purposes.

HOW CAN *YOU* GET RECOGNIZED?

These annual events also provide a forum through which those who make significant contributions to their profession have an opportunity to be formally recognized and their accomplishments acknowledged by their peers and colleagues. Pharmacists and pharmacy technicians may be nominated for a variety of career and service awards, and awardees are recognized during an awards luncheon or dinner.

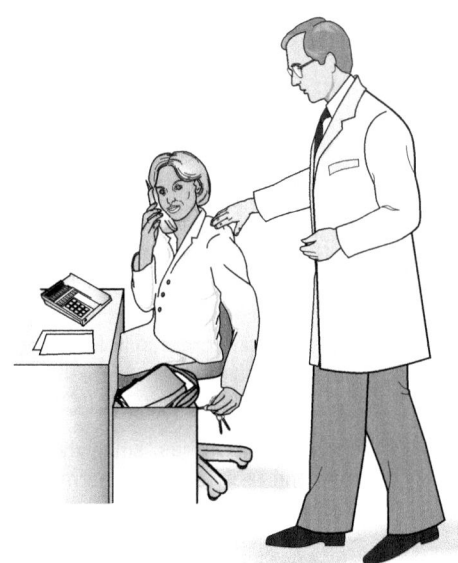

HOW DO YOU *GET* THERE?

These events require paid registration in order to participate; members are offered a lower rate as well as early-bird specials. The significantly lower membership rates provide good incentive for attendees to gain membership, and discount rates for multiyear membership are often offered as well. Registrants may also need to seek out airfare and hotel accommodations. Although there are sponsored meals during each event, participants should be prepared to seek out other sources for evening meals and personal entertainment. A significant expense can be involved; some employers may cover or reimburse part or all of these expenses for a designated number of staff members, both pharmacists and technicians. However, pharmacy technicians should consider planning months ahead for these events (such as by saving paid vacation time) so they will be able to cover the expenses out of pocket if necessary.

Chapter Summary

- Each professional organization has been critical to the development, progression, and vision of the practice and profession of pharmacy.
- One of the best ways to gain a greater appreciation of one's profession is to stay current with the activity of the organizations that help to shape and redefine the practice standards and individual roles of those they represent.
- Pharmacy technicians may gain more credibility within those organizations through membership and may find creative and useful ways to contribute positively.

- Pharmacy technicians should seek out ways to *advocate* for their own practice by joining the ranks of those who have the authority and influence to enact change at the local, state, and national levels of practice.
- The area of practice a technician wishes to pursue will determine which organization he or she may wish to join or engage.
- Students should consider the information provided and contemplate which organizations may best suit them, considering their short- and long-term career goals.
- There are a variety of councils, committees, task forces, and campaigns on which pharmacy technician representation would be valuable.

REVIEW QUESTIONS

Multiple Choice

1. The first national organization formed for pharmacy technicians by pharmacy technicians was:
   a. American Association of Pharmacy Technicians
   b. National Pharmacy Technician Association
   c. Pharmacy Compounding Centers of America
   d. Pharmacy Technician Certification Board

2. This organization's Student Pharmacist Scholarship Program awards 10 scholarships annually to pharmacy technician members who are enrolled full time in a pharmacy technician training program:
   a. American Pharmacists Association
   b. National Community Pharmacists Association
   c. American Society of Health-System Pharmacists
   d. National Association of Chain Drug Stores

3. This organization has, since its formation, focused on setting best practice standards across the profession of pharmacy:
   a. American Society of Health-System Pharmacists
   b. American Pharmacists Association
   c. National Association of Chain Drug Stores
   d. National Community Pharmacists Association

4. This organization was the first to publish a model curriculum for pharmacy technician training programs:
   a. National Pharmacy Technician Association
   b. American Society of Health-System Pharmacists
   c. Pharmacy Technician Educators Council
   d. American Pharmacists Association

5. This organization was the first established organization for pharmacy technicians:
   a. American Association of Pharmacy Technicians
   b. National Community Pharmacy Technician Association
   c. National Pharmacy Technician Association
   d. Pharmacy Technician Educators Council

6. This organization offers specialized training at its in-house training facilities in Houston, Texas:
   a. American Society of Health-System Pharmacists
   b. National Community Pharmacy Association
   c. Pharmacy Compounding Centers of America
   d. American Pharmacists Association

7. Survey data from this organization indicated that pharmacists recognize how better educated and trained technicians advance patient safety:
   a. Pharmacy Technician Certification Board
   b. American Society of Health-System Pharmacists
   c. Pharmacy Technician Educators Council
   d. American Pharmacists Association

8. This organization provides the Educator Bulletin to Pharmacy Technician educators:
   a. American Society of Health-System Pharmacists
   b. Pharmacy Technician Educators Council
   c. Pharmacy Technician Certification Board
   d. Pharmacy Compounding Centers of America

9. Following the completion of the PTCE test takers may receive their pass or fail result:
   a. Immediately
   b. Within 14 days
   c. Within 30 days
   d. Within 60 days

10. This pharmacy technician organization is a member of the Council on Credentialing:
   a. Pharmacy Technician Educators Council
   b. Pharmacy Technician Certification Board
   c. American Association of Pharmacy Technicians
   d. National Pharmacy Technician Association

TECHNICIAN'S CORNER

1. Name two national organizations that have state- and local-level chapters to which pharmacy technicians may gain membership.
2. What value does the PTCB add to the pharmacy technician's career path?
3. Name two pharmacy organizations that offer scholarships annually to technician members who are attending a full-time pharmacy technician training program.

Bibliography

American Association of Pharmacy Technicians. (2009). Retrieved 8/15/2010, from www. pharmacytechnician. com: http://www.pharmacytechnician.com/index.cfm

American Pharmacists Association. *Pharmacy Principles for Health Care Reform Press Release from February 12, 2009.* Retrieved 8/7/2010, from www.Pharmacist.com/AM/Template.cfm?Template=/CM/ ContentDisplay.cfm&ContentID=18677

American Pharmacists Association. (2010). *Government Affairs–APhA's Advocacy Agenda.* Retrieved 8/7/2010, from American Pharmacists Association: http://www.Pharmacist.com/AM/Template.cfm?Section= Government_Affairs&TEMPLATE=/CM/ContentDisplay.cfm&CONTENTID=15744

American Society of Health-System Pharmacists. (2010). *ASHP Mission and Vision.* Retrieved 8/10/2010, from www.ashp.org: http://www.ashp.org/mission-vision

Bethune, J.A., Zellmer, W.A., Sage-Gagne, W (compilers). (2002). *The Early Years of ASHP: A History.* Retrieved 8/10/2010, from www.ashp.org: http://www.ashp.org/DocLibrary/AboutUs/History/AboutASHP_Early Years.aspx

Joint Commission of Pharmacy Practitioners. (2007, Revised January 31, 2008). *An Action Plan for Implementation of the JCPP Future Vision of Pharmacy Practice.* Retrieved 9/15/2010, from American Society of Consultant Pharmacists (ASCP): http://www.ascp.com/advocacy/coalitions/jcpp.cfm

Menighan, T. (2010). *Medication Therapy Management Digest.* Retrieved 8/7/2010, from American Pharmacists Association: http://www.Pharmacist.com/AM/Template.cfm?Section=MTM&TEMPLATE=/CM/Content Display.cfm&CONTENTID=22674

NACDS. (2010). *NACDS: Health IT Vital to Helping Patients Take Medications Correctly.* Retrieved 8/16/2010, from www.nacds.org: http://www.nacds.org/wmspage.cfm?parm1=6885

NACDS. (2010). *Who We Are.* Retrieved 8/15/2010, from www.nacds.org: http://www.nacds.org/wmspage. cfm?parm1=373

National Association of Chain Drug Stores (2010). *NACDS Mission.* Retrieved 8/15/2010, from www.nacds. org: http://www.nacds.org/wmspage.cfm?parm1=372

National Community Pharmacists Association. (2009). *2009 Press Releases: Pharmacy Organizations Brief Congress on Medication Therapy Management.* Retrieved 8/11/2010, from www.ncpa.org: http://www.ncpanet. org/media/releases/2009/pharmbriefonmtm.php

National Community Pharmacists Association. *NCPA's Mission.* Retrieved 8/15/2010, from ncpa.org: http:// www.ncpanet.org/aboutncpa/mission.php

National Pharmacy Technician Association. (2010). *About NPTA*. Retrieved 8/16/2010, from http://www. pharmacytechnician.org

NCPA. (2008). *Project Destiny Executive Summary*. Retrieved 8/12/2010, from www.ncpanet.org: http://www. ncpanet.org/pdf/projectdestinyexecsummary.pdf

NCPA. (2010). *Independent Pharmacy Today*. Retrieved 8/11/2010, from www.ncpanet.org: http://www. ncpanet.org/aboutncpa/ipt.php

PCCA. (2010). *About Us*. Retrieved 8/13/2010, from www.pccarx.com: http://www.pccarx.com/aboutus.aspx

Pharmacy Technician Certification Board. (2010). *Mission and Vision*. Retrieved 8/13/2010, from www.ptcb.org: https://www.ptcb.org/AM/Template.cfm?Section=Mission_and_Vision&Template=/CM/ HTMLDisplay.cfm&ContentID=3561

Pharmacy Technician Educators Council. (2010). *PTEC Position & Goals*. Retrieved 8/14/2010, from http:// www.rxptec.org: http://www.rxptec.org/163/Position–Goals.htm

Pharmacy Technician Educators Council. (2010). *PTEC Position Statement [and] Goals*. Retrieved 9/16/2010, from http://www.rxptec.org/163/Position–Goals.htm

PTCB. (2010). *Figure Indicating Active PTCB CPhTs and State Regulations as of June 30, 2010*. Retrieved 8/14/2010, from www.ptcb.org: https://www.ptcb.org/AM/Template.cfm?Section=Regulations& Template=/CM/HTMLDisplay.cfm&ContentID=3758

The Council on Credentialing in Pharmacy (CCP). *Pharmacy Technician Credentialing Framework. Pg 2*. Approved by CCP Board of Directors in August, 2009. Available at: http://www.rxptec.org/163/Position– Goals.htm (Retrieved 9/15/2010). Page 2.

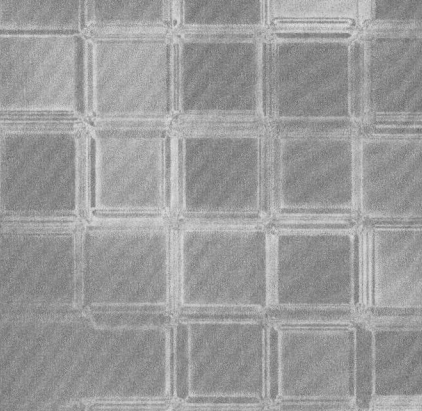

5 Medical Terminology: Learning the Language of the Medication Order

KEY TERMINOLOGY

Combining form: Occurs when a word root is followed by a combining vowel.

Combining vowel: Vowel sound that is used to join these various parts of a medical term when the suffix starts with a consonant.

Prefix: Attached before or in front of (the first segment of) the medical term and indicates the number of parts, location, position, or direction of movement of the organ or body part, or time or frequency.

Root: Denotes the basic anatomical structure.

Suffix: Added to the end of a word or stem.

Introduction

Medical terminology may be defined as the vocabulary, or *language*, of the practice of medicine. Most medical terms are derived from Latin, as many of the ancient manuscripts describing the practice of medicine were transcribed in Latin over the centuries. There are medical terms that define the study of a disease, various aspects of human anatomy and physiology, or a medical procedure. Specific to the practice of pharmacy, medical terminology often describes how a physician has directed a patient to take a prescribed medication. There are specific phrases in Latin that are still used today to describe how often a medication is to be taken, what time of day, whether with or without food, and conditions under which medication therapy should be continued or discontinued. Because these phrases would be quite long if spelled out, they were reduced to abbreviations, which are meant to allow the physician to more efficiently document medication therapy on a prescription pad. Those abbreviations, also known to the pharmacist and pharmacy technician, may then be translated into a common language that patients should be able to understand and follow concerning how and when to start and stop taking their medication.

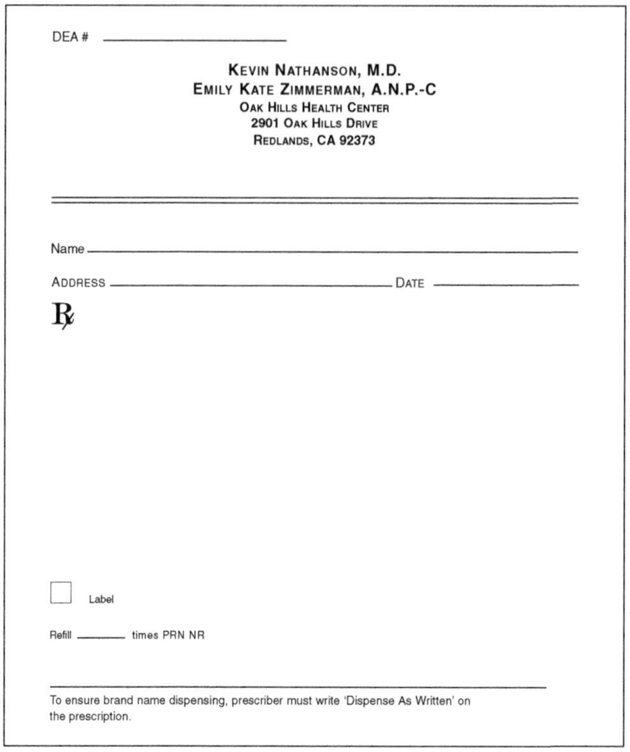

DEA # ____________

KEVIN NATHANSON, M.D.
EMILY KATE ZIMMERMAN, A.N.P.-C
OAK HILLS HEALTH CENTER
2901 OAK HILLS DRIVE
REDLANDS, CA 92373

Name ____________

ADDRESS ____________ DATE ____________

℞

☐ Label

Refill ______ times PRN NR

To ensure brand name dispensing, prescriber must write 'Dispense As Written' on the prescription.

FIGURE 5-1 Example of a prescription pad order form. (From McKenry L: *Pharmacology in nursing,* ed 22, St. Louis, 2006, Mosby.)

Refer to Figure 5-1 for an example of a prescription pad. Did you notice the Rx symbol in the top left corner of the sheet? The Rx symbol is derived from the Latin word *recipere,* which means "to take." The word *prescription* broken down is *pre* or "before" and *script* or "write," which literally translated means that a prescription must be "written before" a patient may receive and begin taking the medication. Other references have further translated Rx in the context of the old English phrase "take thou."

Pharmacy technicians are responsible for entering prescription data in the community pharmacy practice setting, which accounts for a large part of their duties and time spent in that setting. Pharmacy technicians may be allowed to perform limited order entry in the hospital pharmacy setting, depending on the laws and rules established by individual state boards of pharmacy. Interpreting a medication order is much like learning a new language. Unfamiliar medical terminology will be involved, as well as a wide range of clinical, pharmaceutical, and industry-related abbreviations that must be accurately translated and transcribed.

A number of textbooks have been written on the subject of medical terminology, with application in a variety of health care settings. There are literally thousands of medical terms that may be used in health care settings as part of the manual or electronic medical record/patient profile, which health care providers must memorize, translate, and properly utilize. Realistically, pharmacy technicians' practical application of medical terminology is generally limited to that which may be noted on an outpatient prescription or a hospital medication order. However, pharmacy technicians' exposure to and working knowledge of medical terminology is critical to their ability to accurately perform their tasks in a manner that will protect the health, welfare, and safety of patients. Incorrect transcription or translation of medication orders is one of the greatest contributors to medication fill errors in health care. Pharmacy technicians who are familiar with medical terms *should* be less likely to transcribe a medication order incorrectly, if they are using a high degree of attention to detail, gathering appropriate data from patients related to their medication history, and adhering to established workflow processes.

In order to comprehend medical terminology, start by learning how medical terms are structured: each *part* of a medical term has meaning. There are **roots**, **prefixes**, and **suffixes** that are common to a variety of terms. Once one learns how the terminology is structured, learning individual terms is simply a matter of putting together the components to decode the meaning of the word. Additionally, this chapter presents several common abbreviations—many derived from Latin—that may be used by physicians on a medication order or in the practice of pharmacy. Lastly, this chapter also discusses abbreviations that, because of their similarity to other abbreviations, could be easily misinterpreted. These abbreviations should never be used, at the risk of harming patients because an order has been misinterpreted or incorrect medication given. The Joint Commission, a regulatory body that accredits hospitals, set forth a list of unapproved abbreviations because of the high risk of misinterpretation or incorrect transcription. This list can be found online at http://www.jointcommission.org/PatientSafety/DoNotUseList/facts_dnu.htm.

Learning the Basics of Medical Terminology

Knowledge of medical terminology will help a technician better relate to the goals of medication therapy, as the terminology will help define the following:
• What the patient is being treated for
• What other types of treatment the patient is receiving
• What parts of the patient's body are being affected
• What types of symptoms and reactions a patient may experience as a result of treatment

This knowledge may prove very useful when planning workflow processes. For example, if a patient suffers from a heart condition, such as congestive heart failure (CHF), there are a number of drugs that the patient may receive. Technicians may be able to use that knowledge to anticipate filling certain types of prescriptions, particularly in the hospital setting. Additional knowledge concerning common or special handling and storage of certain types of medication used to treat certain conditions may also be gained and used for planning work activities.

The Building Blocks of Medical Terminology

As shown in Figure 5-2, medical terms may have up to three main parts:
• The central segment of the word is called the *root:*
  ◦ The root defines a basic anatomical or physiological system or structure, such as the heart, lungs, or kidneys
• The first segment of the word is called the *prefix*; the prefix modifies the root word and may indicate the following:
  ◦ Number of parts
  ◦ Location, position, or direction of movement of an organ or body part
  ◦ Time or frequency
  ◦ Reverse meaning of root

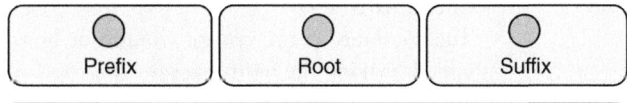

FIGURE 5-2 Example of the three main components of medical terms.

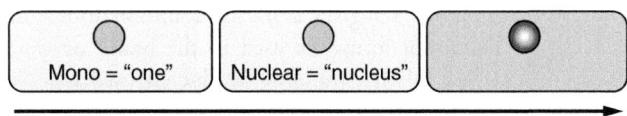

FIGURE 5-3 Defined, *mononuclear* pertains to an organism or cell with one nucleus.

TABLE 5-1   **Medical Term Prefixes**

a-	No, lack of, absence of	**hypo-**	Below; deficient or under
aer(o)-	Air	**intra-**	Within
ang-	Distress; choke	**macro-**	Large
ante-	Before	**muta-**	Mutation [cell]
anti-	Against (to prohibit or prevent)	**peri-**	Around
bi-	Two	**poly-**	Many; much
brady-	Slow	**post-**	After
circum-	Around	**pre-**	Before
contra-	Opposite/against	**pro-**	Before; in front of
di-	Two	**semi-**	Half
diplo-	Double	**sub-**	Under; below
dis-	Away from; separated or apart	**sym-; syn-**	Together; with; joined; in connection with
dys-	Pain; painful; difficult		
geri-	Old age; elderly	**tachy-**	Fast
hemi-	Half	**tri-**	Three
hyper-	Excessive; above		

Table 5-1 contains a list of commonly used terminology prefixes. As an example, consider the term *tachycardia*. Using the building block diagram shown in Figure 5-3, the word would be broken down as follows:

- The last part of the word is called the *suffix:*
  - The suffix modifies the root word and may indicate a condition, disease, or procedure

Table 5-2 contains a list of commonly used suffixes. For example, consider the term *esophagitis*, using the building block diagram shown in Figure 5-4.

There are also vowel sounds that are used to join these various parts of a medical term. The vowel sound is also called a combining vowel. The combining vowel is used when the suffix starts with a consonant. If the suffix starts with a vowel, the combining vowel is not needed.

For example, when considering the word *pericardial*, the suffix -al starts with a vowel, and no combining vowel is needed.

Let's examine another medical term, *cytology*, which is the study of cells and cell structure:

- The root is *cyt-*
- The suffix is *-logy*
- The combined form, *cytlogy*, would not be easy to pronounce, so the combining vowel, -o, is added, making the term *cytology*

When a word root is followed by a combining vowel, this is termed the combining form. The combining form is written with a forward slash between the root and the combining vowel, as shown:

Gastr/o

In medical language, roots are usually written in the combining form.

Table 5-3 gives a list of common root combining forms. Students may see how many of these root forms are used in the brand or generic names of drug products, which will provide a clue to what the drug product is used for. Note that several terms seem to be duplicates. The context or body system will determine which of the combining forms is the most appropriate.

TECH NOTE!
-o is the most common combining vowel that is used in medical terminology.

TABLE 5-2 **Medical Term Suffixes**

-algia	Pain	-megaly	Abnormal enlargement
-ase	Enzyme	-metry	Measurement
-blast	Immature stage; growing thing	-osis	Process; condition
-centesis	Surgical puncture to remove fluid	-partum	Delivery; birth
-crine	Secrete	-pathy	Disease process
-cyte	Cell	-penia	Deficiency; decrease
-cytosis	Abnormal increase in the number of cells	-phagia	Eat; swallow
		-phasia	Speech
-derm	Skin	-phil	Love; attraction (as in cell)
-ectomy	Removal by cutting	-phobia	Fear
-edema	Swelling	-physis	Grow
-emesis	Vomiting	-plasty	Surgical repair or reconstruction
-emia	Condition of the blood	-plegia	Paralysis
-genic	Producing	-pnea	Breathing
-gram	Record, writing or image	-scopy	Process of visual examination using a scope instrument
-graph	Instrument used for writing or recording	-spas/m	Sudden; involuntary muscle contraction
-graphy	Process of recording/writing		
-ia/-ac/-al/-ose	Pertaining to	-sclerosis	Thickening or hardening
-itis	Inflammation	-stenia	Strength
-logy	Study of	-tomy	Cutting; incision
-lysis	Breakdown; separation	-trophy	Nourishment

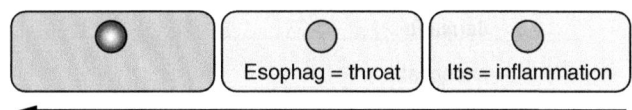

FIGURE 5-4 Defined, *esophagitis* is an inflammation of the esophagus (throat).

ADDITIONAL ENDINGS AND WORD STRUCTURE

Medical terms have evolved over the centuries, and there will always be exceptions to the previously stated rules, particularly when a term has been commonly used for a long period of time. The following are some examples of rule exceptions:

- There may be occasions in which the combining vowel of -a is used; for example:
  - An elevated heart rate would not be termed *tachycardio*—but rather *tachycardia*.
  - A cancerous tumor would be termed a carcinoma**.**
- When forming a term that relates to an anatomical structure, the suffixes -**al**, -**ic**, -**ory**, -**ary,** or -**ac** may be more appropriate than ending with the combining vowel. Examples may include the following:

TABLE 5-3   **Medical Term Combining Forms**

aden/o	Gland	**erythr/o**	Red
adip/o	Fat	**gastr/o**	Stomach
andr/o	Man	**geront/o**	Old age/elderly
angi/o	Vessel	**glyc/o**	Sugar
anter/o	Front; forward	**gynec/o**	Female
arteri(o)	Artery	**hem/o; hemat/o**	Blood
arthr/o	Joint	**hepat/o**	Liver
audi/o	Hearing	**heter/o**	Another; different
aur/o	Ear	**hom/o**	Same
aut/o	Self	**hydr/o**	Water
bi/o	Life	**hyster/o**	Uterus
blephar/o	Eyelid	**later/o**	Side
bucc/o	Cheek	**lith/o**	Stone; calcification
carcin/o	Cancer	**lys/o**	Breakdown; dissolution
cardi/o	Heart	**medi/o**	Middle
cephal/o	Head	**muc/o**	Mucus
cerebr/o	Brain	**myc/o**	Fungus
chol/e	Bile; gall	**my/o**	Muscle
chondr/o	Cartilage	**nephr/o**	Kidneys
cili/o	Hair	**ocul/o**	Eye
crani/o	Skull	**onc/o**	Tumor; mass
cyan/o	Blue	**path/o**	Disease
cyst/o	Bladder	**phleb/o**	Vein
cyt/o	Cell	**tensi/o**	Blood pressure
dent/o	Tooth	**thromb/o**	Blood clot
dermat/o	Skin	**vas/o**	Vessel
encephal/o	Brain		

- cardiac, celiac
- renal, adrenal, buccal
- hepatic, gastric
- biliary, respiratory

IN THE EXAM ROOM

Referring to Table 5-4, medical terminology may be used for a variety of purposes. Health care providers use medical terminology as part of the documentation of a patient's visit for treatment. These terms allow prescribers to formally document the reason for a patient's visit, the diagnosis, and any treatment to be prescribed—including medication.

There are a variety of terms that relate to the treatment a patient receives as part of the examination by the health care provider. There are a couple of terms that specifically relate to medication

TABLE 5-4   **Common Medical Terms**

Acute	Severe, but of short duration
Adipose	Pertaining to fat
Afebrile	No fever
Anemia	Lack of red blood cells
Angina	Distress pain (usually in the chest)
Angioplasty	Widens areas of constriction
Antibiotics	Drugs used to prevent the growth or life of a disease-causing microorganism
Antiemetics	Drugs used to treat or prevent vomiting
Apnea	Absence of breathing or breathing sounds
Arteriography	Process of producing an x-ray image of an artery following injection of a contrast medium
Arthritis	Inflammation of the joint
Biopsy	Microscopic examination of living tissue for abnormalities
Bisection	Cutting into two parts
Buccal	In the cheek
Carcinogenic	Agent that produces cancer
Cardiologist	Physician who specializes in the study of heart disease
Chronic	Recurring or ongoing, of varying degrees of severity
Contraindication	A term often used in pharmacology to refer to a disease or condition that makes the use of certain drugs harmful to the patient
Cyanosis	Abnormal bluish discoloration of the lips, skin, and mucous membranes resulting from the lack of oxygen in the blood
Cystitis	Inflammation of the bladder
Cytology	Study of cells
Dysphagia	Difficulty swallowing
Dyspnea	Difficulty breathing
Embolus(i)	Clot, as in blood that travels through the bloodstream
Encephalitis	Inflammation of the brain
Endocarditis	Inflammation of the inner lining of the heart
Erythroblast	Immature red blood cell
Erythrocyte	Red blood cell
Excision	Surgical removal of an organ or part by cutting
Gastrectomy	Surgical removal of part or all of the stomach
Gerontology	Study of medicine particular to the elderly/aged
Glycolysis	Breakdown of sugar
Hematemesis	Vomiting of blood
Hyper/Hypotension	Abnormal elevation or drop of arterial blood pressure
Incision	The process of cutting into a structure with a sharp instrument
Mycosis	Disease caused by a fungal infection

administration as well. All health care professionals, including pharmacy technicians, should be aware of the following terms and how they are used to document the patient's health record:

- Diagnosis—the process of recognizing a disease by its signs or symptoms.
  - Example: Based on the symptoms of soreness around the ear, runny nose, and a cough, the pediatrician diagnosed the small child with an upper respiratory infection.
- Indication—the clinically proven and approved purpose or use for a medication or medical equipment (recall that this approval is granted by the Food and Drug Administration [FDA]).
  - Example: The drug Lipitor is indicated for the treatment of hyperlipidemia (elevated lipids).
- Prognosis—the process of predicting the outcome of a disease or the likelihood that a patient will recover.
  - Example: Based on the effectiveness of his sustained intravenous chemotherapy drug regimen, the osteochondroma patient was given positive prognosis.
- Sign—a detectable visible indication of a disease or medical condition.
  - Example: Drooping of one side of the face, pain in the left arm, and slurred or unclear speech may all be signs of an impending stroke.
- Symptom—a sign of disorder or disease, usually the human body's reaction to that disease or disorder.
  - Example: Fever, chills, and nasal congestion may be symptoms of an influenza infection.
- Syndrome—a combined set or pattern of symptoms that indicates a medical disorder or disease.
  - Example: A patient may present with a cluster of specific clinical signs and symptoms that may assist a diagnostician in identifying a syndrome, such as Down's syndrome, acquired immune deficiency syndrome (AIDS), or severe acute respiratory syndrome (SARS).
- Contraindication—a factor or consideration that would render the administration of a drug or clinical procedure inadvisable, inappropriate, or unsafe.
  - Example: Many drugs are contraindicated for use during pregnancy, as they may be transferred through the mother's bloodstream and could be toxic to the fetus.
- Side effect—a known response to a medical treatment, often unpleasant.
  - Example: Dizziness and drowsiness are common side effects associated with the use of pain medication.
- Adverse reaction—an unexpected/unforeseen and usually negative physiologic response to a medical treatment.
  - Example: Swelling of the throat following ingestion of a medication would be considered an adverse reaction, one that would require immediate medical attention.

IT'S JUST WHAT THE DOCTOR ORDERED

Up to this point, the structure of general medical terms has been introduced, as well as terms that are commonly used in the general health care setting. Specific to the pharmacy practice, some medical terms and abbreviations are used by prescribers to order a patient's medication. In community pharmacy practice, the outpatient prescription is the means by which a prescriber may indicate the medication therapy, or medical equipment in some cases, that is necessary for the patient to manage his or her medical condition. Federal law requires that authorized prescribers provide patients with a prescription for any medication that must be taken under the supervision of a physician or other prescriber. The necessary fields that must be present on a noncontrolled medication order include the following:

- Prescriber's name, address, phone number
- Date written
- Rx—known as the superscription, indicating the prescription as a recipe
- Patient name
- Drug name, dosage form, strength—also known as the inscription, or drug to be dispensed
- Quantity to be dispensed
- Instructions to the patient—also known as the signa, or sig
- Instructions to the pharmacist—also known as the subscription
- Prescriber's signature
- Special instructions, such as the number of refills authorized or if the medication must be *dispensed as written (or if generic substitution is allowed)*

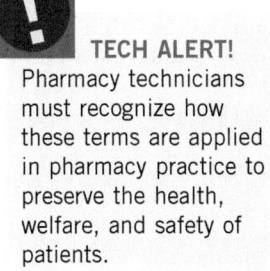

TECH ALERT!
Pharmacy technicians must recognize how these terms are applied in pharmacy practice to preserve the health, welfare, and safety of patients.

- Prescriber's Drug Enforcement Agency (DEA) number is also required on prescriptions for controlled substances
- For DEA schedule II drugs, a triplicate copy prescription may also be required, and no prescription refills may be given

Pharmacy technicians must carefully review each prescription received from a patient to ensure that the prescriber has noted all necessary information and that the prescription is legal and valid. Failure to do so may result in harm to the patient or the inability to fill the prescription until the patient or prescriber provides additional information to validate the prescription. Specific items that must be checked to validate a prescription will be discussed in greater detail in a following chapter.

PRESCRIPTION SHORT-CODES AND ABBREVIATIONS

Abbreviations describe how often the medication should be self-administered, what time of day, and under what conditions. It is extremely important that pharmacy technicians demonstrate the ability to differentiate between various dosage frequency intervals, as failure to do so may result in a patient receiving too much or too little medication. Table 5-5 lists common abbreviations used on written prescriptions for medication. Just like other medical terminology, these abbreviated terms may be used in combination or by themselves. A phrase or sentence composed of these abbreviated instructions is commonly referred to as "short-code" or a "sig code."

For example, the sig code "T 1 TAB PO BID x14 UD" would be translated and transcribed as "Take one tablet by mouth twice daily for 14 days as directed."

Let's take a look at some other examples of order entry short codes, referring to Table 5-5:

Sig Code	Translation
T 1 CAP PO Q6H PRN PAIN	Take one capsule by mouth every 6 hours as needed for pain.
T 1 TSP PO Q12H x7	Take one teaspoonful by mouth every 12 hours for 7 days.
A UNGOU QD UD	Apply ointment to each eye daily as directed.
2 GTT AU* x7	Instill two drops into both ears for 7 days.
Apply BID x3 UD Tx Head Lice	Apply twice daily for 3 days as directed for the treatment of head lice.
1-2 TABS PO PC, NTE 8 PER DAY	Chew one to two tablets by mouth after meals, not to exceed eight tablets per day.

Reading between the Prescription Lines

Oftentimes information is not clearly or specifically articulated, or "spelled out," on the prescription, although it is *understood* that it must be included in the more detailed directions to the patient. The following are some examples of medication dosage forms for which implicit directions must be added to the information written by the prescriber:

- *Oral dosage forms.* Consider the sig code "1 PO QD*." The patient's directions should not simply read, "1 by mouth daily," as both the word *take* as well as an indication of the dosage form should be included. So the entry technician would add in the implied words "Take one [dosage form] by mouth daily." Further, when transcribing medication that will be administered to a child or elderly person, or otherwise administered by a caregiver, the word *take* may need to be changed to *give*. So the previous sig code "1 TSP PO Q12H X 7D" would be translated, "Give one teaspoonful by mouth every 12 hours for 7 days," when appropriate.
- *Dosage forms for the eye or ear.* When entering medication orders for either otic or ophthalmic medications, the action instruction "instill" must be included to direct the patient to place the prescribed number of drops into the indicated area or areas. So the sig code "2 GTT AU* BID

---

*These abbreviations are found on the TJC Do Not Use List and ISMP's List of Error-Prone Abbreviations, Symbols, and Dose Designations due to medication safety issues. They should not be used. These are listed in this text because you may still see them used in practice.

TABLE 5-5   **Sig Code Abbreviations**

AAA	Apply to affected areas	**NKDA**	No known drug allergies
A	Before	**NPO**	Nothing allowed by mouth
AC	Before meals	**OD***	Right eye
AD*	Right ear	**OS***	Left eye
AM	Morning	**OU***	Both eyes
AS*	Left ear	**Oz**	Ounce
AU*	Both ears	**P**	After
BID	Twice daily	**PC**	After meals
C	With	**PO**	By mouth
CAP	Capsule	**PR**	Rectally (per rectum)
cc*	Cubic centimeter	**PRN**	As needed
DAW	Dispense as written	**Q, q**	Every
D/C*	Discontinue	**Q__H**	Every_____hours
Dx	Diagnosis	**QD***	Every day—must be spelled out on prescription
G, gm	Gram		
Gr	Grain (apothecary unit of measurement)	**Qh**	Every hour
		QHS	Every night (evening)
GTT	Drop	**QID**	Four times daily
H, hr	Hour	**QOD***	Every other day—must be spelled out on prescription
HS*	At bedtime		
H₂O	Water	**QS**	Sufficient amount
IM	Intermuscular	**S**	Without
INJ	Injection	**Sc, sq***	Subcutaneous
IV	Intravenously	**Sl**	Sublingual, under the tongue
l, L	Liter	**SS**	Sliding scale, a means for patients to determine the amount of insulin to be administered based on their blood glucose levels
Kg	Kilogram		
MDI	Metered dose inhaler		
MEq	Milliequivalents		
Mcg	Microgram	**STAT**	Immediately
Mg	Milligram	**Susp**	Suspension
Min	Minute	**Tea, tsp**	Teaspoonful
Neb	Nebulizer	**TBSP**	Tablespoonful
N/V	Nausea and vomiting	**TID**	Three times daily
N/V/D	Nausea, vomiting, and diarrhea	**Tx**	Treatment (of)
		UD*	As directed
Nare	Nostril	**Ung**	Ointment
NKA	No known allergies	**V, Vag**	Vaginally

*These abbreviations are found on the TJC Do Not Use List and ISMPs List of Error-Prone Abbreviations, Symbols, and Dose Designations due to medication safety issues. They should not be used. These are listed in this text because you may still see them used in practice.

x7" must be read, "Instill two drops into both eyes twice daily for 7 days." Further, the patient should be informed that any medication given for the eye must be remain sterile to prevent the infection from spreading into the delicate conjunctiva, so care should be taken not to contaminate the applicator dropper or ophthalmic ointment tube tip.

- *Dosage forms to be administered rectally or vaginally.* When entering medication orders for rectal or vaginal suppositories, it is important to recognize that some patients (particularly those who have not previously received one of these dosage forms) may not be aware that there is a protective wrapper surrounding the suppository, which must be removed prior to insertion. Failure to do so may cause great discomfort or injury and could possibly spread the infection to these sensitive areas. Therefore, additional instructions must be included with the prescriber's directions. So the sig code "1 SUPP PR Q6H N/V" must be transcribed, "Unwrap and insert one suppository rectally every 6 hours for nausea and vomiting."

UNAPPROVED MEDICAL TERMINOLOGY ABBREVIATIONS

In 2001, The Joint Commission published a list of abbreviations that were found to be unsafe because of the high volume of documented medication errors resulting from misinterpretation or incorrect transcription of the abbreviation. This list has been modified continually, as many high-risk abbreviations—particularly those that have resulted in serious injury to a patient or patients—have been added over the years. Each of the abbreviations is noted in the Joint Commission's Do Not Use list, which can be accessed by going to www.jointcommission.org. A prescriber may not use these abbreviations while handwriting a prescription or entering a prescription into a computer system; alternatively, the entire word or phrase must be printed *legibly* and spelled out in its entirety to avoid and prevent misinterpretation. For example, insulin is prescribed in units. Rather than writing an order that indicates "10u per SS," the order must be written as "10 *units* per SS," and interpreted as 10 units per sliding scale. A few of the unapproved abbreviations have been included in the tables of this text, as those abbreviations/short codes may still be used during the process of entering orders. Computerized order entry systems typically auto-translate sig codes into clear instructions to the patient, although care should still be taken when using codes that may include an unapproved abbreviation.

Chapter Summary

- Pharmacy technicians use medical terminology during the process of medication order interpretation and entry, whether they are working in a community or hospital pharmacy setting.
- There are key medical expressions that are commonly found on a medication order or used in drug references, such as diagnosis, indication, contraindication, and adverse effect.
- Several medical terms relate to a patient's treatment as part of the examination by his or her health care provider.
- Some medical abbreviations derived from Latin expressions are used in the transcription of a medication order, which pharmacy technicians must learn to accurately interpret into language that a patient will understand and follow.
- These abbreviations describe how often the medication should be self-administered, what time of day, and under what conditions.
- Students should review each of the "short code" abbreviations listed in Table 5-5 until they have memorized and mastered how these terms are commonly applied.
- Pharmacy technicians should also maintain knowledge of the list of abbreviations that were found to be unsafe because of the high volume of documented medication errors resulting from misinterpretation or incorrect transcription of the abbreviation.
- A medical term is structured in two or more parts, including the root, prefix, and suffix.
- Pharmacy technicians should be familiar with common root combining forms, as well as the prefixes and suffixes that modify these roots and give them additional or more specific meaning.

REVIEW
QUESTIONS

Multiple Choice

1. The prefix that relates to old age is:
   a. Geri-
   b. Pedi-
   c. Poly-
   d. Post-

2. A medical term that indicates *distress* or *choking* would contain the prefix:
   a. Ang-
   b. Dys-
   c. Anti-
   d. Macro-

3. A medical term that indicates *conjoining* would contain the prefix:
   a. Diplo-
   b. Sym-
   c. Poly-
   d. Muta-

4. A medical term that defines a *process* or *condition* would contain the suffix:
   a. -megaly
   b. -osis
   c. -itis
   d. -logy

5. A medical term that defines a record, writing, or image would contain the suffix:
   a. -gram
   b. -metry
   c. -graph
   d. -centesis

6. A medical term that defines a *disease process* would contain the suffix:
   a. -algia
   b. -osis
   c. -logy
   d. -pathy

7. A medical term that relates to the heart would contain the word root:
   a. angi/o
   b. cardi/o
   c. cili/o
   d. cephal/o

8. A medical term that relates to the bladder would contain the word root/combining form:
   a. Cyst/o
   b. Bladd/o
   c. Cili/o
   d. Cyt/o

9. A medical term that relates to the blood would contain the word root/combining form:
   a. Erythr/o
   b. Hem/o
   c. Hepat/o
   d. Ren/o

10. A medical term that relates to a vessel would contain the word root/combining form:
    a. Arteri/o
    b. Vas/o
    c. Myc/o
    d. Lith/o

1. Give an example of how knowledge of medical terminology might help pharmacy technicians plan their workflow processes.
2. State the difference between the prefixes **anti-** and **ante-**. Give an example and interpretation of each.
3. How would one change the expression of the combining form cardio/o from a noun to an adjective?

Bibliography

The Joint Commission. (2010). *Facts About the "Do Not Use" List*. Retrieved 9/28/2010, from http://www. jointcommission.org/PatientSafety/DoNotUseList/facts_dnu.htm

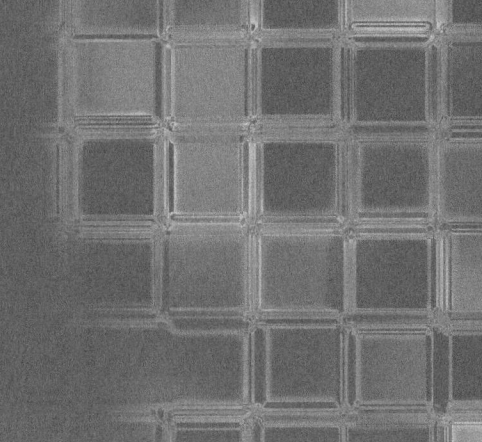

6

The Structure and Workflow Processes of the Community Pharmacy Practice

---

LEARNING OBJECTIVES

By the end of this chapter, students will be able to competently:

1. Recognize the general layout of a community pharmacy practice setting and identify common technician workspaces.
2. Describe each of the critical tasks associated with the prescription order entry, fill, and refill processes.
3. State the components of a complete prescription/medication order, including prescription/medication orders for controlled substances.
4. Name key components of a medication stock bottle label.
5. Discuss and evaluate appropriate strategies for minimizing fill errors caused by look-alike/sound-alike drugs during the medication order entry and filling process.
6. Given various fill counter and telephone scenarios, formulate appropriate responses to customer inquiries or concerns.
7. Describe the processes currently performed for inventory management within a community pharmacy practice setting, including quality control, stock level adjustment, and procedures for shipping/receiving using a purchase order requisition.

KEY TERMINOLOGY

Adjudication: Electronic processing of a patient's prescription benefit claim to an insurance company for processing.

Amber vials: Small plastic (or, rarely, glass) containers that are generally used to dispense solid oral medication.

Auxiliary labels: Small labels affixed onto drug dispensing containers that provide additional instruction to the patient, such as how the medication should be taken, handled, or stored.

Counseling area: A separate patient counseling area that is far enough away from the dispensing counter to allow patients the privacy they need to discuss their questions or concerns with a pharmacist.

Counting trays: Manual devices with a flat surface onto which solid drugs are poured out for counting. A spout at one end allows the drug to be transferred to the dispensing container without being contaminated.

Cycle counts: Ongoing inventory management process that involves manually counting the quantity of all medication and medical devices currently in stock.

Dispense as written (DAW): Line on the outpatient prescription where a prescriber may enter his or her signature to indicate that a prescription must be dispensed for exactly the product indicated.

Drug profile: Computerized listing of the formulary of the products available for dispensing through that pharmacy.

Empathy: Identifying with a patient's situation, feelings, or motives.

Inscription: Area on an outpatient prescription where the name, strength, dosage form, and dispense quantity of medication prescribed is indicated.

Insurance/payer profile: Database within a pharmacy management system that indicates the fee schedule set up to bill a patient, based on how the patient is set up to pay. Payment is generally structured based on whether the patient has pharmacy benefits, pays privately (in cash), or uses some type of drug discount plan.

Medication therapy management: The process whereby pharmacists, in collaboration with other members of the health care and prescribing team, continuously evaluate a patient's prescribed medication for clinical appropriateness and optimal therapeutic benefit.

Patient profile: Computerized database where multiple patient identification factors, such as date of birth or social security number, are entered, along with the prescriber information; additionally, any information related to the patient's medical history should be documented.

Pharmaceutical elegance: Refers to techniques for preparing a product for dispensing in a way that gives it a clean and professional appearance; includes placing a clean label in an appropriate location on the dispensing container in a neat fashion, as well as removing spills or drug residue from the outside of the dispensing container prior to labeling.

Prescription refill: Days' supply allowed in addition to the amount dispensed on a prescription, which the patient may receive following a designated time frame of a medication that may be safely dispensed for long-term use; the type of medication will determine how many refills are allowed.

Production area: Area within a community pharmacy where medication fill processes take place.

Signa: Area on an outpatient prescription that indicates the prescriber's directions to the patient, specifies how the medication is to be administered, and uses various abbreviations to make better use of the limited inscription space on a prescription label.

Stock bottle: Container/bottle that the drug is shipped in.

Superscription: Rx symbol on an outpatient prescription that indicates the area where the drug information will be notated.

Warning labels: Small labels affixed to drug dispensing containers that alert the patient to specific warnings about the administration and storage of the medication, as well as potential food and drug interactions.

Introduction

In the first few chapters, students learned about the foundational principles of the pharmacy practice forged by human development and the changing face of modern health care. The role of both the pharmacist and the pharmacy technician continues to evolve across the practice of pharmacy. The workflow processes of the community versus hospital pharmacy environment are quite different, although there are many shared skill sets that are universally applicable. For this reason, this book offers chapters dedicated to community pharmacy practice and institutional (hospital) pharmacy practice exclusively, although these chapters may compare and contrast the two. By the end of this chapter, students should have a strong sense of the general structure of the community pharmacy as well as the roles and responsibilities of the pharmacy technician within that environment.

Population growth, as well as growth in the number of citizens who require medication therapy of some sort, has continued to elevate the demand for pharmaceutical services in the United States. According to IMS Health data reported by Reuters, U.S. prescription drug sales increased by 5.1% from 2008 to 2009, up to $300.3 billion—despite challenging economic times. The availability of more generic drug products was cited as one of the drivers behind the increase. Another noted contributing factor was a 7.5% rise in the demand for specialty drugs that are used to treat complex chronic health conditions such as cancer. The increasing need for top-selling drugs—the top three being lipid reducers, antipsychotics, and acid reflux drugs—places a growing burden on the pharmacists and pharmacy technicians who work to safely prepare and dispense those medications in the community pharmacy practice setting.

When one hears the word *pharmacy*, he or she is likely to envision one of the large drugstore chains that occupy retail corners in every city across the country. As students learned in Chapter 1, the historical roots of the pharmaceutical practice in the United States may be found in privately owned corner drugstores, which were established long before the population necessitated pharmacy chain stores. In addition to a variety of chain drugstores, many long-standing pharmacist-owned community pharmacies continue to thrive in both rural and metropolitan communities across the United States. Many community pharmacies—both chain and independent—also offer the following:

- Nutrition services
- Immunizations
- Outpatient clinical services, often provided by a nurse practitioner or physician assistant
- Detailed explanations of pharmacy benefits and coordination of benefits
- Home health medical equipment
- Sterile and nonsterile compounding of specialty medication (compounding pharmacies are often still referred to as *apothecaries*)
- Homeopathic and alternative medication therapy
- Mail-order services
- Nonpharmaceutical consumer products
- Veterinary medicine

Retail pharmacies may be stand-alone businesses or part of another business, such as a grocery store, nursing home, or hospital. The area surrounding a pharmacy may determine its majority patient demographic and influences the types of drugs carried and other services offered. For example, a community pharmacy in a retirement community would likely carry a variety of geriatric medications, medical equipment, and other support services for elderly patients. A community pharmacy in a growing residential community may offer services to pediatric and other family-oriented products and services. Pharmacies in younger single-adult communities (such as contemporary uptown areas) may offer products and services related to general wellness and nutrition, athletics, and preventive medicine.

Pharmacy technicians should gain a sense of the pharmacy's surrounding community in order to better appreciate the types of skills that may be useful in that pharmacy. Pharmacies located in culturally diverse areas may seek pharmacists and pharmacy technicians who speak other languages in addition to English. Pharmacy technicians should also consider the general health literacy of the patients they serve. Elderly patients, those who speak English as a second language, or patients in low-income areas may have varying degrees of understanding when it comes to technical medical language. Communication skills are essential to ensure that these patients leave the pharmacy with not only the correct medication but also a clear understanding of how the medication must be safely administered to achieve the maximum health benefit.

This chapter teaches students the essentials of community pharmacy practice in:

- General physical layout
- Typical daily workflow processes
- Individual tasks that pharmacists perform
- Individual tasks that pharmacy technicians may perform
- Types of drugs stocked in a community pharmacy and how each is dispensed
- The components of a written prescription and how prescription information must be interpreted and transcribed in a pharmacy's order entry management system
- Prescription intake, order entry, fill, and dispensing scenarios in which pharmacy technicians must think critically and employ problem-solving skills

There are five primary areas of focus for pharmacy technicians, and this chapter has been arranged to discuss each one in detail. At the conclusion of this chapter, students should have a greater appreciation for the pharmacists and technicians who staff community pharmacies across the United States. Retail pharmacy practice has come a long way from "count-and-pour-and-lick-and-stick." With that in mind, students may also consider their own personal mission statements and how those ideals might best be upheld and actively demonstrated while serving patients in the community practice setting.

Examining General Pharmacy Workstations

Let's take a closer look at the various workstations that make up a retail practice setting. The dispensing counter is the front line, where most of a technician's contact with patients takes place. The counter should always be kept tidy and free of patients' protected health information.

INTAKE AND DISPENSING COUNTERS

In general, the following items will be located in the intake/dispensing counter area:

- Cash register or computer system
- Multiple-line telephone system with prescription refill features
- Prescriptions on file
- Dispensing bags
- General office supplies, such as pads of paper, pens, rubber bands, staplers, scissors, tape, highlighters, and permanent markers

There are generally counter areas designated for customers to drop off and pick up prescriptions. The computer where orders are entered will likely be near the drop-off point, whereas the cash register will likely be near the pick up point. When drive-up services are offered, customers will drop off and pick up their prescriptions at the same drive-up location.

Pharmacy Telephone Customer Service

Call volume in a community pharmacy can be high, as patients may call in with questions as well as refill requests. The staff should utilize the following customer service tips when answering the pharmacy phone:

- Try to answer the phone within three rings
- Greet the caller, then state the name of the business and your name—for example, "Good afternoon. Joe Smith's Neighborhood Pharmacy. This is Anne. How may I help you today?"
- Have a pen and paper handy to jot down key information so that callers will not have to repeat themselves
- Once the patient gives his or her name, write it down and call the patient by name when addressing him or her during the call—for example, "What prescription would you like to have refilled today, Mr. Anderson?"
- Repeat the information to the caller for clarification—for example, "So for clarification, Mr. Anderson, you need a refill on your Lipitor. Is that correct?"
- Let patients know when they can expect services to be rendered or how soon they should expect follow-up.
- Ask if you have assisted the caller adequately and if you can offer any other assistance.
- Thank the patient for calling and say good-bye before disconnecting.

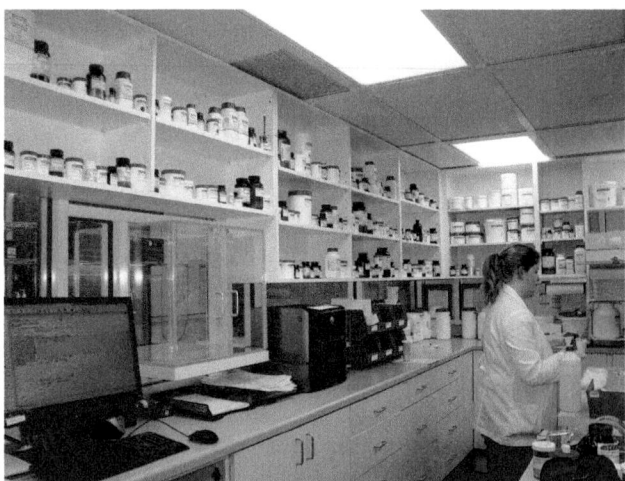

FIGURE 6-1 Pharmacy technician working in the pharmacy setting. (From Hopper T: *Mosby's Pharmacy Technician: Principles and Practice*, ed 3, Philadelphia, 2011, Saunders.)

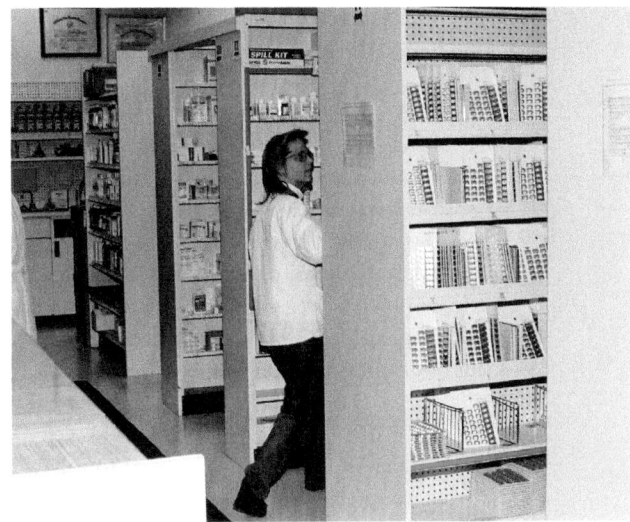

FIGURE 6-2 Pulling medication from the shelf. (From Hopper T: *Mosby's Pharmacy Technician: Principles and Practice*, ed 3, Philadelphia, 2011, Saunders.)

PRESCRIPTION FILL (PRODUCTION) AREA

Once a prescription has been validated, it can be entered into a prescription order entry system. Once the order has been entered, a prescription label that contains all of the dispensing information must be generated. The pharmacy fill area (also referred to as the production area) is where fill processes take place (Figure 6-1). Before any prescriptions are prepared for dispensing, it is important that the fill area is kept clean and clear to prevent fill errors and to keep from introducing contaminants into the products being prepared. Hygienic hand washing must be part of this process.

Hygienic Hand Washing

- Before preparing or dispensing medication, it is vital that pharmacy technicians demonstrate effective hand-washing techniques.
- Gloving may be necessary while preparing compounded drugs and drugs that could be dangerous or irritating.
- Fingernails should also be kept short, and acrylic or other false fingernails should be avoided.

MEDICATION STORAGE AREAS

Medication is generally stored on shelves (Figure 6-2) in the rear of the pharmacy or under refrigerated conditions when appropriate. Drugs are generally stored alphabetically, by either their generic or brand names, and are separated according to their routes of administration. It is critical that the correct drug route is selected during the prescription filling process; separation of various routes helps to prevent medication fill errors. Drugs are available via the following routes and are separated accordingly:

- Internal (oral medications)
  - May be in solid or liquid form
- External
  - Topical
  - Transdermal
  - Rectal
  - Vaginal
- Injectable
- Refrigerated
  - Internal
  - External
- Controlled medication (usually kept in a locked cabinet or vault)
  - Internal, external, and injectable medications are separated

- Refrigerated controlled medications are stored either in a narcotic storage vault or in a locked box in the general storage refrigerator

PATIENT COUNSELING AREA

Once a patient is ready to pick up his or her medication, the pharmacist or pharmacy technician will assist the patient at the front counter in the prescription pickup area. If the patient wishes to or must receive counseling concerning the medication, there is generally a separate patient counseling area that is far enough away from the dispensing counter to allow the patient the privacy needed to discuss questions or concerns with a pharmacist. As pharmacists begin to provide more consultive services to patients regarding their medication therapy, the patient counseling area may also include an office or cubicle space where the pharmacist and patient can sit while discussing the patient's medication therapy in greater detail.

PHARMACY WORKFLOW THROUGH WORKSTATIONS

The pharmacy workflow process tends to follow a linear model:
- Front counter prescription drop-off area
  - Greeting patient and accepting prescription
  - Verifying patient profile, prescription, and third-party billing information
  - Entering prescription order
- Medication storage areas
  - Drug selection
- Production area
  - Medication preparation, packaging, and labeling
  - Auxiliary/warning labeling
  - Final verification by pharmacist
- Front counter prescription pickup area
  - Dispensing and accepting payment from patient
- Patient counseling area
  - Counseling of the patient by the pharmacist

The physical arrangement of workstations may vary by location.

A Closer Look at Daily Pharmacy Operations

Pharmacy staff must work well together every day to accomplish the variety of tasks associated with the community pharmacy practice. Often the size of the pharmacy determines what the pharmacy technician staff will be tasked with on a daily basis. Smaller pharmacies generally call upon all staff to perform all aspects of the job that are legally allowed or required. Larger pharmacies may rotate staff technicians through various workstations, or individuals may be assigned a specific task or tasks on a routine basis. The following subsections detail the individual tasks performed as stages of a process.

STAGE 1: INTAKE AND THE PATIENT INTERVIEW

One of the most important interactions in the community pharmacy setting is the initial conversation between the pharmacy technician and a new patient. Many patients come to the pharmacy prescription intake window with a preconception of the level of customer service they will receive based on past experiences. It is up to each pharmacy technician to uphold a patient's expectation of excellent customer service. It is critical that pharmacy technicians emphasize to new and existing patients that it is not just an option for them to meet with the pharmacist for consultation on their medication. Rather, pharmacy technicians should assert the importance of consultation with the pharmacist as a means for patients to not only gain the greatest therapeutic benefit from the new medication but also to establish a history of medication therapy and learn ways to use medication therapy to better manage their health.

Gathering Vital Information

The pharmacy technician is responsible for ensuring each patient's medication profile is current. This will allow the pharmacist to review each of the medications a patient is taking and to verify

TECH ALERT!
Be sure to ask the patient if he or she is taking any other medications, including over-the-counter medicines, vitamins, and herbal or alternative medicinal products.

that there are no interactions between medications, that no duplicate therapy has been prescribed, and that the prescribed medication is appropriate based on the patient's known medical conditions. Many patients may also self-medicate with over-the-counter medicine as well as herbal and alternative medicinal products; it is important to gather that information from a patient, as the pharmacy technician will need to enter it into the patient's medication history profile.

It is not enough to accept the prescription; a critically thinking pharmacy technician will carefully look over each prescription for completeness and accuracy. It is valuable to ask patients questions about their prescriptions to ensure that they are aware of the medications that have been prescribed. The patient should also be given any relevant information related to pricing. Asking patients a few questions about their prescriptions may bring to light possible prescribing errors or discrepancies, which can be addressed immediately.

Prescriptions for controlled medications should be reviewed with particular care and attention to detail to ensure that the prescription is valid and does not bear any signs of tampering, forgery, or lack of authenticity. If at any time a pharmacy technician suspects that a prescription may be invalid, the prescription should be immediately brought to the attention of the pharmacist.

Once a pharmacy staff member has accepted a prescription, every member of the pharmacy team should ensure that the prescription is reviewed, filled, checked for accuracy, and packaged appropriately.

STAGE 2: PRESCRIPTION ORDER REVIEW AND ENTRY

Part of the patient interview process is the review and acceptance of a patient's prescription. Each prescription must contain specific information to be deemed legitimate and to be legally filled and dispensed by the pharmacy. This is a good point at which to reinforce the need to verify the *five rights of medication administration*:
- Right patient
- Right drug
- Right route
- Right dose
- Right time

Chapter 5 discussed how medication is noted on a prescription. It is vital that key information is verified *before* the patient finishes the intake process, as failure to verify the information may result in significant delays in processing the prescription. The following information must be present on a prescription.

Prescriber Name, Address, and Telephone Number
- This information may need to be verified in the event that the legality of a prescription or prescriber is ever called into question or if the prescriber needs to be contacted for questions.

Date Prescription Written
- The period of time during which a prescription may be filled is determined by the date when the prescription was originally written, so it is very important that the date be verified in order to determine if a prescription may be filled.

Superscription
- The Rx symbol, or superscription, indicates the area where the drug information (or recipe) will be written.

Signa
- Directions to the patient indicate how the medication is to be administered.
- Various abbreviations, such as those indicated in the previous chapter, can be used to make better use of the limited inscription space on a prescription label.
- As indicated in the previous chapter, The Joint Commission (along with the AOA and NCQA) has published and regularly updates a list of unapproved abbreviations because of the high probability of misinterpretation/mistranslation. Prescribers have become increasingly aware of the risks involved with using these abbreviations and more frequently spell out these risky terms. However, for the purposes of medication order entry, short codes that are used to abbreviate directions to

the patient or pharmacist are still regularly utilized during the prescribing process. It is important that pharmacy technicians know these abbreviations, what they stand for, and how to most appropriately translate them during the medication order entry process. Students may wish to review the subsection "Reading between the Prescription Lines" presented in the previous chapter, in which specific information is detailed about how sig codes should be translated given patient-specific variables.

- Pharmacy technicians should carefully review the signa for correctness; handwriting that is unclear or illegible should be brought to the attention of a pharmacist so that the prescriber can be contacted for clarification.

Inscription

- Name, strength, dosage form, and dispense quantity of medication.
- There might be several different strengths as well as dosage forms for any given medication; it is vital that medication has been verified for the correct name, strength, *and* dosage form.
  - Additionally, if a particular strength—given the frequency of the dose indicated in the inscription—seems higher than usual, this information should be brought to the attention of a pharmacist so the prescriber can be contacted for clarification.

Signature Lines

- The prescriber will sign *either* that the medication needs to be dispensed exactly as written or that substitutions are allowed.
- Dispense as written (often abbreviated DAW).
  - There are a variety of reasons why a prescriber may enter his or her signature to indicate that a prescription must be dispensed for exactly the product indicated.
  - Table 6-1 gives a listing of common DAW codes.
  Note that although a physician may signify that substitution is not allowed, a patient's particular prescription benefit plan may not cover a particular medication, brand name, strength, or dosage form (or any combination of these variables). In the event that a patient's benefits cannot be applied, the pharmacist should be notified so that the prescriber can be contacted for consultation.
  For the claims processing procedure, it is extremely important that the most appropriate DAW code is indicated in the order entry screen.

Substitutions

- In the event that the prescriber signs to indicate that substitutions may be made, patients should be made aware, during the intake interview, of any alternatives in terms of generic product substitution. It is *essential* that patients be made aware (particularly if a patient has been taking the brand name product for any period of time) that generic products may look very different than the brand name product the patient is accustomed to seeing. Additionally, patients should be educated concerning the product's generic name, because this is the name that will be printed on the dispensing label.

Refills

- Generally, a prescription may be refilled if the medication prescribed is a drug that the patient will be taking long term (often referred to as *maintenance medication*). Maintenance medications are generally prescribed to manage a disease state that is incurable and must be managed utilizing medication therapy. Common examples would include medications that are used to treat high blood pressure or diabetes. Conversely, products that will be taken for a short duration—or if the patient must be more closely monitored by the care provider while taking the medication—are often not refilled. For example, if a product commonly produces toxic side effects, a patient may be subject to frequent lab testing to ensure that there are no signs of toxicity and will be given a new prescription each time.
- The prescriber must indicate if refills are allowed and if so, how many. The type of medication determines how many refills are allowed. In general, the Drug Enforcement Agency (DEA) allows noncontrolled medication to be refilled for up to a 12-month supply, as determined by the date

TABLE 6-1   **Common Dispense as Written (DAW) Codes**

Common DAW Codes	Description
0	No product selection indicated—default when only one product name is available for a particular product [only one brand or generic product available]
1	Substitution not allowed by prescriber
2	Substitution allowed—brand name requested by patient
3	Substitution allowed—pharmacist-selected product dispensed [multiple appropriate brands or general products might be available]
4	Substitution allowed—generic drug not in stock
5	Substitution allowed—brand product dispensed as the generic product
6	Override
7	Substitution not allowed—brand name drug mandated by law
8	Substitution allowed—generic drug not available in marketplace
9	Other

Source: www.medicaid.state.al.us/documents/News/ALERTS_2009/ALERT_09-6_DAW-2_Audits_3_16_09.pdf.

that the prescription was originally written; controlled medications that fall in DEA schedules III through V may be refilled up to five times over a 6-month period; DEA schedule II medications may not be refilled.

Once all of the prescription information has been verified, the prescription is ready for entry into the computer system. Although various pharmacies utilize different computer systems, much of the functionality is common to most systems.

Many pharmacies utilize a pharmacy management system. An image of the actual drug is shown when the product is selected, to assist the user with product selection later in the fill process. Each field on the screen may link to other screens where other types of information must be entered and stored.

The following discussion describes common pharmacy management system functions and offers examples of how each is used.

New Prescription Entry

This function is used for a brand-new prescription. Often, warnings are set up in the background of a system to alert the user when duplicates are being entered (either duplicate drug names or drugs that fall into the same therapeutic class) or if a drug conflicts with information provided in the patient's profile (such as a drug allergy or an incompatibility with another medication the patient may be already taking). When alerts occur, a pharmacist should be notified immediately so that a solution can be identified.

Refill Prescription Processing

This function is used either to process existing authorized prescription refills or to process a request for a prescription renewal in the event that refills are exhausted or a prescription expires.

Patient Profile

It is important to ensure that the correct patient is selected during the order entry process. This is why the collection of multiple patient identification factors, such as date of birth and insurance number, is important. It is also important to ensure that the correct prescriber is selected. Additionally, any information related to the patient's medical history should be documented in the patient profile. Examples include the following:
- Prescription or over-the-counter medications taken currently or in the past
- Any known seasonal, food, or drug allergies or sensitivities
- Any known documented medical diagnosis

This information greatly impacts the pharmacist's ability to make informed clinical decisions regarding the therapeutic appropriateness of the prescribed medication.

Prescriber Profile

Current information regarding a prescriber must be kept on file; new prescribers must be entered into the pharmacy management system before their prescriptions can be processed. New prescriber information should be carefully reviewed; any suspicious information should be brought to the attention of a pharmacist for further review and investigation as necessary.

Drug Profile

Pharmacy management systems are generally supplied with a formulary of the products available for dispensing through that pharmacy. Drug information is also generally supplied so that the patient can receive detailed information about the drug product. That detailed information is sometimes referred to as a drug monograph. The drug monograph generally prints along with the dispensing label, and the patient is given this monograph during the prescription dispensing process.

The drug profile is often tied to inventory management processes, so the profile should also indicate whether that drug product is in stock and available for dispensing. Drug products are generally listed alphabetically by generic name, along with a unique identifier such as the National Drug Code (NDC) number. Great care and attention to detail must be taken to ensure that the correct product is selected during the new prescription order entry process.

Insurance/Payer Profile

Pharmacy management systems have a fee schedule that is set up to bill a patient based on how the patient is set up to pay (referred to as the insurance/payer profile). Payment is generally structured based on whether the patient has pharmacy benefits, is a private pay (cash) customer, or uses some type of drug discount plan. Thousands of pharmacy benefit plans exist, many of which are automatically set up by the pharmacy management system. The system sends information to an insurance company electronically, based on specific insurance plan information that has been set up under the patient's profile. Care must be taken to enter a patient's insurance plan information accurately; incorrect or incomplete information may result in failure to complete the electronic insurance claim submission—which will create delays that may prevent the patient from receiving the medication in a timely manner.

Reports

There are a variety of activity reports that a pharmacy may need to generate in order to maintain operations, which are generally supplied by the pharmacy management system. Pharmacy technicians should be aware of the types of reports that need to be generated and how to troubleshoot their functionality.

Retaining Prescription Records

Most modern pharmacies create a database of scanned prescriptions, which allows the pharmacist to readily access any prescription without the often-arduous process of looking up the filed hard copy. Most pharmacy management systems include a scan function that allows the prescription to be scanned as part of the order entry process. Pharmacy technicians should ensure that they have a clear understanding of how to use all of the functionalities of the pharmacy management systems, and they should learn how to troubleshoot in the event that there are system-related issues. All pharmacy staff should be made aware of what technical support is available and how to access this support during store hours.

Loaning and Borrowing

Pharmacies have a long-standing tradition of supporting and assisting one another in terms of loaning and borrowing drugs when there is a stock shortage. Legend drugs and controlled drugs that fall within DEA Schedules III through V may be loaned or borrowed. Each pharmacy has a standard form that must be completed in order to create a record of the drug information as well as to project a date for when the borrowed product will be replaced.

Generally, staff members provide copies of the loan/borrow form to the purchasing pharmacist/technician, which allows that individual to follow up on the status of the product's replacement or acquisition.

If a pharmacy needs to borrow a Schedule II controlled drug, a borrow transaction should be handled as though the pharmacy were purchasing rather than "borrowing" the drug. The transfer of drugs must be documented using DEA form 222. The "borrowing" pharmacy will then be billed for the product and will not be required to replace the supply received.

STAGE 3: MEDICATION FILL, PACKAGING, AND LABELING
Selecting the Right Drug

Once the fill area has been cleaned and hygienic hand washing performed, the pharmacy technician may proceed to the pharmacy drug storage area to select (or to "pull") the correct drug from the stock area. As noted earlier, every drug has at least a generic drug name and many drugs come in multiple drug dosage forms. Part of the drug order entry process is selecting the most appropriate product in the order entry system. Computerized order entry systems contain a listing, or formulary, of the drugs carried by the pharmacy. Every drug is assigned a National Drug Code (NDC) number, and each NDC number is unique to a particular product. Therefore, selecting a drug by its NDC number is a nearly failsafe method for selecting the correct drug from stock. Generally, the hard-copy prescription is placed in the fill area, and the pharmacy technician brings the prescription label bearing the entered drug NDC number to the drug storage area in order to ensure that he or she selects the correct product. Care should be taken to select the correct product, particularly as there are a variety of products whose names are spelled or pronounced similarly. The Institute for Safe Medicine Practice (ISMP) has issued multiple listings of look-alike/sound-alike (LASA) drugs in an effort to alert the medical community about drugs that might be easily mistaken for other products. Pharmacy technicians should gather this information so that they know which LASA drugs to be on the alert for in order to prevent medication fill and dispensing errors.

Filling Prescriptions for Controlled Medications

Patients may have a variety of medically necessary reasons for receiving prescriptions for controlled medication. Because of the abuse potential associated with controlled medication, care must be taken to ensure that the prescription is valid prior to filling. According to the DEA, a pharmacy is not legally required to fill any prescription, including those for controlled substances. In fact, pharmacists are ethically and legally required to exercise sound professional judgment when dispensing controlled medication. Pharmacy technicians must readily alert a pharmacist if a prescription for a controlled medication appears questionable. An individual who is found to have knowingly dispensed a questionable or invalid prescription for a controlled medication may be subject to professional discipline (loss of one's license to practice) as well as felony criminal prosecution. To avoid such severe consequences, it is crucial that pharmacy technicians demonstrate proper legal and ethical behavior in the handling of controlled medications and prescriptions.

Prescriptions for controlled medication should be carefully reviewed, just as with any other type of prescription order. Prescriptions for controlled medication must contain the same necessary information as was cited previously. There are additional requirements that must be verified in order to fill a prescription for a controlled medication. The Valid Prescription Requirements issued by the DEA's Office of Diversion Control permit the issuance of prescriptions for controlled substances by a physician, dentist, podiatrist, veterinarian, midlevel practitioner, or other registered practitioner who is:

1. Authorized to prescribe controlled substances by the jurisdiction in which the practitioner is licensed to practice, and
2. Registered with DEA or exempted from registration (e.g., Public Health Service, Federal Bureau of Prisons, military practitioners), or
3. An agent or employee of a hospital or other institution acting in the normal course of business or employment under the registration of the hospital or other institution which is registered in lieu of the individual practitioner being registered, provided that additional requirements as set forth in the C.F.R. are met."

Prescriptions for controlled medication may be issued in writing (written in ink or indelible pencil) or electronically—so long as the pharmacy and its order entry system has demonstrated conformance with the Controlled Substances Act and the order management system has the capability to store all necessary controlled drug prescription information required for DEA reporting and audit requirements. A pharmacist may accept prescriptions from Schedules III through V in writing, by fax, electronically, or verbally. Schedule II drugs may also be received by fax for processing, so long as the original hard-copy prescription is presented to the pharmacist and verified against the fax copy at the time of dispensing.

A licensed pharmacy must have a DEA number in order to fill a prescription for controlled medication; if the store is owned by a pharmacist, that pharmacy must have had a DEA number issued to it individually in order to accept and dispense controlled medication.

DEA NUMBERS

The Drug Enforcement Agency (DEA) may issue a DEA number to an authorized prescriber, site, or pharmacy/pharmacy owner. The DEA registration number is encoded with two letters, followed by seven numbers. Pharmacy staff members should be prepared to verify the validity of a DEA registration number as provided by the medication prescriber. There is a formula whereby a DEA registration number can be verified, as shown in the following example.

Let's use the number BJ1424326 for Dr. Tom Jones.

1. The first letter indicates the DEA number registrant type. See Table 6-2 for a listing of the registrant types.
2. The second letter is the first letter of the prescriber's last name.
3. Add the first, third, and fifth numbers:

$$1 + 2 + 3 = 6$$

4. Add the second, fourth, and sixth numbers:

$$4 + 4 + 2 = 10$$

5. Double the sum of the second, fourth, and sixth numbers:

$$10 \times 2 = 20$$

6. Add the above sum to the sum of the first, third, and fifth numbers:

$$20 + 6 = 26$$

7. The last digit of that sum should be the last number of the DEA number. Because the last number is 6, this is likely a valid DEA number

Students may recall from Chapter 2 that controlled substances are regulated by DEA schedules based on abuse potential. Students may refer back to Table 2-3 for a listing of DEA schedules and examples of drugs that fall into each of those categories.

When removing controlled drugs from bulk containers, it may be helpful to count them more than once to ensure that the correct quantity is being dispensed. Generally, at least Schedule II drugs are maintained with perpetual inventory—that is, the drug quantity on hand is counted before and after the dispensed quantity has been counted or measured. Each controlled medication prescription is generally documented in a fill log as well as a controlled substances inventory log.

The Community Pharmacy Label

The pharmacy label encompasses more than one might expect. Labels include multiple pieces of information that have many different functions. Figure 6-3 shows an example of all of the information that must be contained on a retail prescription label, including the following:

- Pharmacy name, address, phone number
- Pharmacy-generated prescription number
- Date prescription filled
- Patient's name and address
- Directions for use
- Drug name, strength, and dosage form
- Dispense quantity

TABLE 6-2   **DEA Registrant Types**

DEA Registrant Type	Description
A	Now depreciated (for DEA numbers issued prior to 1985, no longer currently issued)
B	Hospital/clinic
C	Practitioner
D	Teaching institution
E	Manufacturer
F	Distributor or practitioner
G	Researcher
H	Analytical lab
J	Imported
K	Exporter
L	Reverse distributor
M	Midlevel practitioner
N–U	Various narcotic treatment programs

Dr. Tracy Crum
DEA#AC1243170
LIC#44550

11287 E Villanova Drive
Aurora, CO 30358
Phone: 303-555-1212

Date: *12/12/07*

Patient's name: Billie Jones   Age: *83 yrs*
Address: 125 Grand Canyon Drive, Tucson, Arizona 85707

Rx:

K-Dur 20 mEq tab
1 daily   #90

Substitution permitted Y N
Refills 1 2 3 4 5 6 7 8 9   Signature_____Tracy L Crum, MD

FIGURE 6-3 Sample of information on a medication label. (From Hopper T: *Mosby's Pharmacy Technician: Principles and Practice*, ed 3, Philadelphia, 2011, Saunders.)

- Prescriber name
- Refills authorized

As this example shows, some types of information might be highlighted on a label, such as when a generic product has been substituted for a particular brand name product.

Preparing a Drug for Dispensing

A solid drug, such as a tablet or capsule, must be placed in the most appropriately sized container for dispensing to the patient. Amber vials are generally used for dispensing solid oral medication. Some drugs, such as birth control pills, may be dispensed in containers or devices supplied by the manufacturer. Drugs manufactured in dispensing devices must be kept in the original containers. Additionally, some drugs must be dispensed in their original manufacturer containers because of their chemical composition. For example, nitroglycerin must be dispensed in the original small, airtight glass vial in which it has been manufactured, as the drug breaks down when exposed to air.

The bottle that the drug is shipped in is generally referred to as the stock bottle. Drug stock bottles come in a variety of sizes and accommodate both large and small dispense quantities. Solid drugs must be carefully counted to ensure that the correct quantity is dispensed (without being touch contaminated), placed in the amber dispensing container, and secured with the appropriate lid. Pharmacists and pharmacy technicians use counting trays to pour out solid drugs for counting, which allows the drug to be transferred to the dispensing container without being contaminated. Drugs are generally counted out in denominations of five using a pharmacy spatula. The counted drug is dragged over into the spouted reservoir at the end of the tray. Once the counting is completed, a funnel on the opposite end of the tray is used to return the uncounted drugs back to the source stock bottle. Then, the dispensing spout allows the counted drug to be transferred into the amber vial. Counting trays should also be cleaned before and after use. Additionally, there may be designated counting trays that are used for hazardous drugs, such as oral chemotherapy drugs. Pharmacy technicians must ensure that they use the appropriate counting tray when counting and pouring solid oral medications.

Recall that the Poison Prevention Packaging Act of 1970 requires that childproof caps be placed on dispensing containers *unless* a patient specifically requires non-childproof lids. At the time of dispensing, these patients must complete documentation stating that they consented to non-childproof caps, are aware of the risks, and will ensure that this packaging is kept out of the reach of children.

Liquid drugs may be dispensed in their original containers or transferred from a large bulk stock container into a smaller dispensing liquid container (also known as an oval vial). A clean measuring device, such as a graduated cylinder, must be used to measure the correct volume of the liquid medication. It is often appropriate to wear gloves when transferring liquid drugs from bulk containers into dispensing containers. There may also be instances in which a drug may come in a powder form that must be reconstituted (purified deionized water added) before it is dispensed to the patient. A pharmacy may use various types of liquid reconstitution systems. These devices also serve as measuring devices for the liquid volume; additionally, some products feature filtration systems that remove possible contaminants from the water that could affect the stability (and taste) of dispensed oral medications. Generally, a drug that must be reconstituted is packaged and bagged in dry powder form and is not reconstituted until the patient arrives to pick up the prescription.

Dispensing Container Labeling

Once the drug has been pulled from stock, counted/measured, and poured into the final dispensing container, the product is then ready for labeling. Drugs that have been manufactured in boxes or cartons must be labeled in such a way as to ensure that the patient will not likely dispose of the prescription information. If a product is likely to be stored in its carton, the prescription label may be affixed to the carton. Care should be taken to position the prescription label in a way that does not conceal any of the product information. Labels should be placed in a neat and professional manner; labels affixed in a crooked or haphazard way may give a patient the perception that the prescription was filled in a hurried or careless and possibly incorrect way. The demonstration of pharmaceutical elegance entails placing a clean label in an appropriate location on the dispensing container in a neat fashion. Spills or drug residue should be removed from the outside of the dispensing container prior to labeling if a product was transferred from another container prior to dispensing. Professionally dispensed drugs boost a patient's confidence in the professional competence of pharmacy staff members and increase the likelihood that the patient will use the product.

Additional Labeling

As part of the order entry fill process, a pharmacy technician affixes additional labels on medication dispensing containers, which provide critical information about the drug being dispensed and how the patient should administer it:

- Warning labels alert the patient to specific warnings concerning the administration and storage of the medication, as well as potential food and drug interactions.
- Auxiliary labels provide additional instruction to the patient, such as how the medication should be taken.

Visit www.pharmex.com for a comprehensive list of commonly used auxiliary and warning labels. Note that many of the labels are shown in English and Spanish; today's technician, particularly those who practice in culturally diverse areas, should become familiar with Spanish-language labels in addition to those printed in English. Many pharmacies use a label template that contains the dispensing label, drug information monograph, and any applicable auxiliary or warning labels.

For accountability purposes, the final step of the label process requires that the person filling the prescription signs his or her initials on the container label to identify that he/she filled the prescription.

STAGE 4: PHARMACIST VERIFICATION

Once the technician has prepared a prescription, a pharmacist must verify it for accuracy before it can be dispensed to a patient. The pharmacist will compare the original prescription against the bottle label, as well as the information on the hard-copy label. The product NDC number will be verified, and the pharmacist will visually inspect the product for correctness. The pharmacist will have checked the patient's profile to verify therapeutic appropriateness. If a pharmacy technician has any concerns or reservations about a prescription, he or she should bring it to the attention of the pharmacist during the order entry, fill, or check processes. This ensures that the pharmacist has an opportunity to investigate whatever issue or concern exists *before* the patient comes to pick up the prescription.

If a prescription could not be filled because of concerns about its validity, then that prescription information must be placed aside so that it can be reviewed with the patient upon his or her arrival. In some cases, the pharmacist may be in the process of contacting the patient's prescriber and may be awaiting a callback. Or the staff may have been unable to contact the patient's pharmacy benefit provider. If it is feasible to call the patient to seek clarification or gain additional information, then pharmacy staff should take that extra step. Additionally, pharmacy technicians should seek to take ownership of prescription fill-related issues. For example, if there was an issue with the third-party billing of a prescription and a particular technician was working on that issue, that technician should take all necessary steps to resolve the issue, rather than leave the issue to be handled by another staff member. At the end of a shift, incoming shift members should receive pass-down information related to any pending issues with prescriptions, along with any relevant background information needed to follow up and serve the patient's needs.

Once the fill process has been completed, checked medications are generally placed in a dispensing bag with a label affixed to the outside that bears the patient's name for identification. Legend and controlled drugs may be stored in different locations, as well as prescriptions that require additional action such as reconstitution, compounding, or consultation by the pharmacist.

STAGE 5: DISPENSING MEDICATION TO THE PATIENT

The last stage of the order entry and fill process is dispensing medication to the patient and collecting payment as required. When a patient comes to pick up a prescription, the pharmacist or pharmacy technician should perform the following steps:
- Greet the patient.
- Clarify what type of prescription the patient has come to pick up (new, refill, and narcotic prescriptions may be stored in different areas).
- Ask for the patient's name; if the patient has a common name, an additional identifier (such as a middle name or address) should be requested.
- Ask if the patient knows what type of medication he or she has come to pick up.
- Ensure that the patient signs the privacy acknowledgment label.
- Ensure that the patient signs the waiver of childproof packaging, as applicable.
- If a particular drug or pharmacy benefit (such as Medicare) requires counseling by the pharmacist, the pharmacy technician must inform the patient of this requirement and show the patient to the counseling area (Figure 6-4).
- Particularly if it is a new prescription, the patient should be encouraged to speak with the pharmacist concerning the administration of that drug.
  - If a pharmacy technician knows of a warning or precaution that a patient needs to be aware of, the technician should use that knowledge as a cue to *strongly encourage* the patient to speak with the pharmacist concerning the medication.

TECH NOTE!

If a pharmacy technician has any concerns or reservations about a prescription, he or she should bring it to the attention of the pharmacist during the order entry, fill, or check processes.

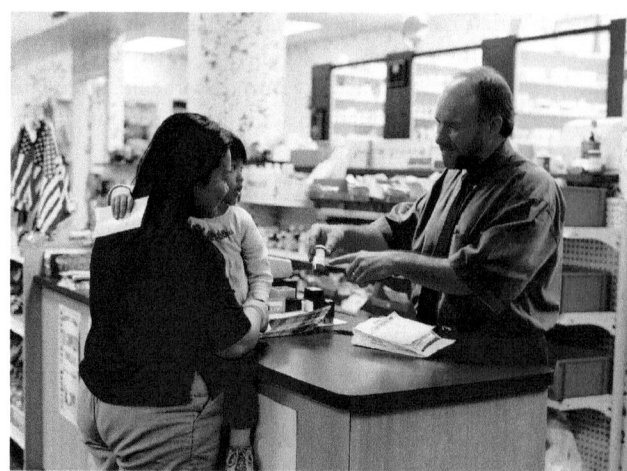

FIGURE 6-4 Patient consultation. (From Hopper T: *Mosby's Pharmacy Technician: Principles and Practice*, ed 3, Philadelphia, 2011, Saunders.)

- Remember, pharmacy technicians must act within their legal scope of practice and should *never* provide clinical information—the patient must *always* be directed to a pharmacist in order to receive that information!
- If a drug must be compounded or reconstituted immediately prior to dispensing, then the pharmacy technician should complete that process, if allowed. Or the pharmacy technician should notify a pharmacist concerning the product compounding or reconstitution so that the pharmacist may perform the action and check the product prior to dispensing.
- Patients with disabilities: It is important to be sensitive to patients' needs in the event of a temporary or permanent physical or mental disability. Every patient should be treated with respect and dignity, and every attempt should be made to address and treat patients with disabilities the same as other patients. There are reasonable accommodations that may be appropriate, including the following:
  - If a patient is deaf and speaks through an interpreter, it is important to speak to the patient directly using direct eye contact, rather than speaking to the interpreter.
  - Pharmacy staff members should disregard service animals and should not treat a service animal as one would treat a pet (service dogs have been specially trained to assist a patient and should not be distracted or interacted with).
  - If it would be more comfortable for a patient to be seated during the dispensing process, then that request should be accommodated whenever possible.
  - Always ask before making physical contact with a patient; additionally, many patients with physical disabilities have learned to be self-sufficient, so it is important to *ask the patient* if he or she would like assistance.
  - Patients often regard permanent wheelchairs and other assistive devices as an extension of their own bodies; therefore, it is important to *ask permission* before coming into physical contact with the patient's chair or other assistive device.
  - It is not necessary to speak more loudly or slowly to an individual with a visible physical/mental disability, such as autism or Down syndrome—and doing so will likely offend the patient. Instead, the patient should be spoken to in a normal voice.
- Cashiering: Ensure that cashiering is performed accurately, and that the patient's payment is correctly processed.
  - If the patient is using cash, the correct change should be correctly counted out.
  - If the patient is using a credit, debit, or flexible spending account card, it is important to ensure that the card is returned at the conclusion of the transaction.

The manner in which pharmacy technicians interact with patients during the dispensing process will help to define or reinforce that patient's view of pharmacy services at large. Every member of the pharmacy team should interact with patients in a way that honorably represents the profession. Professionalism and courtesy should be demonstrated at all times.

OTHER PHARMACY DUTIES AS ASSIGNED

In addition to the tasks noted in the workflow model, other tasks may be required on a daily or routine basis, such as those discussed in the following sections.

Per Shift or Daily Adjunct Tasks

- Returning used medication to shelves
- Maintaining perpetual inventory of all controlled medication
  - The quantity on hand must be verified and documented before, during, and after the dispensing of controlled medications
- Returning designated prescriptions to stock if the patient did not pick them up
- Stocking/restocking shelves following the shipment and receipt of a drug order
- Filing hard-copy prescriptions (written prescriptions must be filed by prescription number or date and retained in a secure record-keeping location)
- Replenishing pharmacy supplies, such as pill bottles, oval liquid bottles, and childproof bottle caps
- Performing a general cleanup, such as wiping down counting trays and countertops and emptying waste baskets

Monthly/Routine Adjunct Tasks

- Cycle counts—manually counting the quantity of all medication and medical devices currently in stock
- Checking expiration dating on all medication in stock, marking items that are due to expire within 60 days, removing expired items from stock and destroying them or setting them aside to be returned to the manufacturer for credit

  The type of pharmacy business may determine other adjunct tasks that the pharmacy technician staff must perform. Although these adjunct tasks may not be among the most popular, they are important and vital to the efficiency and tidy upkeep of the pharmacy environment. It is every pharmacy technician's obligation to perform these and other tasks; demonstrating a key soft skill like a positive attitude will make performing these tasks far less unpleasant!

RECOGNIZING LEGAL LIMITS: WHO DOES WHAT?

Although these duties may vary depending on the state, Box 6-1 provides a list of common tasks that may be legally performed by a pharmacy technician, as well as the related tasks performed by the pharmacist. This list highlights the degree to which the responsibilities of the pharmacist are dependent on the pharmacy technician, and vice versa. Each role is vital to serving the patient and is dependent on the other. Officially, pharmacy technicians may perform any task that does *not* require a clinical judgment/decision, for which an appropriate level of education and credential is legally required. So a pharmacy technician must *never* perform any of the tasks that are to be performed by the pharmacist. A pharmacy technician might be tempted to offer clinical judgment, particularly if he or she has heard a pharmacist provide patient information concerning how a medication should be taken. No matter how many times pharmacy technicians hear clinical information being disseminated, it is not legally permissible for them to provide that information themselves (not even if the patient is in a hurry or the pharmacist is busy with other tasks).

Given the U.S. economy and the volatility of various industries, there has been a surge in the number of individuals seeking the pharmacy technician career path who possess other industry credentials. There may even be situations in which a pharmacy technician does possess other health care credentials (perhaps the technician served as a medical assistant or a licensed vocational nurse, or perhaps he or she acquired a medical credential in another country) and may truthfully possess the education or clinical background to competently answer a question or

TECH ALERT!
Failure to act within the legal technician's scope of practice is not only a violation of federal or state law but creates a heightened risk of providing information to a patient that may be incorrect or therapeutically inappropriate.

BOX 6-1   Technician and Pharmacist Tasks

Technician Duty	Pharmacist Duty
Take prescriptions, collect medication usage history from patients	Create and maintain patient medication and health history database for the purpose of engaging medication therapy management
	Verify medication for therapeutic appropriateness, based on patient's condition and other types of medication currently being used
Verify patient's prescription benefit eligibility	Consult with patient's caregiver to verify medication to be used based on patient's available prescription benefit restrictions
Enter prescriptions into computerized order entry system	Verify order entry accuracy against written prescription for final check
Pull medication from shelf	Verify that correct medication was pulled from stock and used to fill prescription
Perform pharmaceutical compounding	Verify compounding logs, mix sheets, and ingredients to ensure that the proper process was followed and that all required ingredients were used and documented
Fill medication dispensing container and affix prescription and warning labels, if allowed by the state	Verify that all required information is noted on the prescription label, including drug, patient name, directions to the patient, fill quantity, and refill information
Encourage patients to seek out the pharmacist for counseling	Counsel patient on the use of the medication, including any precautions or warnings that should be adhered to; verify medication use history to ensure patient profile is up to date
Answer patient questions related to benefits	Answer patient questions related to benefits
	Answer questions related to how patients should correctly administer their medication and any side effects or possible adverse effects to watch for
Explain product packaging	
Gather vital information regarding immunization records and patient consent to receive immunizations; prepare immunization doses after required training	Administer immunizations after required training
	Answer questions related to the necessity of medical devices
Control the inventory of medication, including processing purchase orders, receiving medication orders, and stocking medication on shelves	Control the inventory of medication, including processing purchase orders, receiving medication orders, stocking medication on shelves
Perform certain supervisory functions, such as the oversight of other technicians, staff scheduling, staff training	Provide ultimate oversight and management of all pharmacy staff and verification of tasks performed for accuracy and safety
Direct patients to the location of various types of over-the-counter products stocked by the pharmacy	Recommend the most appropriate over-the-counter medication or medical devices.
Accept a valid prescription number over the phone for a refill request by a patient	Accept a verbal order
Refer a patient to the pharmacist in the event that a prescription or refills have been exhausted and the patient needs an emergency supply until he or she can see the health care provider	Determine the medical necessity for dispensing a temporary medication supply
Call security and notify a pharmacist if a patient displays behavior that may threaten the patient, pharmacy staff members, or other patients	Contact law enforcement to detain a patient

provide clinical information. From a legal and ethical standpoint, however, pharmacy technicians *must act within their scope of practice.* Failure to do so not only violates federal and state law, but it creates a heightened risk of providing a patient with information that may be incorrect or therapeutically inappropriate given other patient-specific variables.

If a technician wants to serve patients on a more clinical level, he or she should contemplate the educational requirements necessary to earn a doctor of pharmacy degree and explore opportunities for continuing his or her education. Some employers even offer options for tuition assistance or reimbursement if the employee agrees to continue working with that organization for a specified period of time. For individuals who have practiced pharmacy in another country and would like to practice in the United States, there are agencies that evaluate foreign degrees for U.S. equivalency. These credential evaluation agencies may be able to provide any additional educational or licensing requirements that must be fulfilled in order for the individual to practice as a pharmacist in the United States.

PATIENT COUNSELING AND MEDICATION THERAPY MANAGEMENT

Half a century ago, pharmacies were considered social gathering places where patients maintained regular contact with their pharmacist. The soda fountain environment kept pharmacists connected to the patients they served, which increased their familiarity with patients' individual health concerns and medication therapy. Today's community pharmacy environment is very different, although many privately owned pharmacies do offer a greater level of personal attention to their customer base. Chain store pharmacies can be found on nearly every corner of most residential communities, and pharmacies often compete over the same patient population. The volume of prescriptions filled on a daily basis creates a considerable challenge for pharmacists in terms of building and maintaining relationships with their customer base. In light of this challenge, pharmacists have been charged with protecting the health of patients and must seek more opportunities to consult with patients concerning the appropriateness of their medication therapy for managing their health issues.

Medication therapy management (MTM) is the process whereby pharmacists, in collaboration with other members of the health care and prescribing team, continuously evaluate a patient's prescribed medications for clinical appropriateness. MTM is accomplished through the prospective review of the patient's medical history, diagnoses, other medications/supplements being taken, and other patient-specific variables that influence medication use (such as gender, age, or ethnicity). Pharmacists are required to provide consultative service to patients receiving medication therapy that is covered by the Centers for Medicare and Medicaid Services (CMS), as per OBRA '90 legislation (see Chapter 2 to review detailed information on the provisions of OBRA '90). However, many professional pharmacy organizations have speculated about the overwhelming benefits of MTM for improving patients' clinical outcomes and lowering health care expenditures in the United States, if provided to a wider segment of the population. The American College of Clinical Pharmacy published a critical review of MTM in community practice. This report suggested several benefits of MTM:

- MTM can reduce and improve health outcomes, especially in elderly patients
- Many patients consider pharmacists to be approachable and better prepared to take the time to answer questions about their medications
- Improved health outcomes may lessen the need for additional medications when current medications are taken correctly
- Pharmacist interventions may reduce federal expenditures on hospital stays by preventing drug-related adverse events

Optimizing MTM would also help pharmacists to recapture operational expenses, as consultive sessions could be billable to insurance companies just like any other type of patient consultative service or office visit. Recommendations of the above-cited report were "intended to serve as a resource for individuals charged with designing and implementing a Medicare Medication Therapy Management program under the Medicare Modernization Act of 2003 (MMA) as well as those interested in expanding MTMs in both the public and private sectors." The evolution and implementation of medication therapy management has been a subject of great interest and visibility with several state boards of pharmacy and will continue to be so in the coming years, especially in light of health care reform legislation in the United States.

Troubleshooting Prescription Processing Issues

Various factors can upset the medication order entry and fill process, such as prescription drug benefit eligibility issues or drug availability. If a drug is out of stock, it may be possible to borrow the fill quantity from another store location. If a drug is subject to a national shortage, then another product may need to be prescribed. In this instance, the pharmacist may call the patient's prescriber to recommend an alternative product.

Pharmacy technicians may be required to call insurance companies to resolve issues concerning drug benefit coverage or to provide additional information so that the patient's insurance company approves the prescription. This task alone encompasses a large part of a technician's workday. For this reason, it is important for technicians to understand how third-party plans are set up in a patient's profile and to be aware of common issues that may affect the successful processing (also called adjudication) of a patient's benefit claim. Many benefit claims can be successfully processed by providing the following:
- Specific pieces of patient information that were not up to date in the patient's profile
- Updated insurance information in the patient's profile

Many claims and benefits issues that are the most upsetting to customers involve simply educating patients about their pharmacy benefit plan details. For example:
- Many plans are structured with pricing based on the type of drug product to be dispensed
- Patients may simply not have a clear understanding of stairstep (or tiered) medication pricing
  - It may be necessary to take the time to explain how a benefit plan is structured and encourage patients to speak with their benefit providers about the types of medication covered and to find out if there are other eligibility criteria that must be met before benefits are extended

Demonstration of Empathy

Empathy occurs when the pharmacy technician identifies with a patient's situation, feelings, or motives. When a patient arrives at the pharmacy to discover that the needed medication is not ready or is unavailable, the experience can be frustrating. It is important for pharmacy technicians to separate themselves from a patient's emotional response, as it is usually not intended as a personal attack. Instead, a patient should be comforted, reassured, and assisted.

Active Listening and Probing Questions

Pharmacy technicians should learn to ask probing questions that will allow them to better assist the patient and promptly resolve the issue. Often it is useful to ask patients what their understanding of their benefit plan is. The pharmacy technician may need to clarify some issues in order to better educate patients about their pharmacy benefits.

If a patient does need to return to the provider to follow up on an issue, a call to the provider to secure an appointment may be possible by the pharmacy staff; or the pharmacist may be able to speak directly with the provider and resolve the issue without the patient having to return to the caregiver.

If a patient is taking medication that requires a visit to the provider for diagnostic testing to ensure that the dose is therapeutically appropriate, this information should be communicated to the patient from the standpoint of making the patient's health the priority.

In given situations, it is important to personalize patients' issues:
- How would *you* wish to be treated and served in this situation?
- What if the patient was your loved one?
- What would be your fears or reservations in this situation?

Often, personalizing a situation will help to clarify how a pharmacy technician should proceed. Regardless, it is important to:
- Only offer information that a pharmacy technician is legally authorized to provide
- Tell the patient the truth—don't misrepresent an expectation or make a promise that cannot be delivered

- Collect as much information as possible from the patient to avoid multiple visits or phone calls while the issue is being resolved
- Follow through on the issue to resolution
- Refer matters appropriately to the pharmacist

Communicating Issues Involving the Validity of a Prescription

Prescriptions should be carefully examined for evidence of tampering, particularly of the date and medication strength. If a pharmacy technician suspects intentional tampering, he or she should immediately bring those concerns to the attention of a pharmacist, rather than confront the patient directly. The pharmacist will determine the next step.

A patient who is attempting to fill an altered or illegitimate prescription may have chemical dependency issues that may cause the patient to be erratic or aggressive— behavior that could quickly escalate to violence if the situation is not approached carefully. Rather than telling the patient that the medication cannot be filled, it may be more appropriate, for the safety of all, to simply tell the patient to have a seat and that the pharmacist will assist him or her shortly. The pharmacist can then decide whether law enforcement needs to be involved from a safety standpoint.

Legal and Ethical Dilemmas in the Community Pharmacy Environment

There have been situations in which pharmacy staff have knowingly filled fraudulent prescriptions or filled prescriptions provided by prescribers who are involved in illegal activity. The Drug Enforcement Agency works with local state boards of pharmacy to investigate claims, and it is important that suspected illegal activity be reported immediately. Anonymity may be upheld in cases that do not require the state board to reveal its reporting source. Also, most organizations have a fraud, waste, and abuse hotline where suspected illegal activity can be reported securely.

Recall the ninth principle of the Code of Ethics for Pharmacy Technicians, which states, "a Pharmacy Technician does not engage in any activity that will discredit the profession, and will expose, without fear or favor, illegal or unethical conduct in the profession." Pharmacy technicians have a legal and ethical obligation to report illegal/unethical behavior; failure to do so may result in professional or criminal disciplinary action.

Final Note

One reality check that pharmacy technicians should be aware of is the amount of time they will spend on their feet, in light of the structure of workflow processes. The pharmacy practice, particularly retail pharmacy, does not involve many long periods of inactivity. Be prepared to do a lot of standing and bending, and a good pair of comfortable shoes can often be the difference between a good and a bad day!

Because a pharmacy technician's day encompasses many tasks, it is important to:

- Know your role on the pharmacy team
- Know the tasks that technicians may and may not legally perform within your state
- Know your job, and be able to perform tasks proficiently and with efficiency and accuracy
- Know your resources for gathering information to serve the patient and the pharmacist

Chapter Summary

- Pharmaceutical practice in the United States originated with the privately owned corner drug-store, which existed before the rising population necessitated pharmacy chain stores.
- Community pharmacies offer a variety of services aside from traditional prescription drug dispensing.
- Retail pharmacies may be stand-alone businesses or part of another business, such as a grocery store, nursing home, or hospital.
- The area surrounding a pharmacy may determine its patient demographic and it influences the types of drugs carried and other services offered.

- Pharmacy technicians should gain a sense of the surrounding community to get a better idea of the types of skills that may be useful in that pharmacy.
- Communication skills are essential to ensuring that patients leave the pharmacy with not only the correct medication, but also a clear understanding of how the medication must be safely administered so that they achieve the maximum health benefit.
- All pharmacy technicians should be familiar with the legal tasks that may or may not be performed by pharmacy technicians, as detailed in Box 6-1.
- Pharmacy technicians should find productive ways to support and assist the pharmacist in their performance of medication therapy management (MTM).
- Pharmacy technicians fulfill several key roles at various workstations within the community pharmacy environment, including prescription intake and patient interview at the front window.
- Prescription order review and entry into a computer-based medication management system must utilize the five rights of medication administration.
- Prescription order review entails a knowledge of the key required components of a prescription, including:
  - Prescriber information
  - Date the prescription was written
  - Dosage form and dispense quantity of medication
  - Directions to the patient (signa)
  - Signature lines
  - Number of refills authorized
  - Instructions related to whether a product may be substituted or must be dispensed as written by the prescriber
- Pharmacy technicians must be familiar with the types of information that must be entered or updated in the pharmacy's medication management system.
- Pharmacy technicians must be mindful of each of the legally required fields on a prescription drug label, including:
  - Pharmacy name, address, phone number
  - Pharmacy-generated prescription number
  - Date prescription filled
  - Patient's name and address
  - Directions for use
  - Drug name, strength, and dosage form
  - Dispense quantity
  - Prescriber name
  - Refills authorized
- *Warning labels* alert the patient to specific warnings on the administration and storage of the medication, as well as potential food and drug interactions.
- *Auxiliary labels* provide additional instruction to the patient, such as how the medication should be taken.
- Pharmacy technicians may be required to troubleshoot prescription drug benefit eligibility issues or drug unavailability.
- Because of the abuse potential associated with controlled medication, care must be taken to ensure that a prescription for a controlled substance is valid prior to filling.
- Once the technician has prepared a prescription, a pharmacist must review and check it for accuracy before it can be dispensed to a patient.
- Pharmacy technicians then perform the steps associated with dispensing medication and collecting payment from patients.
- Every patient should be treated with respect and dignity, and every attempt should be made to address and treat patients with disabilities the same as other patients.

REVIEW QUESTIONS

Multiple Choice

1. The prescribed drug strength should be noted in which portion of the prescription?
   a. Inscription
   b. Signa
   c. Superscription
   d. DAW

2. Instructions to the patient are noted on which part of the prescription?
   a. Inscription
   b. Signa
   c. Superscription
   d. Subscription

3. A Schedule II drug may be refilled a maximum of _____times.
   a. 0
   b. 2
   c. 6
   d. 11

4. For insurance claims processing, DAW code ____ would be used if the law does not allow use of a generic product.
   a. 3
   b. 7
   c. 5
   d. 2

5. Who is allowed to answer general questions about a patient's drug benefits?
   a. Pharmacy technician
   b. Pharmacist
   c. Pharmacist or pharmacy technician
   d. Pharmacist and pharmacy technician

6. Who may legally answer questions related to the necessity of medical devices?
   a. Pharmacy technician
   b. Pharmacist
   c. Pharmacist or pharmacy technician
   d. Pharmacist and pharmacy technician

7. Who may answer questions related to how patients should correctly administer their medications and any side effects or possible adverse effects to watch for?
   a. Pharmacy technician
   b. Pharmacist
   c. Pharmacist or pharmacy technician
   d. Pharmacist and pharmacy technician

8. Who controls the inventory of medication?
   a. Pharmacy technician
   b. Pharmacist
   c. Pharmacist or pharmacy technician
   d. Pharmacist and pharmacy technician

9. Who may accept a verbal order for a new prescription from a patient care provider?
   a. Pharmacy technician
   b. Pharmacist
   c. Pharmacist or pharmacy technician
   d. Pharmacist and pharmacy technician

10. Who is ultimately responsible for the oversight and management of all pharmacy staff and verification of tasks performed for accuracy and safety?
    a. Pharmacy technician
    b. Pharmacist
    c. Pharmacist or pharmacy technician
    d. Pharmacist and pharmacy technician

TECHNICIAN'S
CORNER

1. Give one of the cited benefits of pharmacist involvement in MTM.
2. Describe the type of action that should be taken if a technician suspects that a prescription has been altered.
3. Explain the process for borrowing a DEA Schedule II drug from another pharmacy.

Bibliography

Berkrot, B. (2010). Retrieved 3/24/2011, from Reuters: www.reuters.com/article/2010/04/01/us-drug-sales-idUSTRE6303CU20100401

DaVanzo, J., Dobson, A., Koenig, L., Book, R. (2005). *Medication Therapy Management Services: Executive Summary Report.* Retrieved 4/20/2011, from www.accp.com/docs/positions/commentaries/mtms.pdf

U.S. Department of Justice Drug Enforcement Administration. (2011). *Office of Diversion Control Pharmacist's Manual.* Retrieved 4/20/2011, from Section IX-Valid Prescription Requirements: www.deadiversion.usdoj.gov/pubs/manuals/pharm2/pharm_content.htm#p10b

7

Team Building and Professionalism in Pharmacy Practice: How Pharmacists and Technicians Collaborate to Foster a Multidisciplinary Mindset

LEARNING OBJECTIVES

By the end of this chapter, students will be able to competently:

1. Describe how a pharmacy technician can use effective teamwork to demonstrate professionalism in the workplace.
2. Define *soft skills,* and explain how pharmacy technicians use them to perform daily tasks.
3. Explain how pharmacy technicians use critical thinking to support and assist pharmacists.
4. Recognize the importance of adopting a *multidisciplinary mindset* when approaching the health care team and patient care.
5. Explain the characteristics of collaborative interdepartmental work relationships.
6. Consistently employ a systematic approach to solve problems encountered during one's work as a technician.
7. Explain the concept of workflow management.
8. Explain the role of pharmacy technicians in managing their own work.
9. Formulate a personal mission statement that describes a pharmacy technician's responsibility as a member of the pharmacy and multidisciplinary health care team.

KEY TERMINOLOGY

Collaboration: Working jointly with others to achieve a common goal.

Multidisciplinary mindset: The patient care provider's knowledge of his or her role on the health care team and the recognition of how that role affects other members of the team and their ability to perform their roles.

Soft skills: Behaviors that a person demonstrates based on his or her own personal attributes and ability to interact with others.

Time management: A combination of behaviors that allow individuals to make the overall best use of their time.

Workflow management: Progress of work being done; a sequence of tasks; a series of activities that involve people, business processes, and software; a set of interdependent tasks that occur in a specific sequence.

Introduction

In an article published by the *American Journal for Pharmaceutical Education (AJPE),* the author reflected on the words of a keynote speaker during the 1999 midyear clinical meeting of the American Society of Health-System Pharmacists (ASHP). In that presentation, Kathleen Marie Dixon presented the preceding thought-provoking ideas concerning the pharmacy student's development of professionalism, which is certainly applicable to technician practice. When considering team building, it is astounding how the actions of a few (or even one!) impact the pharmacy team as a whole. As Dixon suggested, a spark of enthusiasm and desire for professional growth in the pursuit of excellence may well ignite that desire in other members of the pharmacy team.

Although it might be challenging for the everyday person to describe the word *professionalism,* the same person might more easily describe the elements of teamwork, such as working together, pursuit of a common purpose, shared accountability, individual reliability, baseline skill, and competence. Several specific skill sets—such as effective communication, troubleshooting, and critical thinking—set apart a professional from someone who simply meets the minimum requirements to keep his or her job.

A critical element of professionalism in the health care environment is the development of a patient focus. A patient focus means that pharmacy technicians approach their work in consideration of the patient's health and safety. Technicians should also direct their patient focus in terms of how their roles impact other members of the health care team and *their* ability to provide exemplary patient care. The demonstration of patient focus fosters a multidisciplinary mindset, which will be discussed later in this chapter.

Soft skills are the behaviors that many employers feel their technician staff lack or do not demonstrate on a consistent basis. As the role of the pharmacist continues to evolve and branch out into more clinical areas, pharmacists will increasingly depend on their pharmacy technician staff members to perform more challenging tasks that will help better serve patients. Pharmacy technicians must rise to that challenge by consistently demonstrating a strong work ethic, a patient focus, and a commitment to serving both patients and other members of the health care team.

The Pathway to Professional Behavior on the Pharmacy Team

The modern health care environment is one in which a team of patient care providers collaborate—or work jointly—to identify a patient treatment plan that will provide the greatest health benefit and clinical outcome for the patient. Although historically the multidisciplinary team dynamic has been volatile—at times quite adversarial as both physicians and pharmacists may feel threatened by each other's role—members of the health care team recognize the value that each adds in terms of better serving patients. This collaborative effort can only be successful when members of the health care team respect and value each other and demonstrate a high level of professionalism.

The aforementioned *AJPE* article cited several key definitions of professionalism as it relates to the experiential training of pharmacy students. Concern was noted about the unprofessional behavior of some pharmacy students, including inappropriate dress, disrespectful behavior, and a low motivation to learn. Today's student is often described as "lazy and apathetic," and it has been noted that many demonstrate a "sense of entitlement" or the expectation that success is something owed to them rather than something that must be earned through hard work. Just as with the formation of a moral or ethical code, behaviors that define professionalism may not come naturally to everyone—they must be defined, practiced, and modeled by those who play influential roles in the lives of these students.

It does not help that many high-profile figures—whether in politics, professional sports, or the media—demonstrate disrespectful, unethical, and unprofessional behavior in full public view. Those who have been cast as role models—whether or not they wish or have the ability to be—may set a flawed perception and expectation in the minds of young people concerning the value of demonstrating professionalism. The pharmacy profession has not been immune to this social malady, considering the number of high-profile cases that involve unethical and illegal behavior on the part of pharmacists and pharmacy technicians. There is a need for a higher standard of quality and professionalism throughout the pharmacy industry, as employers often communicate to educators in both schools of pharmacy and pharmacy technology training programs.

THE LOOK OF PROFESSIONALISM

The physical appearance of a pharmacy technician is a critical factor for projecting an image of professionalism that will reflect positively on one's employer and the profession in general. Every pharmacy technician should project an outward appearance that sends the message "I am a skilled, responsible professional who can be trusted with patients' protected health information."

Professional Attire

Pharmacy technicians should always present themselves in work attire that is clean and tidy. Descriptions of appropriate attire include the following:

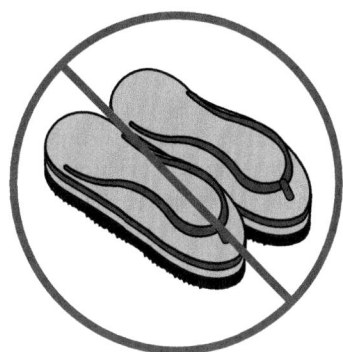

- A clean, neatly pressed, and properly fitting work uniform or business casual style of dress—whichever the employer prescribes
- Slacks and button-up shirt, with or without a tie unless required, for males
- Slacks or knee-length skirt and top with an appropriate neckline for females, with conservative use of jewelry and cosmetics
- Comfortable, close-toed shoes, as the pharmacy technician's job often requires prolonged periods of standing or walking
  Inappropriate attire includes the following:
- Jeans and other casual wear
- Open-toed shoes, including flip-flops or other sandals
- Shirts that display graphics of any sort
- Any clothing that is ill fitting or revealing

Personal Appearance and Hygiene

Maintaining personal hygiene not only sustains a positive work environment but also minimizes the risk of spreading germs on the skin and clothing, which may result from poor personal hygiene. Hair should be styled neatly; purposely distracting hair color or hairstyles may be perceived negatively by patients and should be avoided. Although it is at the discretion of an individual pharmacy, hair length for men may be restricted, so men with longer hair may wish to confirm that this style is acceptable when seeking job opportunities. Generally, heavily scented body lotions and sprays or colognes/perfumes should be avoided because of issues they may raise for patients with respiratory disease.

Cosmetics should be applied conservatively and may actually be restricted in some hospital environments (such as intravenous [IV] preparation clean rooms), so pharmacy technicians may wish to take that into consideration when seeking job opportunities. Body piercings should not be visible except on the ears; piercings on display elsewhere on the body may be inappropriate for the workplace. Lastly, the visual appearance of tattoos should be minimized. Those with tattoos on the forearms should consider wearing long-sleeved shirts or perhaps a long sleeved technician jacket. Some employers may even require this accommodation.

In addition to personal appearance and hygiene, several key behaviors clearly describe professionalism, both in terms of individual behavior and as part of the pharmacy and health care teams. As the author of the *AJPE* article noted, "pharmacy has often focused on more behavioral aspects of professionalism, such as initiative, empathy, appearance, courtesy, lifelong learning, responsibility, exceeding expectations, and pride in the profession" (Dana Hammer, 2006). These key behaviors may be characterized as *soft skills*.

DEFINING SOFT SKILLS

Soft skills are learned behaviors that a person demonstrates based on one's own personal attributes and ability to interact with others. One's chosen profession will often lead demonstrate certain soft skills over others. This is one reason why students should carefully consider whether they wish to pursue the pharmacy profession, in terms of the various hard and soft skills that the pharmacy technician practice and patient care demand. Not every individual possesses strong communication skills or the ability to anticipate a patient's needs based on certain verbal and nonverbal cues. However, when one can clearly define the individual skills that will be necessary, it may be easier to identify whether those attributes can be further developed and effectively utilized in day-to-day practice.

The following section lists several soft skills that are particularly critical in the practice of pharmacy, provides a simple definition of each one, and gives a few practical examples related to the pharmacy technician practice. A degree of overlap exists, and some examples may apply to multiple soft skills. Later on in the chapter, students may revisit these soft skills in reflective role-play scenarios.

Skill: Common Sense

DEFINITION

The ability to apply practicality to a situation, based on factors that are commonly known, visible, or easily identifiable.

EXAMPLES
- Offering a more suitable pickup time or a courtesy follow-up call to patients who have communicated that they are in a hurry
- Offering a person whose writing hand is in a cast assistance with completing forms
- Not asking multiple open-ended questions to someone who has just experienced oral surgery and has difficulty speaking
- Not asking to take a lunch break right in the middle of a busy time of day

Skill: Motivation/Initiative

DEFINITION

The identification of factors in a situation that may drive a person to action without prompting.

EXAMPLES
- Asking if there are additional training opportunities within the department or store as a means to increase skill level and job security
- Actively asking busy co-workers *how*—rather than if—you may give them a helping hand, recognizing that often individuals will avoid asking for assistance for fear of being perceived as ineffective
- Assisting a patient with a billing issue by gathering information rather than simply referring the patient to a pharmacist or the patient's insurance company which will likely expedite the resolution and the patient's ability to receive the needed medication
- Seeking out a floor nurse to ask questions concerning doses that a patient may need urgently rather than waiting for the patient to call the pharmacy as a way to better serve the patient
- Taking the stairs to deliver an urgent medication instead of waiting for a busy hospital elevator (if one possesses the physical capability to do so)

Skill: Integrity

DEFINITION

Firm adherence to a code of moral values; the quality or state of being complete or undivided. May be characterized as the demonstration of making the right decision or choice, given opposing viewpoints; "doing the right thing."

EXAMPLES
- Utilizing ethical decision-making steps to arrive at the most appropriate decision after witnessing a co-worker stealing medication
- Turning in money or credit cards left behind by a patient
- Notifying a pharmacist if an error is discovered after a medication has been dispensed
- Avoiding participation in workplace gossip

June						
S	M	T	W	T	F	S
					1	2
3	4✗	5	6	*Meeting*	8	9
10	*Appointment* 11 *@ 2:00*	12	✗13	14	15	16
17	18	19	20	21 ✗	22	23
24	25	26	*Meeting @ 3:00* 27	28	29	30

Skill: Time Management

DEFINITION

Time management describes a combination of behaviors that allow individuals to make the overall best use of their time.

EXAMPLES

- Returning from lunch and breaks on time (this is also an accountability issue) so that workflow does not suffer in your absence
- Arriving on time to work and staying until the end of scheduled time
- Spending time on the most important work and completing it in a timely manner, rather than stretching it out to avoid having to perform other tasks
- Avoiding personal phone calls or computer use during work hours
- Planning work at the start of a shift

Skill: Optimism

DEFINITION

A personal attitude or perspective that focuses primarily on the most desirable or positive aspects of a person, place, or situation.

EXAMPLES

- Seeking to recognize the positive value of required workplace training, such as fire safety or sexual harassment
- Viewing the busy time of the day as an opportunity to streamline processes and identify barriers to workflow efficiency
- Finding ways to connect with a co-worker who has a challenging personality, such as by identifying common interests or values
- Using predictions of pay cuts or layoffs as motivation to do one's best work to increase one's sense of job security, or expressing appreciation for continued employment
- Focusing on the strengths, rather than shortcomings, of other pharmacy staff members

Skill: Good Manners/Social Skills

DEFINITION

A set of behaviors, often defined by cultural traditions or social trends, that defines the most appropriate manner in which to treat other individuals or approach a given situation.

EXAMPLES

- Holding a door open for an elderly or physically challenged patient or co-worker
- Using verbal salutations, such as "good morning/evening"
- Listening intently to a patient or co-worker during dialogue, without interrupting or diverting attention

- Formally addressing a patient (i.e., Mr., Mrs., Ms.)
- Saying "please" and "thank you"
- Avoiding the use of slang or profanity in the workplace

Skill: Accountability

DEFINITION

An individual's sense of duty or obligation to a commitment or expectation.

EXAMPLES

- Assisting a customer 5 minutes before the pharmacy is scheduled to close for the evening instead of sending the customer away and delaying his or her ability to begin taking the medication
- Informing staff members for the following shift of tasks that are still pending to allow them to better manage their workflow and avoid delays
- Following through on commitments made to co-workers and patients, such as following up on a patient issue until it has been resolved or covering a shift as agreed
- Taking responsibility when involved in an error, rather than placing blame on others or making excuses
- Taking the time to gather all of the necessary information from a patient while taking an order to avoid delays in processing the prescription (particularly if the patient does not wait)

Skill: Empathy

DEFINITION

The ability to identify with another person's perspective or recognize the value of another person's perspective.

EXAMPLES

- Attempting to view a situation from a patient's perspective, whether or not you agree with that perspective
- Affirming and validating a patient's concern or emotional response: "I hear your frustration and will do what I can to help"
- Saying, "I recognize that you are in pain and will do what I can to get your medications filled quickly"
- Saying, "I understand how frustrating it can be to call an insurance company and try to make sense of the language—let me help"

Skill: Sense of Humor

DEFINITION

A subjective means of evaluating a situation in terms of its humorous or comedic context.

EXAMPLES

- Taking oneself lightly (i.e., not seeking opportunities to take offense or view criticism as a personal attack)
- Using a humorous example to explain medication use to a patient, ensuring that the example is culturally/socially sensitive and workplace appropriate
- Making light humor of circumstances outside of one's immediate control—such as a power outage, system server downtime, or inclement weather—as a means to lighten a tense or difficult moment and raise morale

Skill: Critical Thinking/Problem Solving

DEFINITION OF CRITICAL THINKING

Utilizing a step-by-step (systematic) approach when taking action, in light of possible variables.

DEFINITION OF PROBLEM SOLVING

Evaluating a situation to determine the appropriateness of addressing the situation personally as opposed to referring the matter to a more skilled individual.

EXAMPLES

- Knowledge of a pharmacy technician's legal scope of practice in order to determine the appropriateness of providing information to a patient (it is never okay to provide clinical information or a clinical judgment to a patient, even if you have heard a pharmacist recite that information a thousand times!)
- Anticipating third-party billing issues that one may have encountered previously and applying what was learned to other patients' situations in order to resolve their issues more efficiently
- Evaluating a workflow process to identify ways that the work could be performed more efficiently
- Recognizing patterns or trends in the workplace environment that may create opportunities for improvement or better customer service
- Navigating through various aspects of ethical decision making requires troubleshooting skills as well as a focus on caring for the patient and preserving the integrity of the pharmacy profession and one's individual organization

Skill: Effective Communication

DEFINITION

Proficient demonstration of sending and receiving information using verbal, nonverbal, written, and electronic forms of communication.

EXAMPLES

- Active listening: listening to understand and without interruption
- Recognizing and accurately interpreting inferred/implied context in a form of communication
- Speaking clearly and with an appropriate tone and volume
- Using audience-appropriate technical language
- Clarifying that a message was sent/received in the context in which it was intended in order to avoid confusion or misinterpretation
- Providing open, honest, and respectful feedback

Demonstrating each of the described soft skills will increase the capacity of a pharmacy technician to perform more successfully—whether alone or as part of a team. The next section explores how personal attributes may be applied to situations in which technicians must work well as members of the pharmacy and other health care teams.

What Is a Multidisciplinary Mindset?

Management of the health and welfare of a patient involves a collaborative team approach rather than the use of individual knowledge and skills. Medication management databases are designed to tap into various sources of clinical data via an electronic interface; health care providers across multiple clinical areas share information and thus increase each other's ability to make the most informed and appropriate clinical decisions.

Pharmacy technicians may interact with several members of the health care team, including surgeons, physicians, nurses, physical therapists, or social workers. Each member of this team contributes a valuable component of patient care that is dependent on the contributions of other members of that team. Setting expectations regarding individual work performance alone is no longer an effective means of striving for career success in the pharmacy practice. Rather, recognizing one's role as part of a greater team should serve as a greater motivator to achieve higher-quality results.

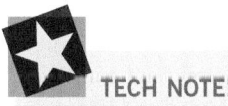
TECH NOTE!
Developing a multidisciplinary mindset requires a health care professional to know his or her role on the health care team and recognize how that role affects other team members and their ability to perform their roles as well.

Building and Sustaining Workplace Relationships

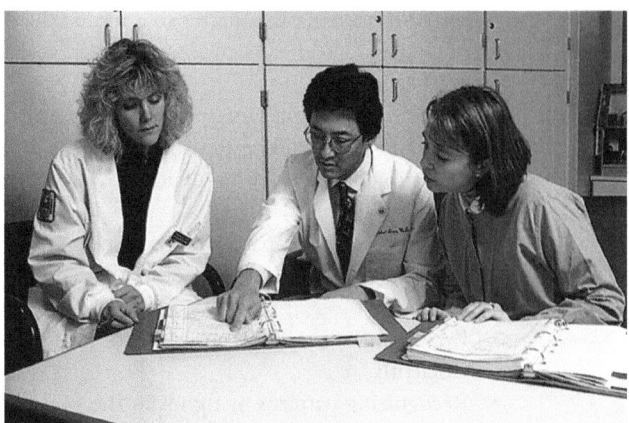

FIGURE 7-1 Working together with your colleagues can lead to new ideas while building lasting professional relationships. (From Purtilo R: *Ethical dimensions in the health professions,* ed 5, Philadelphia, 2011, Saunders.)

Building and sustaining workplace relationships is like planting and maintaining a garden. One cannot simply plant seeds and hope that plants rise from the soil unassisted. In the same way, workplace relationships require intentional action and specific behaviors that will build trust and cohesion. Pharmacy technicians may begin the process of building successful workplace relationships by doing the following:

- Developing a team-oriented mindset
- Seeking their ideal place in an organization (or where they wish to go)
- Learning the personalities and skills of co-workers
- Conducting a personal inventory of one's own strengths and weaknesses
- Increasing one's awareness of behaviors that detract from successful workplace relationships
  Let's examine each of these areas in greater detail.

1. DEVELOP A TEAM MINDSET

Pharmacy technicians must develop or adapt a mindset that will best prepare them for their work environment and the types of workplace relationships in which they will be involved. For example, if a technician came from a background or work environment in which he or she worked alone, it would be useful for the technician to consider how different it will be to work as part of a multi-person team. One will need to utilize communication skills, demonstrate cooperation, be willing to contribute equally, and "feed" a positive attitude into that new environment.

2. FIND YOUR PLACE IN THE ORGANIZATION

A new pharmacy technician must consider the skills/aptitudes he or she possesses and how those skills are best suited for various areas within the pharmacy. Depending on the size of the organization, technicians may be designated to certain areas, or they may be required to cross train in several areas in order to perform a variety of job tasks. No matter where a new pharmacy technician is placed, he or she should approach each new job as an opportunity to learn, grow, and contribute to the profession. No job is too great or too small—and every technician's role is vital and important to each pharmacy organization.

3. BEGIN RELATIONSHIP BUILDING: LEARN YOUR AUDIENCE

A new pharmacy technician should seek opportunities to build relationships with co-workers—fellow technicians and pharmacists alike. Experienced technicians and pharmacists possess workplace and industry experience that will be useful to a technician who is new to the practice of pharmacy. One should ask questions related to the skills and experience that each pharmacy staff member possesses, so that a new technician will know whose expertise to seek out in given situations. Not only should new technicians seek out experienced technicians and their pharmacists as resources, but they should also learn where information might be found within the pharmacy to answer their questions. Technicians should also conduct home Internet research to find out the types of services offered by their new employers and then find ways to learn how to best perform their jobs and contribute to that organization.

Relationship Building Starts with You

It is valuable to take a personal inventory. If there are areas where a technician might be challenged, it is important for every individual to consider how best to overcome those challenges. For example, if a person is naturally introverted and has difficulty approaching a co-worker or supervisor with questions, it might be useful to seek out another person with similar characteristics or plan to have questions answered before the start of a shift, perhaps before other staff members arrive. People who are challenged with remembering instructions should keep a small notepad and pen with them to take notes. That simple act may avert the embarrassment of having to return to staff members multiple times to have instructions repeated—which may not reflect positively on that technician.

It is important to recognize how one learns and processes information, or if there are medical conditions that may present a barrier to learning and retaining information. Many adults struggle with career success because of undiagnosed learning disabilities and other conditions that may be addressed and treated by a physician. If a student is unduly challenged with learning/absorbing or retaining information—and if this has been a challenge in previous job situations—it may be wise to speak to a physician to find out if there are medical reasons for this behavior and what treatment options are available.

4. CONTINUE TO LEARN AND GROW WITH YOUR EMPLOYER

Once a new pharmacy technician gets settled within his or her new environment, there can be a tendency to fall into a rut of complacency and the comfort of a predictable routine. Too many technicians become territorial over time concerning their job tasks, or they become so used to their routine that change of any kind leaves them fearful and unsettled. A high level of skill in only one or two dedicated areas does not equate to job security; rather, a technician's ability to shift and function in a variety of settings will be more useful to an employer in terms of job retention. New pharmacy technicians should posture themselves with the expectation that there will always be new things to learn and adapt to within any pharmacy environment.

Technicians may stay fresh and adaptable by seeking ways to continue to develop themselves professionally. Many organizations offer continuing education workshops, and some may host seasonal or annual community outreach events where staff may contribute and participate on a voluntary basis. These events may create unique opportunities to get to know co-workers outside of the immediate work environment and may allow individuals to further develop their professional relationships and rapport with each other.

5. PULL UP THE WEEDS!

Be aware of workplace behaviors that detract from positive morale and team building. These behaviors include, but are not limited to, the following:

* Repeated tardiness, both at the start of the shift and after lunches and breaks
* Poor or careless work performance, which creates work for others and presents patient safety issues
* Bringing negative attitudes and personal problems to the workplace
* Expressing resistance to helping others or waiting to be asked to do so
* Engaging in nonproductive workplace politics, such as gossip or "cliques"
* Demonstrating any form of dishonesty

New technicians should avoid these and many other behaviors that can place them at odds with their co-workers and become barriers to sustaining workplace relationships. *Trust* is an important "feed and fertilizer" for any interpersonal relationship; one builds trust by displaying behavior that gives co-workers a sense that one can be relied on to perform the job well and that one will consider the pharmacy as a team—a team whose top priority is to serve patients— over one's own personal comfort or routine. Trust also serves to build a sense of *respect*, which one must *earn* from co-workers by producing quality work and demonstrating positive workplace behaviors.

Healthy and productive workplace relationships make it possible for a pharmacy to provide patient care through the management of pharmacy workflow. The next section details several definitions of workflow and how a pharmacy technician can fulfill various roles within the pharmacy setting.

Effective Workflow Management

Workflow can be defined in a variety of ways, depending on one's perspective. Common industry definitions with applications to health care would include the following:

- Progress (or rate of progress) of work being done
- Sequence of tasks; a workflow describes the order of a set of tasks performed by various agents to complete a given procedure within an organization; repetitive workflows are often automated, particularly in organizations that handle high volumes of forms or documents according to fixed procedures
- A series of activities that involve people, business processes, and software that achieve a business goal
- A set of interdependent tasks that occur in a specific sequence

    Workflow management involves people, processes, and technology in today's pharmacy setting—both community and institutional. Out of each of these definitions, we may extract the following elements that relate to the pharmacy technician practice. Pharmacy workflow encompasses the following:

- Daily tasks that must be performed, and in a particular sequence or order
    - Workflow tasks are interdependent, and the performance of individual tasks has an effect on other sequential tasks
- Processes that involve technology—such as computerized order entry or a pharmacy robotics system—that streamline those processes and increase both efficiency and patient safety
- Established standards or expectations concerning the rate at which those tasks should be performed in order for the pharmacy to run efficiently

    Pharmacy technicians must gain a sense of the tasks that technician staff may perform as part of the workflow of a particular pharmacy organization. If a process has been mapped, or documented with great detail, technicians must ensure that the process is followed according to established guidelines (i.e., aseptic IV admixture or batch compounding). If there are deadlines by which tasks must be completed or an average expected time by which certain tasks may be reasonably and safely performed, it is important to know that information so that one may measure performance against that standard and seek to meet or exceed it.

    If technology is involved, pharmacy technician staff will generally receive training; one must have a firm understanding of how to use various forms of pharmacy technology and should know basic troubleshooting techniques in the event that there is equipment failure or an error occurs in a computer application. Pharmacy technicians should know whom to call when dedicated technical support is appropriate and should ensure that staff members who may be impacted by equipment or computer failure are notified in a timely manner.

    The expression "a chain is only as strong as its weakest link" applies when considering pharmacy workflow processes. Because pharmacy tasks are interdependent, pharmacy staff members—pharmacists and technicians alike—should ensure that the performance of their work does not negatively impact, impede, or prevent other members of the pharmacy team from performing their tasks. The driving force behind people who take responsibility for their own productivity and the quality of work they produce is *accountability*.

PERSONAL ACCOUNTABILITY: HOW TECHNICIANS TAKE CHARGE OF THEIR OWN WORK

One of the most frustrating phrases a manager hears is "that's not my job." Depending on the type of pharmacy organization and how workflow is structured, many technicians may be required to train in all job tasks that involve technicians. One of the main reasons why a pharmacy technician may defer a job task to another technician or a pharmacist is because they have either not been adequately trained on how to perform their job, or they do not have a firm enough understanding of their job to feel that they can perform it with confidence. That apprehension may lead a pharmacy technician to push off a task that they feel could be better performed by another member of the pharmacy team. Confidence in one's ability to perform a job is so critical in the health care setting, as apprehension or impaired comprehension of an aspect of the job (such as dosage calculation) may place a patient's health at risk. Pharmacy technicians must be brave enough to address training needs with their pharmacy supervisors and/or managers, to ensure that they are tooled with all the necessary knowledge, understanding, and hands-on skills to perform their jobs with proficiency and confidence.

Poor work ethic may be another common driver behind poor job accountability in the workplace among staff technicians. Unfortunately, that poor work ethic may affect not only that individual's effectiveness, but other members of the pharmacy [and health care] team with tasks that are dependent upon that technician's work. Those who enter the profession of pharmacy must do so with the understanding that poor work ethic translates into compromised patient safety. It *is our job* to constantly perform our job tasks well, and always in the best interest of the patient.

Problem Solving in the Pharmacy Environment

One particular professional soft skill is worth categorizing and discussing on its own—the skill of *problem solving.* Because of inherent opportunities for problematic situations in the workplace, a critical component of team building is problem solving. There are various *types* of problems that a pharmacy technician may encounter on a regular basis in the pharmacy environment; it is important to employ a systematic—or step-by-step—approach to problem solving. Generally speaking, problem solving may be approached in basically the same way, regardless of the variables. A problem may refer to a person, situation, or equipment used as part of the job. Writer Okojie Pedro presented five very basic clear steps to problem solving, which are easily adaptable to the pharmacy technician practice:

1. *Identify the problem. This is critical: you must try to solve the right problem… Identify the right problem by asking the right questions and observing.*
2. *Analyze the problem. How often does the problem occur? How severe is it? Are there any special circumstances that are present when it occurs? What might be the causes of the problem? Can you rule out any causes? How long has it been going on? Has it gotten worse? How is the problem affecting other processes or people?*
3. *Identify decision criteria. How will you and the customer make decisions when it is time to decide? How will you weigh the criteria? Can you identify independent standards that can be used?*
4. *Develop multiple solutions. Don't stop at the first solution that you or others identify. It may be good, but much better ones may exist. Evaluate alternative scenarios. As objectively as possible, assess the pros and cons of each.*
5. *Choose the optimal solution. Use the criteria you developed in the third step of this problem-solving process to choose the best solution. Develop a base of support that will ensure you can implement the solution. Prepare for contingencies.*

Okojie Pedro, 2006

Let's apply these five steps to a few common problems that may occur in a typical pharmacy setting.

PROBLEM 1

A new pharmacy technician has encountered an issue with one of the senior technicians. Every time she approaches her with a question, the senior technician appears annoyed or frustrated. She answers each question curtly then quickly walks away and busies herself with another task, which makes the new technician very uncomfortable. How should the new technician approach this problem?

Step 1: Identify the Right Problem, Setting Apart the Person from the Behavior

Identify why the senior technician is behaving in this manner toward the new technician. There could be a variety of reasons:
- Perhaps she has been frequently approached with questions during a busy time, which frustrates her.

- She may be a natural introvert and is uncomfortable with the interaction required during questioning.
- Perhaps she is uncomfortable with answering questions because she is afraid of giving out the wrong information or being perceived as unknowledgeable if she cannot answer a question.
- She may be insecure about sharing information she has learned over time, feeling that her knowledge base gives her a competitive edge over other technicians and may guarantee more job security.

Step 2: Analyze the Problem

- How often does this happen?
- Are there any common variables that exist each time the new technician approaches the senior technician?
- Is the new technician the only staff member who is treated this way, or has the new technician observed this behavior being projected on other members of the pharmacy staff?

Step 3: Identify Decision Criteria

- What will happen if the new technician chooses to do nothing and hopes that the situation gets better?
- What if the situation worsens?
- What if the new technician is placed in a position where she is working alone with that senior technician during a shift, and they must be able to work together to make sure that the pharmacy workflow processes do not suffer?
- How might patient care suffer as a result of her not addressing this issue?
- What ethical or business principles should be taken into consideration?

Step 4: Develop Multiple Solutions

- Address questions during a slower time of the day, such as the beginning or ending of the shift, to see if the senior technician's general behavior changes.
- Share the behavior observations with the senior technician, using "I" statements and without placing blame or making accusations.
- Ask a supervisor if he or she would be willing to mediate a meeting between the new technician and the senior technician.

Step 5: Choose the (Optimal) Decision Option That Has the Highest Likelihood of Bringing about Resolution

In this instance, it might be useful to employ all three possible solutions. It may be a useful fact-gathering exercise to observe how this technician treats other members of the pharmacy team. This may help to rule out whether this is a general performance issue, or if perhaps one technician is being singled out for inappropriate behavior. Once that is identified, it may become clearer how to approach the individual directly. When approaching someone for the purpose of problem solving, it is important to stick to the facts and focus on the behavior rather than the person. Consider this example:

> "Excuse me, _____. I have noticed that since I began working here, you appear annoyed or unhappy when I approach you with questions. With all of your experience, I value your perspective. Since we're part of the same team, it's important that we are able to work together and gain information from each other. Is there something I am doing that is causing this response from you? Is there something that you would like me to do differently?"

Hopefully, these probing questions will stimulate conversation and allow the two technicians to discuss the issue and find a solution that will work best for both of them. If not, the final mediation option may be the best strategy to bring about resolution.

Let's apply the problem-solving steps to the next scenario involving a patient issue.

PROBLEM 2

Mr. Robinson brought his prescription bottle to the pharmacy to request a refill. The technician behind the counter noted the prescription number on a piece of paper, intending to process the refill later on. The patient indicated that he would return later to pick up his refill. Minutes later, the technician pulled up the prescription number and discovered that the prescription had no refills remaining. What should he do?

Step 1: Identify the Problem(s)

- The patient is returning to pick up his refill, although he does not have any remaining.
- The patient will likely be upset that this information was not verified before he left.
- The patient's medication may be delayed, which could present health concerns.

Step 2: Analyze the Problem

- The preceding problems also describe how this issue may affect the patient by interrupting his medication regimen.
- If the medication is a CII-controlled substance or a medication that requires careful monitoring, the patient may have to return to his care provider to be examined before obtaining a new prescription.

Step 3: Identify Decision Criteria

- What may a technician legally do to help remedy this situation? What tasks must be performed by a pharmacist?
  - Depending on the state, a pharmacist may be required to place a phone call to the patient's health care provider to authorize a new prescription.
- What should be communicated to the patient?
- What, if anything, should be communicated to other members of the pharmacy team?

Step 4: Develop Multiple Solutions

- If allowed, call the physician to request new refills via a new prescription number.
- Explain the situation to the pharmacist, and ask if he or she will call the patient's health care provider.
- Call the patient ahead of time to let him know the situation—whether the pharmacist was able to have new refills generated or if the patient must return to his care provider in order to receive a new prescription.

Step 5: Choose the Optimal Decision

- In this situation, any or all of the preceding steps may need to be taken based on the type of medication.
  - The pharmacist may need to call to request refills; if authorized, the patient could simply pick up the medication as expected and experience no actual delays.
  - If the patient needs to return to his care provider, he should be informed of that requirement in a timely manner to avoid further delays in his medication therapy.
  - If the patient cannot be contacted, it may be wise to inform other members of the pharmacy staff of the issue in the event that the patient returns at a time when the technician who had originally assisted him is not available.

Stand by Your Pharmacist!

This may seem like an odd statement, but it is vital to a new pharmacy technician's development of a multidisciplinary mindset. As students learned in Chapter 3, the Code of Ethics for Pharmacy Technicians charges technicians with the ethical obligation to support, assist, and value the role and position of their pharmacist, along with other members of the health care team. Let's review the third and fourth principles of the code:

- A pharmacy technician assists and supports the pharmacists in the safe and efficacious and cost-effective distribution of health services and health care resources.
- A pharmacy technician respects and values the abilities of pharmacists, colleagues, and other health care professionals.

Assisting and supporting the pharmacists means that technicians should perform their job in a way that allows the pharmacists to better serve patients. Personal ego can become a barrier in this area of pharmacy technician practice. It is important to recognize the level of education and specialized training that a pharmacist has. Pharmacists are the medication experts on the health care team and should be regarded as such. A pharmacy technician should always seek to direct patients as well as other members of the health care team to seek out the pharmacist as that expert and should never cast the role of the pharmacist in a light that would undervalue or discredit the position. As mentioned earlier in this chapter, no matter how many times a technician may have heard a pharmacist explain a clinical process or dispense a clinical judgment to a patient, a pharmacy technician does not possess the knowledge base or the legal right to perform such a task. Every member of the health care team is valuable and needed, and each member must know his or her role, legal responsibilities, and scope of practice.

GETTING TO KNOW YOUR PHARMACIST

Pharmacy technicians should always seek opportunities to build positive working relationships with the pharmacists they have been charged to support and assist. Pharmacists are, of course, human beings with different personalities, varying degrees of management experience, and varying viewpoints concerning the value and role of pharmacy technicians in practice. Although no person should be subject to behavior that would be considered inappropriate or illegal, pharmacy technicians should always seek to provide support and service to their pharmacist in whatever capacity is required of them. Whenever faced with threatening, inappropriate, or unlawful behavior, a pharmacy technician may communicate concerns to other leaders in the organization or convey them through a fraud, waste, and abuse hotline that may allow anonymous reporting of inappropriate or unlawful behavior.

EVOLVING PERCEPTIONS OF TECHNICIANS

The relationship between pharmacists and technicians may at first seem a bit adversarial. Many pharmacy technicians are initially intimidated by the thought of approaching their pharmacists for questions—particularly when the work environment is fast-paced and very busy. There was a time when many pharmacists viewed technician staff as cashiers or support personnel who functioned independently of their roles as pharmacists. The structure, workload, rigor, and increasing pharmacist roles across the profession have prompted a real shift in the perception of pharmacy technician practice.

Pharmacists today generally recognize how critical the technician is to their ability to perform their jobs, as well as to the overall success of any pharmacy organization. There are two primary levels of support that a pharmacy staff provides: clinical and administrative. Pharmacists fulfill the clinical support roles and thoughtfully engage the aspects of medication therapy management for each patient they serve. Pharmacy technicians fulfill the administrative support roles by performing order entry, preparing the medication, and engaging patient care through thoughtful and attentive customer service. No pharmacy could function without both the clinical and administrative aspects of pharmacy practice, and each skill set is dependent on the other.

COLLABORATION IS KEY

Collaborative spirit must exist between pharmacists and technicians—one that transcends age, background, educational level, or experience. Pharmacists greatly value and trust technicians that are knowledgeable, skilled, and seek opportunities to assist them and anticipate their needs. In turn, many pharmacists will avail more opportunities for career advancement to high-performing technicians, allow them more technical or leadership responsibilities, and afford them more independence to perform their jobs. There are many advantages to forging positive working relationships with pharmacists, particularly those who advocate for the technician practice and seek opportunities to advance the careers of the technician staff members who have proven themselves.

Final Thoughts: Formulating a Personal Mission Statement

As has been a theme throughout this text, every student is empowered with choices when deciding whether to pursue a career in pharmacy—in light of the knowledge and hands-on skills that the student will have gained at the conclusion of a training program. Part of the decision-making process should be the formation of a personal and professional mission statement. Many organizations use mission statements to publicly articulate their values, goals, and intended contribution to their internal and external customer base (as any highly effective organization must be as committed to serving its employees as it is to serving its external customers). Mission statements are designed to provide direction and thrust to an organization, an enduring statement of purpose. It is valuable for pharmacy technicians to formulate a personal mission statements concerning the direction they wish to take their career and the value that they bring to a health care team and pharmacy organization. The statement could be posted on a résumé, so that potential employers will know the applicant's goals, values, and intended contributions. A personal mission statement also allows job seekers to identify companies that have similar values and beliefs and helps them better assess the costs and benefits of any new career opportunity.

The noted author, public speaker, and educator Dr. Randall S. Hansen articulated a five-step plan for formulating personal mission statements:

Step 1: Identify Past Successes. Spend some time identifying four or five examples where you have had personal success in recent years. These successes could be at work, in your community, at home, etc. Write them down.

Try to identify whether there is a common theme—or themes—to these examples. Write them down.

Step 2: Identify Core Values. Develop a list of attributes that you believe identify who you are and what your priorities are. The list can be as long as you need.

Once your list is complete, see if you can narrow your values to five or six most important values.

Finally, see if you can choose the one value that is most important to you.

Step 3: Identify Contributions. Make a list of the ways you could make a difference. In an ideal situation, how could you contribute best to:

the world in general

your family

your employer or future employers

your friends

your community

Step 4: Identify Goals. Spend some time thinking about your priorities in life and the goals you have for yourself.

Make a list of your personal goals, perhaps in the short-term (up to three years) and the long-term (beyond three years).

Step 5: Write Mission Statement. Based on the first four steps and a better understanding of yourself, begin writing your personal mission statement.

Randall S. Hansen, 2011

A sample mission statement for a pharmacy technician might be something like this:

To learn, grow, and contribute to the profession of pharmacy in a manner that will allow me to serve patients with compassion, perform my tasks to the best of my ability and with the right attitude, and uphold the ideals and values of my local, national, and global health care team—using a combination of knowledge, skills, and information technology.

Once a personal/professional mission statement has been constructed, it may be evaluated periodically and modified as one's personal and career goals shift and evolve over time.

Chapter Summary

- Success in a team-driven environment is often measured by one's contribution to the collective goals of the team, which in this case is the delivery of exemplary patient care.
- Pharmacy technicians must begin to view their role as a part of something greater than themselves in order to take on the shared values and responsibilities of the health care team.
- Pharmacy technicians must develop a multidisciplinary mindset, in which they recognize how their work habits and contributions affect other members of the team and their ability to serve patients.
- One who productively contributes to a team demonstrates several key qualities of professionalism and team building, often referred to as soft skills.
- Effective pharmacy technicians then take those qualities and apply them to workplace situations and their interactions with others on the internal pharmacy team.

- Functioning as part of the pharmacy team requires building and sustaining healthy and productive professional relationships with fellow pharmacy technicians and staff pharmacists. Technicians should also identify and avoid any workplace behaviors that would detract from the effectiveness of the pharmacy team.
- Pharmacy team members must individually and collectively contribute to pharmacy workflow—which involves people, processes, and technology in today's pharmacy setting. Workflow entails a series or sequence of tasks that must be performed in a particular order or following an established process in order for tasks to be completed in an efficient manner. Pharmacy technicians must be *accountable* to their job tasks, recognizing how the sequence of their tasks impacts the job tasks of others on the pharmacy team.
- Pharmacy workflow is inevitably slowed or diverted by a variety of problems involving patients, technology, other members of the health care team, and even co-workers. Every pharmacy technician must be equipped with problem-solving skills to address each problem directly and seek the most appropriate resolution in as timely a manner as possible. One may employ the stated problem-solving steps:
  - Identify the problem.
  - Analyze the problem.
  - Identify decision criteria.
  - Develop multiple solutions.
  - Choose the optimal solution.
- A pharmacy technician must acknowledge and respect the education, role, and leadership position of the pharmacist. The Pharmacy Technician Code of Ethics establishes this as an ethical responsibility, and the success of the pharmacy team depends on every technician's ability to establish a positive rapport with the staff pharmacists. There are many advantages to building successful working relationships with pharmacists in terms of job satisfaction, harmony in the workplace, and opportunities for career advancement. So once again, stand by your pharmacist—both you and the pharmacist will be glad you did!
- The pharmacy technician's understanding of and commitment to professionalism and team building—and how those behaviors translate to the delivery of patient care—may be embodied in one's personal mission statement.

REVIEW QUESTIONS

Multiple Choice

1. Workflow may be defined as:
   a. Working jointly with others to achieve a goal
   b. A sequence of tasks to be performed in a particular order
   c. Behaviors that reflect one's ability to interact with others
   d. Behaviors that allow individuals to make the best use of their time

2. The following would *not* be a description of professional attire:
   a. Comfortable sandals
   b. Pressed khaki slacks
   c. Blouse with conservative neckline
   d. Buttoned shirt without a tie

3. The ability to apply practicality to a situation would refer to the use of which soft skill?
   a. Initiative
   b. Common sense
   c. Integrity
   d. Optimism

4. Taking action without prompting describes:
   a. Initiative
   b. Time management
   c. Accountability
   d. Empathy

5. Utilizing a step-by-step approach when taking action is to use _____ skills
   a. Common sense
   b. Sense of humor
   c. Critical thinking
   d. Empathy

6. This soft skill is often subjective and should only be used when appropriate in the workplace:
   a. Manners
   b. Empathy
   c. Sense of humor
   d. Problem solving

7. Adherence to a code, given opposing viewpoints demonstrates:
   a. Motivation
   b. Common sense
   c. Time management
   d. Integrity

8. Behaviors that allow people to make best use of their time are_____ skills.
   a. Accountability
   b. Time management
   c. Problem solving
   d. Effective communication

9. This soft skill requires the use of active listening:
   a. Empathy
   b. Effective communication
   c. Critical thinking
   d. Common sense

10. This soft skill allows a person to focus on the most desirable aspects of a situation:
    a. Empathy
    b. Common sense
    c. Effective communication
    d. Optimism

TECHNICIAN'S CORNER

1. Give an example of how one might demonstrate time management in the pharmacy environment.
2. Explain the expression, "Find your place in your organization."
3. Write a personal/professional mission statement to share with your instructor.

Bibliography

Hammer, D. (2006). *Improving Student Professionalism During Experiential Learning, American Journal of Pharmaceutical Education*, 70(3):59.

Kuali Foundation. (2010). *Glossary.* Retrieved 3/14/2011, from oleproject.org/overview/ole-reference-model/data-dictionary

Managing Enterprise Content Glossary. (n.d.). Retrieved 3/14/2011, from www.managingenterprisecontent.com/myweb/Glossary.htm

Pedro, O. (2006). *The Five Step Problem Solving Approach.* Retrieved 3/15/2011, from http://e-articles.info/e/a/title/The-Five-Step-Problem-Solving-Approach

Procullux Media Limited. (2010). *Loosely Coupled.* Retrieved 3/14/2011, from http://www.looselycoupled.com/glossary/workflow

Randall, S., Hansen, P. (2011). *The Five-Step Plan for Creating Personal Mission Statements.* Retrieved 3/18/2011, from Quintessential Careers: Your Job Search Starts Here: http://www.quintcareers.com/creating_personal_mission_statements.html

WordNet Search 3.0. (2011). *WordNet Search 3.0.* Retrieved 3/14/2011, from http://wordnetweb.princeton.edu/perl/webwn?s=workflow

8

Pharmacology: The Study of Drugs and Their Effects

LEARNING OBJECTIVES

By the end of this chapter, students will be able to competently:

1. Explain the five primary rationales for medication therapy and the ways pharmacy technicians use this information to provide patient care.

2. Differentiate between pharmacognosy and biopharmaceuticals with regard to the pharmaceutical products currently available.

3. Identify and describe the four phases of the pharmacokinetic drug cycle.

4. List the basic pharmacodynamics of drugs that affect each of the 10 major body systems.

5. Give examples of circumstances in which a drug may become toxic, either as the result of the absorption, distribution, metabolism, and elimination (ADME) process or because of a reaction caused by concomitant administration of another drug.

6. Give examples of key risk factors in pharmacotherapy that may lead to medication fill errors and list the steps pharmacy technicians can take to prevent such errors.

KEY TERMS

Absorption: The process by which drug molecules move from the site of administration into the circulatory system.

Bioavailability: The extent to which a drug reaches the site of action and is available to produce its effects.

Biotransformation: The chemical alteration of a substance (e.g., a drug) in the body, such as by the actions of enzymes.

Distribution: The process of movement of a drug from the circulatory system across barrier membranes to the site of action.

Dosing schedule: The established intervals between drug dosages that maintain a drug concentration in the circulatory system at a desired level.

Drug: A substance used to diagnose, treat, cure, prevent, or mitigate disease in humans or other animals.

Drug delivery system: The dosage form or device designed to release a specific amount of drug.

Duration of action: The time between the onset of a drug's action and its discontinuation.

Efficacy: The measurement of the effectiveness of a drug in a specified dosage range.

Enteral: A drug dosage form meaning any oral route of administration.

Homeopathic medicine: A system of healthcare in which drugs are administered in small quantities to stimulate the body's natural healing processes.

Hydrophilic: Having a strong affinity for water.

Hydrophobic: Lacking an affinity for water.

Legend drug: A drug that can be dispensed only with a valid prescription, as required by federal law.

Metabolism: The biochemical process by which active drugs are transformed into a compound that can be easily eliminated.

Metabolite: A product of drug metabolism; it may be an inactivated drug or a drug with an activity level equal to or greater than that of the parent drug.

Onset of action: The time required for a drug to reach the concentration necessary to produce a therapeutic effect.

Parenteral: A drug dosage form administered by injection or infusion.

Pathophysiology: The study of structural and functional changes produced by disease.

Pharmacognosy: The study of the biologic and biochemical features of natural drugs and their constituents (i.e., drugs of plant and animal origin and their chemical and physical properties, toxicology, and therapeutics).

Pharmacokinetics: The dynamic process that drugs undergo to produce their therapeutic effects.

Pharmacology: The study of the use of drugs in the treatment of disease.

Physiology: The study of the human body and the functions of each of its systems.

Toxicology: In pharmacology, the study of a drug's adverse effects on the body.

This chapter explores the key principles and concepts of pharmacology. Pharmacology is the study of drugs—their origin, composition, pharmacokinetics, therapeutic use, and toxicology (Merriam-Webster, 2010). It is the study of drugs' effects on the human body, and the body's effect on drugs and the ways they are used.

This chapter answers the following questions:
- What is a drug?
- From where or what materials are drugs derived?
- What is medication therapy?
- How are drugs used by the body?
- How do drugs affect the body?
- What makes a drug toxic?

The answers to these questions are important to the pharmacy technician, because a working knowledge of the clinical basis of medication therapy improves the technician's ability to help the pharmacist safely and effectively provide pharmaceutical care to patients. A pharmacy technician who understands the function of a medication, its effects on the body, and the reason it is prescribed may be more likely to recognize a situation in which a medication should *not* be given and why. Such knowledge is useful when:
- Gathering healthcare information from a patient
- Selecting a product from stock from among a variety of drug formulations
- Preventing look-alike and sound-alike entry errors in medication orders
- Catching a prescribing error
- Performing the steps in filling a medication order (e.g., applying the appropriate auxiliary or warning labels)
- Directing patients to a pharmacist for consultation about their medications, when warranted

As each of these topics is covered, the relevance or application to pharmacy technician practice is briefly discussed. Pharmacy technicians should continually learn more about drugs. This enables them to use that information to streamline their work and anticipate the pharmacist's needs. It also fosters a greater sense of appreciation for the clinical contributions of the pharmacy technician to the healthcare process.

Origin of Drugs

Pharmacognosy is the study of the natural origin of drugs and of the constituents of natural drugs that are responsible for their effects. Thousands of substances in our environment may be considered drugs. In general, drugs are derived from natural or synthetic sources. Nearly 80% of the drugs currently available, both prescription and nonprescription, may have been derived from natural sources, such as plants, microorangisms, and animal sources. If drugs do not come from a natural source, they are synthetically compounded and referred to as biopharmaceuticals.

How Drugs Affect the Human Body

MEDICATION THERAPY

Medication therapy is the process by which natural or biopharmaceutical products are administered to diagnose, treat, cure, prevent, or mitigate disease; these are the five primary rationales for medication therapy. With some drugs, therapy must be administered and monitored by a team of healthcare providers; with others, the drug may be safe enough for self-administration by a patient. Prescribers now rely on the expertise of other providers to help determine the best course of therapy for a patient. A body of clinical information about the patient now is collected from a variety of sources:

- The patient's medical history is generally documented by the primary or specialty healthcare providers (or both).
- If laboratory tests are required, laboratory technologists and pathologists also collect information based on the results of the tests. If the patient requires x-ray imaging, radiology technologists and radiologists collect imaging data.
- Pharmacy technicians and pharmacists collect information on the patient's use of medications, past and present.

Medication therapy is best managed when this comprehensive body of clinical data is shared among the members of the multidisciplinary team treating the patient.

Once the treatment options have been identified, a variety of patient-specific factors must be taken into consideration, such as:

- Gender
- Age
- Weight
- Current and past history of disease
- Immune responses
- Kidney and liver function
- Allergies
- Physical or psychological limitations

These and other factors must be considered in determining the most appropriate course of medication therapy. The amount of one or more drugs that may be safely administered is determined, and a prescription or medication order is written that specifies the following five elements for each drug:

- Product name
- Strength in units
- Quantity to be administered in each dose
- Route of administration
- Duration of therapy

Once patients have begun medication therapy, it is important that they check in with their healthcare providers regularly so that the patient's health status and the effects of the prescribed medication can be monitored. In fact, many insurance companies will approve certain medications only as long as the patient maintains contact with the prescriber (see Chapter 12). Some medication orders cannot be refilled until the medication benefit provider has documentation that the patient has undergone diagnostic procedures confirming the safety and effectiveness of the treatment.

How the Human Body Processes and Uses Medication

In general, the medication therapy process may be categorized into three primary phases.

- *Phase 1:* This phase encompasses the medical office or hospital visit, when the medication therapy first is prescribed. The prescriber must determine the most appropriate medication dosage form, based on the patient-specific variables. It is important that patients be given a drug dosage form and dosing regimen that make it more likely they will take the medication exactly as prescribed. The dosage form should ensure ease of drug delivery; the frequency of dosing is determined by the drug's effect in the body. Often medication must be taken at intervals to maintain the appropriate amount of drug in the circulatory system and thus achieve therapeutic results. Dosing frequency should also be considered in terms of the patient's ability to administer doses consistently at the prescribed interval and dose.

- *Phase 2:* A period of time is required for a drug to travel from the site of administration (i.e., a drug is applied to the skin, given orally, or injected) to the site of action. A drug can be absorbed only in a liquid state, so drugs in solid or semisolid form must undergo phase 2 (the pharmaceutical phase), which involves disintegration (breakdown) and dissolution (liquefaction) of the drug so that it can be absorbed by the body. The drug must reach certain concentrations at the site of action to provide a therapeutic effect. The time required for a drug to reach the concentration necessary to achieve a therapeutic effect is called the onset of action. Once the maximum drug concentration has been reached in the patient's bloodstream, the drug achieves its peak effect. The duration of action is the total amount of time the drug provides a therapeutic effect, from the onset of action until the therapeutic effect stops and the drug is eliminated from the body.

- *Phase 3:* This phase, which follows a drug's onset of action, is marked by a four-step process: absorption, distribution, metabolism, and elimination (also called the *ADME process*). Pharmacokinetics is the study of the time course of this process. The ADME process is important, because a major goal of medication therapy is to provide a drug's maximum therapeutic effect while minimizing the risk of toxicity and the severity of side effects.

Pharmacokinetics

ABSORPTION

Absorption is the first step of the pharmacokinetic process. As mentioned, drugs must be in liquid form to be carried to the site of action and absorbed by the body. A drug's route of administration determines the rate and site of absorption. In the pharmaceutical phase, a solid drug must undergo complete dissolution before it can be absorbed into the vascular lining of the stomach or moved into the intestines.

Absorption is the movement of drug molecules across the skin and across or through cell membranes into the body's circulatory system (i.e., blood vessels). Plasma cells are composed primarily of lipids, proteins, and water-filled channels. Drug molecules may pass through the membrane of these cells, if they are lipid-soluble, or through one of the water-filled protein channels; this is called drug transport. The two forms of drug transport into cell membranes are active transport and passive transport.

Passive Transport

Matter tends to flow naturally from an area of higher concentration into an area of lower concentration to create a balance, or *homeostasis*. This is also the principle of passive transport. Initially no drug is present in the plasma cell; however, if the drug has solubility with the cell, molecules of the drug may pass through the plasma membrane into the red blood cell. Because the cell membrane is composed primarily of lipid compounds, lipid-soluble drugs may pass naturally through the membrane into the plasma cell. Drugs that are water-soluble may pass through the cell membrane by means of the water-filled protein channels. Drugs that are lipid-soluble and un-ionized (uncharged) have the highest rate of passive transport.

Active Transport

Active transport allows a drug to be transported across the plasma cell membrane regardless of the drug concentration. Special "carrier proteins" or pumps use the internal and external cell charges to generate energy that transports the drug molecule across the cell membrane.

Factors That May Influence Drug Absorption

The following factors can affect the absorption of a drug.

- *Drug pH:* pH is an expression of the acidity or alkalinity of a compound. The range indicating acidity is 1 to 6.99. A pH of 7 is considered neutral, and a pH value greater than 7.01 and less than 14 indicates alkalinity (base). Most drugs are either weak acids or weak bases. When a weakly acidic or weakly basic drug is dissolved in an aqueous solution, it dissociates (releases positively or negatively charged atoms) and becomes ionized. The more ionized a solution, the more difficult it is for the drug to diffuse across a plasma cell membrane. Weakly acidic drugs become less ionized in acidic solutions, and weakly basic drugs become less ionized in basic solutions. This explains the ability of acidic solutions to cross the membranes in the stomach, where the acidic concentration is high because of the presence of hydrochloric acid. Absorption of the same drug is reduced once the drug reaches the intestines, which have a less acidic environment.

- *Blood flow:* The greater the blood flow, the greater the availability of plasma cells for drug absorption.
- *Drug concentration at the site of absorption:* The longer a drug is present for absorption, the greater the absorption. Drugs that are not intended for absorption in the stomach are coated to delay disintegration and dissolution until the drug has been transported into the intestines.
- *Tissue thickness:* The greater the distance a drug must travel to cross the plasma cell membrane, the lower the absorption. The rate of absorption is slower in a variety of tissues, such as the muscles in the extremities, than at other sites.

DISTRIBUTION

Distribution is the second step of the pharmacokinetic process. Distribution is the movement of a drug from one location in the body to the site of action. The molecular structure and properties of various drugs determine where they are distributed and used. Lipid-soluble, un-ionized drugs are most likely to be absorbed into plasma and transported rapidly to the site of action. Some drugs have a special attraction to (or *affinity* for) certain types of cells, which are better able to retain the drug for metabolism. Drugs continue in their distribution to the absorbing cells until homeostasis has been achieved between the amount of absorbed drug in the plasma cells and the amount of drug outside the cell, which is affected by the constant elimination of the drug after metabolism.

Most drugs are lipid-soluble and best absorbed and distributed when they are non-ionized and small enough to pass through the capillaries of the body's natural barriers. For example, the capillaries to the brain, placenta, and testicles are extremely small; therefore, only drugs with a small enough molecular size that are un-ionized and highly fat-soluble may pass through the capillary plasma cell walls into these anatomic structures for distribution to the site of action.

The clinical significance of the blood-placenta barrier is to protect the fetus. Because a variety of drugs can cross the blood-placenta barrier, studies have been done to determine the safety of drugs for use during pregnancy. The findings have resulted in a categorization system:

- *Category A* drugs have been tested and have proved to be safe for administration.
- *Category B* drugs have been tested in the laboratory, but their safety in humans has not been fully validated.
- *Category C* drugs have not undergone clinical trials, or no data are available on their use in humans during pregnancy; therefore, the therapeutic benefits must be carefully weighed against the possible risks.
- *Category X* drugs that have been clinically proven to cause birth defects, and *must not* be used during pregnancy

Distribution may be significantly affected by blood flow; areas of the body where blood flow is generally higher show greater distribution. The areas of greatest blood flow tend to be organs with smooth muscle and structures controlled by the "fight or flight" system, which is designed to sustain structures that keep the body alive:

- Heart
- Lungs
- Liver
- Kidneys

Areas of varying blood flow or a naturally lower rate of absorption and distribution to the site of action include:

- Skeletal (striated) muscle
- Skin
- Bone
- Fatty tissues

Plasma Binding

Many drugs have a natural affinity for blood plasma proteins and bind to those proteins for a time. The greater the concentration of protein-binding drug in the bloodstream, the fewer the number of unbound free drug molecules for distribution. As the free molecules are distributed and the overall drug concentration decreases, more protein-bound molecules are released and subsequently distributed. In this way, blood plasma acts as a reservoir for certain types of drugs and maintains the overall blood concentration of these drugs for a prolonged period.

The following are some examples of the clinical significance of plasma binding.

- Drugs that may be toxic at therapeutic levels may be retained longer. For example, renal disorders, in which fluids are retained rather than eliminated properly, pose a risk of drug toxicity because of a prolonged and accumulating drug concentration in blood plasma.
- Multiple drugs with an affinity for plasma proteins may compete for plasma binding, affecting the availability of each other's free unbound molecules. This could result either in lowering of the therapeutic concentration needed from a particular drug or in increased unbinding and release of one of the drugs, causing an unsafe and potentially toxic blood serum concentration as the drug is rapidly distributed.

Drugs that are lipid-soluble are generally hydrophobic and tend to concentrate in fatty tissues for absorption and distribution. Therefore, patient-specific factors such as obesity may affect the storage of lipid-soluble drugs. Water-soluble drugs tend to stay in the blood and the aqueous fluid that surrounds cells (extracellular fluid), where they are absorbed and used. Such drugs tend to be distributed to "water compartments" of the body.

Still other drugs have a very narrow range of cells for which they have an affinity, and these drugs generally remain free and unbound for rapid distribution directly to their intended location. For example, iodine concentrates primarily in the thyroid gland; therefore, molecules of iodine in the bloodstream are carried directly to the thyroid without a great degree of plasma protein binding.

METABOLISM

Metabolism is the third step of the pharmacokinetic process. After drugs have been absorbed at their site of action in a concentration necessary for the onset of action, they must be broken down for storage, use, or elimination. The process by which a drug is broken down into a form that is either more or less active than the drug alone is known as metabolism, or biotransformation. Although metabolism usually takes place in the liver, it also may occur in the intestines, lungs, kidneys, or other cellular structures. This process is assisted by enzymes. The drug, known as a substrate when subject to the action of enzymes, is broken down into either an active or an inactive metabolite.

Enzymes are special protein compounds produced by the body (they are also naturally occurring in other sources). Enzymes act as catalyzers that speed up the chemical reactions that sustain life. The body has more than 1,000 types of enzymes, which act upon specific substrates (Table 8-1). Enzymes catalyze chemical reactions that serve the following body functions:

- Breakdown (digestion) of nutrients or drugs for elimination
- Production of energy
- Production of hormones and other human secretions
- Destruction of foreign substances

In drug metabolism, enzymes break down drugs into metabolites that are used and then eliminated by the kidneys. Often *microsomal enzymes* produced in the liver are responsible for

TABLE 8-1   **Enzymes and Their Corresponding Substrates**

Enzyme	Substrate	Site of Production
Protease	Proteins	Pancreas
Lipase	Lipids	Pancreas
Rennin or pepsin	Proteins (proteolytic)	Stomach
Trypsin or chymotrypsin	Proteins (proteolytic)	Pancreas
Amylase	Carbohydrates	Salivary glands, pancreas, lining of small intestine

transforming lipophilic (lipid loving) drugs into compounds that may be more easily eliminated by the kidneys. A particular enzyme system, cytochrome P-450 (or CYP450), is an example of a microsomal enzyme.

Factors That Influence Enzyme Metabolism

The action of enzymes on their drug substrates may create complications in medication therapy when certain enzyme groups act on multiple drugs taken concurrently. Some drugs may induce increased enzyme metabolism of other types of drugs, whereas other drugs may decrease or inhibit the enzyme metabolism of certain drugs. If one drug increases the metabolism of another drug, the second drug may be eliminated too quickly, which diminishes the therapeutic effect of that drug. If a drug inhibits the metabolism of another drug, the second drug may remain active in the bloodstream for a prolonged period. Depending on the drug, either action could be harmful to a patient.

The process of metabolism does not necessarily inactivate every drug. Some drugs may not be metabolized in their original form; the action of the enzyme on its substrate may activate the drug, which may then be metabolized by its designated site of action. Drugs that must be catalyzed from an inactive to an active form are called *prodrugs*. An example of a prodrug is the glaucoma medication dipivefrin. This drug has been formulated to be metabolized in the eye rather than the liver. Another common example is the antiparkinsonian drug levodopa. Levodopa more easily crosses the blood-brain barrier in its inactive form than does its active metabolite, dopamine. The active metabolite is more readily metabolized in the nerve cells of the brain. It is crucial to ensure that prodrugs are not administered concurrently with drugs that inhibit their metabolism, because prodrugs remain inactive until converted into an active form through the process of biotransformation.

First-Pass Effect

Before an orally administered drug can reach the circulatory system for delivery to its site of action, it must be metabolized by the liver. Once a drug has been absorbed, either by the stomach or by the lining of the intestines, it is delivered to the hepatic portal system and carried by the portal vein to the liver. The liver converts many drugs into a nearly inactive metabolite state before recirculation into the bloodstream. This can be a problem if not enough drug is bioavailable to provide a therapeutic effect at the intended site of action. Drugs subject to first-pass inactivation may be formulated for administration to bypass the digestive system and liver entirely, such as by the sublingual or parenteral routes. A common example is the sublingual drug nitroglycerin. Nitroglycerin is 90% cleared during a single pass through the liver. However, a high concentration of blood vessels is present under the tongue; therefore, sublingual administration of nitroglycerin allows the absorbed drug to be delivered directly to the bloodstream and allows opening of the veins, which can decrease the intensity of a cardiac event. Many other drugs are formulated in injectable form to avoid the first-pass effect.

Many of the factors that influence metabolism involve the body's ability to eliminate the drug after it has performed its therapeutic action. In a patient with certain clinical factors, drug metabolism may be compromised, which may result in ineffective drug therapy or impaired elimination of the drug, leading to systemic toxicity. In such cases the healthcare team may need to monitor the patient's serum blood levels frequently to measure the amount of drug being eliminated and thus minimize the risk of toxicity. The following are examples of clinical factors that must be considered during medication therapy.

- *Compromised liver function:* In patients with compromised liver function, drug metabolism is decreased; therefore, drug dosing generally is reduced to minimize the chance of toxicity.
- *Lung and kidney disease:* Lung and kidney diseases reduce the body's ability to metabolize, absorb, and/or eliminate drugs, in terms both of the production of enzymes and of absorption rates.
- *Congestive heart disease:* Decreased blood flow to the liver reduces drug metabolism, partly because of the compromised production of microsomal enzymes.
- *Infants and elderly patients:* Both infants and elderly patients have decreased liver function compared with adult patients. Elderly patients have higher body fat ratios, which may increase the absorption of lipophilic drugs. Infants have underdeveloped metabolizing enzyme systems.

TABLE 8-2   **Some Food and Drug Interactions That Affect Drug Metabolism**

Food	Drug	Interaction
Vitamin K–rich foods (e.g., broccoli, spinach)	Warfarin (blood thinner)	These foods increase warfarin's blood-thinning effect, thereby increasing the risk of life-threatening bleeding.
Tyramine (found in chocolate, avocados, beer, and wine)	Monoamine oxidase inhibitors (MAOIs)	These foods slow metabolism of MAOIs, which can result in a dangerous rise in blood pressure.
Natural licorice	Blood pressure medications and diuretics	Natural licorice reduces the effectiveness of blood pressure medications and diuretics.
Antacids and dairy products	Ciprofloxacin	These foods block the absorption of ciprofloxacin, diminishing its therapeutic effects.

In both of these patient groups, lower doses generally are required to produce therapeutic effects.

- *Genetic defects:* Patients genetically may lack or have a deficiency of a metabolic enzyme, reducing the body's ability to metabolize drugs that are substrates of that enzyme.
- *Nutrition:* Many foods may either induce or inhibit the metabolism of a variety of drugs (Table 8-2), to the extent that these foods must be avoided entirely during medication therapy. A common example of this is grapefruit juice. A growing list of pharmaceutical products are either inhibited or induced by grapefruit juice. It may take up to 4 days for the body to metabolize drugs inhibited by grapefruit juice, and it can take that length of time for the effects of a single glass of grapefruit juice to wear off. It is crucial that patients be informed about the types of foods they must avoid, because this prevents adverse reactions and diminished therapeutic effects of the drugs they take.
- *Gender:* Males may metabolize certain drugs more rapidly than women (e.g., propranolol, a blood pressure medication). Women, on the other hand, metabolize other drugs (e.g., acetaminophen, an analgesic) more rapidly than men. This suggests that gender hormones may influence drug metabolism.

ELIMINATION

Elimination is the fourth and final step of the pharmacokinetic process. Once a drug has been biotransformed into a metabolite, some inactive metabolites may be excreted and others may be reabsorbed into bloodstream and recirculated through the body. In general, the organs that excrete drug metabolites excrete the hydrophilic metabolites rather than the lipophilic metabolites. Nonionized lipophilic drug metabolites are more likely to be reabsorbed across the fatty protein surfaces of blood plasma. Sites of drug excretion include:

- Lungs
- Urine
- Saliva
- Tears
- Perspiration
- Bowel and feces (generally consists of orally ingested metabolized drugs excreted in the bile)
- Breast milk (can result in fetal toxicity because of the fetus's limited enzyme systems)
- Hair

Drug elimination by the kidneys generally is performed by the nephrons. Drugs are transported through the bloodstream to Bowman's capsule, where the blood is filtered by the glomerulus. Much of the water filtered through the kidneys is reabsorbed by the kidneys and recirculated through the body. A drug that does not bind to plasma proteins for reabsorption, along with body water, generally remains in the kidneys for excretion.

Elimination is measured clinically in terms of the *elimination half-life;* that is, the time required for 50% of the drug to be cleared completely from the bloodstream. Eliminating a drug from the body takes about four or five half-lives. A drug's half-life can be as short as a few minutes or as long as several days. Measuring a drug's half-life is important for determining the length of time the drug has a pharmacologic effect on the body.

Clinical Significance of Elimination

As with metabolism, several clinical factors can influence the excretion of drugs. If drug A induces the biotransformation of drug B, the rate of elimination of drug B is increased, diminishing its pharmaceutical effects. Conversely, if drug A inhibits the biotransformation of drug B, drug B may remain in the bloodstream longer, which increases its concentration and potential for toxicity.

Because drugs may be excreted as a result of the activity of bile in the liver and the nephrons in the kidneys, disease that compromises kidney or liver function affects the excretion of drugs. Diseases of the bowel, particularly those that cause severe, chronic diarrhea, may cause more rapid elimination of drugs and thus a diminished therapeutic effect.

Pharmacodynamics

We have seen the way drugs are processed through the human body. Now, let's examine the ways the body responds to drug therapy. Pharmacokinetics is the study of the time course over which drugs are processed by the body; pharmacodynamics, then, is the study of the time over which the body responds to the drugs. Every drug has a method of action, which describes how that drug produces an effect on various body systems.

Recall that the five rationales for medication therapy are diagnosis, treatment, cure, prevention, or mitigation of disease.

*   *Diagnosis:* Drugs may be administered to identify body responses that may indicate disease or malfunctioning of a system.
*   *Treatment:* Drugs may be administered to activate, deactivate, or stimulate normal body processes that are compromised in some way and need the assistance of the drug to function as intended.
*   *Cure:* In the event of a pathogenic invasion, drugs may be used to destroy the pathogens' cell walls to prevent the development of or to cure infection.
*   *Prevention:* To prevent disease, drugs may be administered to elicit an immunologic response that enhances the body's ability to fight off specific organisms that can be life-threatening. Prevention may also include the prevention of pregnancy through the application of chemicals or devices that block conception.
*   *Mitigation:*

Through absorption and distribution, drugs are delivered via the circulatory system to their intended site of action. The site of action is also called the *receptor site.* Drugs and their receptor sites may be compared to a lock and key or to the conjoining pieces of a puzzle. Drugs with an affinity for a particular receptor (i.e., they fit well in a molecular sense) have a greater chance of binding. Cells may have primary or secondary receptor sites that activate to produce the desired drug effect. Drugs may have various effects, based on the action they perform at the receptor site. A drug at a receptor site may act as an agonist or an antagonist.

AGONISTS

Agonist drugs bind to the receptor site and perform their intended action either by activating a receptor that had been in a resting state or by turning off a receptor that had been activated. If more than one agonist drug is administered, the drugs compete for binding with receptors, and the drug or drugs with the greatest affinity for binding successfully bind and produce their intended effect. Drug-receptor binding may stimulate the release of a normal body chemical to produce the drug's effect, or the binding may mimic the effects produced when normal body chemicals bind to their corresponding receptors. For example, the drug-receptor binding of the drug amantadine results in the release of the neurotransmitter dopamine, which in turn reduces the symptoms of Parkinson's disease.

ANTAGONISTS

Antagonist drugs bind to receptor sites to block or prevent another drug or natural body chemical from binding to or activating the receptor site. For example, an antihistamine binds to the body's histamine receptors to block the histamines released by allergens from binding and causing the symptoms associated with allergic reactions. Antagonist drugs may also block the actions of agonist drugs. *Noncompetitive antagonists* bind to alternative sites on the receptor site as agonist drugs, resulting in inactivation of the receptor of the site. *Partial agonists* act as agonists in some conditions and as antagonists under other conditions.

DOSE-RESPONSE RELATIONSHIP

The body's response to a drug is linked to the amount and potency of the dose administered in several ways. This relationship may be considered in terms of the drug's efficacy, potency, ceiling effect, and therapeutic index.

- *Efficacy* is a measurement of the effectiveness of a drug in a specified dosage range. In terms of drug action, agonists typically have the greatest efficacy. The efficacy of an antagonist drug is measured in terms of how effectively the drug interferes with the effect of an agonist (natural or synthetic drug).
- Drug potency is measured by the amount of a drug that must be administered to achieve the intended response. If only a small amount of a drug is required to produce an effect, the drug is considered very potent; conversely, if a large amount of a drug is required, the drug is considered to have low potency.
- The ceiling effect of a drug is measured by the dosage at which the drug does not provide any greater response, regardless of how much more is administered (and continued administration and an increased blood concentration may result in toxicity).
- Many drugs may be toxic at therapeutic doses or near the normal therapeutic dose. The relationship between a drug's therapeutic dose and a lethal dose is referred to as the drug's therapeutic index. Drugs with a wide therapeutic index may allow for greater variance in dosing with minimal risk of overdose or severe side effects; conversely, drugs with a narrow therapeutic index must be administered precisely to minimize the risk of a toxic or lethal dose. The drug lithium, which is used to treat manic depression, can be toxic at near therapeutic levels; therefore, these patients must be monitored by blood tests to ensure normal elimination of the drug by the kidneys to prevent toxicity and overdose.

PATIENT-SPECIFIC FACTORS THAT AFFECT PHARMACODYNAMICS

As mentioned previously, a number of patient-specific factors must be taken into consideration when medication therapy is prescribed. Besides age, gender, and genetics, these factors include:

- Weight
- Disease state
- Pregnancy
- Immune response
- Desensitization
- Idiosyncratic reactions
- Psychological factors
- Adverse reactions

Weight

The patient's weight may be used to calculate the drug dose; an obese patient or a small child may require a significantly higher or lower dose. For some patients whose weight is abnormal, the body surface area (BSA) may be used to determine the dose, as is done with chemotherapeutic drugs.

Disease State

A disease state influences the degree to which a drug takes effect at its site of action. Diseases that alter body system functioning affect a drug's rate of absorption, speed of distribution, rate of metabolism, and degree and speed of elimination.

Pregnancy

Because many drugs can cross the blood-placenta barrier, pregnant women may be limited in the number of medications they may take safely.

Immune Response

A patient may have a hypersensitivity or an allergic reaction to a particular drug or class of drugs, requiring alternate forms of drug therapy. Many drugs may have molecular similarities or methods of action similar to those of a drug to which a patient is allergic. In addition, patients with certain diseases or conditions that diminish the immune response may be limited in the types of drugs they can take. Examples of such patients include those with acquired immunodeficiency syndrome (AIDS) or burns.

Desensitization

As a result of repeated or prolonged therapy, a patient may become desensitized to a particular drug. Desensitization may result in changes to the drug-receptor binding ability or loss of a drug's ability to block other agonist drugs after a prolonged period.

Idiosyncratic Reactions

Idiosyncratic reactions are unexpected adverse drug reactions.

Psychological Factors

Patients' perceptions of a drug's effect often prompt what they report as tangible responses to the drug's activity. These perceptions also may affect patients' compliance and consistency with their medication therapy. Because a patient's perception of the benefit of medication therapy can be subjective, drug studies may be performed to collect data on a patient's response to receiving a medication. In a blind study, patients do not know whether they are taking an active drug or a *placebo* drug (i.e., a drug that contains only inert ingredients, such as sugar). In a double-blind study, neither the patient nor the provider knows whether the patient is taking an active drug or a placebo.

Adverse Reactions

Expected side effects are reported during clinical trials before a drug is approved by the U.S. Food and Drug Administration (FDA). However, after a drug is put on the market, some patients may experience unexpected adverse reactions. Adverse drug reactions (ADRs) account for a significant percentage of healthcare costs from hospital stays, and some result in permanent damage, coma, and even death. Common adverse reactions may include the following:

- *Drowsiness or dizziness:* The body's reaction to the drug produces undesired depression of the central nervous system (CNS).
- *Respiratory depression:* The body's reaction to the drug results in a life-threatening inability to breathe independently.
- *Hepatotoxicity or nephrotoxicity:* These conditions often occur when a drug accumulates in the body, because the body is unable to biotransform or eliminate it or because another drug inhibits its ability to biotransform or bind to a receptor.
- *Teratogenicity:* The drug causes fatal defects in the fetus.
- *Carcinogenicity:* The drug causes mutation of human deoxyribonucleic acid (DNA), causing cells to become cancerous or to form cancerous tissue.
- *Dependence or tolerance:* The drug (usually a narcotic) has abuse potential or carries the risk of chemical dependence.

Adverse drug reactions must always be documented so that the cause of the reaction can be investigated; this helps prevent future ADRs. Figure 8-3 is an example of the Med Watch Form, the FDA's Safety Information and Adverse Event Reporting Program.

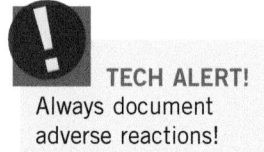

TECH ALERT!
Always document adverse reactions!

Pharmacology and Pathophysiology: the Relationship Between Human Body Systems, Human Disease, and the Drugs Used to Treat Them

Living things seek to achieve and maintain a state of internal balance. Maintaining health involves a balance of diet, exercise, and monitoring of individual-specific risk factors. Disease or any impairment of the body's normal functioning compromises health and wellness. Disease can arise from many sources:

- Genetic predisposition
- Injury
- Physical or psychological trauma
- Poor or destructive lifestyle habits, such as an unhealthy diet, little or no exercise, excessive alcohol consumption, cigarette smoking, illicit drug use, or adverse effects of medication therapy.

Imbalance may occur at every level; molecular components on up to an entire body system may not function normally or may fail to function at all. The extensive medical education of healthcare professionals such as physicians, surgeons, nurses, and pharmacists includes the study of the human body and its functions. Physiology is the study of the human body and the workings of each of its systems; pathophysiology is the study of the diseases and conditions that can affect the body and its systems. With regard to pharmacology, pathophysiology concerns the ways the chemical makeup of various drugs may affect body systems affected by disease or some degree of imbalance.

Recall the five rationales for medication therapy. These rationales are applied to the use of drug therapy in the following ways.

- *Diagnosis:* A drug may help reveal symptoms or signs of disease in the body. For example, radioactive drugs may be injected to delineate how well the heart functions, or an allergy titer can help reveal substances that produce a significant allergic response.
- *Treatment:* A drug may be used to recreate balance by triggering or mimicking the body's own chemical processes, which are impaired or not functioning. For example, a drug may stimulate the release of hormones or provide a synthetic replacement for the body to use to restore balance.
- *Cure:* A drug may be used to target a disease-causing organism that is attacking healthy cells. For example, a drug can be used to treat an upper respiratory infection.
- *Prevention:* A drug may be used to create conditions in the body that help prevent disease. For example, vaccinations help prevent hepatitis B infection and chickenpox.
- *Mitigation:* A drug may be used to help manage the symptoms of a disease that has no known cure. For example, an oral medication can help a patient with chronic obstructive pulmonary disease (COPD) breathe better.

Pharmacy technicians, too, may find ways to apply the principles of pathophysiology to their work. Although pharmacy technicians cannot legally provide information that requires a clinical judgment, they certainly may use a working knowledge of pathophysiology to anticipate the types of drugs that may be used to treat certain conditions. Also, a knowledge of the chemical structure of a drug helps technicians understand how it must be prepared, handled, or stored to maintain its potency, purity, and chemical and physical stability.

The next sections provide general information on each of the 10 systems of the human body. The basic anatomy and physiology of each system and its encompassing parts (e.g., organs and glands) are presented, followed by a brief summary of the types of disease that may occur in each system.

AUTONOMIC AND CENTRAL NERVOUS SYSTEM

The central nervous system (Figure 8-1) acts as the communication center for all the body's systems. It consists primarily of the brain and spinal cord. These components work together to detect any changes in the internal or external environment and then process that information to produce the appropriate response by initiating signals to muscles or glands. Neurons transmit these responses by means of neurotransmitters, which are amino acids divided into the following classes:

- Amino acids
- Monoamines
- Peptides and others

Some neurons release norepinephrine and epinephrine; these are known as *adrenergic neurons.* Adrenergic neurons bind to specialized adrenergic receptors, affecting the activity of smooth muscle.

When norepinephrine binds to alpha-adrenergic receptors in the smooth muscle of blood vessels, it stimulates the muscle, causing the muscle to constrict. When norepinephrine binds to beta-adrenergic receptors in cardiac muscle, its stimulating effect results in a faster and stronger heartbeat.

Cholinergic neurons release acetylcholine and bind to cholinergic receptors.

Peripheral and Autonomic Nervous Systems

The peripheral nervous system (PNS) is made up of 31 pairs of spinal nerves that emerge from the spinal cord and 12 pairs of cranial nerves that emerge from the brain. The PNS has two function divisions: sensory and motor.

The autonomic nervous system (ANS) regulates involuntary actions, such as the heartbeat, smooth muscle contraction, and glandular secretions, to produce and maintain homeostasis. The

TECH NOTE!
A drug's name often provides a clue to its use. For example, the *chol*inergic drug bethane*chol,* or the brand name for the anti*hy*pertensive drug terazosin (i.e., *Hy*trin). Look for name clues, especially in drugs that belong to a particular class. Drugs of the beta-blocker class, for example, commonly end in the suffix *-lol.*

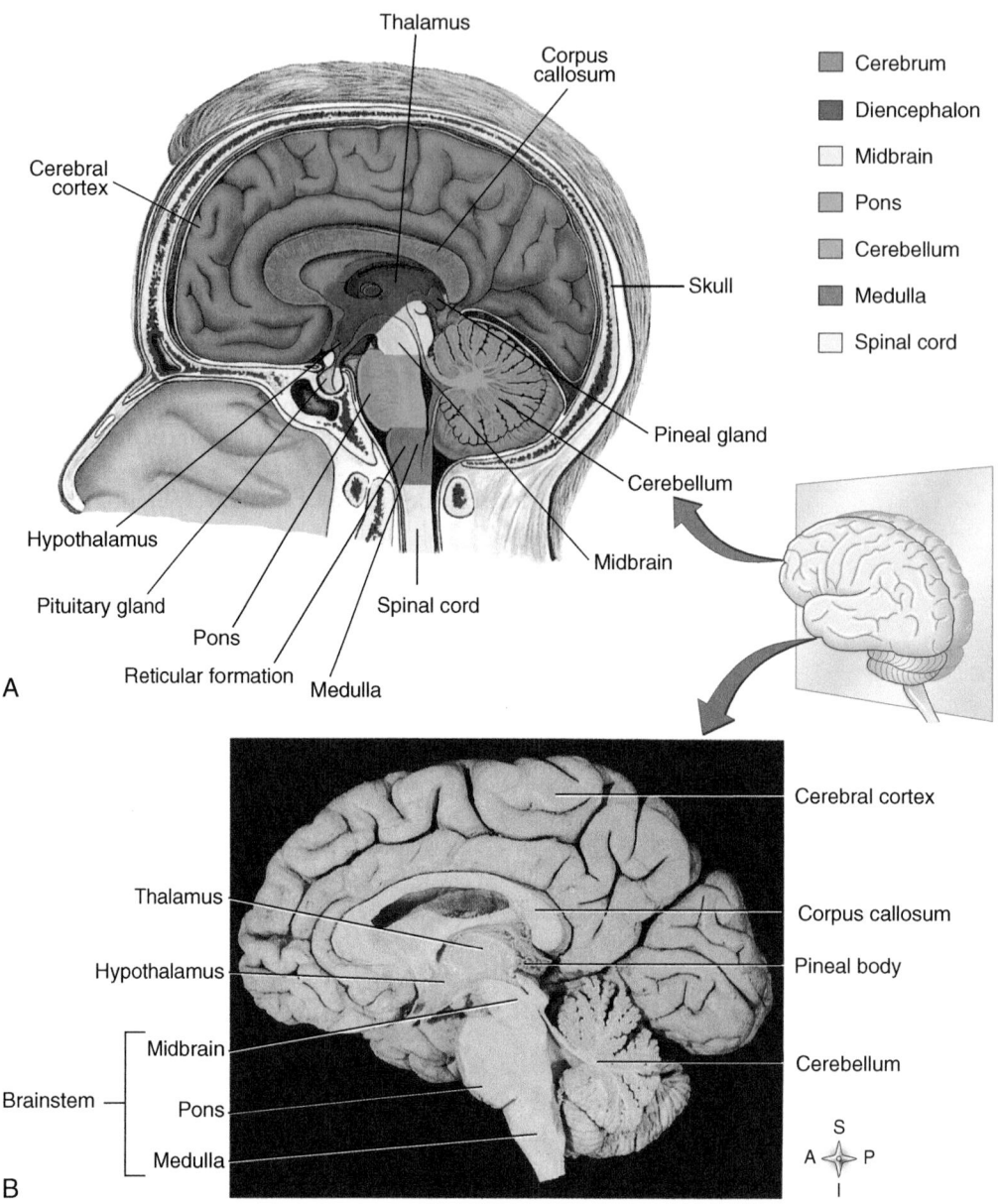

FIGURE 8-1 Major regions of the central nervous system. **A,** Sagittal sections of the brain and spinal cord. **B,** Section of preserved brain. (From Thibodeau G, Patton K: *Structure and function of the body,* ed 13, St Louis, 2008, Mosby.)

ANS is divided into two main divisions, the sympathetic system and the parasympathetic system, which have opposite effects.
- The sympathetic system is the emergency system that creates the "fight or flight" response. When the body experiences physical or psychological stress, outgoing sympathetic signals increase greatly.
- The parasympathetic system is the dominant controller of autonomic systems, particularly during times of "rest and digest."

Technician Connection: How to Use This Information

Several drugs are used to treat depression and anxiety. Recall that drugs that are uncharged and highly lipid-soluble generally are absorbed more quickly, achieve a more rapid onset of action, and are more likely to be reabsorbed (also referred to as *reuptake*) back into the general circulation after the first pass through the kidneys. For this reason, benzodiazepines (e.g., alprazolam and lorazepam) have a faster onset of action and a longer duration of action than do some other classes of antianxiety drugs.

The benzodiazepines are associated with two points of concern:

- The potential for their abuse as a result of long-term CNS depression
- The potential for look-alike/sound-alike medication fill errors

During the fill process, therefore, it is vital that pharmacy staff members be on the lookout for signs of chemical dependence and that they alert the pharmacist immediately if they note such signs. Also, care must be taken when filling prescriptions for these medications to ensure that multiple product identifiers are used to prevent a fill error. Such identifiers include comparing the bottle label to the prescription hard copy and ensuring that the product National Drug Code (NDC) numbers match.

The selective serotonin reuptake inhibitors (SSRIs) do not have the same mechanism of action as the benzodiazepines. The SSRIs interfere with the reuptake of serotonin produced by the body; over time, this produces the therapeutic action in the treatment of anxiety and obsessive-compulsive behavior. In fact, patients may not realize the maximum therapeutic benefits of these drugs for 1 to 3 weeks. Patients who are just beginning therapy with an SSRI must be informed. In some cases patients who do not see an immediate improvement in their condition assume that the drug is not working and stop taking it. A pharmacy technician who knows the mechanism of action (MOA) of the SSRIs should direct a patient beginning therapy with one of these drugs to speak to the pharmacist about the drug's therapeutic benefits and onset of action.

MUSCULOSKELETAL SYSTEM

The human skeletal system consists of two main divisions: the axial skeleton and the appendicular skeleton (Figure 8-2, *A*).

- The *axial skeleton* consists of the cranium, bones of the face and ear, vertebral columns, ribs, sternum, and hyoid.
- The *appendicular skeleton* consists of the bones of the upper extremities and lower extremities.

The muscular system consists of more than 600 muscles, which are divided into three major categories: smooth muscle, skeletal muscle, and cardiac muscle (Figure 8-2, *B*).

- *Smooth muscle* cells form the walls of the digestive, urinary, and reproductive tracts and the walls of large blood vessels.
- *Skeletal muscle* facilitates the excitability of the muscle tissue to allow for muscle extension and movement.
- *Cardiac muscle* is found only in the heart. The specialized cells of this type of muscle work in unison to rhythmically and continuously provide the pumping action necessary to maintain circulation in the body.

In general, muscles require energy to contract; energy is supplied by the nucleotide adenosine triphosphate (ATP). Glucose and oxygen are required for efficient catabolism within muscle fibers. If glucose and oxygen are not present in the muscle cells, lactic acid is produced, causing pain and stiffness in the joints.

Common Diseases of the Musculoskeletal System and Current Drug Treatment

Skeletal muscle movement occurs when the neurotransmitter acetylcholine (ACh) activates communication between nerve cells and muscle cells. Drugs that reduce the production of ACh, therefore, cause the relaxation of muscles. A variety of drugs used during surgery block the neuromuscular response. These drugs are particularly dangerous because improper product selection, storage, or dosing, can result in permanent injury, respiratory arrest, and death.

Autoimmune diseases also can affect the musculoskeletal system, including:

- Multiple sclerosis
- Myasthenia gravis
- Rheumatoid arthritis
- Lupus

Drugs used to treat these diseases (and also those used to treat pain from muscle strain or injury) act primarily by suppressing inflammation, pain, and the immune system response. Some

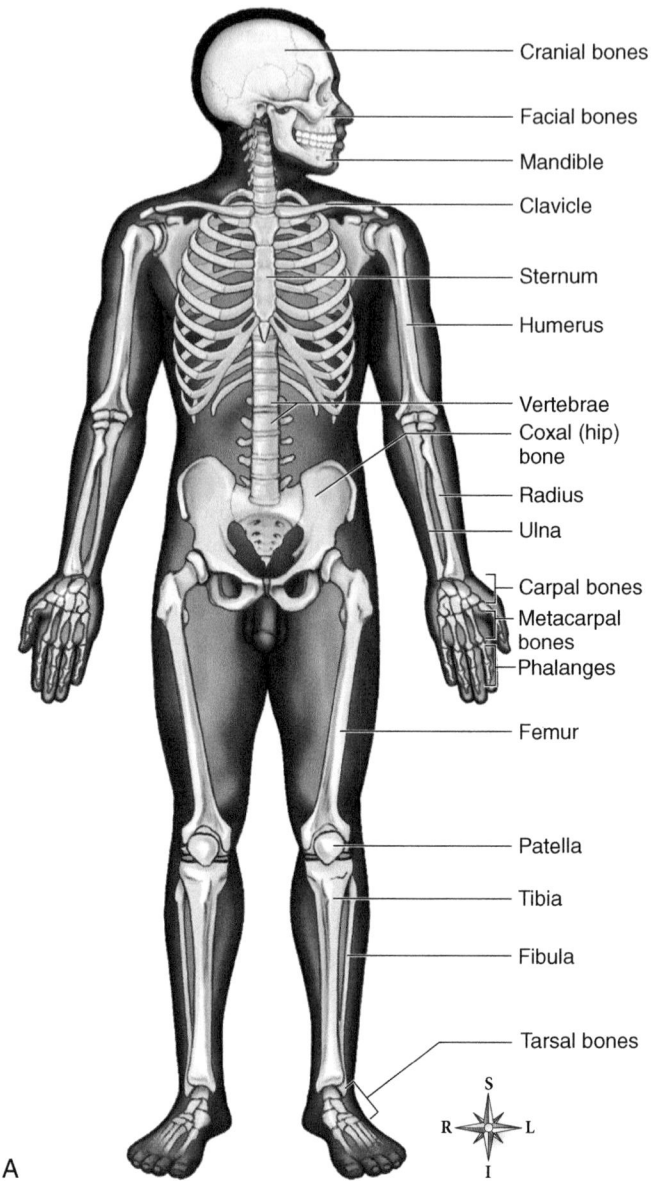

FIGURE 8-2 A, The skeleton. (From Patton K, Thibodeau G: *Anatomy and physiology,* ed 7, St Louis, 2010, Mosby.)

glucocorticoids, such as prednisone and methylprednisolone, are used to treat these and other musculoskeletal conditions involving inflammation. Other drugs used include skeletal muscle relaxants and nonsteroidal antiinflammatory drugs (NSAIDs).

Technician Connection: How to Use This Information

Pharmacy technicians who work in a surgical setting (e.g., a satellite pharmacy in a surgical suite) must exercise great care when gathering neuromuscular blocking drugs for dispensing by the pharmacist. Table 8-3 presents a list of common neuromuscular blocking agents and how each should be handled and stored by pharmacy technicians. Important points in the dispensing of neuromuscular blocking agents include the following:

- Watch out for look-alike/sound-alike drugs in this category!
- Neuromuscular blocking agents should be stored separately from other drugs, whether under refrigerated conditions or in patient care dispensing areas.
- These drugs should be appropriately labeled as paralyzing agents so that patient caregivers are more aware of the dangers and risk involved in their use.

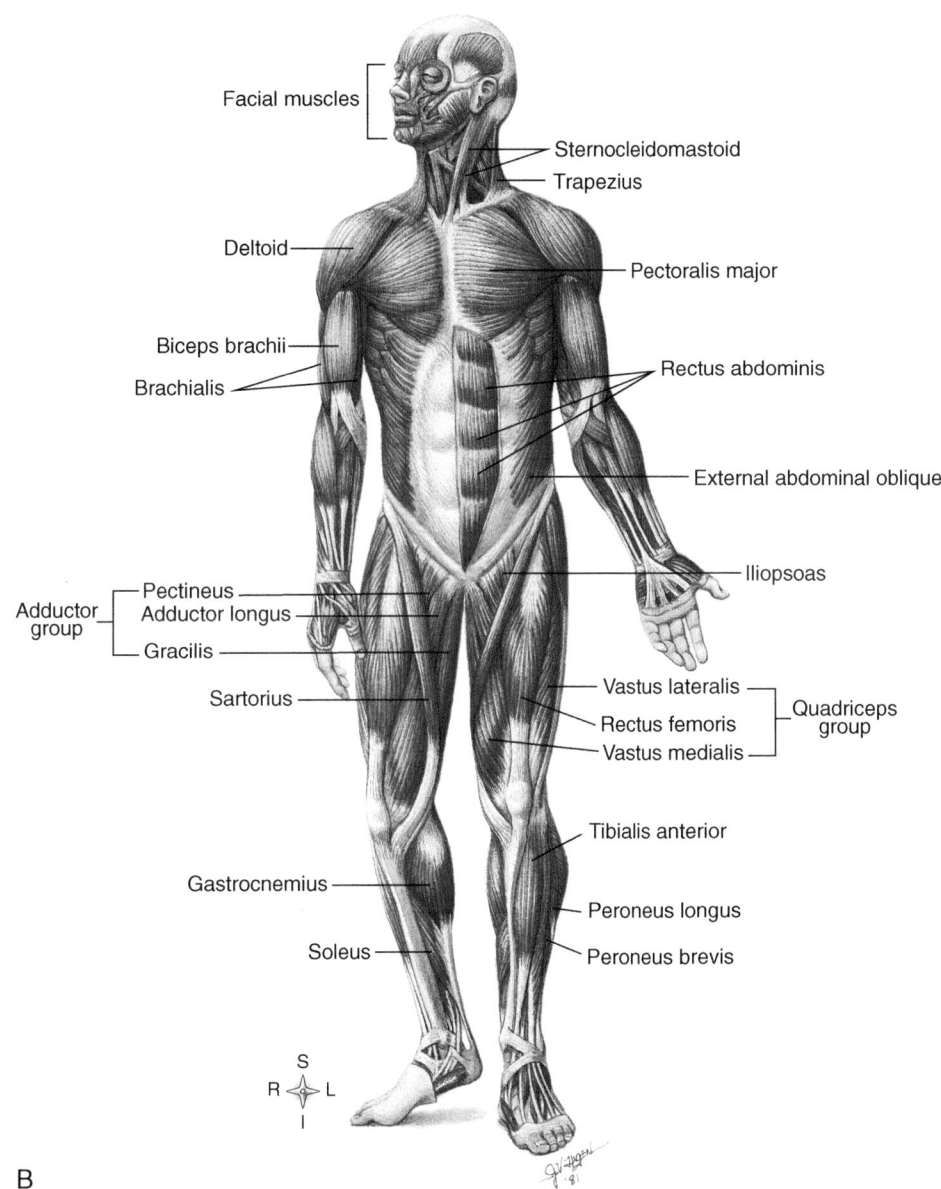

B

FIGURE 8-2, cont'd B, Anterior view of the body's musculature. (From Thibodeau G, Patton K: *Structure and function of the body,* ed 13, St Louis, 2008, Mosby.)

OPHTHALMIC AND OTIC SYSTEMS

Ophthalmic Structure

The human eye (Figure 8-3) has three primary layers.
- Fibrous layer
  - Sclera and cornea
- Vascular layer
  - Choroids, ciliary body, and iris
- Inner layer
  - Retina, optic nerve, and retinal blood vessels

Accessory Structures

- Conjunctiva lines each lid and continues over the surface of the eyeball.
- The lacrimal apparatus secretes tears and drains them from the surface of the eyeball. It consists of the lacrimal glands, lacrimal ducts, lacrimal sacs, and nasolacrimal ducts.

TABLE 8-3   **Neuromuscular Blocking Drugs**

Generic Name	Brand Name	Warning Label/Handling Instructions
Succinylcholine	Quelicin	• Keep refrigerated.
Atracurium	Tracrium	• Keep refrigerated.
Botulinum toxin	Botox	• Keep refrigerated. • After dilution, refrigerated solutions must be used within 4 hours of preparation.
Mivacurium	Mivacron	• Store at room temperature.
Pancuronium	Pavulon	• Keep refrigerated. • Do not store in plastic syringe.
Rocuronium	Zemuron	• Keep refrigerated. • Protect from freezing. • Use within 24 hours of reconstitution.
Vecuronium	Norcuron	• Store unreconstituted at room temperature. • Protect from light. • Reconstitute with bacteriostatic water and use within 5 days. • Reconstitute with other solutions, then refrigerate and use within 24 hours.

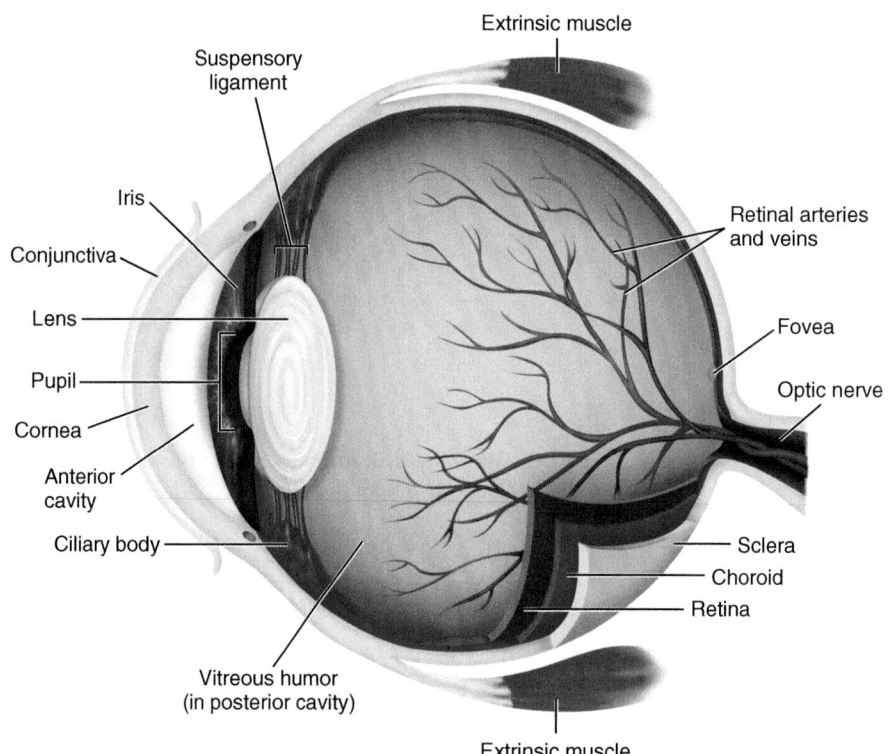

FIGURE 8-3 Structure of the eye. Light passes through the eye to photoreceptor cells in the retina. In this lateral view, the eye is shown partly dissected to show its internal structures. (From Solomon E: *Introduction to human anatomy and physiology,* ed 3, Philadelphia, 2008, Saunders.)

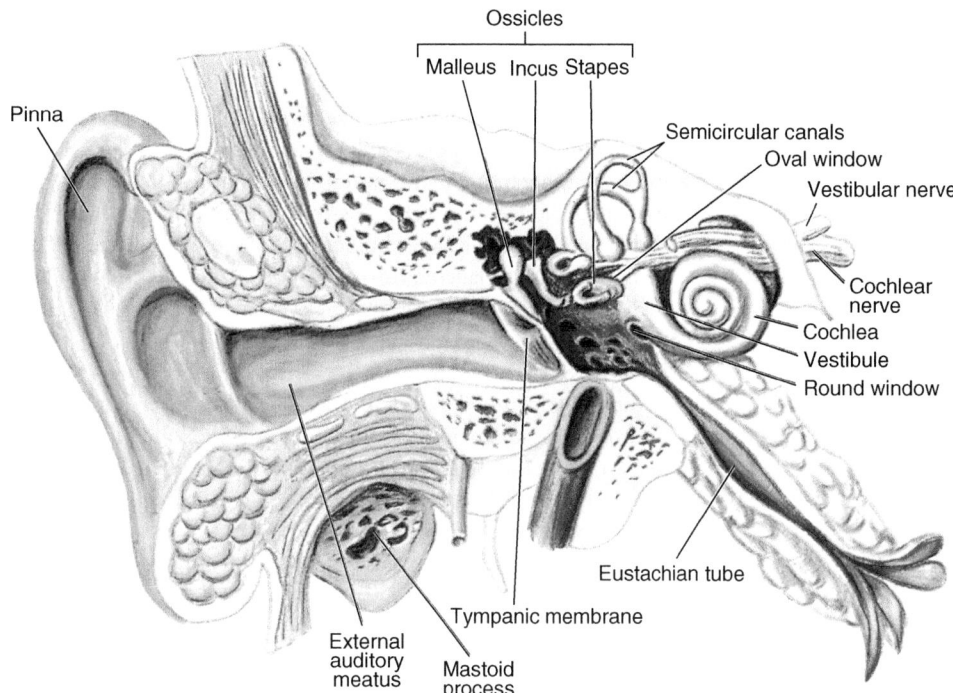

FIGURE 8-4 Structure of the ear. The ear is adapted to direct sound waves from outside the body to receptors in the inner ear. (From Solomon E: *Introduction to human anatomy and physiology,* ed 3, Philadelphia, 2008, Saunders.)

Ear (Otic) System

The ear (Figure 8-4) has three parts that work together to perform the sensory functions of hearing and equilibrium.

- External ear
  - Auricle (pinna)
  - Auditory meatus (ear canal)
    - Extends into the temporal bone, ending at the tympanic membrane
    - Site of cerumen secretion
- Middle ear
  - Three auditory ossicles
    - Malleus (hammer)
    - Incus (anvil)
    - Stapes (stirrup)
  - Eustachian tube, composed of bone, cartilage, and fibrous tissues; extends from the middle ear into the nasopharynx and equalizes pressure between the inner and outer surfaces of the tympanic membrane
- Inner ear—labyrinth consists of:
  - Bony labyrinth
    - Vestibule
    - Cochlea
    - Semicircular canals
  - Membranous labyrinth
    - Utricle
    - Saccule
    - Cochlear duct
      - The organ of Corti contains sensory neurons that extend to form the cochlear nerve, which conducts impulses to the brain and produces the sensation of hearing.
      - Hearing results from the stimulation of the auditory area of the cerebral cortex.

Common Diseases of the Ophthalmic and Otic Systems and Current Drug Treatment

OCULAR DISEASE

Glaucoma is a worldwide disease, with predictions of greater than 60.5 million people suffering from symptoms of the disease. Glaucoma results in excessive intraocular pressure (IOP), which causes degeneration of the optic nerve and eventually may lead to blindness. Several drugs are used to treat elevated IOP. These drugs act on alpha- and beta-adrenergic receptors to reduce the formation of vitreous humor or to promote increased drainage of those fluids. The most commonly used glaucoma drug, now considered the first-line treatment, mimics prostaglandin, relaxing the ciliary muscle of the eye and allowing for drainage of the vitreous humor.

DISEASES AND DISORDERS OF THE INNER EAR

Because the components of the inner ear act to create equilibrium for movement, the primary disorder associated with the otic system involves impaired perception of motion. This condition is known as *vertigo*. Benign paroxysmal positional vertigo (BPPV), and Ménière's disease are the most common causes of vertigo. Meclizine, which also acts on the central nervous system, is used to treat the symptoms of vertigo.

Other conditions may cause inner ear pain, including swimmer's ear and bacterial infections of the inner ear. Otic analgesics and antibiotics may be used to treat these conditions.

Technician Connection: How to Use This Information

Pharmacy technicians can best help patients with glaucoma by teaching them how to prevent contamination of the optic mucosal areas. Technicians should remind patients to wash their hands before instilling eye drops and to make sure the tip of the eye drop dispenser does not touch the hands or the eye. Also, patients who wear contact lenses should be instructed to remove the lenses before instilling eye drops and then wait 15 minutes before reinserting the lenses. Prostaglandin drugs must be stored in the refrigerator.

CARDIOVASCULAR SYSTEM

The cardiovascular system is responsible for transporting food, oxygen, and water to every system of the body through a complex matrix of blood vessels (Figure 8-5). It consists primarily of the heart, blood vessels, and lymphatic system. Blood is composed of plasma (a straw-colored fluid), erythrocytes (red blood cells), leukocytes (white blood cells), and thrombocytes (platelets). About 90% of blood volume is water, and the other 10% consists of dissolved substances that must be circulated through the body. These critical solutes include:

- Proteins—Amino acids, globulin
- Albumin
- Nutrients derived from food sources—Glucose, amino acids, lipids
- By-products of metabolism—Urea, uric acid, creatinine, and lactic acid
- Respiratory gases—Oxygen and carbon dioxide
- Regulatory substances—Hormones and enzymes

Whole blood constitutes about 8% of total body weight. Blood volume is 4 to 5 liters for women and 5 to 6 liters for men.

Heart

The human heart consists of four chambers encased in an outer sac known as the *pericardium*. The heart wall consists of three layers:

- Epicardium
- Myocardium
- Endocardium

The four chambers of the interior of the heart are:

- Atria: Two upper chambers, which receive blood from the veins
- Ventricles: Two lower chambers, which receive blood from the atria

When the heart is functioning normally, its valves permit blood flow in only one direction. The two sets of valves are the *atrioventricular valves* and the *semilunar valves*.

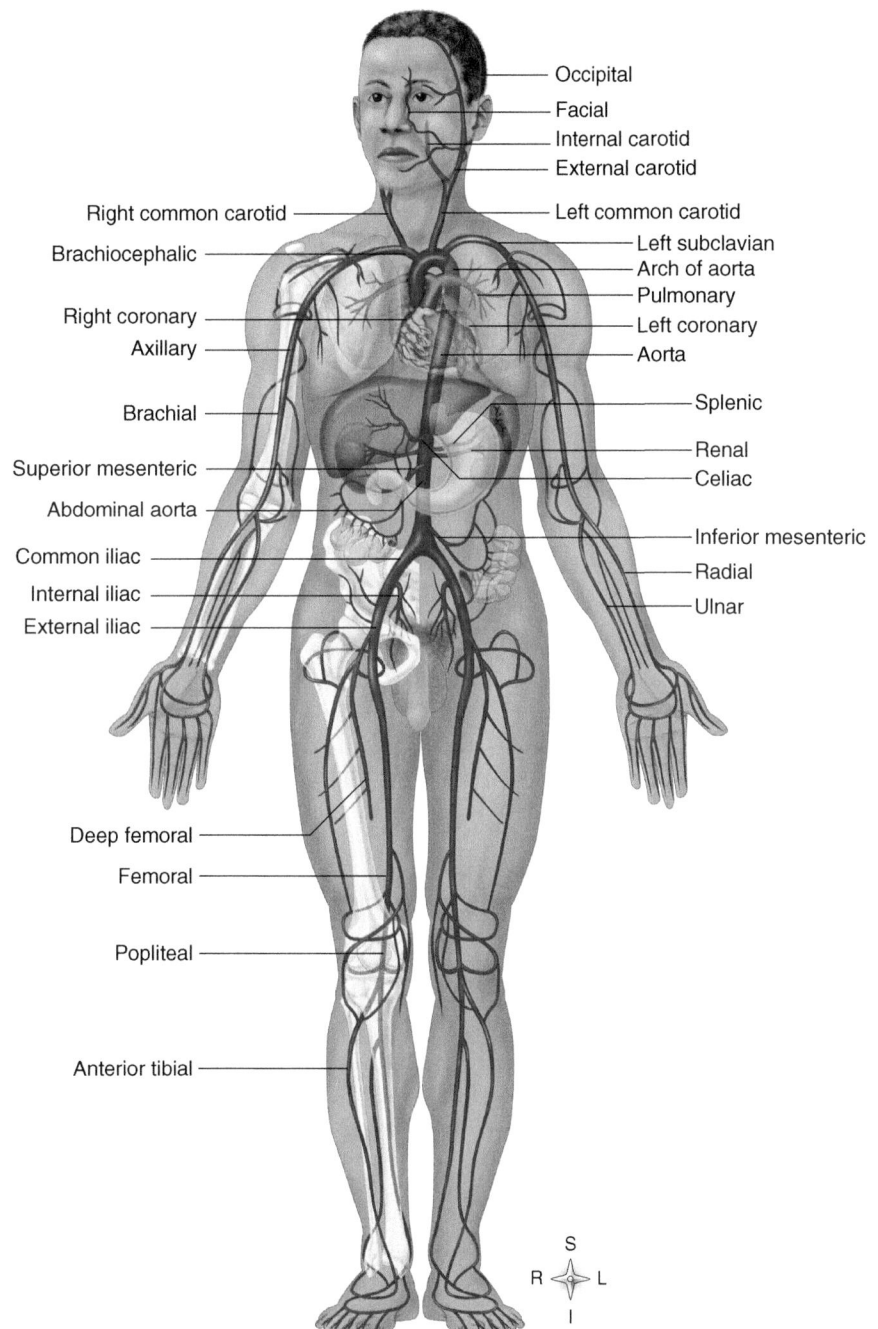

FIGURE 8-5 Principal arteries of the body. (From Patton K, Thibodeau G: *Anatomy and physiology,* ed 7, St Louis, 2010, Mosby.)

The heart circulates the blood by means of three types of transport vessels:
- Arteries (large vessels that carry blood away from the heart)
- Veins (smaller vessels that carry blood toward the heart)
- Capillaries (microscopic vessels that transport nutrients between blood and tissue cells)

Common Diseases of the Cardiovascular System and Current Drug Treatment

A variety of diseases can affect the cardiovascular system. These can involve the production of blood and blood constituents, the blood vessels and the way they transport blood, or the muscle and tissue of the heart. The following are diseases associated with the cardiovascular system:

- Blood disorders
  - Leukopenia (low white blood cell count)
  - Bone marrow disorders (which result in other blood disorders)
  - Hemophilia (failure to create any of a variety of blood clotting factors)
- Heart disease
  - Endocarditis/pericarditis (inflammation of inner or outer linings of the heart) caused by bacterial infection
  - Arteriosclerosis (loss of elasticity of blood vessels)
  - Thrombophlebitis (blood clots in the veins)
  - Angina (symptom of ischemic heart disease characterized by severe, pressurized chest pain)
  - Coronary heart disease (hardening and narrowing of the arteries, resulting in a reduced blood supply to the heart and body tissues)
  - Dysrhythmia (irregular heartbeat)
  - Hypertension (abnormally high blood pressure, which may be caused by a variety of patient-specific factors or by various drugs and organic compounds that increase cardiac output)
- Heart failure: Inability of the heart to pump blood at a rate that allows the body's metabolic functions to be sustained with oxygen and other needed nutrients transported by the blood; may include:
  - Stroke
  - Myocardial infarction

Drugs used to treat diseases of the cardiovascular system have various effects on the tissues of the heart and the blood vessels. Drugs used to treat hypertension work at the various sites in the body where blood pressure is regulated, such as:

- Kidneys
- Heart
- Blood vessels
- Brain
- Sympathetic nerves

Technician Connection: How to Use This Information

Several classes of drugs are used to treat the various forms of heart disease. It is extremely important for pharmacy technicians to become familiar with each product and to make sure that multiple product identifiers are used to verify correct product selection.

A trait that most pharmacists particularly appreciate in technicians is the ability to anticipate the patient's needs and the best way to support the pharmacist. For example, a pharmacy technician working in a cardiac or intensive care unit should make an effort to learn the cardiac medications that sustain a patient's life and that need to be prepared and ready for delivery. Other products are prepared in the event of a cardiac or respiratory crisis but may not need to be filled right away unless requested. Such *as needed,* or PRN, medications may be expensive, and a technician who knows when to inquire about when a dose should be prepared, based on the patient's condition, is a great asset to the pharmacist.

GASTROINTESTINAL SYSTEM

The gastrointestinal (GI) system (Figure 8-6) prepares food ingested orally for absorption and distribution to cells of the body. The constituents of the oral cavity allow for chewing, swallowing, and speech. The oral cavity contains three pairs of salivary glands that secrete enzymes and mucus, which facilitate the breakdown of food before swallowing. The pharynx, which passes from the mouth to the esophagus, is the passageway for air and food. The esophagus extends from the pharynx to the stomach and serves as the passageway for food.

The digestive system consists primarily of the stomach, liver, gallbladder, pancreas, and small intestine.

The stomach performs the following functions:

- Serves as a reservoir for food while it is being broken down for absorption and delivery to the intestines

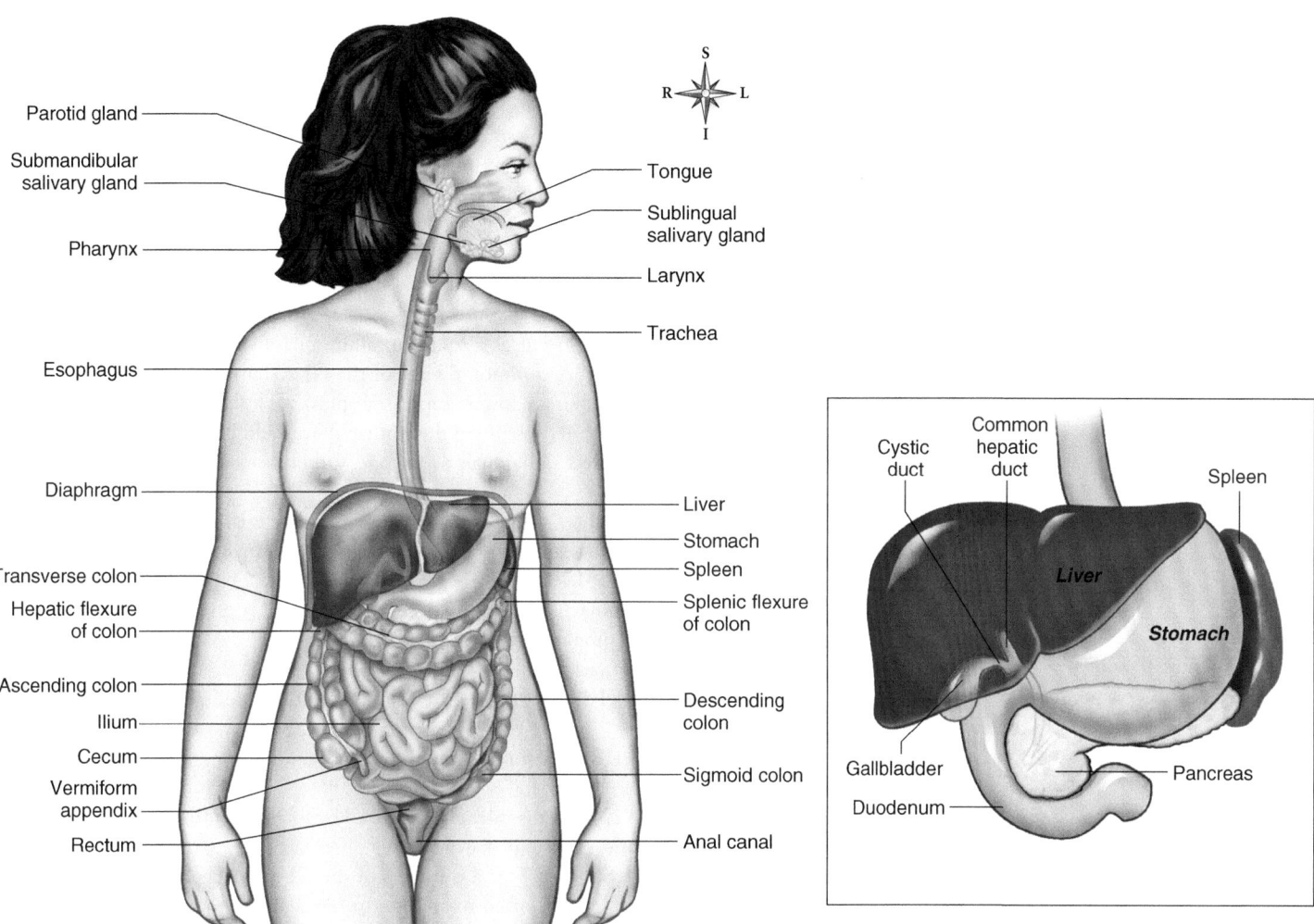

FIGURE 8-6 Location of the digestive organs. (From Patton K, Thibodeau G: *Anatomy and physiology,* ed 7, St Louis, 2010, Mosby.)

- Secretes gastric juice and hydrochloric acid to break down food and destroy pathogenic bacteria that may have been ingested
- Secretes intrinsic factor
- Produces the hormone gastrin to regulate digestion and ghrelin (endocrine cells) to increase appetite

The intestinal system consists primarily of the small and large intestines, the appendix, liver, gallbladder, and pancreas. The small intestine consists of the duodenum, jejunum, and ileum; the lining of the intestines contain tiny projections, called *villi,* that create additional surface area for absorption of nutrients broken down during chemical digestion in the stomach.

The large intestine consists of the cecum, colon, rectum, and anal canal. This portion of the intestinal system facilitates the transport of digestive by-products and waste for excretion externally. The appendix, which is just behind the cecum, is thought to cultivate nonpathogenic intestinal bacteria that aid digestion or the absorption of nutrients. The liver, the largest gland in the body, consists of two lobes; it performs the following functions:

- Accomplishes detoxification
- Secretes bile
- Metabolizes proteins, fats, and carbohydrates
- Contains phagocyte cells that remove bacteria, worn red blood cells, and other particles from the bloodstream

- Stores vitamins A, B₁₂, and D
- Produces plasma proteins
- Serves as the site of blood production during fetal development

The gallbladder, which is beneath the liver, stores, concentrates, and ejects bile into the duodenum.

The pancreas consists of both endocrine and exocrine cells, which produce insulin and glucagon, hormones that control carbohydrate metabolism. Exocrine cells secrete the digestive enzymes found in pancreatic juice.

Common Diseases of the Gastrointestinal System and Current Drug Treatment

Disease of the gastrointestinal system may occur as a result of failure or impaired function of any of the organs associated with the GI tract. A common disease of the GI system is gastroesophageal reflux disease (GERD), which develops when the lower esophageal sphincter leaks stomach contents into the esophagus as a result of a buildup of pressure in the stomach. This ailment may or may not involve pre-existing factors, and it can affect individuals of any age. Other diseases of the GI system include:

- Ulcers (open wounds or sores in the tissue); these are caused by bacterial infection or over-production of stomach acids or by weakening of the stomach or intestinal mucosa (or both). The three types of GI ulcers are:
  - Gastric ulcer: Ulcer in the stomach
  - Duodenal ulcer: Ulcer in the upper portion of the small intestine
  - Peptic ulcer: Ulcer of the stomach or duodenum
- Crohn's disease: An irritable bowel disease that causes GI inflammation and impairs the body's ability to absorb nutrients.
- Inflammatory bowel syndrome (IBS): A condition in which abdominal stress results in diarrhea and/or constipation.
- Irritable bowel disease (IBD): A chronic disorder characterized by intestinal inflammation that leads to abdominal cramping and persistent diarrhea.

A variety of drugs can be used to treat diseases and disorders of the GI tract. These drugs generally act on the smooth muscle of the GI tract, often to counter or block the production of gastric juices that can be damaging to the tissues. Many of these products interact with other drugs or food (or both), and the patient should avoid these other drugs and foods while taking GI medications.

Technician Connection: How to Use This Information

Because of the number of interactions and side effects associated with many of the GI drugs, pharmacy technicians must make sure the appropriate auxiliary and warning labels are affixed to the dispensing containers of these products. Although clinical symptoms may not be discussed, a pharmacy technician may direct the patient's attention to the information noted on these labels. This information is crucial to achieving the medication's therapeutic effect. These critical labels include:

- Avoid antacids, dairy, and iron products before and after taking
- Avoid alcohol
- Shake well
- Swallow whole (when indicated)
- May cause drowsiness
- May cause discoloration of urine or feces
- Avoid prolonged exposure to sunlight
- May decrease effectiveness of oral contraceptives while taking
- Take on an empty stomach
- Drink plenty of fluids
- Do not discontinue abruptly
- Take with food

Patients taking GI medications, particularly those receiving the prescription for the first time, should be directed to speak with the pharmacist to learn additional clinical information on how these products work best and on key lifestyle changes that should be made to enhance wellness and the efficacy of the medications.

RESPIRATORY SYSTEM

The primary function of the respiratory system (Figure 8-7) is to distribute air, supply oxygen to the blood and cells of the body, and remove carbon dioxide from the cells. This is accomplished through internal respiration (gas exchange in the pulmonary capillaries of the lungs), transport of gases by blood, and external respiration (breathing).

The respiratory system is divided into upper and lower tracts.
- The upper respiratory tract includes the nose, nasopharynx, oropharynx, laryngopharynx, and larynx.
- The lower respiratory tract includes the trachea, all segments of the bronchial tree, and the lungs. The bronchioles divide into alveolar ducts. The alveoli are the structures that exchange carbon dioxide and oxygen in the capillaries with which they come in contact through the thin walls of the respiratory membrane.

Common Diseases of the Respiratory System and Current Drug Treatment

Diseases of the respiratory system may include damage to or dysfunction of the lungs or respiratory airways and impairment of their ability to allow for respiration that transports oxygenated blood to the heart and other tissues of the body. Common diseases include asthma, which produces inflammation, irritation, and obstruction or tightening of the airways; and chronic obstructive pulmonary

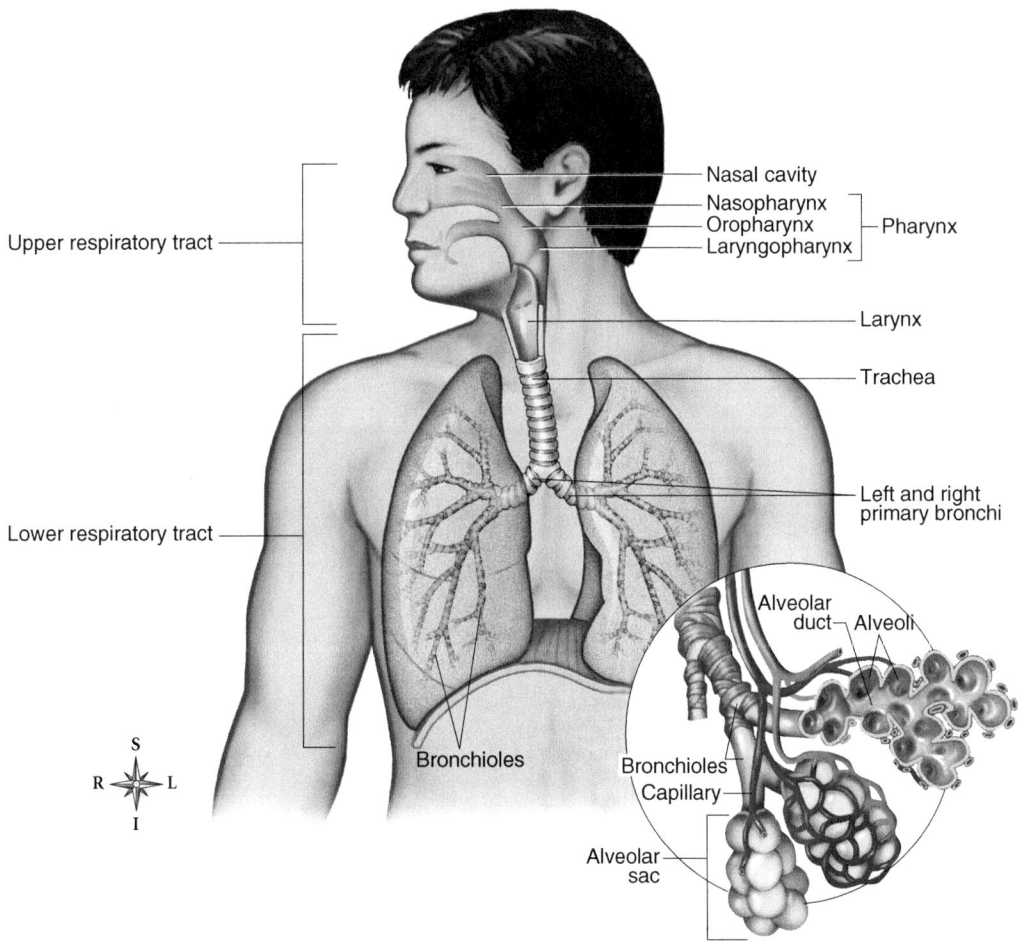

FIGURE 8-7 Structure of the respiratory system. (From Patton K, Thibodeau G: *Anatomy and physiology,* ed 7, St Louis, 2010, Mosby.)

disease (COPD), which produces a gradual loss of overall pulmonary function. Respiratory disease also may occur as a result of allergies or contraction of a bacterial infection in the lungs or bronchioles.

Drugs used to treat respiratory disease attack and destroy bacterial and viral pathogens, or they may act on the smooth muscle tissues of the lungs to relax and open constricted airways, allowing for easier breathing. Drugs for constricted airways may be used in an acute respiratory crisis, such as an asthma attack, in which rapid airway obstruction can be life-threatening. Some medications act on the muscle and tissues of the lungs and bronchioles, reducing inflammation and irritation over a prolonged period, thus keeping the airways open.

Technician Connection: How to Use This Information

Many of the products used to treat pulmonary disease have a variety of side effects. Patients who take these medications should be directed to speak to the pharmacist about possible adverse effects. Patients also must be taught to use the devices that may accompany these medications, such as oral inhalers and spacers. If the device is not used properly, the efficacy of the drug is compromised, and respiratory symptoms may not be controlled.

GENITOURINARY SYSTEM

The primary function of the urinary system (Figure 8-8) is to maintain body fluid homeostasis through the filtration of waste for excretion and water for reabsorption. The nephrons of the kidneys specifically reabsorb fluid and electrolytes, filter the blood, and excrete urine. Urine is eliminated

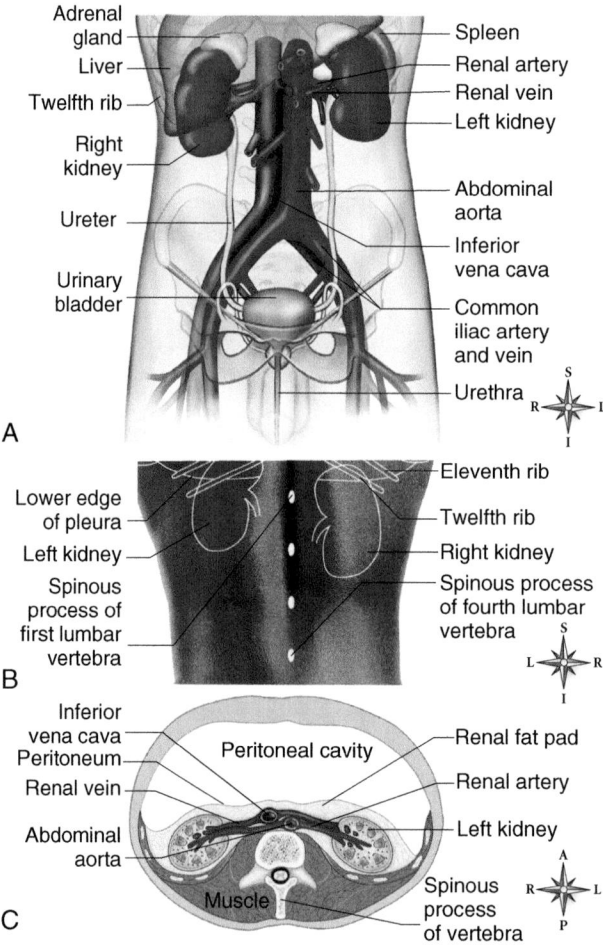

FIGURE 8-8 Location of the urinary system organs (anterior view of the urinary organs with the peritoneum and visceral organs removed). (From Patton K, Thibodeau G: *Anatomy and physiology,* ed 7, St Louis, 2010, Mosby.)

through the accessory organs (i.e., ureters, urinary bladder, and urethra). Each kidney has approximately 1.25 million nephrons.

The process of filtration and reabsorption begins when the renal artery brings blood to each kidney, which branches off into a network of capillaries in the Bowman's capsule (the *glomerulus*). Extending from the glomerulus are the proximal tubule, loop of Henle, and distal tubule, where the secretion of waste products and reabsorption of water and nutrients take place. The ureters are two tubes that transport urine from the kidneys to the urinary bladder. The urinary bladder is anterior to the vagina and in front of the uterus in women and rests on the prostate in men. The bladder acts as a reservoir for urine, which is expelled through the urethra, a small tube that leads from the bottom of the bladder to the exterior of the body.

Common Diseases of the Genitourinary System and Current Drug Treatment

Diseases of the urinary system often involve compromised functioning of the kidneys' ability to:
- Filter impurities
- Sustain the fluid and electrolyte balance in the body
- Allow for reabsorption of nutrients or drugs after passage and filtration

Treatment of dysfunction of the male genitourinary system has gained momentum, and more treatment options are becoming available. Several products for erectile dysfunction are among the top 200 drugs used in the United States. Treatments associated with the female genitourinary system most frequently involve contraception, or the prevention of pregnancy.

Technician Connection: How to Use This Information

Many of the drugs used to treat genitourinary conditions may interact with other medications or may themselves cause unpleasant side effects or adverse reactions; patients should be informed of this possibility. Patients also should be directed to speak with the pharmacist to make sure they know how to take these drugs properly and the types of other drugs to avoid while taking genitourinary medications.

ENDOCRINE SYSTEM

The endocrine system (Figure 8-9) is a network of glands that perform regulatory functions much like the central nervous system. The chemical transmitters are hormones that diffuse into the blood and are carried throughout every major system of the body (Table 8-4). The key components of the endocrine system are the pituitary gland, thyroid gland, parathyroid glands, thymus, adrenal glands, pancreas, ovaries, and testes.

Hormones must target specific receptors for which they have a high degree of affinity. In fact, hormones bind only with receptor sites that "fit" them exactly; consequently, they often remain free in the bloodstream until they are delivered to their highly specific site of action.

Pituitary Gland

The pituitary gland is sometimes referred to as the "master gland." Its activity in conjunction with the central nervous system may allow for CNS control of all body cells during times of crisis, when the body's survival is threatened. The pituitary gland is divided into two parts, the adenohypophysis and the neurohypophysis. During stress, the hypothalamus of the brain may take over the adenohypophysis and in doing so send signals to every cell in the body.

Thyroid Gland

The hormones released by the thyroid primarily control calcium levels in the body by increasing the activity of osteoblasts, which are specialized cells that form bone. Some cells help whittle down bone tissue for shaping and resorption, a normal body function. However, to maintain balance and prevent excessive bone loss, the thyroid gland also inhibits or controls bone breakdown by osteoclasts.

Parathyroid Glands

The parathyroid glands are embedded in the surface of the thyroid. Hormones released by the parathyroid glands act on bone and kidney cells to cause the release of calcium into the blood, which results in less bone formation and more old bone dissolution.

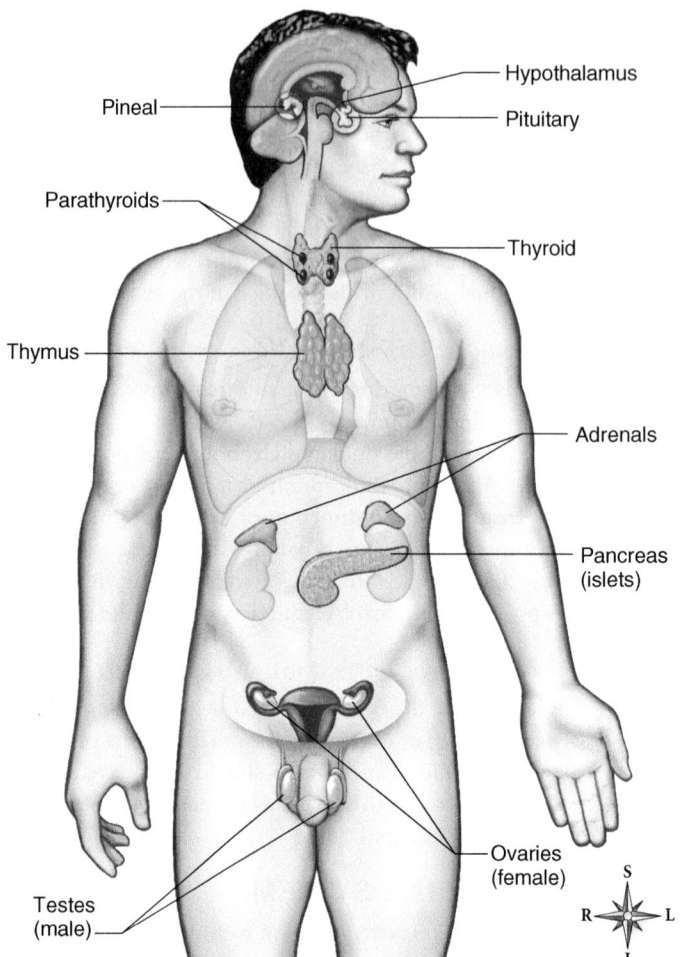

FIGURE 8-9 Locations of some major endocrine glands. (From Patton K, Thibodeau G: *Anatomy and physiology,* ed 7, St Louis, 2010, Mosby.)

Adrenal Glands

The two adrenal glands are situated on top of the kidneys. Each gland consists of two parts, the adrenal cortex and the adrenal medulla. The adrenal cortex secretes several hormones, including sex hormones. The adrenal medulla secretes two vital hormones, epinephrine and norepinephrine.

Pancreas

The pancreas is located at the beginning of the small intestine, behind the stomach. The pancreas secretes several vital hormones, including insulin and fluid containing digestive enzymes that drain into the small intestine.

Gonads

The gonads are the primary sex organs in both males and females. In males, the testes consist of coils of tubules that produce sperm. In the area between the tubules, special interstitial cells produce the male hormones, androgens; testosterone is the primary androgen. In females, the ovaries, a pair of glands in the pelvis, produce the sex hormones estrogen and progesterone.

Common Diseases of the Endocrine System and Current Drug Treatment

Hormones are involved in so many metabolic processes that their overproduction or underproduction may produce many signs of disease. Numerous drugs are used to treat diseases of the endocrine system, either by synthetically replacing hormones the body cannot produce or by acting on

TABLE 8-4   **Classification of Tropic and Non-Tropic Hormones of the Endocrine System**

Classification	Hormone
Steroid hormones	Aldosterone Cortisol Estrogen Progesterone Testosterone
Nonsteroidal hormones	Parathyroid hormone (PTH) Growth hormone (GH) Prolactin (PRL) Calcitonin (CT) Glucagon Adrenocorticotropic hormone (ACTH)
Nonsteroidal glycoprotein hormones	Follicle-stimulating hormone (FSH) Luteinizing hormone (LH) Thyroid-stimulating hormone (TSH) Human chorionic gonadotropin (hCG)
Nonsteroidal peptide hormones	Oxytocin Antidiuretic hormone (ADH) Melatonin-stimulating hormone (MSH) Somatostatin (SS) Thyrotropin-releasing hormone (TRH) Gonadotropin-releasing hormone (GnRH) Atrial natriuretic hormone (ANH)
Nonsteroidal amino acid derivative hormones	Epinephrine Norepinephrine Thyroxine (T_4) Triiodothyronine (T_3)

organ receptors to block actions that cause overproduction of hormones, such as occurs in hyperthyroidism.

A common hormone deficiency disease that affects millions of Americans each year is diabetes mellitus. Insulin is essential to the regulation of carbohydrates, fats, and proteins in metabolism, and it enables glucose to be carried out of the bloodstream and used in various cells. Absence or underproduction of insulin results in blood glucose levels that increase the risk of heart disease and other serious health problems. Type 2 diabetes accounts for 90% to 95% of cases of diabetes.

Technician Connection: How to Use This Information

Because metabolic hormones are essential to just about every major body system, treatment of endocrine system disorders is crucial to these patients' overall health and ability to maintain quality of life despite their disease. Patients should be directed to any auxiliary or warning label information, because adherence to these directives has a significant impact on the therapeutic efficacy of the drugs.

IMMUNOLOGIC (LYMPHATIC) SYSTEM

The lymphatic system is a network of glands composed of cells that function integrally to support the immune response to foreign bodies and to maintain fluid balances. Lymphatic vessels in the intestinal walls also absorb fats from the intestines. Lymphatic vessels lead to tissue masses known as *lymph nodes,* which are located in various areas in the body along the pathway of the lymphatic vessels. Figure 8-10 shows critical points in the lymphatic system and the locations of lymph nodes.

Lymph is a clear to white fluid that contains fats and proteins from the intestines and a variety of specialty cells that target and destroy foreign bodies, known as antigens. Specialized cells called *macrophages* are located in the lymph nodes; macrophages surround and destroy antigens in a process

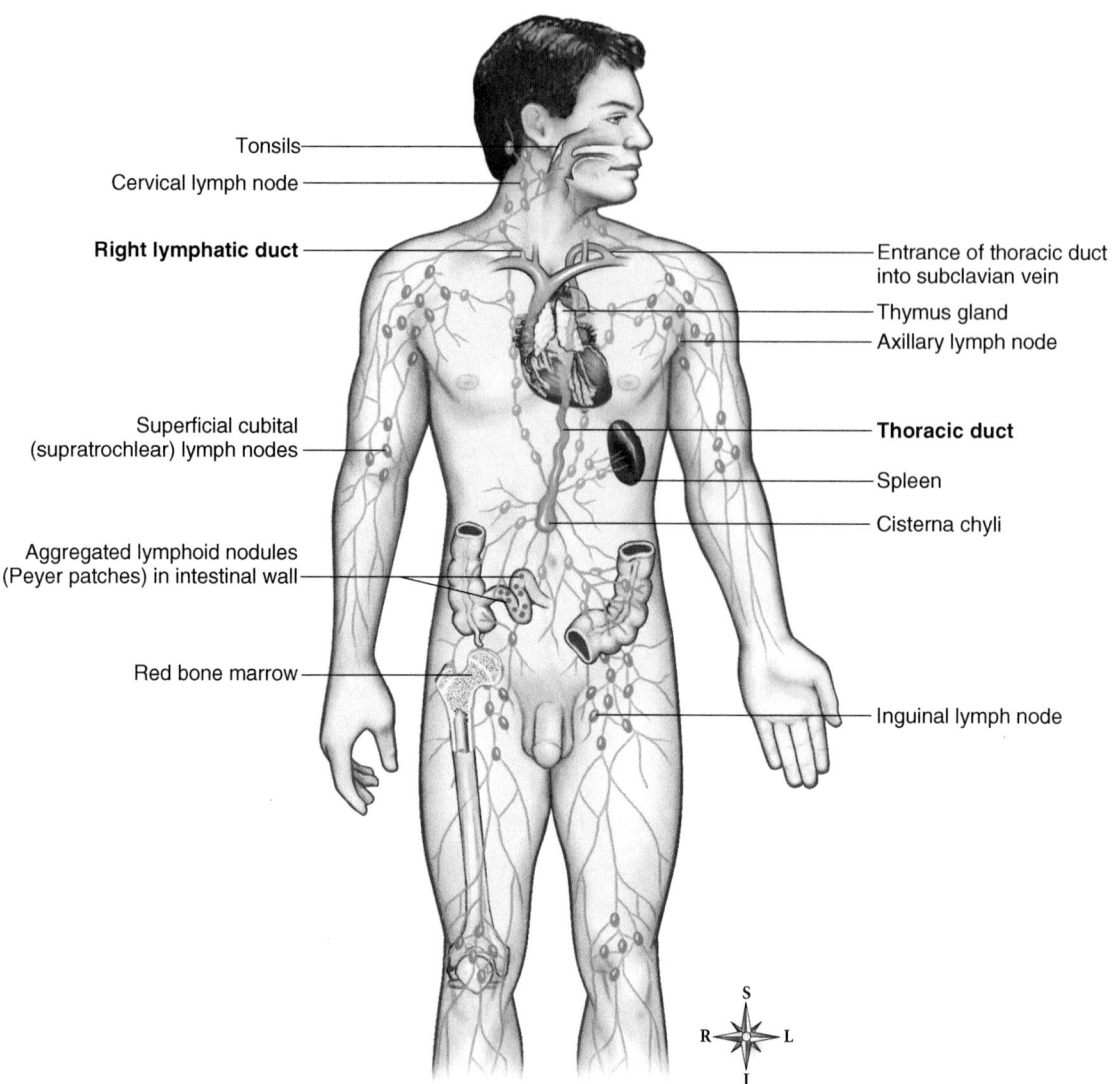

Tonsils

Cervical lymph node

Right lymphatic duct

Superficial cubital
(supratrochlear) lymph nodes

Aggregated lymphoid nodules
(Peyer patches) in intestinal wall

Red bone marrow

Entrance of thoracic duct
into subclavian vein

Thymus gland

Axillary lymph node

Thoracic duct

Spleen

Cisterna chyli

Inguinal lymph node

FIGURE 8-10 Principal organs of the lymphatic system. (From Patton K, Thibodeau G: *Anatomy and physiology,* ed 7, St Louis, 2010, Mosby.)

known as *phagocytosis.* The two main types of lymphocytes are B cells, which produce antibodies, and T cells, which directly attack bacterial and foreign cells by attaching to them and destroying them.

The specialized cells of the lymphatic system help create two levels of defense against invading pathogens and any microbes or substances that these cells identify as foreign to that body. The first level of defense, *innate immunity,* is created by any of the following mechanisms:

- *Species resistance:* Lymphocytes recognize genetic materials of certain pathogens and automatically mount an immune response.
- *Mechanical and chemical barriers:* The skin and mucosa form a barrier that separates the internal environment from the external environment.
- *Inflammatory response:* This response isolates infecting agents and stimulates intervention by a number of inflammatory mediators, such as:
  - Histamines
  - Kinins
  - Prostaglandins
  - Leukotrienes
  - Interleukins

- *Phagocytosis:* Phagocytes (e.g., neutrophils and macrophages) ingest and destroy pathogens.
- *Natural killer (NK) cells:* This group of lymphocytes kills various types of cancer cells and virus-infected cells.
- *Interferon:* Interferon inhibits the spread of a viral infection.
- *Complement:* This dedicated group of plasma protein enzymes catalyzes chemical reactions that result in the destruction of pathogens.

Adaptive Immunity

Adaptive immunity is called *specific immunity* primarily because lymphocytes recognize specific pathogenic agents and mount an immune response at them directly through the activity of either B-cell lymphocytes or T-cell lymphocytes. B-cell lymphocytes produce antibodies that attack the pathogens (this action is also referred to as *humoral immunity*). T-cell lymphocytes attack the pathogenic cells directly and mediate an immune response. The humoral immunity response may be created artificially through immunization, which provides the immune system with an inactive pathogen against which an antibody may be produced.

Common Diseases of the Lymphatic System and Current Drug Treatment

Diseases of the lymphatic system often involve the contraction or development of disease through introduction of a disease-causing microorganism. A variety of drugs have been produced to treat bacterial, viral, fungal, and parasitic infections. For prevention (one of the five rationales), vaccinations can be administered to produce an immunologic response that promotes antibody production, creating disease immunity.

A number of cancer drugs can target cancer cells. These drugs inhibit protein synthesis of the cancer cell wall, producing lysis, or act on the cancer cell's DNA, slowing its production. Other cancer drugs inhibit cell mitosis in cancer cells, which slows the progression of the disease.

Technician Connection: How to Use This Information

Pharmacy technicians should become familiar with both oral and injectable antiinfective drugs to minimize the risk of a medication fill error. A serious health concern in the United States is the overuse of antibiotic therapy, which has resulted in widespread microbial resistance to drug treatment. Patients' medication profiles should always be checked for multiple prescribed drugs in the same therapy class, and instances of such should be brought to the attention of a pharmacist.

Also, patients should be directed to their pharmacist when they indicate an allergy to a particular product that requires the use of an alternative product. In many cases, what the patient believes to be an allergic response is actually a known side effect that the patient may consider too unpleasant to manage. Such misinterpretation of a variety of known (and often quite undesirable) clinical side effects may lead to unnecessary overuse of products of various classes, which may cause a progression of drug resistance in patients over time.

One of the great drivers of drug resistance is failure to complete a drug therapy regimen. Patients often stop taking their antibiotics once they start to feel better. It is important that patients be reminded, as indicated on auxiliary labeling, that the entire regimen of drug therapy must be completed to avoid the possibility of the infection returning, with increased resistance to the prescribed drug.

INTEGUMENTARY SYSTEM

The skin itself (Figure 8-11) can be considered a natural defense against disease, because it creates a physical barrier between the internal and external environments. The skin may also be considered the largest and thinnest organ of the body. The skin is divided into two primary layers, the superficial layer, known as the epidermis, and the deeper and thicker layer, the dermis. The dermis, which supplies a layer of capillaries for nourishment of the outer layer, contains several key structures.

The dermis (often referred to as the "true skin") acts as a reservoir for water and necessary electrolytes. Sensory receptors in the dermis produce information to protect the integrity of both the dermis and the epidermis. The sensory receptors signal pain, pressure, touch, and temperature. Other appendages of the skin include the hair, nails, and skin glands. Skin glands include:

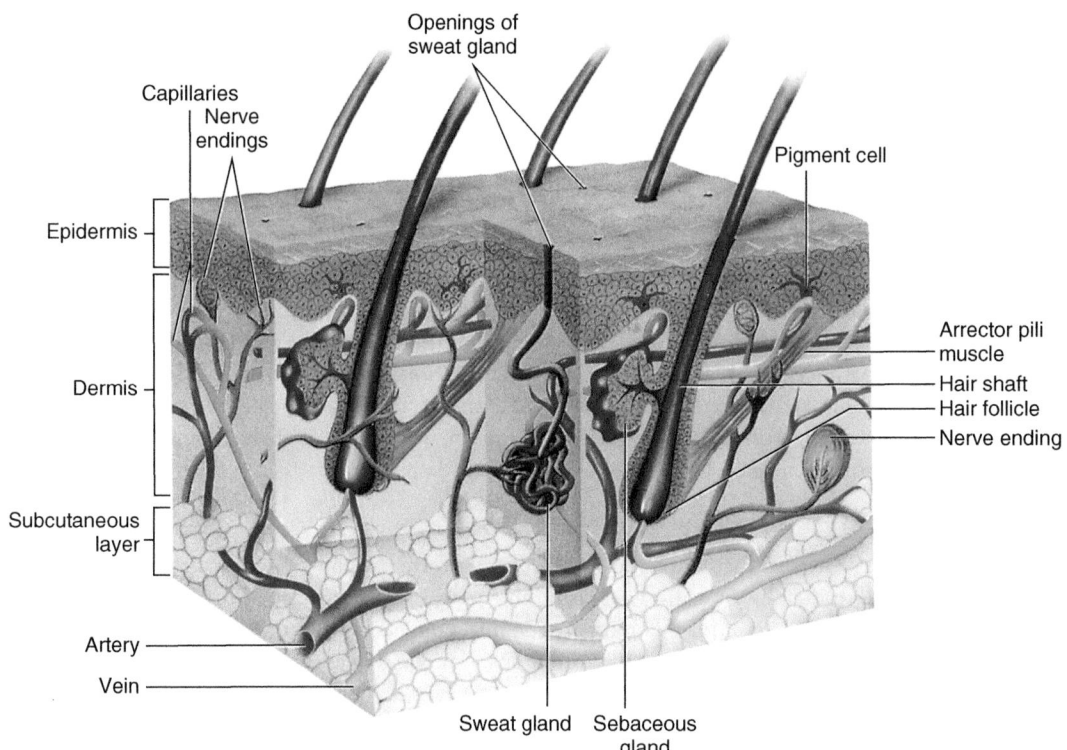

FIGURE 8-11 Microscopic structure of the skin. (From Solomon E: *Introduction to human anatomy and physiology,* ed 3, Philadelphia, 2008, Saunders.)

- Sweat glands, which produce perspiration that contains salts, ammonia, uric acid, urea, and other wastes
- Sebaceous glands, which secrete oil for the hair and skin
- Ceruminous glands, which secrete a waxy substance that protects the skin of the ear canal from dehydration

Common Diseases of the Integumentary System and Current Drug Treatment

Diseases of the skin and skin structures result from bacterial, viral, fungal, or parasitic infection or infestation. Fungal infections of the skin are generally referred to as *mycoses.* Common fungal infections include candidiasis of the skin or vaginal area and ringworm of the scalp, body, feet, fingernails, or toenails.

Technician Connection: How to Use This Information

Treatment options for fungal infections are available both by prescription and over the counter, depending on the severity of the infection. The antifungal classes of drugs also have a broad variety of interactions with other drugs, so it is imperative that pharmacy technicians gather information from patients about all other medications taken (including over-the-counter and herbal varieties). This gives pharmacists a more accurate medication profile, which allows them to validate the clinical appropriateness of the product or products prescribed.

Chapter Summary

This review of the body's systems should have made it clear how a working knowledge of the clinical basis for medication therapy improves a pharmacy technician's ability to support and assist pharmacists in the safe, efficacious delivery of pharmaceutical care. Pharmacy technicians should seek opportunities to increase their clinical knowledge and ways to use it in their day-to-day routines. A pharmacy technician should never use clinical knowledge to provide a patient with information that requires an independent clinical decision, because that is outside a technician's legal scope of practice. Rather, a pharmacy technician may use that clinical knowledge to:

- Gather information from a patient that a pharmacist needs to know to determine the clinical appropriateness of a drug in light of patient-specific variables and other drugs the patient takes.
- Select a product from stock, considering the variety of drug formulations, packages, and routes of administration available.
- Avoid look-alike/sound-alike errors in medication order entries.
- Catch a prescribing error.
- Perform the medication order fill processes, such as applying appropriate auxiliary and warning labels.
- Recognize the clinical appropriateness of directing patients to a pharmacist for information on the use of their medications.

REVIEW QUESTIONS

Multiple Choice

1. Bioavailability refers to a drug's:
   a. Movement from the circulatory system
   b. Ability to produce its effect at the site of action
   c. Route of administration
   d. Time frame for reaching its maximum concentration

2. The study of the biologic features of natural drugs refers to the science of:
   a. Biopharmaceuticals
   b. Pharmacognosy
   c. Pharmacodynamics
   d. Pharmacokinetics

3. The time required for a drug to reach the concentration necessary to produce a therapeutic effect is the:
   a. Onset of action
   b. Metabolism
   c. Duration of action
   d. Dosing schedule

4. Most prescription drugs are generally:
   a. Weak acids
   b. Strong acids
   c. Weak bases
   d. A and C

5. This category of drugs has been determined to cause birth defects when used during pregnancy:
   a. A
   b. B
   c. C
   d. X

6. Multiple drugs with an affinity for plasma protein binding:
   a. Compete for receptor binding sites
   b. Oppose each other, preventing both drugs from binding
   c. Destroy each other
   d. Bind to an equal number of receptor sites

7. Drugs that are activated during metabolism are known as:
   a. Enzymes
   b. Activites
   c. Prodrugs
   d. Substrates

8. The following are sites of drug excretion except:
   a. Hair
   b. Urine
   c. Saliva
   d. Perspiration

9. The maximum amount of drug that may be administered to achieve its peak effect is known as the:
   a. Ceiling effect
   b. Drug potency
   c. Efficacy
   d. Therapeutic index

10. An adverse effect characterized by the accumulation of a drug (and an increased concentration) because the body is unable to biotransform the drug is:
    a. Hepatotoxicity
    b. Teratogenicity
    c. Dependence
    d. Respiratory depression

TECHNICIAN'S CORNER

1. Explain how congestive heart disease affects liver metabolism.
2. Give an example of a food that affects drug metabolism.
3. Why is it important to verify the medications a patient is already taking when antifungal therapy is prescribed for a disease of the skin?

Bibliography

American Society of Health-System Pharmacists. (2006). *A Summary of Medication Therapy Management Programs in Medicare.* Retrieved 11/27/2010, from www.ashp.org/s_ashp/docs/files/GAD_Summaryof MTMP0806.pdf

American Society of Health-System Pharmacists. *Concepts in Clinical Pharmacokinetics—Lesson 1: Introduction to Pharmacokinetics and Pharmacodynamics.* Retrieved 7/23/2011, from www.ashp.org/DocLibrary/ Bookstore/P2418-Chapter1.aspx

American Society of Health-System Pharmacists. (2004). *Medication Therapy Management Services Definition and Program Criteria.* Retrieved 11/27/2010, from www.ashp.org/s_ashp/doc1c.asp?CID=738&DID=4069

Best, C.T. (1966). *The Physiological Basis of Medical Practice.* Baltimore: Williams & Wilkins.

Biology Online: Prion. (2011). Retrieved 7/26/2011, from www.biology-online.org/dictionary/Prion

Disease.com. (2010). *First Pass Metabolism.* Retrieved 7/24/2011, from http://disease.disease.com/Metabolism/ First-Pass-Metabolism.html

Forcon Forensic Consulting. (2004). *Excretion.* Retrieved 7/24/2011, from www.forcon.ca/learning/excretion. html

Freehealthandnutrition.com. (2011). *Enzymes: The Whole Story.* Retrieved 7/24/2011, from www.freehealthand nutrition.com/enzymes.html

Gilman, A.G. (1985). *Goodman and Gilman's the Pharmacological Basis of Therapeutics.* New York: Macmillan.

Medline Plus. (2010, November 14). *Lymph System.* Retrieved 6/26/2011, from www.nlm.nih.gov/ medlineplus/ency/article/002247.htm

Merriam-Webster Online. (2010). *Pharmacology.* Retrieved 11/16/2010, from www.merriam-webster.com/ dictionary/pharmacology

Moscou, K.S. (2009). *Pharmacology for Pharmacy Technicians.* St. Louis: Mosby/Elsevier.

Siegel, J.D., Rinehart, E., Jackson, M., et al. (2007). *Guideline for Isolation Precautions: Preventing Transmission of Infectious Agents in Healthcare Settings.* Retrieved 7/26/2011, from www.cdc.gov/ncidod/dhqp/pdf/ isolation2007.pdf

U.S. Army Medical Department Center and School, Academy of Health Sciences. (2011). *Lesson 1: Communicable Diseases*. Retrieved 7/27/2011, from www.tpub.com/content/armymedical/MD0540/MD05400005. htm

Webb, D. (2010). *When Foods and Drugs Collide: Studies Expose Interactions Between Certain Foods and Medications, Today's Dietitian*, 12:26. Retrieved 7/24/2011, from www.todaysdietitian.com/newarchives/121610p26. shtml

Your Dictionary. (2010). *Biotransformation Medical Definition*. Retrieved 7/22/2011, from http://medical. yourdictionary.com/biotransformation

9

Introduction to Pharmaceutical Dosage Forms

LEARNING OBJECTIVES

By the end of this chapter, students will be able to competently:

1. Describe the drug dosage forms.
2. Describe the different drug delivery systems and their uses.
3. Describe the physical properties of solid drug dosage forms.
4. Identify the solid and semisolid dosage forms, along with their uses.
5. Describe the physical and chemical properties of various liquid drug dosage forms.
6. Differentiate drug dosage forms that provide either local or systemic effects.
7. Discuss the advantages and disadvantages of the different drug dosage forms.
8. Describe the packaging and storage requirements of drug dosage forms used in the pharmacy and healthcare environments.

KEY TERMS

Buccal: A term referring to a solid drug dosage form that is held between the cheek and gum and allowed to dissolve slowly.

Dosage form: The form in which a medication is provided (i.e., solid, semisolid, or liquid).

Drug metabolism: The process by which the body breaks down and converts medication into active or inactive chemical substances, primarily in the liver.

Local effect: The body's response to a drug dosage form in which the therapeutic action of the drug generally occurs at the site of administration.

Parenteral: A term referring to the route of administration by which a drug enters the vascular system by a means other than through the gastrointestinal system. The term generally refers to drugs administered subcutaneously or intravenously.

Pharmacokinetics: The science of mathematically determining a drug's plasma concentrations based on the length of time since the dose was administered and other clinical factors, such as the patient's disease state.

Sublingual: A term referring to the route of administration in which a solid or liquid medication is placed under the tongue for dissolution and absorption into the oral mucosa.

Systemic effect: The body's response to a drug dosage form in which the drug must be transported via the bloodstream and metabolized by the liver.

Troche: A solid dosage form (also known as a *pastille*) that is administered buccally.

By now you should be familiar with the variety of different drugs available to treat disease in the human body. The term dosage form means different things to different people, depending on perspective, clinical exposure, or experience. Patients may view a drug's dosage form in terms of their ability to self-administer the medication. To healthcare providers, dosage forms are drug delivery systems that help them manage each patient's treatment plan. In addition, the dosage form can dictate the conditions under which the medication must be stored in patient care areas.

By definition, a drug delivery system refers to:
- A physical device used to administer a drug
- A physical characteristic (or the makeup) of a drug that affects the way the body breaks down (metabolizes) the drug
- A means by which a drug is delivered into the body (also known as the *route of administration*)

An aspect of medication therapy management is ensuring that a patient receives the most appropriate medication, given the patient-specific variables, such as:
- Age
- Weight
- Gender
- Ethnicity
- Disease state/metabolic functions
- Disease-driven risk factors

Pharmacists may make recommendations on the most appropriate medication in light of these factors. A drug's effect on the body, from the standpoints of stability and of action at the cellular level, must be taken into consideration when selecting the most appropriate route of administration.

Some of the factors that determine the most appropriate route of administration include:
- The condition being treated
- The drug's active ingredient
- The amount (or rate, if infused parenterally) of active ingredient to be delivered
- Which administration sites may be used for delivery
- The total duration of the medication therapy

Time is a critical factor in medication administration. The length of time a drug remains in the body weighs heavily in the determination of the most appropriate drug delivery system, especially when patient-specific variables are taken into consideration.

Chapter 8 discussed medications in terms of pharmacokinetics. To review, pharmacokinetics refers to the way a drug is:
- Absorbed into the body
- Distributed to body systems and cell structures
- Metabolized and used on a cellular level
- Eliminated by the body after metabolism

This chapter discusses the various dosage forms that are dispensed and administered to patients in a variety of healthcare settings. Pharmacy technicians generally dispense, stock, and deliver medication to patients and drug storage areas. They are also involved in the medication order entry processes. Technicians who are knowledgeable about the most therapeutically appropriate use of drug delivery systems will be more alert to possible errors in drug prescribing, order entry, or fill processes. For example, a patient with third-degree burns over 80% of his body is not likely to receive pain medication through a transdermal delivery system (i.e., one that is placed on the surface of the skin). Therefore, an order for a pain medication patch probably is the result of a medication error and should be questioned.

Patients' health and welfare depend on the healthcare team's observance of the six rights of medication administration:
- Right patient
- Right drug
- Right dose
- Right route
- Right time
- Right documentation

We must strive to get it RIGHT, every time.

General Classification of Drug Dosage Forms

Drugs are manufactured in three main dosage forms that influence their packaging, storage, and administration:

- Solid
- Semisolid
- Liquid

TECH NOTE!

Carelessness in filling prescriptions for liquid dosage forms presents a specific hazard. Liquid formulations have a faster systemic action, which may mean less time to reverse the effects of taking the wrong medication.

LOCAL AND SYSTEMIC MECHANISMS OF ACTION

When a person takes a drug, two actions occur:

- The drug acts on a cellular level in the body structures with which it comes in contact.
- The drug has an *effect;* that is, an observable consequence results from the drug's action.

Depending on the condition being treated, symptomatic relief may be achieved without the drug having to cycle through the gastrointestinal (GI) tract into the bloodstream and be broken down by various systems to take action. Drugs that elicit an external response have *local action.* Drugs that must be transported via the bloodstream and metabolized (broken down and converted) into cellular building blocks by the liver or other system elicit *systemic action.*

Any solid oral drug dosage form generally provides systemic action, because it must be ingested and then broken down in the stomach or intestines before transport to the liver for metabolism. Oral liquid dosage forms take the same pathway but tend to act more quickly, because the GI system does not have to break them down before absorption. See Figure 9-1 for a diagram outlining drug absorption and distribution.

Systemic action also is generally seen with drugs administered by the parenteral route (i.e., a route other than through the GI system). This may be done using a needle to penetrate the topmost layer of the skin into deeper skin layers, muscle, or the vascular system or internal structures. Because the drug is not processed by the GI system for absorption, the systemic effect occurs quickly. For this reason, greater risk is involved in the use of injectable drugs. Prescribers and pharmacists must carefully weigh the risks, in light of the drug's therapeutic benefit and the patient-specific variables.

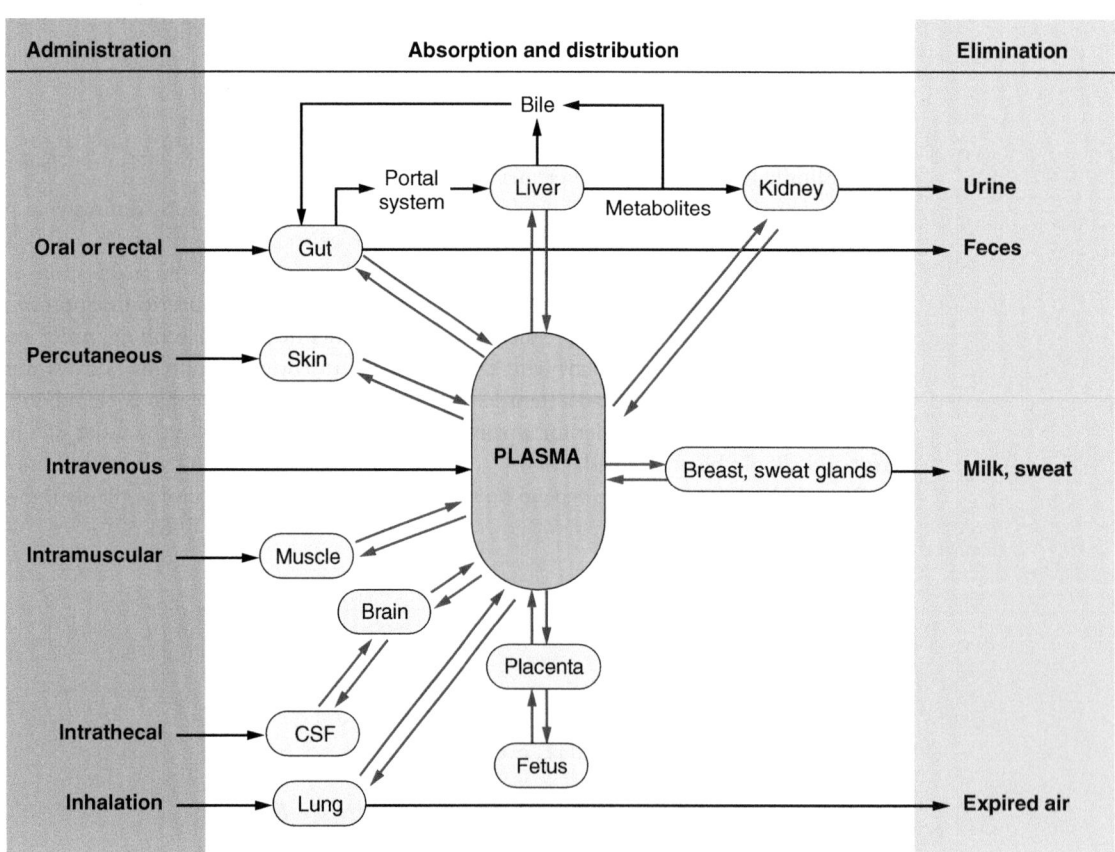

FIGURE 9-1 Routes of drug administration. (From Key JL, Hayes E, McCuistion L: *Pharmacology: a nursing process approach,* ed 6, Philadelphia, 2009, Saunders.)

Solid Drug Dosage Forms

A variety of solid drug dosage forms currently is manufactured (or manually compounded in pharmacies) and dispensed to patients, including:
- Tablets
- Capsules
- Powders and crystals
- Granules

Semisolid dosage forms include:
- Lotions
- Ointments
- Creams
- Pastes and plasters

Specialized solid dosage forms include:
- Transdermal systems
- Intranasal and oral inhalers
- GI therapeutic systems
- Ocular inserts

DISPENSING AND ADMINISTERING SOLID DRUG FORMS

Oral solid drugs are the most commonly dispensed drug dosage form. In the community pharmacy setting, pharmacy technicians can easily package oral solid drugs in amber vials or label their stock bottle containers or foil blister packs for dispensing. The quantity generally represents an entire course of therapy for an acute condition, or an approved days' supply for long-term treatment of a chronic condition.

In the inpatient hospital setting, drugs are packaged and dispensed in individual, or unit-dose, containers. Because doses generally are packaged for distribution to various drug storage areas, labeling is usually not patient-specific. Individually packaged doses are labeled with all necessary drug information to reduce medication errors and preserve product integrity. Bar codes on the packaging allow for scan verification of the correct drug to ensure safety when the package is opened and administered at the patient's bedside. A patient's medication therapy may be adjusted frequently, based on the person's condition; therefore, doses generally are dispensed only in a 24-hour supply.

In the outpatient setting, solid oral drug dosage forms are easily self-administered by patients, provided the individual has no problems with swallowing. Auxiliary labeling on oral solid dosage forms generally recommends that patients take these medications with an adequate amount of water or other specified fluids to allow for easy swallowing, to prevent esophageal irritation, and to aid dissolution in the stomach (i.e., the process by which enzymes and stomach acids break down and dissolve the solid drug).

Some oral medications that *must not* be swallowed, but rather must be held in the mouth and allowed to dissolve slowly. Such dosage forms include troches (pronounced tro-keys) and sublingual tablets.
- A clotrimazole troche prescribed for the treatment of an oral fungal infection must be administered by the buccal (pronounced like buckle) route; that is, held between the cheek and gum and allowed to dissolve slowly.
- A nitroglycerin tablet prescribed for the treatment of angina (severe acute chest pain) is a sublingual drug; that is, it is held under the tongue and allowed to dissolve slowly.

The oral mucosa makes an excellent route of administration because of the speed with which drugs delivered in this manner are absorbed into the bloodstream for transport to the liver for metabolism. Drugs formulated for the buccal and sublingual routes of administration must be manufactured with materials that can be easily broken down by the digestive enzymes in saliva. This route of administration is also ideal for drugs that were not designed to be absorbed through the GI tract because of their molecular structure:

Pharmacy technicians should always make sure oral solid drugs are packaged with all the information required for caregivers to administer the product safely to patients in the hospital or long-term care setting.

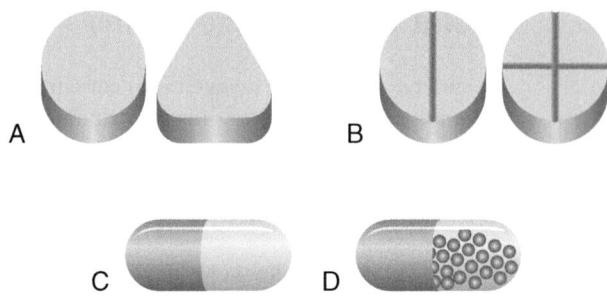

FIGURE 9-2 Shapes of tablets and capsules. **A** and **B,** Tablets. **C** and **D,** Capsules. (From Kee JL, Hayes E, McCuistion L: *Pharmacology: a nursing process approach,* ed 6, Philadelphia, 2009, Saunders.)

TABLETS

Tablets are the most common oral solid dosage form for medication (Figure 9-2, *A* and *B*). Tablets are available in a variety of forms:

- *Chewable*—Usually flavored, such as for children's medication, antacids, some vitamins, and antiflatulents.
- *Buccal*—Placed between the gum and the cheek to allow slow dissolution and absorption through the buccal mucosa.
- *Sublingual*—Placed and absorbed under the tongue (for drugs that must be dissolved rapidly and absorbed quickly into the bloodstream).
- *Vaginal*—Inserted into the vagina with an applicator; dissolves and is absorbed through the vaginal mucosa.
- *Implant* or *pellet*—Small cylinders placed intradermally (under the skin) or in the subcutaneous tissue for prolonged and continuous absorption of potent hormones, such as testosterone or estradiol. Implants are ideal for long-term and controlled release of medication (e.g., long-term contraception). They are very convenient, but some complications can occur, such as patient discomfort, dislodgment of the implant, or infection at the insertion site.
- *Lozenge* (also known as a *troche* or a *pastille*)—A dosage form containing active ingredients and flavorings that is dissolved in the mouth to exert a local effect.

To form a tablet, a drug's active ingredient and other ingredients, known as *excipients,* are pressed together in a mold. The following are types of excipients:

- *Diluent* (or *filler*): Adds bulk volume to the tablet (e.g., sucrose, microcrystalline cellulose, corn starch, whey, yeast).
- *Binder:* A sticky substance that helps ingredients adhere to each other (e.g., xanthan gum, Carbopol)
- *Disintegrant:* Assists in the breakdown process of ingredients at the site of absorption, establishing a drug's release rate (e.g., crospovidone, croscarmellose sodium, gellan gum)

A drug's *release rate* influences how the active ingredient takes action in the body. An immediate-release drug is designed to break down in the stomach for absorption and transport for metabolism; this type of drug generally takes effect quickly and does not remain in the bloodstream for an extended period.

An extended-release drug is designed to break down more gradually, for slower absorption. The disintegrants in extended-release drugs allow for uniform absorption of the drug in the GI tract over an extended period. This dosage form is ideal for the treatment of chronic conditions.

Often drug manufacturers formulate extended- or sustained-release drugs with higher concentrations of the active ingredient, designed for delivery over a longer period. This reduces the frequency with which the patient must administer a dose. Patients taking medication for a chronic condition generally are more likely to take it consistently if they only have to administer it once or twice daily.

Very potent drugs may be formulated for extended release to allow for slower, gradual absorption and metabolism. Patients should be cautioned that chewing an extended-release drug can have dangerous consequences.

TECH NOTE!

Patients should be informed if their drug's release rate has changed, particularly if they previously had taken an immediate-release product and now have been switched to a sustained-release formulation. Failure to recognize this change may result in an overdose. Pharmacy technicians should direct patients to speak to their pharmacist about a change in drug formulation.

Fast-Dissolving Disintegrant Systems

Fast-dissolving drug delivery systems are growing in popularity with patients. Drug manufacturers have been developing these products for years, and many new products have been recently introduced to the market. One such product is a fast-dissolving, freeze-dried tablet that dissolves on the tongue in seconds. Not only is the drug absorbed more quickly, but also no swallowing is necessary, so water is not required. According to Wilmington Pharmaceuticals, "75% of patients expressed a preference for the fast-dissolve formulation compared with a conventional tablet" (Wilmington Pharmaceuticals, 2011).

Another fast-dissolving product for *transmucosal* drug delivery takes the form of a thin film for oral administration. Such products often are marketed for patients who may have a choking hazard or difficulty swallowing (e.g., the elderly, pediatric patients, or patients with conditions that cause dysphagia, or difficulty swallowing). Oral film technology allows for delivery of the active ingredient to provide either a local effect or a systemic effect. In the future, this delivery system may extend to other mucosal routes, such as ocular, dermal, vaginal, or rectal sites.

Drugs are formulated in a particular way for a variety of reasons:

- *Aesthetics:* Manufacturers attempt to make drugs more visually appealing in color and shape.
- *Enteric coating:* An enteric coating allows the drug to travel from the stomach to the intestines or other absorption sites based on the pH level needed to dissolve the coating and allow disintegration of the tablet for absorption. An enteric coating also protects the stomach lining from a drug that might cause irritation, corrosion, and discomfort for the patient.
- *Sugar coating:* A sugar coating masks or improves the flavor of a tablet that otherwise would have an unpleasant taste.
- *Flavoring:* Drugs manufactured in chewable form generally are flavored to make the taste pleasant and palatable. Because of pH and other considerations, some flavors generally are designated for particular liquid products. Some manufacturers of drug flavoring products offer guidelines on their websites concerning the variety of flavors that best mask the taste of various drugs.

CAPSULES

Capsules are manufactured with either a soft or hard shell. In soft-shell capsules, the active drug ingredient has been dispersed in an oil or hydrophilic liquid. Soft-shell capsules usually are commercially made and generally are composed of a single structure (i.e., they cannot be entered without releasing the liquid contents). Hard-shell capsules act as a vehicle for the transport of a powder, granule particle, or very small tablets. The choice of a soft- or hard-shell capsule for a drug helps determine where the drug is absorbed and used by the body. Most soft-shell capsules are coated to prevent stomach acids from fully dissolving the capsule shell. This allows the capsule to be transported farther into the GI tract or to some other location, where the environmental pH allows the coating to be dissolved so that the contents may be absorbed and metabolized at the most appropriate site of action.

POWDERS AND CRYSTALS

Before compressor technology opened the door to the manufacture of solid tablets, drug ingredients were rolled into a crude tablet form or administered orally in powder form. Because of their often unpleasant bitter taste, most drugs are not supplied in powder form for direct oral administration anymore. Instead, a drug powder may be dispensed in a packet or pouch for dissolution in water. Many oral antibiotics prepared for administration to patients with limited swallowing capabilities (e.g., children and elderly patients) are packaged in powder form. When dispensed, a prescribed volume of water is added to the powder to create a liquid suspension, which may be administered by the patient. (The properties and administration methods of liquid drugs are addressed later in the chapter.)

Bulk fibers are also packaged as powders and must be added to water or juice for administration.

GRANULES

The granule drug dosage form is far more coarse than a powder form. Granules may be described as small, irregularly shaped, solid particles. Granules often are pressed into tablets for effervescent drug formulations. The granules generally contain sodium bicarbonate, as well as citric acid, tartaric acid, or sodium biphosphate, in addition to the active ingredients. The introduction of water creates an acid-base reaction, in which the sodium bicarbonate breaks down, and carbon dioxide is released as a by-product. This effervescent action allows for more rapid dissolution of the active ingredient. Often citrus flavoring is used to mask the otherwise bitter taste of most active ingredients. Many over-the-counter antacids and combination cold and flu products are manufactured in this dosage form.

SEMISOLID DOSAGE FORMS

Semisolid is the next most common drug dosage form. Semisolid drugs are too thick to be considered a liquid but are not fully solid. Semisolid drugs generally are formulated for external application. They may be applied to skin surfaces and the mucosa of the eye; they also may be given by certain routes of administration (e.g., nasal, rectal, vaginal). Semisolid dosage forms are actually oil and water dispersions. A dispersion is made through the mechanical mixture of oil-based compounds with water. Tiny droplets of water and oil are uniformly suspended, and neither component is fully dissolved.

Creams and Ointments

The percentage of oil to water determines whether a compound is considered a cream or an ointment. Generally, products with a higher percentage of water (50% or greater) are considered creams. Those with a high percentage of water and other liquid diluents may be considered lotions. Products that contain less than 50% water are generally considered ointments. Most ointments contain 80% oil and 20% water, and some may contain no water at all (anhydrous ointments). These products may or may not contain an active drug ingredient. Active drug ingredients (liquid , solid, or both) are uniformly incorporated into the cream or ointment base. The thickness of a product often defines how the product is used. Semisolid drug dosage forms may be used for any of the following:

- Skin protectant
  - These products are very thick so that they can remain on the surface of the skin to act as a barrier; they are not absorbed.
  - Skin protectants generally are referred to as *pastes* or *plasters.*
- Emollient
  - These products may be in cream or lotion form; they provide moisture that increases the skin's softness and pliability,
- Lubricant
  - These products are even less viscous; they specifically provide moisture and help ease discomfort or irritation caused by dryness in a particular area (e.g., the mouth, eyes, or vagina).
- Active drug delivery
  - Creams or ointments may contain an active ingredient that may provide either a local or a systemic effect.
  - Viscosity may determine the degree to which the ointment base is absorbed.

The U.S. Pharmacopoeia (USP) classifies ointment bases according to their use:

- Absorption bases
  - May be water-based or anhydrous and are designed for absorption through the epidermis
- Emulsions
  - These products are more water-soluble and may be removed with water alone.
- Oleaginous bases
  - These products contain hydrocarbons (petroleum-based products).
- Water-soluble bases
  - These products are mostly water-based and may be dissolved in and removed with water.

Suppositories

Suppositories are manufactured using absorption bases that are either solid or semisolid at room temperature. They are designed for administration by the rectal or vaginal route. After insertion, body temperature dissolves the bases and releases the active ingredients for absorption in these highly vascular areas. Depending on the base formulation, suppositories may need to be refrigerated for storage. Suppositories typically are manufactured or manually compounded in sizes appropriate for either an adult or a child.

SPECIALIZED SOLID DRUG DELIVERY SYSTEMS

A few drugs technically are considered solid drug dosage forms, because they do not exclusively involve liquid drug delivery. As are other solid dosage forms, these forms are a noninvasive vehicle through which active drug ingredients may be transported to the bloodstream.

- *Transdermal patch:* A transdermal patch delivers active drug ingredients through the skin to provide either a local or a systemic effect. The transdermal delivery system requires four key components:
  - External liner (packaging that protects the patch before placement)
  - Active drug ingredient
  - Adhesive (binds together the components of the patch and enables it to adhere to the skin)
  - Membrane (controls the release of the drug; it typically allows for a controlled, sustained release of the active drug ingredient)
- *Intranasal* or *oral inhaler:* The intranasal drug delivery system delivers either an aqueous or a dry-powder drug through a pressurized canister. A metered (measured) dose is dispensed in a fine mist, which is inhaled through the nostrils or orally into the lungs.
- *Ocular inserts:* Intraocular drug delivery systems use a relatively new polymer technology. The system functions in one of two ways: (1) the active drug ingredient is suspended in a polymer material to form a homogeneous solid unit, from which the active drug is transferred, or (2) the drug is placed in a reservoir and covered by a polymer membrane, through which the drug is uniformly released. The benefits of ocular polymeric systems include effective drug delivery, longer contact time for the drug in the cul-de-sac, and sustained drug action. This drug delivery system currently is used to treat dry eye, vascular diseases that affect the eye (e.g., glaucoma), and various eye infections.

ADVANTAGES AND DISADVANTAGES OF SOLID DOSAGE FORMS

Patients generally prefer oral solid dosage forms whenever possible, for the following reasons:

- Easy to store and transport
- Convenient for self-medication
- Largely devoid of taste and odor
- More stable than other solid dosage forms
- Predivided dosage forms that ensure an accurate dose
- Especially suited for drugs that are not stable in liquid form and therefore provide a longer shelf life for such drugs
- Better suited for sustained and delayed release of medication, because controlled-release techniques generally work better in solid than in liquid dosage forms

From a drug safety standpoint, oral solid dosage forms may be administered in any setting, and unless contaminated by touch, they carry minimal risk of introducing contaminants during administration. From a child safety standpoint, solid drug dosage forms must be dispensed in childproof packaging. Patients should be further cautioned to ensure that all prescription drugs be kept out of the reach of children, regardless of the drugs' packaging and place of storage.

Liquid Dosage Forms

The liquid dosage form offers some therapeutic advantages, particularly in the rate of drug delivery. Liquids may not always be the most convenient drug delivery system, because they generally require some instrument of measurement. Nonetheless, in many cases the liquid dosage form is the most clinically appropriate for a patient's needs. Figures 9-3 through 9-5 show various liquid drug delivery devices.

Drugs dispensed in liquid form may be administered by a variety of routes. The following are external routes of administration.

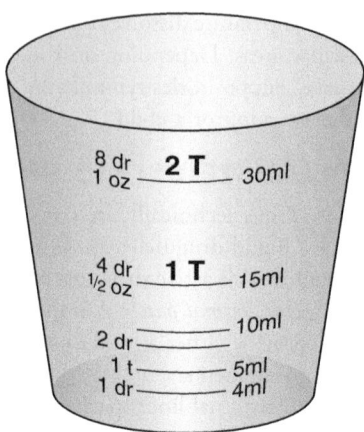

FIGURE 9-3 Medicine cup for liquid measurement. (From Kee JL, Marshall SM: *Clinical calculations,* ed 6, St Louis, 2009, Saunders.)

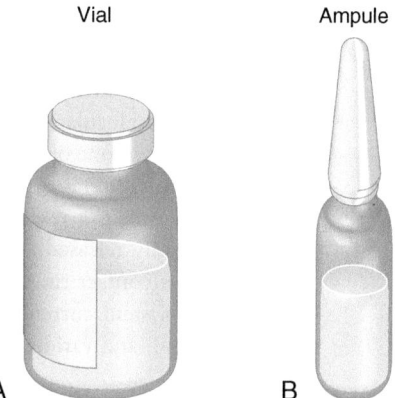

FIGURE 9-4 A, Vial. **B,** Ampule. (From Kee JL, Marshall SM: *Clinical calculations,* ed 6, Philadelphia, 2009, Saunders.)

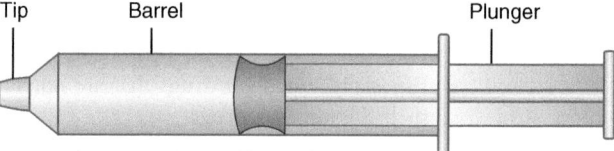

FIGURE 9-5 Parts of a syringe. (From Kee JL, Marshall SM: *Clinical calculations,* ed 6, Philadelphia, 2009, Saunders.)

- *Epicutaneous:* Used for medications that must be applied to the skin to treat superficial skin conditions (e.g., calamine lotion to treat itching and skin irritation from a rash or insect bite).
- *Otic:* Used for drugs instilled (administered) into the ear (e.g., antipyrine/benzocaine earwax flush solution).
- *Ophthalmic:* Used for drugs instilled into the eye or the conjunctival tissues of the eye (e.g., pilocarpine 4% to treat glaucoma).
- *Oral:* Used for drugs administered by mouth for swallowing or for absorption into the oral mucosa (e.g., liquid ibuprofen to relieve pain and inflammation).
- *Rectal:* Used for drugs that may be inserted or administered through the rectum (e.g., soap suds liquid enema for constipation).
- *Urethral:* Used for drugs that may be inserted or administered through the urethra (e.g., alprostadil to treat erectile dysfunction).

- *Vaginal:* Used for drugs that are inserted or administered through the vagina (e.g., miconazole or clotrimazole to treat vaginal candidiasis, a yeast infection).

PARENTERAL ROUTE

Many drugs, because of their chemical composition, are not designed for absorption in the stomach or intestines or are intended for immediate delivery. In such cases a variety of injectable routes of administration may be used. Parenteral drugs are injected (1) into or through the skin into the body or (2) into the bloodstream by means of an intravenous (IV) catheter or other sterile medical device. Drugs may be injected for a single dose of therapy or may be administered at set intervals for extended use (e.g., through a peripherally inserted central catheter [PICC]).

Injectable Sites of Administration (Figure 9-6)

The following are injectable routes of administration:

- *Percutaneous:* Used for drugs administered through the skin.
- *Intramuscular:* Used for drugs injected deep into muscle tissues, generally the deltoid or gluteus. Deltoid injections are 2 ml or less; gluteal injections are 5 ml or less.
- *Subcutaneous:* Used for drugs injected to deep layers of the skin but not into the muscle. Injections are 2 ml or less; no more than 1.3 ml is ideal.
- *Intradermal:* Used for drugs injected between the layers of the skin. Injections are 0.1 ml or less.
- *Epidural:* Used for drugs injected into the spinal cord, directly into the cerebrospinal fluid.
- *Intravenous:* Used for drugs administered into a vein.

A few specialized injection routes are designed for the administration of drugs to a specific local site.

- *Intrasynovial:* Used for drugs injected into the joints.
- *Intrathecal:* Used for drugs injected into the subdural space of the spinal cord.
- *Intraarticular:* Used for drugs injected into the space between joints.

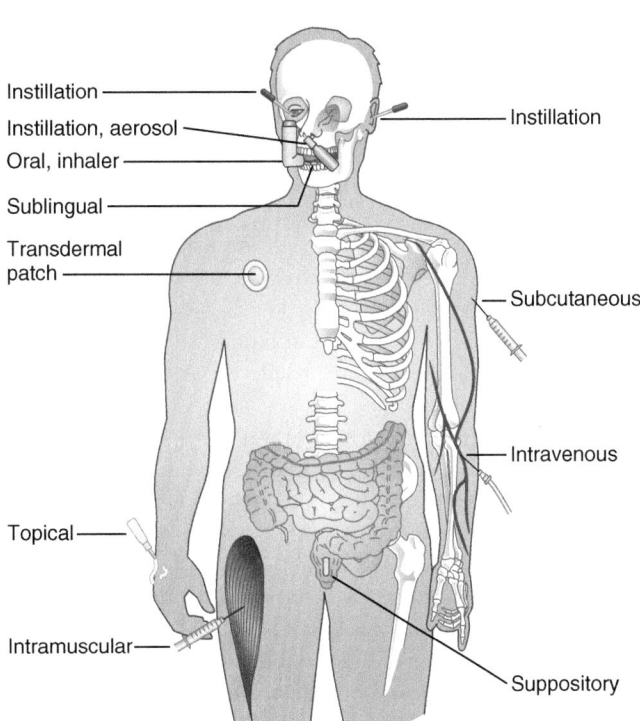

FIGURE 9-6 Some routes for medication administration. (From Kee JL, Hayes E, McCuistion L: *Pharmacology: a nursing process approach,* ed 6, Philadelphia, 2009, Saunders.)

ADVANTAGES AND DISADVANTAGES OF LIQUID DOSAGE FORMS

As mentioned, the liquid dosage forms have considerable therapeutic advantages:

- Rapid delivery to the site of action (no need for dissolution in the stomach or intestines)
- Ease of swallowing
- Ideal for drugs that cannot or should not be delivered orally (e.g., anesthetics)
- A more uniform dosage form

However, carrying a dose of liquid medication in a purse or pocket presents a challenge. The following are other disadvantages of the liquid dosage forms.

- Rapid delivery to the vascular system poses a greater danger if the wrong drug or incorrect dose is administered.
- A measuring device is required to deliver the correct dose safely; this may be inconvenient.
- Storage requirements may be less convenient (e.g., a liquid drug may require refrigeration to maintain its physical or chemical stability).
- Currently, oral formulations present flavoring problems, particularly with the ability of various flavors to mask an unpleasant taste.
- If it does not contain a preservative, a liquid drug may act as a reservoir or vehicle for bacteria; also, it may contain ingredients (e.g., sugar) that create ideal conditions for bacterial growth.

Chapter Summary

- A *drug delivery system* is a device used to administer a drug. It is also a physical characteristic or the makeup of a drug that affects the way the body breaks down or metabolizes the drug.
- The means by which a drug is delivered into the body is the *route of administration.*
- A drug's effect on the body must be taken into consideration when selecting the most appropriate route of administration.
- Pharmacy technicians who are knowledgeable about the most therapeutically appropriate use of various drug delivery systems are more alert to possible errors in drug prescribing, order entry, or fill processes.
- Medications cause two basic bodily responses: drugs applied externally have local action, and drugs that must be transported via the bloodstream and metabolized (broken down and converted) into cellular building blocks by the liver or other system elicit systemic action.
- Medication may be manufactured or compounded in several dosage forms, including solid (tablets, capsules, powders, and crystals), liquid, semisolid (lotions, ointments, creams, suppositories, pastes and plasters, and a few specialized forms).
- Pharmacy technicians should always make sure oral solid form drugs are packaged with all the information necessary for safe administration.
- The percentage of oil to water determines whether a compound is considered a cream or an ointment.
- The thickness of a cream or ointment often determines the product's use.
- Semisolid drug dosage forms may be used for skin protectants, emollients, lubricants, or active drug delivery.
- Drugs dispensed in liquid form may be administered by a variety of routes. External routes of administration include the epicutaneous, otic, ophthalmic, oral, rectal, urethral, and vaginal routes.
- Some advantages of solid dosage forms are that they are easy to store and transport; they have a longer shelf life; and they are convenient for self-medication.
- Parenteral drugs are injected (1) into or through the skin into the body or (2) into the bloodstream through an IV catheter or other sterile medical device.
- The most common injectable routes of administration are the percutaneous, intramuscular, subcutaneous, intradermal, epidural, and intravenous routes.
- Some advantages of liquid dosage forms include rapid delivery to the site of action; ease of swallowing; ideal form for drugs that cannot or should not be delivered orally (e.g., anesthetics); and a more uniform dosage form.
- Disadvantages of liquid dosage forms include the danger of rapid delivery to the vascular system if the wrong drug or incorrect dose is administered; the need for a measuring device to deliver the correct dose safely; less convenient storage requirements; flavoring challenges for oral

formulations; the risk that liquid drugs that do not contain preservatives may act as a reservoir or vehicle for bacteria and may contain ingredients (e.g., sugar) that create ideal conditions for bacterial growth; and the presence of preservatives in some liquid drugs, which may restrict their use in certain patients or prevent administration by certain routes.

REVIEW QUESTIONS

Multiple Choice

1. A drug administered by which route acts directly on the central nervous system (brain) before delivery to the blood plasma?
   a. Intradermal
   b. Inhalation
   c. Intrathecal
   d. Oral

2. This drug dosage form must undergo dissolution before absorption.
   a. Intravenous
   b. Oral
   c. Rectal
   d. B and C

3. This oral dosage form should be held between the cheek and gum for slow dissolution and absorption.
   a. Lozenge
   b. Troche
   c. Sublingual
   d. Buccal

4. This drug dosage form may be dispensed in a packet for dissolution in water.
   a. Capsule
   b. Tablet
   c. Powder
   d. Pellet

5. This solid drug ingredient adds bulk to a tablet.
   a. Diluent
   b. Disintegrant
   c. Binder
   d. Excipient

6. The semisolid drug form with the highest percentage of water is a(n):
   a. Cream
   b. Ointment
   c. Paste
   d. Lotion

7. According to the USP classification, this type of ointment base contains hydrocarbons.
   a. Emulsions
   b. Oleaginous
   c. Water soluble
   d. Absorption

8. This specialty delivery system releases drug through a membrane for absorption.
   a. Pastille
   b. Transdermal
   c. Ocular insert
   d. B and C

9. A 3-ml injection is most appropriately given by which route of administration?
   a. Subcutaneous
   b. Epicutaneous
   c. Intramuscular to the deltoid
   d. Intramuscular to the gluteus

10. A 0.1-ml allergy test injection may be administered:
    a. Subcutaneously
    b. Intradermally
    c. Intravenously
    d. Epidurally

TECHNICIAN'S
CORNER

1. What types of patient-specific factors might be taken into consideration in prescribing a drug dosage form?
2. The suppository dosage form poses what serious risk?
3. What storage considerations apply to liquid dosage forms?

Bibliography

Boradia, S. (2008, March 28). *Oral Film Technology: Quick Dissolving Films—A Novel Approach to Drug Delivery.* Retrieved 6/9/2011, from www.drugdeliverytech.com/ME2/dirmod.asp?sid=&nm=&type=Publishing&mod=Publications%3A%3AArticle&mid=8F3A7027421841978F18BE895F87F791&tier=4&id=1462E9E570724362AF256AB9CEC63126

Ford-Martin, PA. (2011). *Drug Metabolism/interactions.* Retrieved 6/9/2011, from www.healthline.com/galecontent/drug-metabolism-interactions

Gilhotra, R. (2009, April 5). *Polymeric Systems for Ocular Inserts.* Retrieved 6/9/2011, from www.pharmainfo.net/reviews/polymeric-systems-ocular-inserts

Integrated Publishing. (2011). Retrieved 6/15/2011, from www.tpub.com/content/armymedical/MD0809/MD08090092.htm

Orphardt, C. (2003). *Introduction to Drug Action.* Retrieved 4/22/2011, from www.elmhurst.edu/~chm/vchembook/650drugs.html

Pharmacorama. (2011). *Routes of Drug Administration.* Retrieved 6/9/2011, from www.pharmacorama.com/en/Sections/Pharmacokinetics-5.php

Vitamist Spray Vitamins. (2011). *Things to Know: Real Facts about Nutrition.* Retrieved 6/9/2011, from www.vitamist.com/Articles.asp?ID=137&?Click=3634

Wilmington Pharmaceuticals. (2011). *What Is Fast Dissolve?* Retrieved 6/9/2011, from www.wilmingtonpharma.com/what-is-fast-dissolve/

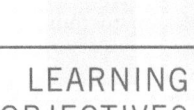

10 Pharmaceutical Calculations

Rick Leyva and LiAnne Webster

LEARNING OBJECTIVES

By the end of this chapter, students will be able to competently:

1. Solve computations using addition, subtraction, multiplication, and division.
2. Solve computations involving weight and volume.
3. Convert between the three main systems of pharmaceutical measurement: the household, metric, and apothecary systems.
4. Calculate prescription quantities and the number of days supply to be dispensed.
5. Make dosage calculations using ratio and proportion.
6. Perform the basic calculations necessary to prepare a weight-to-weight, weight-to-volume and volume-to-volume solution.
7. Use Clark's rule, Young's rule, Fried's rule, and the BSA rule to calculate pediatric medication doses.
8. Calculate the correct drip rate for intravenous (IV) admixtures to deliver the appropriate amount of drug and/or fluid prescribed.
9. Solve pharmaceutical calculations using ratio strength or percentage to prepare compounds or admixtures.
10. Perform pharmaceutical calculations that require conversion between Fahrenheit and Celsius (Centigrade) temperatures.

KEY TERMS

AWP: Average wholesale price.

Fraction: A part of a whole.

Gross profit: The total profit gained from a sale (the selling price minus the purchase price).

Improper fraction: A fraction in which the numerator is larger than the denominator (e.g., $\frac{8}{5}$).

Markup: The selling price minus the purchase price; the cost to purchase.

Markup rate: The markup divided by the cost.

Mixed fraction: A combination of a whole number and a proper fraction (e.g., $2\frac{1}{4}$).

Net profit: The total profit minus the overhead (the selling price minus all costs, including overhead).

Overhead: The costs of doing business (e.g., salaries, rent, taxes).

Proper fraction: A fraction in which the numerator is smaller than the denominator (e.g., $\frac{3}{5}$).

Proportion: The relationship between two ratios (e.g., $\frac{3}{4} = \frac{75}{100}$).

Ratio: A comparison of part of a whole, similar to a fraction (e.g., $2:5$).

Skill, accuracy, and confidence in performing pharmaceutical mathematics are a basic requirements for all pharmacy technicians. The ability to perform a calculation or measure a dose accurately directly affects patients' health and safety. Every precaution must be taken to minimize the chance of human error during dosage calculations. Therefore, in most community pharmacies, many of the calculations are performed electronically by the pharmacy order entry management system. However, this usually is not the case with pharmaceutical compounding. Both sterile and nonsterile compounding generally require the calculation of dosages or quantities.

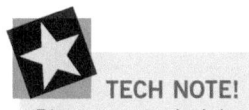

Pharmaceutical calculations are grounded in the six rights of medication (right patient, right drug, right dose, right route, right time, and right documentation). Administration, specifically the *right dose* at the *right time* (because intervals between doses may also be calculated manually).

The competencies covered in this chapter are crucial to the pharmacy technician's effectiveness in protecting patients' safety and health. They also account for a large percentage of the questions on national certification examinations.

Arithmetic Review: Basic Mathematical Operations

Most pharmacy math calculations, whether simple or complex, can be solved if the technician knows how to set up the problem or equation properly. The most common mistakes are caused by improper setup. For this reason, this chapter begins with basic concepts and works up to more complex equations.

FRACTIONS

In the simplest terms, a fraction can be defined as a part of a whole. For example, if you have one tablet and must break it in half (into two equal pieces), each part is half of the whole:

$$1 \div 2 = \tfrac{1}{2}, \text{ or half of the whole}$$

A fraction is composed of two parts, the numerator and the denominator. The numerator is the top part of the fraction, which defines the number of parts you have, and the denominator is the bottom part of the fraction, which defines how many parts make a whole. In the previous example, the tablet is broken in half. Therefore, the fraction $\tfrac{1}{2}$ tells us we have 1 part and that 2 parts make up the whole tablet.

Example 1
A patient is to take 125 mg of a medication. The medication on hand is 500 mg. If the medication on hand is to be used, what part must be given to the patient?

Step 1: 125 mg is the part to be administered, and 500 mg is the whole; therefore, the fraction is:

$$\frac{125}{500}$$

Step 2: Fractions should always be reduced. The fraction $^{125}\!/_{500}$ is an unreduced fraction, meaning the fraction can be reduced by dividing the numerator and denominator by the same number. 125 and 500 can both be divided by (and therefore reduced by) 125.

$$125 \div 125 = 1, \text{ and } 500 \div 125 = 4$$

$$\text{Therefore, the reduced fraction of } \frac{125}{500} = \frac{1}{4}$$

Because both the numerator and denominator cannot be further reduced by the same whole number, we can state that the fraction is reduced.

Types of fractions:
- Proper fraction: A fraction in which the numerator is smaller than the denominator (e.g., 3/5).
- Improper fraction: A fraction in which the numerator is larger than the denominator (e.g., 8/5).
- Mixed fraction: A fraction that contains a whole number and a proper fraction (e.g., $2\tfrac{1}{4}$). When solving problems that contain a mixed fraction, the mixed fraction must be converted to an improper fraction.

Example 2
Convert $2\tfrac{1}{4}$ into an improper fraction.

Step 1: Multiply the denominator by the whole number: $4 \times 2 = 8$.
Step 2: Add the numerator to the number obtained in step 1: $8 + 1 = 9$.
Step 3: Put the answer you calculated in step 2 over the original denominator.
Solution: $\tfrac{9}{4}$

Example 3

Convert $\frac{9}{4}$ back to a mixed fraction.

Step 1: Divide the numerator by the denominator: $9 \div 4$; 4 goes into 9 twice, so the whole number is 2 and the remainder is 1.

Step 2: Put the remainder over the original denominator: $\frac{1}{4}$.

Solution: $2\frac{1}{4}$

Adding and Subtracting Fractions

To add or subtract fractions:

1. Find the lowest common denominator. For example, for the fractions $\frac{1}{2}$ and $\frac{1}{4}$, the lowest common denominator is 4.
2. Multiply the first fraction (both numerator and denominator) by 2, so that the two fractions have the same denominator: $\frac{1}{2}$ becomes $\frac{2}{4}$.
3. Add or subtract the numerators. The denominators always remain the same: if adding, the solution would be $\frac{3}{4}$; if subtracting, the solution would be $\frac{1}{4}$.
4. Reduce the answer to the lowest terms.

Example 4

Add $\frac{1}{3}$ and $\frac{1}{4}$: ($\frac{1}{3} + \frac{1}{4}$).

Step 1: Find lowest common denominator. To find it for 3 and 4, multiply the first fraction (both numerator and denominator) by the denominator of the second fraction and then do the same to the second fraction (multiply the numerator and denominator by the denominator of the first fraction): $\frac{4}{12} + \frac{3}{12}$.

Step 2: Add the fractions. Remember, only the numerator changes; the denominator stays the same: $\frac{7}{12}$.

Step 3: Reduce answer. Because this answer is already in its lowest terms, the problem is complete.

To subtract $\frac{1}{4}$ from $\frac{1}{3}$:

  a. Find the lowest common denominator, as in step 1: $\frac{4}{12} - \frac{3}{12}$
  b. Subtract only the numerators; the denominators stay the same: $4 - 3 = 1$.

Solution: $\frac{4}{12} - \frac{3}{12} = \frac{1}{12}$

Multiplying and Dividing Fractions

To divide fractions:

1. To divide fractions, switch the numerator and denominator of the second fraction (the fraction that results is known as the *reciprocal* of the first fraction).
2. Multiply the numerators.
3. Multiply the denominators.
4. Reduce the answer to its lowest terms.

Example 5

Divide $\frac{8}{9}$ by $\frac{2}{5}$: $\frac{8}{9} \div \frac{2}{5}$.

Step 1: Since this is a division problem, switch the numerator and denominator of the second fraction: $\frac{2}{5}$ becomes $\frac{5}{2}$

Step 2: $8 \times 5 = 40$

Step 3: $9 \times 2 = 18$, so the final fraction is $\frac{40}{18}$

Step 4: Reduce answer: 40 and 18 can both be divided by 2:

Solution: $\frac{20}{9}$

To multiply fractions:

1. Multiply the numerators.
2. Multiply the denominators.
3. Reduce the answer to its lowest terms.

Example 6

Multiply $\frac{5}{6}$ by $\frac{3}{4}$: $\frac{5}{6} \times \frac{3}{4}$.

Step 1: 5×3 = 15
Step 2: 6×4 = 24, the fraction becomes $^{15}\!/_{24}$
Step 3: Reduce answer: 15 and 24 can both be divided by 3:
Solution: $^{5}\!/_{8}$

DECIMALS

Medication orders are most commonly written as decimals.

Converting Fractions to Decimals

To convert a fraction to a decimal, divide the numerator by the denominator. For the fraction $^{2}\!/_{5}$, this would be 2 ÷ 5.

$$2 ÷ 5 = 0.4$$

Converting Decimals to Fractions

1. Move the decimal two places to the right: 0.4 = 40
2. Place the new number over 100: $^{40}\!/_{100}$
3. Reduce the fraction its lowest terms: $^{40}\!/_{100} = {}^{4}\!/_{10} = {}^{2}\!/_{5}$.

Example 7
Convert $1\frac{1}{2}$ to decimal form.
Step 1: Convert the mixed fraction to an improper fraction: $1\frac{1}{2} = \frac{3}{2}$
Step 2: Divide the numerator by the denominator: 3 ÷ 2 = 1.5
Solution: 1.5

Adding and Subtracting Decimals

When adding or subtracting decimals, the decimals in each number must be aligned and carried down. Once the equation has been set up properly, add or subtract.

Example 8
Add: 2.14 + 6.8 + 12.833
Step 1: Align the numbers by decimal point:

$$
\begin{array}{r}
2.14 \\
6.8 \\
+\,12.833 \\
\end{array}
$$

(Hint: It may help to add 0s as placeholders.)
Step 2: Add the numbers.

$$
\begin{array}{r}
02.140 \\
06.800 \\
+\,12.833 \\
\end{array}
$$

Solution: 21.773
  Follow the same steps when subtracting decimals.

Multiplying and Dividing Decimals

With decimals, multiply and divide the numbers as you would normally. The decimal points do not need to be aligned. However, you must move the decimal point one place for each number that is to the right of the decimal for each of the numbers being multiplied or divided.
To divide decimals:
1. Set up the equation properly.
2. Remove the decimal by moving the decimal point in the divisor (the number that is being divided *into*) to the right, counting how many places it is moved.
3. The decimal point in the dividend (the original number that is going to be divided) must be moved the same number of places to the right.

4. Set up the numbers in a traditional division format and move the decimal point up to the same position in the quotient. Solve.

Example 9
Divide: 2.25 into 0.5
Step 1: 2.25 ÷ 0.5.
Step 2: The divisor is 0.5. The decimal point is moved only one place: 5
Step 3: The decimal point in the dividend 2.25 is moved one place to the right, changing the number to 22.5.
Step 4: $5\overline{)22.5}$

Solution: 4.5

PERCENTAGES

Fractions and decimals are commonly written as percentages to describe the strength of a medication.

Converting Fractions to Percentages

To convert a fraction to a percentage:
1. Find the decimal conversion.
2. Multiply the decimal by 100 (move decimal two places to the right).

Example 10
Convert ⅓ to a percentage.
Step 1: Divide 1 by 3: 1 ÷ 3 = 0.333.
Step 2: 0.333 × 100 = 33.3.
Solution: 33.3%. To convert a percentage to a fraction, remember that a number presented as a percentage is to be interpreted as part of 100.

Example 11
Convert 45% to a fraction.

Solution: $\dfrac{45}{100}$. To express $\dfrac{45}{100}$ as a decimal, simply move the decimal point 2 places to the left. $\dfrac{45}{100}$ would be 0.45 in decimal form.

RATIOS AND PROPORTIONS

Most dosage calculations performed by pharmacy technicians can be done using the ratio/proportion calculation method. Most often a conversion must be performed to find the correct strength of medication to administer or to find the dosage to be given. When a formula is not required, setting up the equation into ratios helps in finding the answer.

A ratio expression is a comparison of part of a whole, similar to a fraction. The ratio usually consists of two numbers: the first number is a part, and the second number is the total amount.

Ratio setup: a : b

For example, if a patient is prescribed 2 tablets of amoxicillin, and each tablet has 250 mg of medication, the ratio would be:

500 mg : 2 tablets, or 500 mg/2 tablets

The ratio can be written side by side, connected by a colon (:) or as a fraction.
This ratio tells us that 500 mg of medication are contained in 2 tablets.

Example 12
A 120-ml bottle of medication contains 1,250 mg of active ingredient. Write this as a ratio.
Step 1: Set up the ratio by first selecting the number that contains a part of the whole: 1,250 mg.

Step 2: Write the ratio expression: 1,250 mg: 120 ml, or 1,250 mg/120 ml.

A proportion is the relationship between two ratios. The two ratios in the proportion are unique because they are equal.

Proportion setup: a : b = c : d

Are these two ratios equal: 5 mg: 1 ml = 10 mg: 2 ml? To find out:
1. Multiply the two outer numbers, known as the *extremes:* $5 \times 2 = 10$
2. Multiply the two inner numbers, called the *means:* $1 \times 10 = 10$
3. $10 = 10$, therefore the two ratios are equal.

Another way to solve this problem is to set up the ratios as fractions and then cross-multiply:

a. $$\dfrac{5\ mg}{1\ mg} \diagup\!\!\!\diagdown \dfrac{10\ mg}{2\ ml}$$

b. $5 \times 2 = 10$; $1 \times 10 = 10$

Solution: $10 = 10$, therefore the ratio proportions are equal.

Example 13

If a patient takes 1 tablet of a certain medication, she will receive 150 mg of the active ingredient. If the patient is prescribed 6 tablets daily, how much total active ingredient will she be receiving in 1 day?

Step 1: Begin by creating the first ratio. This ratio should consist of the "known," or the information that has been given. In this case, the known is that a patient will receive 150 mg in 1 tablet:

150 mg : 1 tablet = ? : ?

Step 2: Create the second ratio, setting it up the exact way the first one was set up:

150 mg : 1 tablet = x mg : 6 tablets

x is added in front of the milligrams because the question is how much medication (the unknown) a patient will receive by taking 6 tablets.

Step 3: Solve for *x:*
a. Multiply the extremes: $150 \times 6 = 900$.
b. Multiply the means: $1 \times x = x$.
c. Set up the equation: $900 = x$; the answer is 900 mg.

Solution: The patient will take 900 mg of medication in 1 day.

Conversions Between Systems of Measurement

Pharmacy calculations often involve multiple systems of measurement. Although a prescriber may write a prescription for a drug quantity using a metric measurement, the patient may more easily recognize a household measurement. For example, a pediatric medication dose of 5 milliliters (ml) is equal to the household measurement of 1 teaspoon.

Pharmacy technicians must be knowledgeable about various systems of measurement and the equivalencies among systems. Conversion between various systems of measurement is essential to the order entry and medication fill process; units must be converted based on directions to be provided to the patient or to fill a prescription order based on what is on hand or in stock. The metric system of measurement is used most frequently in both community and hospital pharmacies, although apothecary measurement may be used in a few cases. The most important factor in metric conversions is placement of the decimal point. Misplacement can kill patients—it is that serious.

FLUID MEASURE

Fluid volume measurement is the metric measurement most commonly used. The basic standard unit for fluid measurement is the liter, which is the fluid's volume occupied by 1 kilogram of water at its temperature of greatest density. Any other unit used is a multiple of a liter or a fraction of a liter:

- Liter: One liter, expressed as 1 L
- *Deci*-liter: One tenth of a liter, expressed as 0.1 L

TABLE 10-1   **Systems of Fluid Measurement**

Apothecary	Metric	Household
5 ml	5 ml	1 tsp.
15 ml	15 ml	1 tbsp.
29.57 ml	29.57 ml	1 fl. oz.
473 ml	473 ml	1 pt.
3,785 ml	3,785 ml	1 gal.

fl. oz., Fluid ounce; *gal.*, gallon; *pt.*, pint; *tbsp.*, tablespoon; *tsp.* teaspoon.

- *Centi*-liter: One hundredth of a liter, expressed as 0.01 L
- *Milli*-liter: One thousandth of a liter, expressed as 0.001 L or 1 ml

Table 10-1 presents the fluid volume measurements with which pharmacy technicians must be familiar and the common equivalencies in other systems of measurement.

Example 14
A patient is to be dispensed 12 fluid ounces of a liquid suspension; how many teaspoons would this be?

Step 1: Set up the ratio proportion to first determine how many milliliters are in 12 fluid ounces (fl. oz.).

$$\frac{1 \text{ fl oz}}{30 \text{ ml}} = \frac{12 \text{ fl oz}}{x \text{ ml}}$$

Step 2: Cross-multiply:

$$29.57 \times 12 = 1x$$
$$x = 354.84 \text{ ml}$$

The entire volume of suspension is equal to 354.84 ml.

Step 3: Set up the ratio proportion to determine how many teaspoons there are in the entire volume of suspension.

$$\frac{1 \text{ tsp}}{5 \text{ ml}} = \frac{x \text{ tsp}}{354.84 \text{ ml}}$$

Step 4: Cross-multiply:

$$5x = 354.84$$
$$354.84 \div 5 = 70.968$$

Because teaspoons are a fixed unit of measurement, we may round to the nearest whole number: 71.

Solution: There are about 71 teaspoons of suspension in 12 fluid ounces of solution.

RULES OF ROUNDING
Pharmaceutical dosage calculation must be precise, and rounding can be a very sensitive subject in the performance of pharmaceutical calculations. It is important to recognize that tenths or hundredths of a weight or volume measure constitute a quantity of drug that must be taken into consideration. The drug itself and the patient who will be receiving it are the two factors that generally determine whether rounding a number is appropriate. The best rule of thumb is: Do not round until the very end of the calculation, and even then, round only when necessary to allow for the most accurate measurement of the medication dose.

Example 15
A patient must receive 18 fl. oz. of an oral solution.

TECH ALERT!
Do not round until the very end of the calculation; even then, round only when necessary to allow for the most accurate measurement of the medication dose.

TABLE 10-2 **Systems of Weight Measurement**

Apothecary	Avoirdupois	Metric	Household
1 gr		65 mg	
5 gr		325 mg*	
12 oz	16 oz		1 lb
		1 kg (1,000 g)	2.2 lb
		1 g = 1,000 mg 1 mg = 1,000 mcg	
	1 oz	28.35 g	
	454 g		1 lb

If we rounded to 30 ml instead of dispensing the actual metric volume of 29.57 ml, the patient would be dispensed 540 ml of solution instead of 532.26 ml. This may not seem to be a huge difference; however, if the patient takes 1 teaspoon of medication at a time, that extra volume accounts for nearly two extra doses that the patient may take and should not.

Rounding can make a difference with weight measurement in particular. The metric ounce weight measurement is 28.35 g (Table 10-2)—not 28 g, not 29 g. Referring to the patient in the preceding example, if the patient is to be dispensed an external cream that contains 18 oz of an active ingredient, the actual amount of active drug the pharmacy technician must weigh out is 510.3 g. However, if the technician rounds the metric ounce weight measurement to 29, the amount of active ingredient measured out will be 522 g, a difference of 11.7 g of active ingredient. Depending on the active ingredient, that could mean the difference between a safe drug preparation and an unsafe one.

Tenths of a drug add up; therefore, do not round during dosage calculation! Round only on the final dispensing quantity, and then only when necessary for accurate measurement purposes.

USING DIMENSIONAL ANALYSIS CALCULATION TO SOLVE RATIO PROPORTIONS

Dimensional analysis is a form of comparing conversion ratios that involve several units of measure. Rather than having to set up several ratios and proportions, one dimensional analysis may be set up to help cancel out factors and arrive at the solution.

Example 16

Perhaps you want to know how many grains of acetaminophen are needed to compound 1 pound (lb) of acetaminophen suppositories. Dimensional analysis can be used to answer this question. Using the information in Table 10-2, always start with the units on top and bottom that you will need to find the solution; then position the other proportions in a way that allows you to cancel out like units of measure along the way. Units in a dimensional analysis may be "canceled out" by reducing them to a unit of 1.

Step 1: Set up the ratio of what you need to know.

$$\frac{x \text{ grains}}{1 \text{ lb}}$$

Step 2: You know that 1 lb = 454 g. You also know that 1 grain = 65 mg. That is all you need to set up your dimensional analysis:

$$\frac{x \text{ grains}}{1 \text{ lb}} = \frac{1 \text{ lb}}{454 \text{ g}} = \frac{65 \text{ mg}}{1 \text{ grain}}$$

Step 3: You must make sure that you have **like units** to reduce and cancel them out; therefore, either the grams need to be converted to milligrams, or the milligrams need to be converted to grams. Because the unit of measurement for grains is expressed in milligrams, converting all metric units to milligrams is a necessary step. 1 g = 1,000 mg; therefore, 454 g can be converted to 454,000 mg.

$$\frac{x \text{ grains}}{1 \text{ lb}} = \frac{1 \text{ lb}}{454,000 \text{ mg}} = \frac{65 \text{ mg}}{1 \text{ grain}}$$

The grain and pound measures are already reduced to units of 1. All that is left is the milligram units. To reduce 65 mg to 1, you must divide it by itself; therefore, you would also divide 454,000 by 65.

$$454,000 \div 65 = 6,984.615 \text{ (you can round this measurement)}$$

Solution: There are 6,984.62 grains of acetaminophen in 1 lb.

Example 17

If you needed to know how many 325-mg tablets of acetaminophen would be needed for this formulation, you would perform the following calculation.

Step 1: Set up the dimensional analysis proportions:

$$\frac{x \text{ tablets}}{6,984.62 \text{ grains}} = \frac{325 \text{ mg}}{1 \text{ tablet}} = \frac{1 \text{ grain}}{65 \text{ mg}}$$

Step 2: Cancel out the milligrams: 325 ÷ 65 = 5.
Step 3: Divide 6,984.62 by 5 = 1,396.92. Because tablets can be measured only by unit, you can round to the nearest whole number.
Solution: 1,397 tablets of acetaminophen would be needed to compound 1 lb of suppositories.

ROMAN NUMERALS

Roman numerals are commonly used in pharmacy to prevent confusion (Table 10-3). The following are rules for converting Roman numerals:
Rule 1: Add the numerals when the numeral on the left is larger than the numeral on the right: VI = 6 (only for I, X, and C).
Rule 2: Subtract the numerals when the numeral on the left is smaller than the numeral on the right: iv = 4 (only for I, X, and C)
Rule 3: A numeral can be repeated consecutively only three times: iii = 3 (V, L, and D are not repeated).
Rule 4: Only one smaller numeral can be used before a larger numeral.

Example 18

Convert 14 to a Roman numeral.
Step 1: Find the closest Roman numeral conversion: X, or 10, is the closest to 14.
Step 2: Find the Roman numeral that can be added to the first to get the answer: 5 is the closest.
Step 3: Add other Roman numerals as needed: XV is 15; to obtain 14, place I between X and V. (Recall the rule: a smaller numeral to the left of a larger numeral is subtracted from the larger numeral: IV = 4.)
Solution: The answer is XIV.

TABLE 10-3 **Roman Numerals**

Roman numeral	Numeric value	Roman numeral	Numeric value
I or i	1	C or c	100
V or v	5	D or d	500
X or x	10	M or m	1,000
L or l	50		

Example 19
Convert XIX into Arabic numerals.
Step 1: The first letter is X; therefore, 10 is the first conversion.
Step 2: The second and third conversions are 1 and 10; therefore, you have 10, 1, and 10.
Step 3: The second number, 1, is smaller than the third, 10; subtract 1 from 10.
Step 4: 10 + 9 = 19.
Solution: 19

CALCULATION OF TIME AND DOSING INTERVALS

For prescription purposes, time is written in military time (i.e., according to a 24-hour clock). This prevents confusion and time misinterpretation. For example, a prescription may read, "Take 2 tablets at 8:00." The patient does not know whether the prescriber means 8 AM or 8 PM. This common mistake can be corrected by using military time. Military time begins at 12 AM (written as 2400), continues to 1 AM (0100), and on through the number system for a 24-hour period, ending at 2400 hours (12 AM).

Example 20
Convert 3 PM to military time.
Solution: Begin with 1200 midday and count to 3 PM: The answer is 1500.

CALCULATING TEMPERATURE FOR DRUG STABILITY

Temperature affects the physical and chemical stability of medications. A critical task of the pharmacy technician, in both community and hospital pharmacies, is to check and log refrigerator temperatures, to ensure that products in the refrigerator are stored within the appropriate temperature range. Some medications, such as insulin, must be stored at certain temperatures. Depending on the medication and the measuring device, the required temperature may be stated or measured in Fahrenheit or Celsius (Centigrade). Pharmacy technicians should be familiar with the equivalents between these two systems.

Fahrenheit and Celsius (Centigrade) Standards
- Water boils at 212° Fahrenheit (F) and at 100° Celsius (C).
- Water freezes at 32°F and at 0°C.
  For the Fahrenheit and Celsius temperature scales, there is a difference in:
  - The boiling point of water: 100 : 180, or $\frac{5}{9}$
  - The freezing point of water: °F − 32
  Therefore, the formula for converting from Fahrenheit to Celsius is: °C = 5/9 × (°F − 32)
  However, the most frequently used formula for conversion is: °C = °F − 32/1.8
  The formula for converting Celsius to Fahrenheit is: °F = 9 × °C/5 + 32

Applying Temperature Conversion Formulas
Example 21
Convert 165° F to Celsius.
Step 1: Insert the Fahrenheit degrees to the formula:

$$°C = 165 \; °F − 32 / 1.8$$

Step 2: Solve the equation.
Solution: 165°F = 73.9°C

Example 22
Convert 40°C to Fahrenheit.
Step 1: Insert the Celsius degrees to the formula: °F = [(9 × 40) ÷ 5] + 32.
Step 2: Solve the equation.
Solution: 40°C = 104°F

Metric System

In pharmacy practice two units of the metric system are used: weight and volume. Weight is used to describe a medication's strength; the primary unit of weight measurement in the metric system is the gram. When medications are given in a solid form, such as a tablet or capsule, the strength is the amount of medication in each dose. A patient may be prescribed 250 mg of a medication; this means the patient will be receiving 250 mg of the medication in each dose.

Example 23

For a 25-year-old man, a physician prescribes 375 mg of a medication to be taken three times a day. How much total medication, in milligrams, will the patient take in 1 day? That is, if each dose contains 375 mg of medication, how much medication is provided in three doses?

Step 1: Use the proportion method to set up the problem: 375 mg: 1 dose = x mg: 3 doses

Step 2: Multiply the extremes: $375 \times 3 = 1{,}125$.

Step 3: Multiply the means: $1 \times x = x$.

Solution: $x = 1{,}125$; three doses contain a total of 1,125 mg of medication

Medication can also be administered in liquid form; the measurement for liquids in the metric system is volume, most commonly *milliliters* (ml). For example, the available strength of amoxicillin in liquid form is 250 mg per 5 ml. This means that if a patient is given 5 ml of medication, he will receive 250 mg of amoxicillin.

Example 24

Amoxicillin 125 mg/5 ml is prescribed for a 9-year-old child. The dosage is 10 ml per dose. How much amoxicillin is to be given in a single dose? That is, if each 5 ml contains 125 mg, then how many milligrams are there in 10 ml? You can use the method of proportion to set this up.

Step 1: Set up the proportion: 125 mg: 5 ml = x mg: 10 ml.

Step 2: Multiply the extremes: $125 \times 10 = 1{,}250$.

Step 3: Multiply the means: $5 \times x = 5x$.

Step 4: Solve for x: $x = 1250 \div 5 = 250$.

Solution: The child will receive 250 mg of amoxicillin when given a 10-ml dose.

METRIC SYSTEM CONVERSIONS

The metric system is the most commonly used form of measurement in pharmacy practice. To convert metric units, the decimal is moved in units of 10.

Weight Conversions

The basic unit of measurement in the metric system is the gram for weight and the liter for volume. However, simple conversions are often required. Use Table 10-4 when converting grams.

Conversion Rules

Rule 1: When converting by moving from left to right: increase the number by adding a zero for each move.

Rule 2: When converting by moving from right to left: reduce the number by moving the decimal point one place to the right for each move.

TABLE 10-4 **Converting Grams**

	Kilogram	Hectogram	Gram	Centigram	Milligram	Microgram
Abbreviation	kg	hg	g	cg	mg	mcg
Conversion	1,000 g	100 g	1	0.01	0.001	0.000001

TABLE 10-5 **Converting Liters**

	Liter
Abbreviation	L or l
Conversion	1,000 ml

Example 25
Convert 10 g to milligrams.
Solution: As Table 10-4 shows, 1 mg equals 0.001 of a gram; therefore, add 3 zeros to the number of grams to convert to milligrams: 10,000.

Example 26
Convert 30 mg to kilograms.
Solution: As can be computed from Table 10-4, 1 kg equals 1,000,000 mg; therefore, move the decimal point 6 places to the left to convert the milligrams to kilograms: 0.00003 kg.

Volume Conversions

Use Table 10-5 to convert liters.
One liter equals 1,000 milliliters, and 1 ml equals 0.001 liters.

Example 27
How many milliliters are in 2 L?
Solution: 1 L = 1,000 ml; therefore, 2 L = 2,000 ml.

PRESCRIPTION INTERPRETATION
Dosage Calculations

To dispense the correct amount of medication based on how many doses are needed, use the following formula:

$$\text{Number of doses} = \frac{\text{Total amount}}{\text{Size of each dose}}$$

Example 28
A prescription calls for 25 mg of Ritalin to be given 3 times a day for 30 days. Ritalin 25-mg tablets are available. How many tablets should be given to complete the order?
Step 1: What is the total number of doses? The patient will be taking 1 dose 3 times a day for 30 days, so the total number of doses is 90.
Step 2: What is the size of each dose? Each dose is 25 mg, 1 tablet.
Step 3: Enter the known information into the formula: $90 = \frac{x}{1}$
Solution: $x = 90$; 90 tablets are needed to complete the order.

Example 29
A prescription calls for a child to take Augmentin 250 mg/5 ml liquid. The directions are: Take 10 ml twice a day for 10 days. How many milliliters of the medication should be dispensed?
Step 1: The total number of doses is 20 doses (2 times a day for 10 days).
Step 2: The strength of each dose is 10 ml.
Step 3: Enter the known information into the formula: $20 = \frac{x}{10 \text{ ml}}$
Step 4: Solve for x using cross-multiplication: $20 \times 10 = x$.
Solution: $x = 200$; 200 ml of medication should be dispensed.

PEDIATRIC DOSING

The importance of accuracy in pediatric medication dosing cannot be overstated. An incorrect dosing calculation can have disastrous consequences in a child's life. It is critical that pediatric doses be double-checked by the preparer, in addition to the checking pharmacist's review. As with all medication dosing, ensuring the five rights is essential.

Although pediatric dosing generally is performed electronically or by a pharmacist, pharmacy technicians should be familiar with the four pediatric dosing formulas, which are based on specific factors for that patient. With each of these formulas, the pediatric dose is calculated as a percentage of an adult dose.

- When the child's weight is known, use Clark's rule:

$$Clark's\ rule: \frac{Child's\ weight\ (lb)}{150} \times Adult\ dose = Child's\ dose$$

- When a child is *over 1 year old* and the age is known, use Young's rule:

$$Young's\ rule: \frac{Child's\ age\ (years)}{Child's\ age + 12} \times Adult\ dose = Child's\ dose$$

- When a child is *under 1 year old* and the age is known, use Fried's rule:

$$Fried's\ rule: \frac{Child's\ age\ (months)}{150} \times Adult\ dose = Child's\ dose$$

The most accurate way to determine the strength of a child's dose based on the adult dose is to use the body surface area (BSA) rule. The first step is to use a nomogram that calculates the BSA based on the child's weight and size (Figure 10-1). The BSA from the nomogram then is used in the formula:

$$Body\ surface\ area\ rule: \frac{Child's\ BSA}{1.73m^2} \times Adult\ dose = Child's\ dose$$

Example 30

A nurse practitioner has prescribed cefaclor 250 mg adult strength for a child weighing 25 pounds. What strength should be given to the child?

Step 1: Determine which formula to use. Because the child's weight is known, Clark's rule is used.

Step 2: $\dfrac{25\ lbs}{150} \times 250\ mg$

Step 3: $0.17 \times 250\ mg = 42\ mg$

Solution: The child should receive 42 mg.

Example 31

A 12-year-old is to be given Zantac, based on the adult dose of 150 mg. What is the child's dosage based on his age?

Step 1: Because the child's age is known (and is *over* 1 year), Young's rule is used.

Step 2: $\dfrac{12}{24} \times 150\ mg$

Step 3: $0.5 \times 150\ mg = 75$

Solution: The child should be given a 75-mg dose.

PERCENTAGE CONCENTRATIONS

All medications, whether in solid or liquid form, have a certain amount of active ingredient, known as the *solute.* The percentage of active ingredient in a medication can be calculated as weight to weight, weight to volume, or volume to volume.

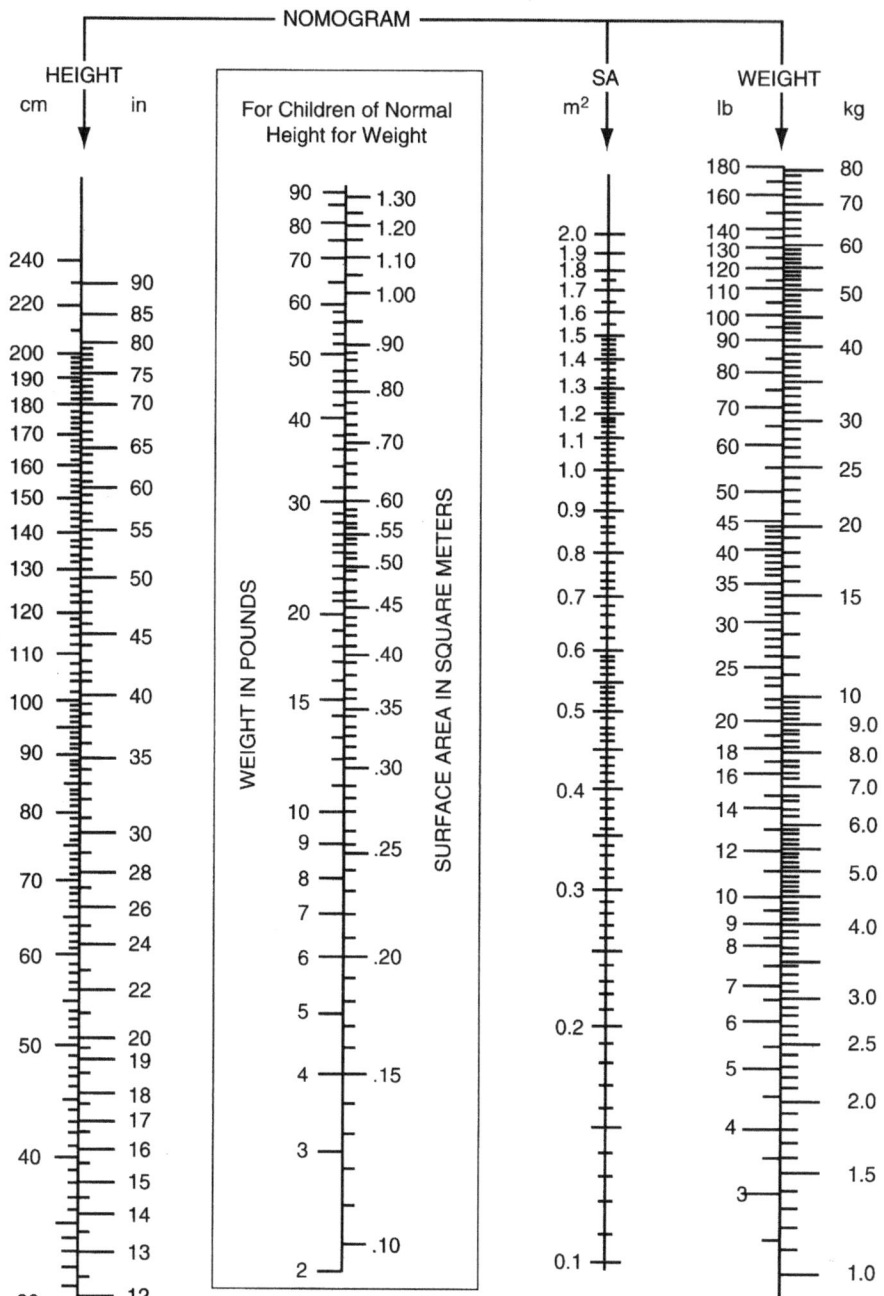

FIGURE 10-1 Nomogram for measuring body surface area for a child. (Modified from data by Boyd E, West CD. In Behrman RE, Vaughan VC: *Nelson's textbook of pediatrics,* ed 14, Philadelphia, 1992, Saunders.)

- **Weight-to-weight percentage:** The units for a solid medication are grams/grams (g/g). Ketoprofen 10% cream contains 10 g of ketoprofen (solute) in each 100 g of cream.
- **Weight-to-volume percentage:** The units for a solid mixed into a liquid are grams/milliliters (g/ml). Amoxicillin 125 mg contains 0.125 g of solute in each 100 ml. Note the metric conversion: the strength of the medication is in milligrams, but the weight-to-volume percentage is calculated in g/ml.

- **Volume-to-volume percentage:** The units for a liquid mixed into a liquid are milliliters/milliliters (ml/ml). The smaller amount of liquid is the *solute,* and the larger amount is the *solvent.*

Example 32
How many grams of hydrocortisone are needed to prepare 500 g of 10% cream?
Step 1: 10% is 10 g/100 g.
Step 2: To prepare 500 g, find out how much hydrocortisone is needed *(x).*
Step 3: Set up the equation:

$$\frac{10 \text{ g}}{100 \text{ g}} = \frac{x \text{ g}}{500 \text{ g}}$$

Step 4: Cross-multiply to solve for *x:* $100x = 5000$; $x = 50$ g.
Solution: 50 g of hydrocortisone is needed to prepare 500 g.

Percentage Strength Calculation

To find percentage strength, use the method of ratio and proportion using the given percent and $x/100$ as the concentration ratio.

Example 33
What is the percentage strength of a zinc oxide cream that contains 45 grams in a 480 gram tube?
Step 1: The 480-g tube has 45 g. This is the first ratio: 45/480.
Step 2: Set up the proportion using $x/100$:

$$\frac{45}{480} = \frac{x}{100}$$

Step 3: Cross-multiply to solve for *x:* $480x = 4,500$; $4,500 \div 480 = 9.38$.
Solution: A zinc oxide cream that contains 45 g in a 480-g tube has a percentage strength of 9.38%.

STOCK SOLUTIONS

Most medications in the pharmacy are manufactured and packaged in a certain strength. However, these stock solution concentrations often need to be diluted to a lower strength.

The following formula is used to dilute stock solutions:

$$Q1 \times S1 = Q2 \times S2$$

where *Q1* is the weight or volume of the stock solution; *S1* is the strength of the stock solution; *Q2* is the weight or volume of the requested solution; and *S2* is the strength of the requested solution.

Example 34
The pharmacy carries a 7% hydrocortisone cream prepackaged in 500-g tubes. How many grams of hydrocortisone 2.5% can be made from the stock?
Step 1: Find the stock medication amounts: $Q1 \times S1 = 500$ g $\times$ 7%
Step 2: Find the requested quantity and strength: $Q2 \times S2 = x$ g $\times$ 2.5%; 500 g $\times$ 7% = x g $\times$ 2.5%.

Step 3: Solve for *x* (remember to convert the percentages to decimals before calculating):

$$500 \times 0.07 = x \text{ g} \times 0.025; \; x = 35 \div 0.025 = 1,400$$

Solution: 1,400 g of hydrocortisone 2.5% can be made from 500 g of hydrocortisone 7%.

 If a prescription calls for a medication strength that falls between two stock solution strengths, the two stock solutions can be combined to make the requested strength. A pharmaceutical alligation calculation may be used to solve this problem.

PHARMACEUTICAL ALLIGATIONS
Alligation

To solve alligation problems, create a diagram based on the stock medications on hand and the amount ordered in the prescription.

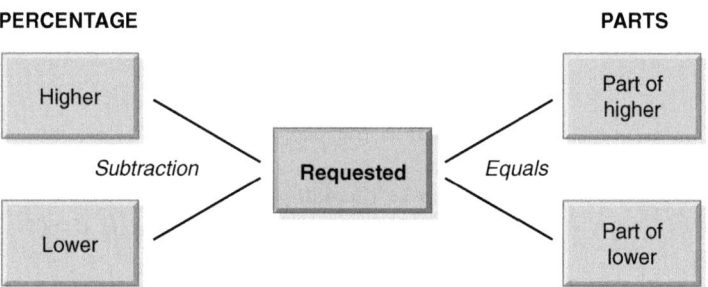

Proceed as follows:
1. Find the two stock solutions (one higher and the other lower than the requested strength).
2. Enter the higher strength value in the HIGHER box in the diagram.
3. Enter the lower strength value in the LOWER box in the diagram.
4. Enter the requested strength in the REQUESTED box in the diagram.
5. Subtract the REQUESTED value from the HIGHER value and enter that number in the PART OF LOWER box in the diagram.
6. Subtract the REQUESTED value from the LOWER value and enter that number in the PART OF HIGHER box in the diagram.
7. Add the two parts to find the total parts required.
8. Multiply the requested amount by the ratio of parts. This gives the amount of the higher strength solution needed..
9. Multiply the requested amount by its ratio of parts. This gives you the amount of the lower strength solution needed.

Example 35
A prescription calls for dextrose 20%. The two dextrose strengths currently stocked in the pharmacy are dextrose 10% and dextrose 50%. What quantity of each should be used to prepare 500 ml of the requested 20% solution?
Step 1: Fill in the appropriate strengths in the alligation diagram.
 a. In the HIGHER box, enter the higher concentration of dextrose in stock: 50
 b. In the LOWER box, enter the lower concentration of dextrose in stock; 10
 c. Enter the REQUESTED amount in the center: 20

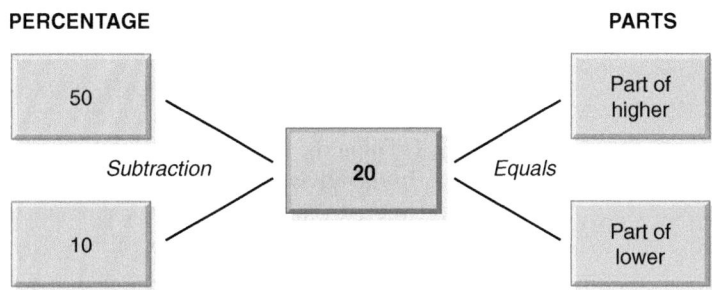

Step 2: Subtract the HIGHER value from the REQUESTED amount and put the result in the LOWER PART box.
Step 3: Subtract the LOWER from the REQUESTED amount and place the number in the HIGHER PART box.

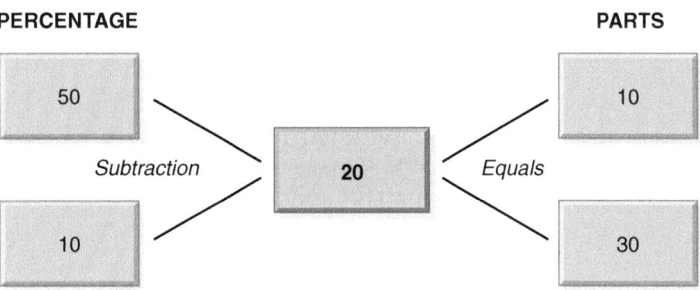

Step 4: Add the two parts.

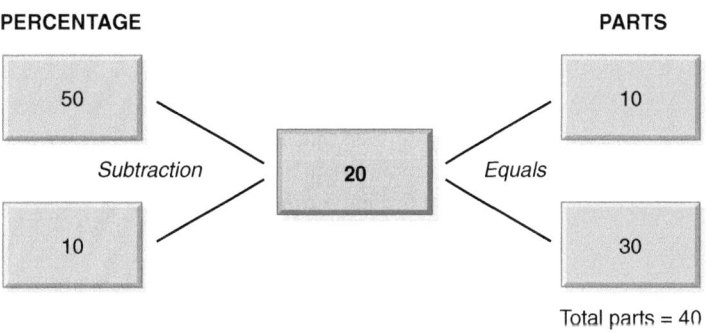

Total parts = 40

Step 5: You now have what you need to make the calculation.
  a. Find out how much of the higher concentration solution is needed first:
    Amount requested: 500 ml; 500 × 10/40 = 125 ml
Step 6: Find out how much of the lower concentration is needed:
    Amount requested: 500 ml; 500 × 30/40 = 375 ml
Solution: 125 ml of dextrose 50% should be mixed with 375 ml of dextrose 10% to prepare 500 ml of dextrose 20%.
  Note: When a solution is combined with a neutral liquid, such as sterile water or a compound base, the lower value is 0, because sterile water contains 0% of ingredient.

Example 36

A prescription calls for 25 g of 10% zinc oxide ointment. The pharmacy has 15% zinc oxide and Eucerin base ointment to prepare the compound. How much of each item is needed to prepare the requested amount and strength?

Step 1: Fill in the appropriate strengths into the alligation diagram.

a. In the HIGHER box, enter the higher concentration of zinc oxide in stock: 15

b. In the LOWER box, enter the lower concentration in stock: because Eucerin ointment does not contain zinc oxide, the number is 0.

c. Enter the REQUESTED amount in the center: 10

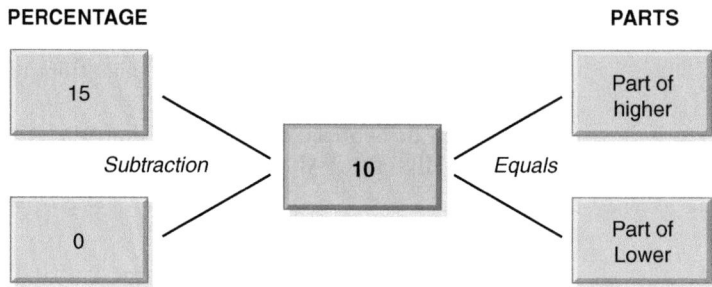

Step 2: Subtract the HIGHER from the REQUESTED amount and put the number in the LOWER PART box.

Step 3: Subtract the LOWER from the REQUESTED amount and put the number in the HIGHER PART box.

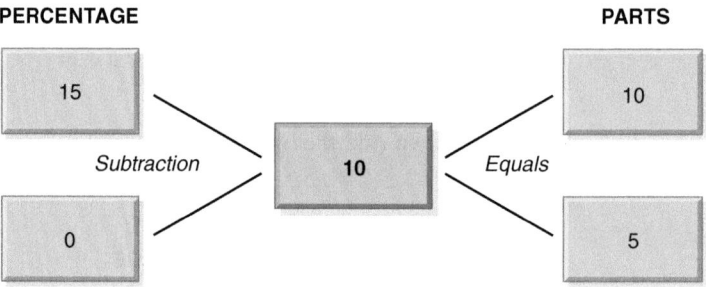

Step 4: Add the two parts: 10 + 5 = 15 total parts.

Step 5: Find out how much of the higher concentration is needed first:

Amount requested: 25 g; 25 × 10/15 = 16.7 g

Step 6: Find out how much of the lower concentration is needed:

Amount requested: 25 g; 25 × 5/15 = 8.3 g

Solution: 16.7 g of zinc oxide 15% should be mixed with 8.3 g of Eucerin ointment to prepare 25 g of zinc oxide 10%.

BUSINESS MATHEMATICS IN COMMUNITY PHARMACY PRACTICE

Business calculations are useful for determining the cost of medications and the pharmacy's profit. The following are some common business terms and the more commonly used business math formulas.

Overhead: The costs of doing business (e.g., salaries, expenses, taxes).

Gross profit: The total profit gained from a sale (Gross profit = Selling price − Purchase price)

Net profit: Profit minus overhead (Net profit = Selling price − All costs, including overhead)

Markup: Selling price minus purchase price

Markup rate: Markup divided by the cost (Markup rate = Markup ÷ Cost)

AWP: The average wholesale price of a medication, including discounts and special costs to the pharmacy

Inventory: The number of medications stocked in the pharmacy at a given time.

Example 37
A bottle of Tylenol 500 mg that contains 100 tablets costs the pharmacy $1.01. The pharmacy adds a 12% markup. What is the selling price of the bottle?
Step 1: The pharmacy is charged $1.01 for the bottle of Tylenol. How much did they mark up the price? $1.01 \times 0.12 = 0.12$
Step 2: Add the markup, 0.12 to the cost to the pharmacy: $1.01 + 0.12 = $1.13.
Solution: The selling price of the bottle is $1.13.

Example 38
What is the AWP of a medication if the original cost of the medication is $39.95, but the pharmacy receives an 8% discount from the wholesaler? (The AWP is the cost of the medication to the pharmacy after all discounts.)
Step 1: Find the discount to the pharmacy: $39.95 \times 8\% = $3.20.
Step 2: Subtract the discount from the cost: $39.95 - $3.20 = $36.75.
Solution: The AWP of the medication is $36.75.

Example 39
A pharmacy purchases Zantac 150-mg tablets in a quantity of 12 for $15.99. The pharmacy sells the medication for $39.99. (A) What is the markup? (B) What is the markup rate?
Step 1: Calculate (A) first: Markup = $39.99 - $15.99 = $24
Step 2: Now find the markup rate: $24 \div 15.99 = 1.50$
Solution: (A) The markup is $24. (B) The markup rate is 150%.

CALCULATION OF IV SOLUTION FLOW RATES AND INFUSION TIMES

Intravenous (IV) flow rates and infusion times are calculated in institutional pharmacy practice. These calculations must be performed to determine how much medication is given through a parenteral solution or to find out how long it will take to administer the medication.

Flow rate: The following formula is used to determine the flow rate (in drops per minute) of a solution:

$$\text{Drops per minute (flow rate)} = \frac{\text{ml of Solution} \times \text{Number of drops/ml}}{\text{Minutes of administration (hours} \times 60)}$$

Example 40
What is the flow rate of a parenteral solution that infuses 1 L of D_5W over 6 hours and the set delivers 10 drops per ml?
Step 1: Enter the given information into the formula:

$$x = \frac{1{,}000 \times 10/1}{(6 \times 60)}$$

Step 2: $x = 10{,}000 \div 360 = 28$
Solution: The flow rate is 28 drops/min.

Infusion time: The following formula is used to calculate how long (time) it takes for a parenteral solution to be administered:

$$\text{Infusion time} = \text{Volume of solution} \times \frac{\text{Drops}}{\text{ml}} \times \frac{\text{Minutes}}{\text{Drops}} \times \frac{1 \text{ hour}}{60 \text{ min}}$$

Example 41
What is the infusion time for an infusion solution of 2 L set to infuse 15 drops/ml at 25 drops/min?

Step 1: Enter the given information into the infusion time formula:

$$x = 2000 \times \frac{15}{1} \times \frac{1\,\text{min}}{25} \times \frac{1\,\text{hour}}{60\,\text{min}}$$

$$x = \frac{2000 \times 15 \times 1 \times 1}{1 \times 25 \times 60}$$

$$x = \frac{30{,}000}{1{,}500} = 20$$

Solution: The infusion time is 20 hours.

Chapter Summary

- Basic mathematical operations, in addition to basic algebraic equations (e.g., ratio/proportion or dimensional analysis) can be used to calculate a patient's medication dosage
- Pharmacy technicians must know the proper order of operation for the addition, subtraction, multiplication, and division of both fractions and decimals.
- Pharmacy technicians also must be familiar with systems of measurement commonly used by caregivers, pharmacists, and patients.
- Students should memorize certain measurements and equivalencies between different systems of measurement to ensure accurate dosing and the patient's safety.
- A fraction is composed of two parts, the numerator and the denominator.
- Most pharmacy dosage calculations can be performed using the ratio/proportion calculation method.
- A ratio expression is a comparison of part to the whole, similar to a fraction. The ratio usually consists of two numbers: the first number is the part, and the second number is the total amount. Ratio setup: a:b
- To dispense the correct amount of medication based on the number of doses needed, the ratio formula used is:

$$\text{Total amount} = \frac{\text{Number of doses}}{\text{Amount per dose}}$$

- A proportion is the relationship between two ratios. The two ratios in the proportion are unique because they are equal. Proportion setup: a:b = c:d
- Conversion must be performed to find the correct strength of medication to administer or to find the amount of dosage to give.
- Dimensional analysis is a form of comparing conversion ratios that involve several units of measure. Instead of setting up several ratio and proportions, one dimensional analysis may be set up to help cancel out factors to arrive at the solution
- Do not round until the very end of the calculation, and even then round only when necessary to allow for the most accurate measurement of the medication dose.
- Pharmacy calculations often involve multiple systems of measurement
- Roman numerals are commonly used in pharmacy to prevent confusion (see Table 10-3).
- The metric system is the system of measurement most frequently used in both community and hospital pharmacies. Occasionally, apothecary measurement may be used.
- The basic standard unit for fluid measurement is the liter, which is a fluid's volume occupied by 1 kilogram of water at its temperature of greatest density.
- For prescription purposes, time is written in military time (24-hour clock time). This prevents confusion and time misinterpretation.
- Equivalence between the Celsius and Fahrenheit systems of temperature measurement can be measured by various devices. The most frequently used formula for conversion is 9°C = 5°F − 160.
- Pharmacy technicians should know the four pediatric dosing formulas, which are based on specific known factors about individual patients:

$$\textit{Clark's rule}: \frac{\text{Child's weight (lb)}}{150} \times \text{Adult dose} = \text{Child's dose}$$

$$\textit{Young's rule}: \frac{\text{Child's age (years)}}{\text{Child's age} + 12} \times \text{Adult dose} = \text{Child's dose}$$

$$\textit{Fried's rule}: \frac{\text{Child's age (months)}}{150} \times \text{Adult dose} = \text{Child's dose}$$

$$\textit{Body surface area rule}: \frac{\text{Child's BSA}}{1.73 \text{ m}^2} \times \text{Adult dose} = \text{Child's dose}$$

- In pharmacy practice, two units of the metric system are used: weight and volume.
- Weight is used to describe medication strength; the primary unit of weight in the metric system is the gram.
- When medications are given in a solid form (e.g., a tablet or capsule), the strength is the amount of medication in each dose.
- Fractions and decimals are also commonly written as percentages to describe medication strengths.
- Any percentage is equal to that number divided by 100.
- All medications, whether in solid or liquid form, have an amount of active ingredient.
- If a prescription calls for a medication strength that falls between two stock solution strengths, the two stock solutions can be combined to make the requested strength. Pharmaceutical alligation calculation can be used to solve this problem.
- Business calculations are useful for determining the costs of medications and pharmacy profits.
- An IV solution flow rate is calculated to determine how much medication is given through a parenteral solution or to find out how long it will take to administer a medication. The formula is:

$$\text{Drops per minute (flow rate)} = \frac{\text{ml of Solution} \times \text{Number of drops/ml}}{\text{Minutes of administration (hours} \times 60)}$$

- To calculate how long it will take for a parenteral solution to be administered (i.e., the infusion time), the formula is:

$$\text{Infusion time} = \text{Volume of solution} \times \frac{\text{Drops}}{\text{ml}} \times \frac{\text{Minutes}}{\text{Drops}} \times \frac{1 \text{ hour}}{60 \text{ min}}$$

REVIEW QUESTIONS

Calculations

1. Convert $\frac{8}{5}$ to a mixed fraction.
2. $\frac{5}{6} \div \frac{1}{5} = $ _____.
3. $0.6 \times 5.8 = $ _____.
4. Convert 0.45 to a fraction.
5. Convert 10 gm to micrograms (mcg).
6. Convert 250 mg to kilograms (kg).
7. A patient weighs 16.7 kilograms. What is the patient's weight in pounds (lb)?
8. A prescription calls for 250 ml. How many liters (L) is this?
9. Convert 1 fluid ounce to minims.
10. Convert 2 teaspoons to ml.

TECHNICIAN'S
CORNER

1. A physician has written a prescription for Hyzaar 25-mg tablets. The directions to the patient read: Take ¼ tablet in the morning, ¼ tablet at noon, and ½ tablet at bedtime. How many milligrams will the patient take in each dose?
2. What fraction of an adult's 150-mg tablet should be given to a 10-year-old child?
3. If a drug is acquired for $45 and sold for $52.50, what is the percent markup?

11 Principles of Nonsterile Pharmaceutical Compounding

LEARNING OBJECTIVES

By the end of this chapter, students will be able to competently:

1. Describe the compounding pharmacy as an institution and the services commonly provided.
2. Review pharmaceutical dosage forms and compound ingredients commonly dispensed.
3. Identify key instruments of measurement used in the preparation of nonsterile pharmaceuticals.
4. Perform mathematical operations necessary for compound preparation.
5. Describe key pieces of equipment used in pharmaceutical compounding.
6. Describe various nonsterile pharmaceutical compounding techniques.
7. Discuss quality assurance measures required for nonsterile pharmaceutical compounding.
8. Describe stability, packaging, and storage considerations for nonsterile pharmaceuticals.

KEY TERMS

Aromatic waters: Clear, saturated aqueous solutions of volatile oils or other aromatic or volatile solutions.

Class A balance: A two-pan device that can be used for weighing small amounts of drugs (i.e., at least 120 mg, but no more than 120 g).

Compounding slab: A plate made of ground glass with a hard, flat, nonabsorbent surface that is used for mixing compounds.

Conical graduates: Devices used for measuring liquids; they have wide tops and wide bases and taper between the top and the bottom.

Counter balance: A device capable of weighing larger quantities, up to about 5 kg; often a double-pan device.

Cylindrical graduates: Devices used for measuring liquids; they have a narrow diameter that is the same from top to base.

Dispersions: Liquid preparations in which active ingredients are undissolved and dispersed evenly in the liquid with a suspending vehicle.

Electronic balance: A one-pan device that can be used for weighing small amounts of drugs (i.e., 0.001 g up to 300 g).

Elixirs: Sweetened, flavored hydroalcoholic solutions.

Emulsion: Either a small amount of water dispersed in oil (W/O), or a small amount of oil dispersed in water (O/W).

Extracts: Potent substances derived from an animal or a plant source, from which most or all the solvent has been evaporated to produce a powder, paste, or solid.

Fluid extracts: Substances prepared by extraction from plant sources and commonly used in the formulation of syrups and flavorings.

Geometric dilution: A compounding technique in which the active ingredient is mixed with an equal weight or volume of diluent; the process is repeated until all the diluent has been incorporated with the active ingredient to create a homogeneous mixture.

Homogeneous: A volume or quantity of a substance throughout which particles are evenly dissolved or distributed.

Irrigations: Liquids used to cleanse or bathe an area of the body (e.g., the eye or ear) or to irrigate tissues exposed by wounds or surgical incisions.

Levigate: To grind into a smooth substance with moisture.

Meniscus: The curve in the upper surface of a column of liquid (i.e., the level of the liquid is slightly higher at the edges); "moon-shaped body."

Mortar: A cup-shaped vessel in which materials are ground or crushed with a pestle.

Ointment: A semisolid dosage form meant for topical application.

Paste: A semisolid dosage form similar to an ointment but containing more solid materials; stiffer and applies more thickly than ointments.

Pestle: A solid, batonlike device used to crush or grind materials in a mortar.

Solution: A liquid dosage form in which one or more or more chemical active ingredients are dissolved in a liquid vehicle.

Solvent: The liquid substance in which another substance may be dissolved.

Spirits: Alcoholic or hydroalcoholic solutions containing volatile, aromatic ingredients; commonly used as medicine or flavoring.

Syrups: Aqueous solutions saturated with a large amount of sucrose or sugar substitute to which medication, flavorings, colors, or aromatic agents may be added.

Tinctures: Alcoholic or hydroalcoholic solutions of extractions from plants; typically topical preparations.

Triturate: To reduce to a fine powder by friction.

Compounding may be considered closest to the way pharmacy was practiced for thousands of years. Pharmaceutical compounding is the art of mixing raw materials with active drug substances to create a drug product that can be dispensed to the patient. Regulatory agencies, such as the U.S. Food and Drug Administration (FDA), have stated that "compounded prescriptions are ethical and legal as long as they are prescribed by a licensed practitioner for a specific patient and are compounded by a licensed pharmacist. The bulk drug substances used in a compounded medicine must qualify for use in compounding either via FDA-approved lists or via a listing in the U.S. Pharmacopoeia National Formulary (USP/NF), published by an independent standard-setting organization" (FTM Resource Guide, 2011).

The emergence of chain drug stores more than 60 years ago has had a significant impact on the community pharmacy; nevertheless, this longstanding traditional practice site has stood the test of time. Once (and sometimes still) called the *apothecary* or druggist's shop, it now is known as the *compounding pharmacy.* Compounding pharmacies typically provide products and services to patients and customers who need formulations not typically produced by drug manufacturers, or drug products that are infrequently dispensed because of the nature of the product. In addition to standard prescription processing and dispensing, compounding pharmacies may provide a variety of specialty services, including:

- Product flavoring
- Product formulation into custom dosage forms
- Veterinary medicines
- Homeopathic, naturopathic, and other alternative medications
- Durable medical equipment and specialty equipment and supplies (e.g., walkers, canes, compression hosiery, and sports medicine devices)
- Podiatric formulations
- Oncology drugs
- Ophthalmic preparations
- Neurologic products
- Vitamins and supplements
- Sports medicine needs
- Investigational drugs

Compounding pharmacies generally are independently owned by a pharmacist or group of pharmacists who have specialty credentials in the area of pharmaceutical compounding or naturopathic medicine or both. These nonstandard products often are complex formulations requiring multiple ingredients, and compounding pharmacists and technicians must keep up with the most current information on formulating and preparing compounded drugs. A recognized source of information for compounding professionals is the Professional Compounding Centers of America (PCCA). As noted in Chapter 4, the PCCA has become the nation's comprehensive resource for pharmaceutical compounding, including raw materials, equipment, technology, education, and professional resources. Because many compound formulas require specialty raw and active ingredients, it is essential for compounding pharmacies to purchase those materials from a reputable source that makes sure the purity and integrity of the products meets or exceeds the FDA's quality standards. The PCCA has established itself as a trusted source of unformulated compounding chemicals and ingredients. It is registered with (and inspected by) both the FDA and the Drug Enforcement Administration (DEA) as a valid manufacturing and repackaging source.

The PCCA provides an expansive database that includes compound formulations, preparation instructions, product stability data, and packaging and storage requirements. Many compounding pharmacies that use pharmacy technicians allow them access to drug database information only after they have been formally trained in the use of those systems. Staff education and training are other vital resources that the PCCA provides; their training program has been accredited by the American Council for Pharmacy Education (ACPE). A variety of educational symposia, seminars, training courses, and workshops are available throughout the year.

Compounding pharmacies provide a valuable service to the healthcare community, because they create opportunities for healthcare providers to prescribe medications in dosage forms that best suit patients' needs. For example, a child with a chronic disease may require pain management to have a reasonable quality of life. The patient's prescriber may have a compounding pharmacy mix pain medication lollipops or freezer pops that would make taking the medication more appealing to the child. Remember, patients are more likely to take a medication as prescribed if it is dispensed in a dosage form that makes administration easier.

A growing and diverse group of patients is using pharmaceutical compounding services:
- Children and infants who need extremely low doses of potent medications.
- Individuals who need allergen-free medications.
- People who are sensitive to excipients (fillers and binders) in manufactured products.
- Older women who want alternate sources for hormone replacement therapy (HRT).

Health and Wellness

As national healthcare costs continue to rise, more patients are turning to sources of alternative medicine and preparations that help build and sustain wellness and a healthy lifestyle. Many compounding pharmacies offer organic products, which allow patients to manage a variety of health conditions using compounds derived from natural sources. Additionally, many of these pharmacies have consulting physical therapists and nutritionists, who can provide patients with professional advice on selecting products and self-administering them safely and properly.

Pharmacy Technicians in the Compounding Pharmacy

Most compounding pharmacies employ pharmacy technicians; therefore, career opportunities exist in this area of practice. Also, because of the nature of the daily work flow, the technician's base salary in a compounding pharmacy may be higher than in other community pharmacy practices. Compounding pharmacies generally seek technicians with the following workplace skills:
- Strong written and verbal communication skills
- Strong work ethic
- Ability and willingness to learn new processes
- Strong mathematical skills
- Meticulous attention to detail

Often patients of these pharmacies are paying the full cash price for their medications, because specialty drug formulations are not required to carry a National Drug Code (NDC) number, which often makes them difficult to bill through a third-party pharmacy benefits manager. It is essential that compounding ingredients are measured and prepared properly and that those who prepare them do so accurately to ensure the patient's safety and minimize product waste.

This chapter addresses the art and science of pharmaceutical compounding in terms of the types of products mixed, the techniques used during preparation, and the equipment and supplies required. The chapter also covers various mathematical operations commonly used for dosage calculation and product preparation. It is extremely important that technicians in a compounding pharmacy have a strong foundation in mathematics and basic algebra. To ensure that the patient receives the right dose, a pharmacy technician must calculate accurately and then measure the right amount of the right ingredients.

Another important topic addressed throughout the chapter is the industry standards set for pharmaceutical compounding. Individuals involved in the compounding of nonsterile pharmaceuticals must observe regulatory standards established by the U.S. Pharmacopeia (USP). Validation of quality standards is crucial when working with a variety of raw materials; therefore, quality assurance measures used in a compounding pharmacy also are addressed.

Down the Aisle of the Apothecary Shop

As discussed in Chapter 10, a variety of pharmaceutical dosage forms are available commercially, and an even greater variety may be prepared manually in a compounding pharmacy. Many specialty dosage forms may be prepared for a patient using commercially prepared drugs and raw materials (Box 11-1).

SOLID AND SEMISOLID FORMULATIONS

Recall from Chapter 9 that various solid drug forms may be used in the formulation of a compound product, including:

- Tablets
- Capsules
- Powders and crystals
- Granules (generally for drugs that do not need a sustained-release coating)

Any of these dosage forms may be reformulated (e.g., by crushing a tablet or emptying a capsule) into another dosage form, such as a liquid or other form that makes administration easier for the patient.

Semisolid drug formulations include any of the following:

- Creams
- Ointments
- Pastes or plasters

Often commercial preparations may be diluted or may have ingredients added to them.

LIQUID FORMULATIONS

A variety of liquids may be used to formulate a compound drug (Table 11-1) based on the physical and chemical properties of the ingredients to be added. These vehicles allow for other liquid or solid ingredients (whether inert or active drugs) to be either dissolved or suspended in them. A *solution*

TECH NOTE!

Because a special coating is used on sustained- and extended-release formulations, generally only immediate-release tablets are used in compounds.

During the compounding process, if a tablet has a coating, double-check to verify that the correct product was selected.

BOX 11-1   **Specialty Drug Production Formulations**

- New tablet compression
- Reformulation of a solid or a liquid into a cream, ointment, or paste
- Repackaging of a solid drug into a capsule for sustained release
- Lollipops
- Freezer pops
- Rectal suppositories
- Urethral or vaginal suppositories
- Transdermal patches
- Injectable drugs
- Lip balms

TABLE 11-1   **Liquids Used in the Formulation of Compound Drugs**

Liquid	Description	Common Uses	Examples
Aromatic waters	Clear, saturated aqueous solutions of volatile oils or other aromatic or volatile solutions.	Skin care and cosmetics Eyewashes Pain control Burns Gargles	Peppermint oil, USP Camphor water *Hamamelis* water (witch hazel)
Syrups	Aqueous solutions saturated with a large amount of sucrose or sugar substitute (e.g., sorbitol or propylene glycol); may have additional flavorings, colors, or aromatic agents; may be medicated or nonmedicated.	Sweetened vehicle for drugs to mask bitter or other unpleasant flavor.	Ora-Plus or Ora-Blend Compounding Syrup/ Suspension vehicles
Extracts	Potent substances derived from an animal or plant source, from which most or all the **solvent** has been evaporated; produced from fluid extracts.		
Fluid extracts	Prepared by extraction from plant sources.	Commonly used in the formulation of syrups.	
Tinctures	Alcoholic or hydroalcoholic solutions of extractions from plants.	Commonly used as an alternative medicine or dietary supplement.	
Spirits	Alcoholic or hydroalcoholic solutions containing volatile (strong-smelling), aromatic ingredients.	May be used as a medicine or flavoring	
Irrigations	A medicated solution.	Used to cleanse or bathe an area of the body; topically in the eye or ear; or to flush out tissues exposed by wounds or surgical incisions	Antibiotic solutions.

may be classified by its water content or ethanol content (or both). Hydroalcoholic solutions contain both water and alcohol. Oral solutions also may contain:

- Antimicrobial agents to prevent the growth of bacteria, yeasts, and mold
- Sorbitol or glycerin to improve the texture
- Thickening agents (e.g., cellulose gums)
- Sugar-free sweeteners for diabetic patients (e.g., aspartame or sorbitol)

Liquid dosage forms present both flavoring and stability challenges. The compounding pharmacist must ensure continued physical and chemical stability and a final product that satisfies the patient's needs. Because many flavorings are derived from plants that have medicinal properties themselves, it is essential that only an expert, such as a compounding pharmacist, pair a compounded drug with the most compatible and appropriate flavoring.

Pharmaceutical Systems of Measurement

Before performing any compounding technique, the pharmacy technician must make sure to use the most accurate measuring device to measure ingredients, because this ensures that the correct amount of a compound ingredient is used. Depending on the compound formulation, a variety of

TABLE 11-2   **Systems of Weight Measurement**

Avoirdupois	Metric	Household
	35 mg	
	325 mg	
16 oz		1 lb
	1 kg (1,000 g)	2.2 lb
1 oz	1 g = 1,000 mg 1 mg = 1,000 mcg	
454 g		1 lb

TABLE 11-3   **Systems of Liquid Measurement**

Metric	Household
5 ml	1 tsp
15 ml	1 tbsp
29.57 ml	1 fl oz
473 ml	1 pt
3,785 ml	1 gal

Fl oz, Fluid ounce; *gal,* gallon; *pt,* pint; *tbsp,* tablespoon, *tsp,* teaspoon.

measuring devices may be used. Pharmacy technicians must have a working knowledge of common systems of measurement that may be used and also must know how to convert between various systems of measurement. For example, a physician may prescribe a dosage in a unit of measurement that is unfamiliar to the patient. During the order entry process, that unit may need to be converted to a household measurement that the patient understands.

Table 11-2 lists each of the common systems used for solid and semisolid weight measurement. Generally, metric and household units of measurement are most commonly seen in pharmacy practice. Table 11-3 lists each of the common units of liquid volume measurement that a compounding pharmacy technician may encounter.

Medications generally are prescribed and dosed according to patient-specific factors such as:
- Age
- Weight
- Height
- Gender
- Health or disease state

A patient's body weight helps determine how quickly blood serum levels of a drug are reached, safely achieving the drug's therapeutic action. Based on the patient's response to the medication, a prescriber may choose to continue at that dosage range, adjust the dose, or select a different course of therapy. The patient's weight generally is noted in the medical record in metric units, or kilograms. Pharmacy technicians must know how to convert a patient's weight in U.S. standard pounds to kilograms, using the conversion factor 1 kg = 2.2 lb. For example, if a patient weighs 180 pounds, the appropriate calculation is:

$$180 \div 2.2 = 81.81 \text{ kg}$$

MEASUREMENT DEVICES

Compounding pharmacies use a variety of pharmaceutical-grade balances (Table 11-4). Solid drugs are measured by weight, and a balance must be used to measure the solid drug or other compound ingredient accurately. The amount of the substance that must be measured often determines which

TABLE 11-4   **Devices Used for Measuring Solid and Semisolid Substances**

Device	Description
Class A balance	A two-pan device that can be used for weighing small amounts of drugs (not more than 120 g)
Electronic balance	A two-pan device that can be used for weighing small amounts of drugs (not more than 120 g)
Counter balance	A device capable of weighing much larger amounts, up to about 5 kg; often a double-pan device

TABLE 11-5   **Terminology and Devices Used in the Measurement of Liquid Volume**

Device	Description
Conical graduates	Devices with wide tops and wide bases that taper between the top and the bottom.
Cylindrical graduates	Devices with narrow diameters that are the same from top to base.
Meniscus	A term meaning "moon-shaped body"; the curve in the upper surface of a column of liquid (i.e., the level of the liquid is slightly higher at the edges).

balance is most appropriate. USP Chapter <795> states that ingredients must be measured with an accuracy that ensures that each unit of prepared product is no less than 90% and no greater than 110% of the calculated weight. Every pharmacy must have a Class A balance (Figure 11-1, *A*).

Liquids are measured by volume, so a variety of graduated volumetric instruments are used (Table 11-5). Liquid measurement devices are graduated (lined) to reflect units of volume (Figure 11-2). It is important to ensure that the appropriate graduated device is used, because this yields the most accurate measurement of volume. Chemical properties of the drug itself may determine which measuring device is most appropriate. For example, a volatile ingredient may need to be measured in glass rather than plastic, which might degrade (melt or break down) during the measuring process.

The liquid measured must be viewed at eye level to verify accurate measurement. The liquid's surface is concave, rather than level, and appears slightly higher at the edges; this is referred to as the meniscus (a term that means moon-shaped body). To read the measurement accurately, the technician measures to the lowest center point of the meniscus (Figure 11-3). According to USP Chapter <795>, the final volume of a liquid emulsion, solution, or suspension must be no less than 100% and no more than 110% of the labeled volume. As always, accuracy in measurement is crucial.

COMPOUND DOSAGE CALCULATION

Calculating the drug dose is a critical step in the pharmaceutical compounding process. Accurate calculation ensures that the patient receives the right dose at each dosing interval (time) during the course of therapy. As mentioned, medication generally is dosed based on the patient's weight and is often expressed as milligrams per kilogram per day (mg/kg/day). Depending on the course of therapy, a patient's daily dose may be divided and given at set intervals over 24 hours. Once the dosing regimen has been determined, the prescriber may write a prescription for the total amount of drug a patient is to receive to complete a course of therapy or is to continue taking for the length of time specified by the prescriber.

Compound dosage calculation involves measuring out the appropriate amount of each ingredient in the particular formulation of the drug prescribed. The most appropriate balance is used to measure the weight of any solid or semisolid ingredients. The most appropriate graduated device is used to measure out the volume of any liquid ingredients.

Generally, a compound's active ingredient accounts for a relatively small volume or weight. The active ingredient is added to a vehicle that dilutes it into a larger quantity, which may be administered over an established period. To fill such a prescription, four steps must be performed:

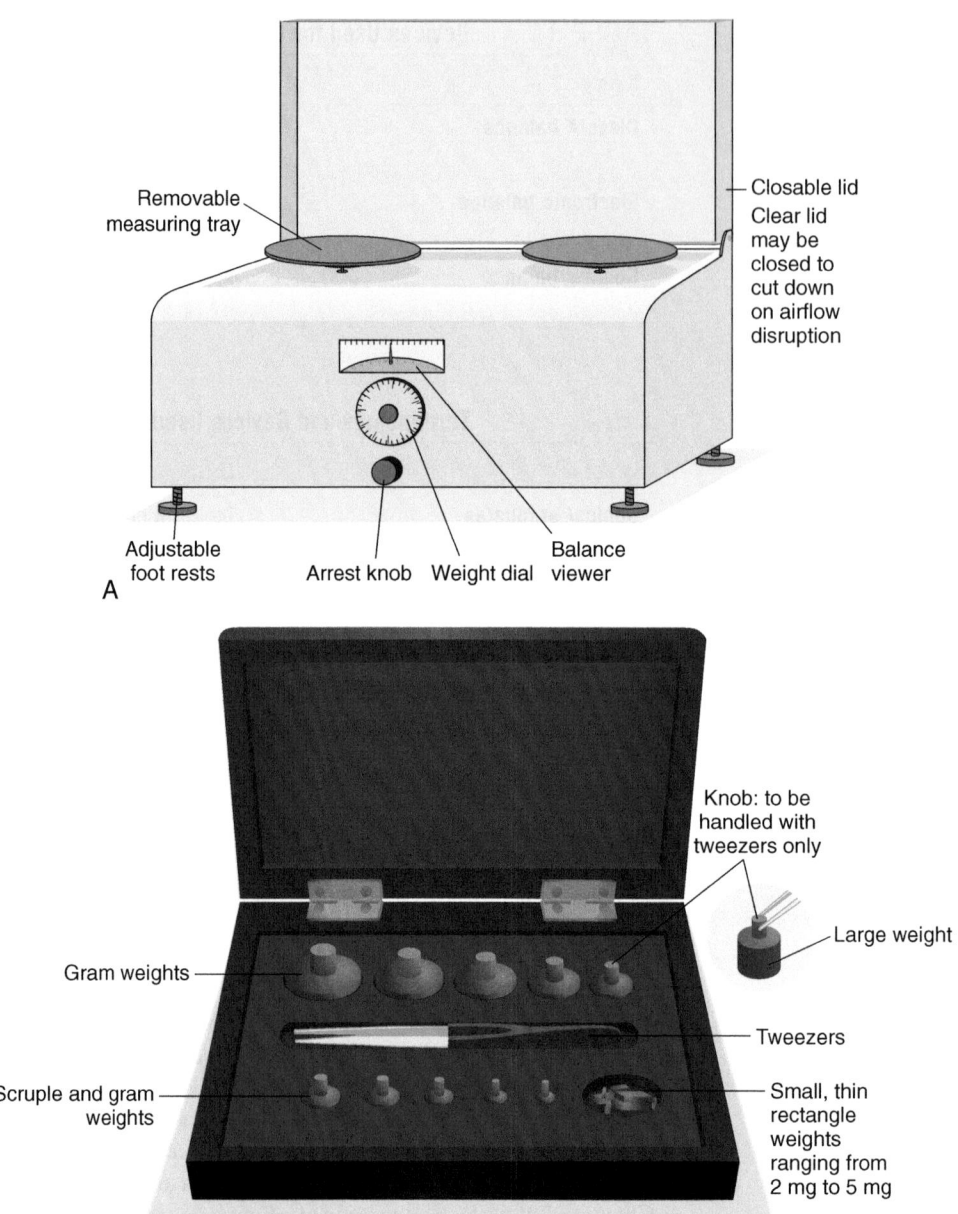

FIGURE 11-1 Class A balance. (From Hopper T: *Mosby's pharmacy technician: principles and practice,* ed 3, Philadelphia, 2011, Saunders.)

1. Determine the total amount of active drug needed.
2. Determine the amount of the solid, semisolid, or liquid vehicle required to allow for reasonable dilution of the active ingredient.
3. Determine the ratio of active drug to vehicle needed (preparation concentration).
4. Calculate how much of the concentration is needed to provide the total amount of active drug the patient must receive.

Let's apply these steps to a sample scenario. A nurse practitioner has prescribed 500 mg of penicillin suspension twice a day for a total of 10 days.

1. *Determine the total amount of active drug needed.*

The patient must be administered 500 mg twice a day for 10 days:

$$500 \times 2 \times 10 = 10,000 \text{ mg}$$

In other words, the patient must be dispensed 10,000 mg for the total prescription.

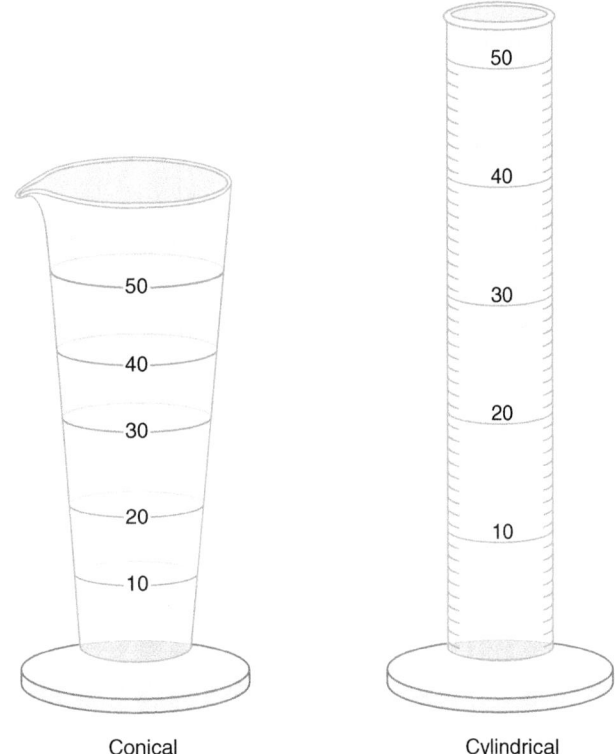

FIGURE 11-2 Graduated cylinders are used for liquid measurement. (From Hopper T: *Mosby's pharmacy technician: principles and practice*, ed 3, Philadelphia, 2011, Saunders.)

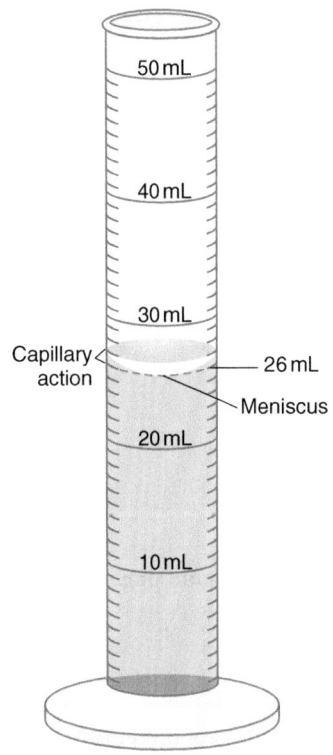

FIGURE 11-3 The meniscus is the level at which liquids are measured and recorded. For accuracy, always have the container at eye level when determining the volume. (From Hopper T: *Mosby's pharmacy technician: principles and practice*, ed 3, Philadelphia, 2011, Saunders.)

Using weight conversion, you know that 10,000 mg equals 10 g. This is a measurement of powder that likely would fit into a household teaspoon; it is a relatively small amount. The 10 g of powder will be mixed with an oral liquid vehicle (likely a flavored suspending vehicle) that will be measured as a volume that allows for equal doses based on the drug-to–suspending vehicle ratio over the entire 10 days of therapy. This concentration ratio typically is expressed as milligrams per milliliter (mg/ml).

2. *Determine the amount of the solid, semisolid, or liquid vehicle needed to allow for reasonable dilution of the active ingredient.*

   If the 10 g of powder is incorporated into 200 ml of suspending vehicle, the ratio of powder to suspending vehicle is 10,000 mg/200 ml. Any ratio must be reduced to its lowest terms; therefore, you perform a ratio-proportion calculation as follows:

$$\frac{10,000 \text{ mg}}{200 \text{ ml}} = \frac{x \text{ mg}}{1 \text{ ml}}$$

To solve:

$$200x = 10,000$$

$$x \text{ mg} = (10,000 \text{ mg}) (1 \text{ ml}) / (200 \text{ ml})$$

$$x \text{ mg} = (10,000 \text{ mg}) / 200 \text{ (ml cross out)}$$

$$x \text{ mg} = 50 \text{ mg}$$

After solving for *x,* it is vital to check your work to ensure that both sides of the ratio proportion are correct:

$$\frac{10,000 \text{ mg}}{200 \text{ ml}} = \frac{50 \text{ mg}}{1 \text{ ml}}$$

$$200 \times 50 = 10,000$$

The formula is balanced, so the solution is correct.

You have determined that this volume of diluting vehicle would provide a concentration strength of 50 mg/ml.

3. *Determine the ratio of active drug to vehicle needed (preparation concentration).*

   The patient is to receive 500 mg in each dose; therefore, you must determine how much the patient must take of this 50 mg/ml suspension.

$$\frac{50 \text{ mg}}{1 \text{ ml}} = \frac{500 \text{ mg}}{x \text{ ml}}$$

$$50x = 500$$

$$x = 500 \text{ mg} \div 50 \text{ mg} = 10 \text{ ml}$$

Check the ratio proportion:

$$\frac{50 \text{ mg}}{1 \text{ ml}} = \frac{500 \text{ mg}}{10 \text{ ml}}$$

The ratio proportion is balanced; the answer is correct.

4. *Calculate how much of the concentration is needed to provide the total amount of active drug the patient must receive.*

   The patient must take 10 ml twice daily for 10 days, which will require a total dispensing volume of 200 ml.

When a solid is added to a liquid, the mass of that solid displaces some of the liquid in the final measurement, and that amount of liquid must be accounted for. Therefore, for pharmaceutical compounding of a liquid, the accepted practice is to add a sufficient volume to equal the total volume needed. The Latin abbreviation *QSAD* may be interpreted as, "Add a sufficient quantity to make____."

The compounding technician would measure out 10 g of penicillin powder and add enough of a flavored suspending vehicle to measure a final dispensing volume of 200 ml.

In hospitals a prescriber often orders medication based on the dosage range per day. The hospital pharmacist or pharmacy technician must calculate how much medication should be dispensed to fill that medication order.

Let's apply this to a sample scenario. A patient weighing 65 kg has been given a prescription for an oral suspension, in which the maximum daily dose is 5 mg/kg/day for 5 days. The dosing interval is every 8 hours.

1. *Determine the total amount of active drug needed.*
   Based on the patient's weight, calculate the total dose:

$$5 \text{ days} \times 65 \text{ kg} \times 5 \text{ mg/kg/day} = 1{,}625 \text{ mg total amount needed}$$

2. *Determine the amount of solid, semisolid, or liquid vehicle needed to allow for reasonable dilution of the active ingredient.*
   The 1,625 mg is a mass of powder equivalent to a little more than a household tablespoon. This could be reasonably added to 500 ml of oral syrup vehicle.

3. *Determine the ratio of active drug to vehicle needed (preparation concentration).*
   The ratio of powder to liquid is 1,625 mg : 500 ml. Perform the ratio-proportion calculation:

$$\frac{1{,}625 \text{ mg}}{500 \text{ ml}} = \frac{x \text{ mg}}{1 \text{ ml}}$$

$$500 \text{ ml } x = 1{,}625 \text{ mg}$$

$$x = 1{,}625 \text{ mg} \div 500 \text{ ml} = 3.25$$

The established concentration strength of this formulation will be 3.25 mg/ml.

4. *Calculate how much of the concentration is needed to provide the total amount of active drug the patient must receive.*
   Based on the prescribed dose of 5 mg/kg/day, the patient should receive 325 mg/day. Now, calculate the daily dose:

$$\frac{3.25 \text{ mg}}{1 \text{ ml}} = \frac{325 \text{ mg}}{x \text{ ml}}$$

$$3.25 \text{ mg } x = 325 \text{ mg}$$

$$x = 325 \text{ mg} \div 3.25 \text{ mg} = 100 \text{ ml}$$

The patient will receive 100 ml/day × 5 days. The total dispensing quantity is 500 ml.

The compounding pharmacy technician would measure out 1,625 mg of drug, and QSAD to 500 ml to flavored syrup vehicle.

In the pharmacy, the amount of diluent (vehicle) will have been predetermined and will be documented on a formula sheet for use by the compounding pharmacist and technician. This formula sheet is known as the *master formula record*. A master formula record is kept on file for every compound a pharmacy dispenses. In the modern compounding pharmacy, computerized compound formulation databases have assembled information and preparation instructions, in addition to stability and storage information, for a variety of compounds. Many compounding pharmacies also have customized formulations for specialty drugs unique to that particular pharmacy.

After the compound ingredient quantities have been determined, compounding technicians must perform specific steps to ensure that the active ingredient is equally distributed throughout the entire volume or quantity of the vehicle. Particular techniques must be performed to accomplish this while ensuring that no contaminants (e.g., microorganisms, foreign particulate matter, or impurities) are introduced into the compound. Compounding technicians must receive adequate training in nonsterile and sterile compounding techniques. Such training may take place in-house or may be provided by an outside agency (e.g., the PCCA).

Nonsterile Compounding Techniques

PREPARING FOR NONSTERILE COMPOUNDING: PERSONAL PROTECTIVE EQUIPMENT AND ASEPTIC HAND WASHING

Even before gathering the materials for the compounding process, pharmacy technicians must put on appropriate attire, which creates a physical barrier between them and the product being mixed. This minimizes the risk of a contaminant (e.g., hair or saliva) entering the product. Also, if a product is volatile (gives off fumes or gas by-product) or corrosive, protective equipment increases the preparer's safety and minimizes the risk of injury during the compounding process.

Every compounding process should begin with proper hand washing with an antiseptic product that can kill bacteria on the surface of the hands. Use of alcohol-based hand rubs is also acceptable and generally encouraged in addition to hand washing. Once hand washing has been performed, any of the following protective gear may be put on, as appropriate:

- Bouffant cap or head cover
- Mask and/or beard cover
- Gown, scrubs, or protective laboratory coat
- Shoe covers
- Goggles
- Gloves (may be sterile or nonsterile, depending on the formulation of the compound)

It also is important to prepare the compounding area before beginning the mixing process. Compounding is best and most safely performed in an area that does not have a great deal of traffic and where airflow does not increase the risk of airborne contaminants being introduced into products. All countertops, compound instruments, and measuring devices should be cleaned with an appropriate antiseptic before the compounding process begins and also after it is completed.

THE TOOLS OF THE TRADE

A compounded drug may be prepared for a single patient, or it may be prepared in a large quantity, packaged, and stored for use by multiple patients. In the outpatient setting, particularly when expensive or specialty ingredients are used, doses are usually prepared for an individual patient based on a written prescription from an authorized prescriber. This type of compounding is known as *extemporaneous compounding*.

A few essential supplies and equipment are used to perform various compounding processes. According to the nonsterile compounding standards in USP Chapter <795>, all compounding equipment and supplies must be used to:

- Reduce solute ingredients to the smallest reasonable particle size
- Ensure that solutions have no visible undissolved matter when dispensed
- Make sure products are homogenized to ensure a uniform final dispersion

The following equipment is commonly used in a compounding pharmacy.

Compounding slab: A plate made of ground glass with a hard, flat, nonabsorbent surface that is used for mixing compounds. Levigation using a compound spatula is performed on a compounding slab. This device is used to perform geometric dilution of creams, ointments, pastes, and other semisolid preparations.

Compounding spatula: A device used to incorporate pharmaceutical ingredients into a homogeneous (evenly distributed) final product.

Extemporaneous compounding: The preparation, mixing, assembling, packaging, and labeling of a drug product based on a prescription from a licensed practitioner for an individual patient.

Geometric dilution: A compounding technique in which the active ingredient is mixed with an equal weight or volume of diluent; the process is repeated until all the diluent has been incorporated, with the active ingredient, into a homogeneous mixture. In manual geometric dilution, a compounding technician uses the surface of the levigation spatula to press the drug ingredients firmly into the semisolid ingredients, using even, constant strokes, to ensure that

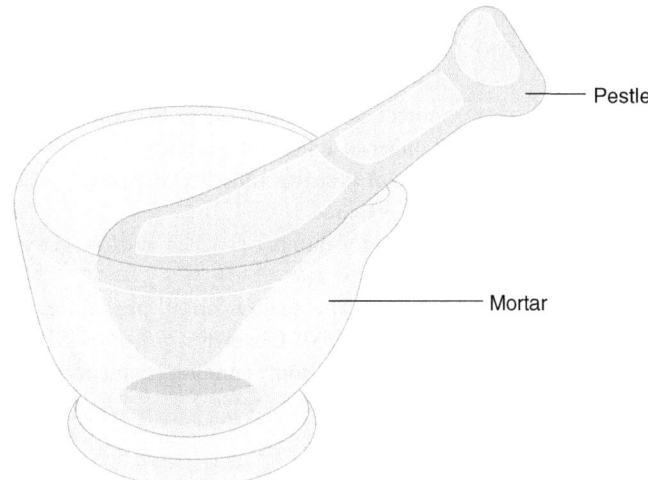

FIGURE 11-4 Mortars and pestles are used to crush solids. Both glass and porcelain types are used in compounding. (From Hopper T: *Mosby's pharmacy technician: principles and practice,* ed 3, Philadelphia, 2011, Saunders.)

a powder ingredient is thoroughly and evenly distributed throughout the entire quantity of the vehicle base.

Homogenizer: A mechanical device used to reduce solid particle sizes uniformly in a compound mixture. A homogenizer is ideal for reducing the particle size of formulations intended for injection.

Levigate: To grind or press into a smooth substance with moisture. This may be done manually using a levigation slab and spatula, or using a mechanical compounding device, such as an ointment mill. Particle size reduction using an ointment mill increases the amount of active drug that may be absorbed through the skin.

Mortar: A cup-shaped vessel in which materials are ground or crushed (Figure 11-4).

Pestle: A solid device used to crush or grind materials in a mortar. After manual incorporation of a solid and a base, a product may further be processed using an ointment mill. This device pushes the base and powder mixture through porcelain rollers, further reducing the particle size of solid ingredients and creating an even, smoother final product. Other electric mortar and pestle devices ensure that vehicles and active drug ingredients are evenly mixed and allow the final product to be transferred to a dispensing container with little or no exposure to the outside environment.

Triturate: To reduce to a fine powder by friction. This generally is accomplished with a mortar and pestle or mechanically with a homogenizer. USP Chapter <795> states that a product containing solid ingredients should be reduced to the "smallest reasonable product size."

MASTER FORMULA RECORD

The master formula record can be considered the recipe or blueprint for each compounded preparation. The following information must be included in the master formula record:

- Names, strengths, and dosage forms of the compounded ingredients
- Compounding supplies and equipment used during preparation
- Compounding instructions
- Order of mixing, including temperature and other environmental controls
- Beyond-use date
- Dispensing container
- Storage requirements
- Any quality control procedures
- Sample label format

Depending on the format of the master formula record, documentation of each individual compound may be placed on the formula record itself, or an extemporaneous or batch compound record may be prepared.

Compounding Record

USP Chapter <795> specifies the information that must be included in the compounding record:
- Name and strength of compounded preparation
- Sources and lot numbers of ingredients
- Number of units compounded
- Name of preparer and checking pharmacist
- Date prepared
- Internal lot number assigned and/or prescription number generated
- Beyond-use date
- Results of any quality control procedures

According to USP Chapter <795>, a USP Monograph Experience Reporting Form must be completed any time compounding problems occur with products prepared according to USP compounding monographs.

Internal Lot Number and Beyond-Use Date

The manufacturer assigns each ingredient an individual expiration date, but the compounding pharmacy establishes an internal lot number unique to each batch of compound mixed. The lot number often consists of the date, a letter that designates the type of drug (e.g., *C* for legend drug, *N* for narcotic drug, *O* for ophthalmic preparation), and the sequential order of compounds mixed on a particular date. Therefore, the sample lot number *C06252011001* indicates a legend drug compound mixed on *06/25/11* that was the first compound of that type mixed on that date.

Expiration (or beyond-use) dating of pharmaceutical products is vital to ensuring that the patient knows the time frame in which a product may be safely administered and considered physically, chemically, and therapeutically stable. Compounding pharmacists consult drug databases for the most current stability information on compound formulations so that they can date a product appropriately before it is dispensed to a patient.

USP Chapter <795> has established requirements for product stability. Five types of stability are specified, along with criteria that define whether a product has acceptable levels of stability:
- *Chemical stability:* Each ingredient retains its chemical integrity and labeled potency.
- *Physical stability:* The product retains its original physical appearance, uniformity, dissolution, and suspendability.
- *Microbiologic stability:* The product retains its sterility and ability to resist microbial growth.
- *Therapeutic stability:* The product's ability to exert its therapeutic effect is unaffected.
- *Toxicologic stability:* The product's toxicity level does not increase.

USP Chapter <795> also details beyond-use dating requirements based on the constitution of the compounded product.
- Solid/nonaqueous semisolid formulations:
  - When a product contains a manufactured product as an active ingredient, the beyond-use date must be no later than 25% of the time remaining until the product's expiration date or 6 months, whichever is earlier,
  - If a USP/NF substance is the active ingredient, the beyond-use date is a maximum of 6 months.
- Water-containing formulations (prepared from ingredients in solid form):
  - The beyond-use date is no more than 14 days with storage at cold temperatures (i.e., 2° to 8°C [36° to 46°F]).
- All other formulations:
  - The beyond-use date is the duration of therapy or 30 days, whichever is sooner (unless documentation substantiates a longer stability for a specific preparation).

! TECH ALERT!
Only one compound should be prepared at a time in the compounding area.

STEP-BY-STEP COMPOUNDING PROCESS

Once a compounding prescription has been evaluated for suitability for the patient, the products' formulation and stability have been verified, and the prescription has been entered and a label generated, the compounding technician is ready to begin the pharmaceutical compounding process.

Using a master formula record or other compounding log (or both) for documentation, the compounder performs the following steps:

1. Perform all necessary calculations and document the quantities of all ingredients in the compounding log.
2. Identify the equipment and supplies needed to complete the compounding process.
3. Put on the proper protective attire and perform hand washing.
4. Clean the compounding area and any equipment to be used.
5. Gather the necessary compounding ingredients.
6. Measure all ingredients using appropriate weighing devices and instruments.
7. Compound the preparation according to the prescribed compound formula and/or prescription.
8. Once the compound is complete, perform the quality control visual inspection and assess the final product for the following:
   a. Acceptable weight variation
   b. Adequate mixing, as evidenced by consistency, texture, and even distribution of all ingredients
   c. Clarity and color (especially observe for any unexpected color changes or cloudiness, which may indicate product instability)
   d. Odor (especially observe for any unexpected odor or gaseous by-product, which may indicate product instability)
   e. pH
9. Record the description of the final product in the compounding log.
10. Attach the product label, which must include the following information:
    a. Name of the preparation
    b. Internal lot number
    c. Beyond-use date
    d. Initials of the compounder
    e. Storage requirements
11. Ask the pharmacist to sign and date the prescription, affirming that all procedures were carried out to ensure uniformity, identity, strength, quantity, and purity.
12. Promptly clean all equipment, store it properly, and return all ingredients to the proper storage areas.

Only when an established process is followed can its effectiveness be assessed. It is important that all pharmacy technicians involved in nonsterile compounding perform each of the critical steps in compounding *exactly* as prescribed on the master formula. Only then can quality assurance measures be applied to ensure that the final product meets the standards of quality, purity, and stability expected by the USP.

Nonsterile Compounding Standards of Practice and Quality Assurance

COMPOUNDING PERSONNEL RESPONSIBILITIES

USP Chapter <795> details the regulatory standards for nonsterile pharmaceutical compounding. Nine key responsibilities have been established for those who perform nonsterile compounding.

1. *Personnel must be capable and qualified.* All individuals must receive adequate training, either in-house or from an accredited outside agency.
2. *Ingredients used must have their expected identity, quality, and purity.* Ingredients should be purchased from a trusted source, and all expiration dates should be checked before use.
3. *Compounded preparations must be of acceptable strength, quality, and purity, with appropriate packaging and labeling, and must be prepared in accordance with good compounding practices, official standards, and relevant scientific data and information.* Any compound prepared first must have been investigated by a pharmacist and determined to be safe for administration, as evidenced by the clinical data available.
4. *Critical processes must be validated to ensure that procedures, when used, consistently result in the expected qualities in the finished preparation.* The compounding process should be established and documented, and every individual who performs compounding should prepare the product exactly as detailed to ensure the same quality in the finished preparation consistently.

5. *The compounding environment must be suitable for its intended purpose:*
   - The compounding area must have low traffic and adequate lighting, airflow, and ventilation.
   - The compounding area should have potable water for proper equipment and hand washing, in addition to adequate detergents, air dryers, and/or paper towels.
   - All compounding supplies and preparation areas must be kept clean and must be disinfected before and after use to prevent cross-contamination.
   - Care must be taken when compounding products commonly associated with allergic reactions (e.g., penicillins, sulfa drugs).
   - Care must be taken to keep separate and adequately label supplies used to prepare chemotherapeutic and other hazardous drugs. Supplies should be decontaminated and disinfected before and after each use.
6. *Appropriate stability evaluation must be performed or determined from the literature to establish reliable beyond-use dating so as to ensure that the finished preparations have the expected potency, purity, quality, and characteristics, at least until the labeled beyond-use date.*
   - Before a master formula record is prepared on a particular product, stability information must be gathered verifying that the finished product will remain physically and chemically stable and that the purity of the ingredients used will sustain the product's therapeutic stability.
7. *Quality assurance processes are always performed as specified.* An established compounding process, as documented on a master formula record, must be followed by all compounding personnel.
8. *Compounding conditions and procedures must be adequate for preventing errors:*
   - Compounding areas must be well lit.
   - Compounding processes must be adequately documented.
   - Compounding ingredients must be properly stored based on their stability requirements and adequately labeled with multiple product identifiers.
   - The process for product selection and preparation should allow for at least three in-process checks to verify that the correct ingredients have been chosen.
9. *Adequate procedures and documentation are required for investigating and correcting failures or problems in compounding or testing, or in the preparation itself:*
   - Standard operating procedures should include a process for examining errors to determine the root cause, such as inadequate training, poor or careless staff performance, inadequate environmental conditions, and inadequate labeling (e.g., look-alike/sound-alike drugs are stored near each other).
   - Once the root cause has been determined, corrective action must be planned, documented, implemented, and assessed for effectiveness.

PHARMACISTS' RESPONSIBILITIES

USP Chapter <795> charges pharmacists with the following six primary responsibilities, in addition to the nine noted previously. Pharmacy technicians can help their pharmacists meet these standards.

1. *Dispense the oldest stock first and observe expiration dates.*
   - *Technician's role:* Technicians may help rotate stock and label drugs within 30 to 60 days of their beyond-use dates (also referred to as *short fills*).
2. *Store products under the environmental conditions noted in their monographs, labeling, or both.*
   - *Technician's role:* Technicians should make sure products are returned to their correct storage location after completion of compound processes.
3. *Observe products for evidence of instability.*
   - *Technician's role:* Technicians should also be alert to product consistency and should notify the pharmacist immediately of anything that appears out of the ordinary or unexpected (e.g., discoloration, rapid separation of a suspension, formation of a particulate in a solution, or formation of gas bubbles or streaks in a preparation).
   - The technician should observe for signs of incompatibility or instability during all steps of the compounding, storage, and dispensing of compound drugs,

4. *Properly treat and label products that are repackaged, diluted, or mixed with other products.*
   - *Technician's role:* Technicians should prepare a product only if it has a proper label verified and generated by a pharmacist.
5. *Dispense products in the proper container with the proper closure.*
   - *Technician's role:* If a technician accepts a prescription, information such as a patient's request for a non-childproof container should be brought to the pharmacist's attention, and the patient's acknowledgement signature must be obtained during dispensing.
6. *Inform and educate patients about the proper storage and use of products, including the disposal of outdated or excessively aged prescriptions.*
   - *Technician's role:* Technicians may point out auxiliary labeling that indicates storage instructions (e.g., Keep Refrigerated) and encourage patients to speak to the pharmacist about safe disposal of their expired medications.

Chapter Summary

- Pharmaceutical compounding is an ancient form of medical practice dating back thousands of years.
- Pharmaceutical compounding is the art of mixing raw materials with active drug substances to create a drug product for dispensing to a patient; this is called *extemporaneous compounding.*
- In addition to standard prescription processing and dispensing, compounding pharmacies may provide a variety of specialty services.
- Compounding pharmacies generally are independently owned by a pharmacist or group of pharmacists with specialty credentials in pharmaceutical compounding or naturopathic medicine (or both).
- Compounding pharmacies must purchase materials from a reputable source that guarantees that the purity and integrity of its products meet or exceed the FDA's quality standards. Such a source is the Pharmacy Compounding Centers of America (PCCA), the nation's most comprehensive data and supply resource.
- Compounding pharmacies look for the following traits in pharmacy technicians: strong written and verbal communication skills, strong work ethic, ability and willingness to learn, strong mathematical skills, and attention to detail.
- Many dosage forms may be reformulated into another dosage form that allows easier administration by the patient.
- Medications generally are prescribed and dosed according to patient-specific factors.
- Pharmacy technicians must know how to convert a patient's weight from U.S. standard pounds to kilograms using the conversion factor: 1 kg = 2.2 lb.
- Compounding should be performed in a low-traffic area of the pharmacy.
- All countertops, compounding instruments, and measuring devices should be cleaned with an appropriate antiseptic agent before the compounding process is started and also at the conclusion of the process.
- The compounding process should begin with proper hand washing with a product that has antiseptic properties.
- Any of the following protective gear may be worn as appropriate: bouffant cap or head cover, mask and/or beard cover, gown, scrubs or protective laboratory coat, shoe covers, goggles, or gloves.
- According to the nonsterile compounding standards established in USP Chapter <795>, the appropriate compounding equipment and supplies must be used to reduce solute ingredients to the smallest reasonable particle size, using any of the following techniques: geometric dilution, levigation, and trituration.
- Solutions should have no visible undissolved matter when dispensed.
- Homogenized products have a uniform final dispersion.
- Compounding equipment and supplies include the compounding slab, compounding spatula, homogenizer, and mortar and pestle.
- The master formula record can be considered the recipe or blueprint for each compounding preparation.

- The compounding pharmacy establishes an internal lot number unique to each batch of compound mixed.
- USP Chapter <795> details the criteria for product stability.
- Expiration (or beyond-use) dating of pharmaceutical products is vital to ensuring that the patient knows the time frame in which a product may be safely administered and considered physically, chemically, and therapeutically stable.
- Before beginning the compounding procedure, the technician must perform the following steps:
  - Determine the total amount of active drug needed.
  - Determine the amount of solid, semisolid, or liquid vehicle needed to allow for reasonable dilution of the active ingredient.
  - Determine the ratio of active drug to vehicle needed (preparation concentration).
  - Calculate how much of the concentration is needed to provide the total amount of active drug the patient must receive.

REVIEW QUESTIONS

Multiple Choice

1. Extemporaneous compounding:
   a. Provides a way to customize prescriptions for the specific needs of the patient
   b. Includes hormone replacement therapy, chronic pain management, and pediatric dosing
   c. Involves combining multiple medications into a single, more convenient dose
   d. All of the above

2. A potent substance derived from a plant source that is in powder form is a(n):
   a. Elixir
   b. Fluid extract
   c. Tincture
   d. Extract

3. A clear alcoholic solution containing aromatic ingredients that is used for flavoring is a(n):
   a. Tincture
   b. Spirit
   c. Aromatic water
   d. Irrigation

4. Solid and semisolid formulations derived from manufactured products have a beyond-use date no later than what percentage of time away from the manufacturer's expiration date?
   a. 10%
   b. 25%
   c. 50%
   d. 75%

5. Irrigations for this wound site must remain sterile:
   a. Skin and skin structures
   b. Ear
   c. Eye
   d. Mouth

6. Which balance would be most appropriate for weighing 2 g of a solid drug?
   a. Counter balance
   b. Electronic balance
   c. Class A torsion balance
   d. B and C

7. The final weight of a solid compound ingredient must be no less than what percentage of the calculated weight?
   a. 75%
   b. 90%
   c. 100%
   d. 110%

8. When measuring liquid, the correct graduation reading should be at the _____ of the meniscus.
   a. Top
   b. Middle
   c. Bottom
   d. Side

9. If a patient is to receive 500 mg of a drug each day, how much of an 85 mg/ml solution would be administered each day?
   a. 7.5 ml
   b. 6.25 ml
   c. 6.67 ml
   d. 6.5 ml

10. The beyond-use date is no more than _____ days with storage at cold temperatures.
    a. 3 days
    b. 7 days
    c. 14 days
    d. 28 days

TECHNICIAN'S CORNER

1. What types of workplace skills might a compounding pharmacist seek in a new compounding technician?
2. Why must many customers of compounding pharmacies pay full price for their prescriptions?
3. Calculate the daily dose for a patient weighing 70 kg who has a prescription for a drug dosed at 15 mg/kg/day.

Bibliography

Chenguang Biotech Group. (2011). *Natural Nutritional and Pharmaceutical Extract.* Retrieved 6/27/2011, from www.cn-cg.com/english/product.asp?dl=2&xl=9

David, B., Troy, E. (2006). Part 5. Pharmaceutical manufacturing: Aromatic Waters. In Remington, JP, editor, *The Science and Practice of Pharmacy,* 21st Edition. Baltimore: Lippincott, Wilkins & Williams.

Dougherty's Pharmacy. (2010). *Compounding: Solving Your Medication Challenges.* Retrieved 6/23/2011, from www.doughertys.com/services/compounding

FTM Resource Guide. (2011). *Compounding Pharmacies.* Retrieved 6/23/2011, from www.ftmguide.org/compounding.html

Hieber's Pharmacy. (2007). *Equipment Used.* Retrieved 6/24/2011, from www.hpharmacy.net/equipment.htm

IREL. (2011). *Pharmaceutical Extracts and Tinctures.* Retrieved 6/27/2011, from www.irelcosmetics.com/en/products/matricariae-tinctura

Maron, J. (2009, October 9). *Compounding Pharmacy Has Many Benefits.* Retrieved 6/23/2011, from www.articlesbase.com/medicine-articles/compounding-pharmacy-has-many-benefits-1320050.html#axzz1Q6wTphIw

Natural Health eZine. (2011). *The Use of Aromatic Water for Your Health.* Retrieved 6/23/2011, from http://naturalhealthezine.com/the-use-of-aromatic-waters-for-your-health/

Specialty Medicine Compounding Pharmacy. (2006). *Compounding Lab Tour: Electronic Mortar and Pestle, Ointment Mill and Homogenizer.* Retrieved 6/25/2011, from www.specialty-medicine.com/Compounding/CompoundingLabTour-EMPOin.html

12

Pharmacy Billing and Claims Processing

LEARNING OBJECTIVES

By the end of this chapter, students will be able to competently:

1. Explain the relevance of accessible healthcare and the benefits to protecting public health.
2. Differentiate private and public sources of health benefit plans.
3. Describe government benefit plans, including pharmacy benefits.
4. Explain the rationale for pharmacy benefits management, and describe how employers commonly implement it.
5. Discuss how the Affordable Care Act of 2010 is expected to impact the delivery of pharmacy benefits to patients and how pharmacy staff should respond to customers' changing needs.
6. Define the role of the pharmacy benefits management (PBM) company and the types of jobs that pharmacy technicians perform within these organizations.
7. Examine common coverage and eligibility issues that may influence successful pharmacy benefits claims processing.
8. Given various insurance scenarios, effectively assess the most appropriate verbal responses and actions to patients concerning their benefits and eligibility.
9. Appreciate the necessity for taking ownership of customers' needs related to claims processing.
10. Consider strategies for troubleshooting pharmacy claim billing issues, including asking probing questions, gathering pertinent information, and sharing resources.
11. Discuss the type of information and industry terminology that a pharmacy technician must utilize to assist patients with pharmacy benefits claims processing.
12. Examine strategies for diffusing an angry or uncooperative customer.

KEY TERMS

Beneficiary: An individual who is eligible to receive health care benefits, which often include pharmacy benefits for medication therapy.

Claim: A paper or electronic invoice that details the medical/pharmaceutical care that was provided, the date on which that service was provided, and the payment required.

Co-insurance: A percentage that the beneficiary must pay for a particular type of care.

Co-pay: An established fixed amount that a beneficiary pays for a particular medical service or prescription.

Deductible: An established dollar amount that a beneficiary must pay out of pocket before the insurance plan pays out any benefits.

Medicare: A national health care plan that provides benefits to citizens age 65 and older, as well as many individuals with qualifying disabilities who are unable to work.

Preexisting condition: Any health issue that the patient had *before* applying for a health insurance plan.

Premium: A monthly rate established by the insurance provider that the beneficiary of medical/pharmacy benefits must pay in order to establish and maintain insurance coverage.

Introduction

Health care is a billion-dollar industry that affects every man, woman, and child in the United States. The only thing that patients need as much as health care is insurance coverage, also known as health care benefits. Health care benefits allow the population greater access to services that will allow them to stay healthy, treat minor illness or injury, and assess risk factors for certain types of diseases for which certain populations may be more susceptible. From the standpoint of public health, the accessibility of health care and immunizations allows for the control of the spread of communicable diseases that would affect the health of the population at large. Additionally, the number of individuals in our society who require multiple levels of health care continues to increase because of a large aging population as well as a sharp increase in the incidence of heart disease, diabetes, and high blood pressure in both children and adults. The accessibility of health care and affordable benefits—for the good of the population at large—is an issue that the United States government has continued to evaluate and improve.

One of the functions of the federal government is to provide resources that serve the citizens and inhabitants of the United States. Because of the cost involved, there is ongoing debate over public health care resources, the benefits they provide, and who should be eligible to receive them. Because of an increasing aging population, more American citizens are eligible for these benefits—and this growing number is rapidly escalating the cost. Because the cost involved exceeds what the rest of the population is paying into the system via taxes, a huge funding disparity exists. The ongoing goal of health care reform is to identify a strategy for managing the health care needs of U.S. citizens and ensuring the accessibility of health care to everyone, regardless of social status. The greatest challenge of health care reform is effectively managing the cost. In addition to general health care, the cost of medication therapy in the United States also continues to rise. At the same time, many pharmacies (particularly those that are privately owned and operated) are challenged with managing their costs and gaining federal reimbursement for the goods and services they provide to patients with both private and public pharmacy benefits.

Much of what pharmacy technicians learn about pharmacy benefits management is gained on the job by collaborating with patients and the insurance companies that administer their pharmacy benefits. This chapter provides a foundation that pharmacy technicians may find useful for serving patients with pharmacy billing issues. In order to do that, pharmacy technicians need to know how insurance *works*, as well as the basic types and structure of health and pharmacy benefits that exist. Further, there is an industry language that technicians must learn, apply, and explain to patients. Pharmacy technicians need to know the law and possess the ability to explain pharmacy benefits as they relate to both federal and state legislation. This chapter highlights the Affordable Care Act of 2010 and explains how this legislation will likely affect the administration of patients' pharmacy benefits over the next several years. There are a number of important changes to the provision of both private and government-sponsored health care and pharmacy benefits; in light of some rather dramatic changes, pharmacy staff members need to be prepared to respond appropriately to patients' questions related to their eligibility and restructured health and pharmacy benefit plans. Box 12-1 details several general provisions of the act, including those that will be discussed in this chapter. Each section provides an explanation or example of how pharmacy technicians may use the information.

Medical Benefit Eligibility: It's a Matter of Your Health

One of the many reasons why many individuals in the United States don't choose to obtain health insurance is because they feel they are healthy enough not to need it or would rather not spend the money on it if they don't have to. The truth is that the best time to enroll in a health insurance plan is *while you are healthy,* in order to gain the greatest benefits for the lowest cost. The healthier a person is, the more affordable the health insurance usually is. In many cases, companies that provide health insurance require individuals to disclose any serious or chronic health care conditions in order to establish whether a person may receive coverage through that provider. Such a condition is known as a preexisting condition. A preexisting condition is any health issue that the patient had *before* applying for a health insurance plan. Examples would include the following:

BOX 12-1   **Affordable Care Act General Provisions**

2010
- Disallows insurance companies from rescinding benefits—declaring them invalid from their original start date—because of an honest mistake concerning information provided or leaving out information that has little bearing on the health care services needed
- $250 rebate for those in drug benefit coverage gap
- In March 2010, the Food and Drug Administration (FDA) may approve generic biological drugs
- Reinsurance coverage for employers providing insurance to retirees over age 55 who are not eligible for Medicare
  - Department of Health and Human Services (DHHS) began accepting applications in June 2010, which will be implemented through January 1, 2014
- Enactment of an insurance coverage plan for individuals with preexisting conditions who have been uninsured for at least 6 months; plan operated either by federal or state government agencies
- Enrollment began July 2010
  - Federal government is operating programs in 23 states and Washington, D.C.; remaining states operating their own programs
  - New plans for 2011 will lower PCIP premiums for enrollees
  - As of March 2011, 18k enrollees in PCIPs
- Adult-dependent coverage through age 26 on new plans and renewals to existing plans that renewed on or after September 23, 2010
- Prohibits insurance plans from placing lifetime limits on the dollar value of coverage, rescinding coverage (except in cases of fraud), and denying children coverage based on preexisting medical conditions or from including preexisting condition exclusions for children; restricts annual limits on the dollar value of coverage (and eliminates annual limits in 2014) for plans or policies beginning on or after September 23, 2010
- Insurance plans must have a process in place whereby consumers may appeal health plan decisions; must be an external review process for appeals submitted on or after September 23, 2010
- Requires new insurance plans to cover at a minimum preventive care services such as the following:
  - Recommended immunizations
  - Preventive care for infants, children, and adolescents
  - Additional preventive care screening for women

2011
- Consumer website with plan and benefit information required of Department of Health and Human Services, launched July 1, 2011
- Closing the gap on pharmacy benefit coverage with 50% discount on prescription drug prescriptions, implemented January 1, 2011—will reduce gap co-insurance payment from 100% in 2010 to 25% in 2020
- Freezes Medicare Part B premiums at 2010 through 2019 for higher-income beneficiaries
- Lowers percentages of fee-for-service rates for Medicare Advantage Plans; freezes 2011 rates at 2010 amounts
- Excludes costs of OTC drugs from reimbursement by health savings accounts
- Requires states to establish an American Health Benefit Exchange, which will provide affordable health care benefit plans to individuals who are currently uninsured; must be created by January 1, 2014
- Requires states to establish a small business health option plan for small businesses with 100 or fewer employees; requires both affordable and competitive health benefit plan options with better quality care options

2013
- Reduces amount of contribution to flexible spending accounts to $2500; implementation by January 1, 2013

BOX 12-1   Affordable Care Act General Provisions—cont'd

- Sets a 2.3% excise tax on any taxable medical device, scheduled for implementation on January 1, 2013
- Creates a consumer-operated and oriented plan (co-op) to foster the creation of nonprofit, member-run health insurance companies by July 1, 2013

2014
- Expansion of Medicaid benefits to all individuals not eligible for Medicaid under the age of 65, including the following:
  - Pregnant women
  - Parents
  - Adults without dependent children

- Asthma
- Heart or circulatory disease (such as high blood pressure or congestive heart failure)
- Diabetes
- Cancer
- Organ failure

Much like any other type of insurer, the companies that provide these services assess the extent to which a consumer will likely need to use their services. A person in poor health, or one with preexisting health conditions that require a great deal of provider care, medication therapy, or other types of treatment, would be considered a higher-risk patient by the company that outlays expenses for those services.

Often a person applying for health insurance may be subject to a physical or psychological examination by a qualifying health care provider to determine coverage eligibility. Insurance companies structure their plans based on the overall health of the consumer seeking coverage; until 2010, individuals with preexisting conditions either did not qualify or were subject to extremely high costs in order to receive those benefits. As a result of the Affordable Care Act, signed into effect by President Obama in 2010, there are emerging federal and state-sponsored insurance coverage plans for individuals with preexisting conditions who have been uninsured for at least 6 months. These are referred to as preexisting condition insurance plans (PCIPs).

Private and Public Health Benefits: Who's Paying What?

Health and pharmacy benefits may be administered either through a private source or through a program funded by either the federal government or a state agency. A beneficiary is an individual who is eligible to receive health care benefits, which often include pharmacy benefits for medication therapy. A beneficiary covered under a benefit plan may be the insured, the person's spouse, or any legal dependents. Each type of benefit plan has established coverage parameters, which clearly set forth the types of benefits that the plan will allow, based on the beneficiaries' eligibility. Benefit plans generally establish the following:
- Detailed information concerning what types of services are eligible for coverage and what is *not* covered
- The portion that the insurance company pays for eligible services
- The portion that the beneficiary or his or her employer pays for eligible services, if applicable
- A maximum dollar amount per service that the insurance provider will pay over the life of the plan policy, as well as the maximum dollar amount that a patient would be required to pay out of pocket per plan year and lifetime maximums for the policy

Pharmacy technicians need to be aware of a few key terms that may apply to both private and government benefit plans, and they should know how to explain those terms to patients concerning their benefits.

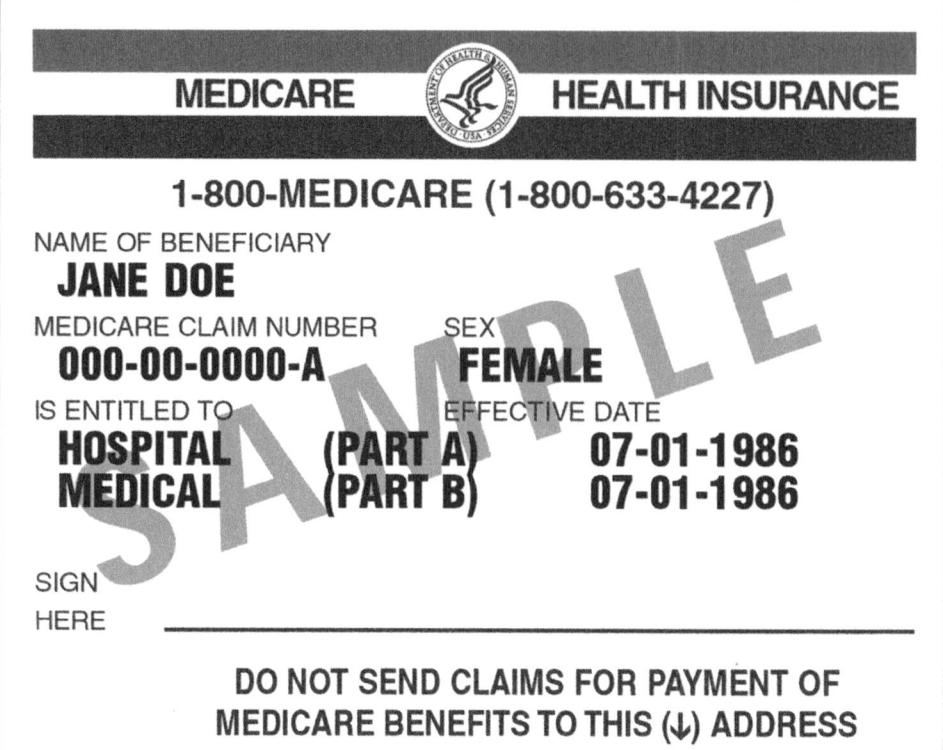

Sample insurance cards. (From DeVore A: *The electronic health record for the physician's office with MedTrak systems,* Philadelphia, 2011, Saunders.)

PRIMARY CARE PROVIDER (PCP)

Patients covered under a medical benefit generally must have an established primary care provider who will attend to the majority of their health care needs. This is typically a family or general practitioner who is qualified to attend to most areas of preventive care and general wellness and to treat minor to moderate conditions. From the standpoint of establishing a comprehensive treatment plan, it is in the best interest of the patient to build and maintain a medical history with a particular provider, thus generating a complete, accurate, and up-to-date medical profile that can be shared with other providers as applicable. This discourages patients from going to multiple providers and receiving several types of medical and pharmaceutical care, which may result in duplicate therapy or create therapeutic conflict between treatments.

If a PCP determines that the patient needs to seek the services of a specialist in a particular medical profession (such as a cardiologist or gastroenterologist), the patient's PCP will generally refer the patient to that specialist. Depending on the structure of the benefit plan, some plans require that the PCP formally refer the patient in writing, whereas others may allow patients to seek specialty services by an approved provider on their own.

DEDUCTIBLES AND PREMIUMS

A premium is a monthly rate established by the insurance provider that the beneficiary of medical/pharmacy benefits must pay in order to establish and maintain insurance coverage. For employer-provided benefits, both the employer and employee generally pay a portion of the monthly premium. A deductible is an established dollar amount that a beneficiary must pay out of pocket before the insurance plan pays out any benefits.

CO-PAYS

A co-pay is an established fixed amount that a beneficiary pays for a particular medical service or prescription. For example, each time the patient goes to the PCP, he or she may be required to pay $20 as the office visit co-pay, regardless of the service provided. Depending on how the benefit plan is structured, fixed co-pays are established for a variety of services, such as urgent/emergency care, laboratory/radiology diagnostics, or specialist doctor visits.

CO-INSURANCE

A co-insurance is a percentage that the beneficiary must pay for a particular type of care. For example, a patient who must have a hospital stay may be required to pay a co-insurance of 20% of the total amount that is billed to the insurance company. The insurance provider would then be responsible for the remaining 80%.

How Pharmacy Technicians Use This Information

As this information relates to pharmacy benefits, patients may be unaware of the fixed co-insurance or co-pay amounts that have been established by their medical/pharmacy benefit provider. In communicating with a benefit provider, pharmacy techs should verify prescription co-pay or co-insurance amounts, which may then be communicated and explained to the patient.

Private Health Insurance

Private health insurance may be provided by an individual's employer or by companies that provide stand alone health care insurance benefit plans based on the type of health care services that a person and his or her dependents may need. Employer-provided medical/pharmacy benefits were initially structured 60 years ago as an incentive to attract the best employees to a particular company. These early plans were structured based on an established, fixed "fee for services" that was determined by physicians. A patient would pay for services at the time they were rendered and forward the bill to the insurance company. The company would then evaluate the bill and reimburse the patient for an established portion of the costs. As the cost of medical and pharmaceutical care continued to rise in the 1980s and 1990s, employers sought ways to better manage expenses, with the help of outside organizations that could negotiate better pricing by establishing a network of health care providers. What is now known as *managed care* is administered by establishments known as health maintenance organizations (HMOs), preferred provider organizations (PPOs), or high-deductible health plans.

HEALTH MAINTENANCE ORGANIZATIONS

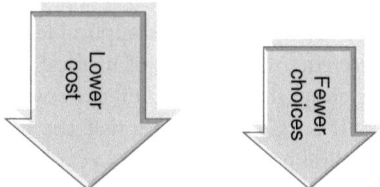

The focus of a health maintenance organization (HMO), as the name implies, is the maintenance of health through preventive care that should preserve a patient's overall health and wellness. Patients who regularly maintain their health are less likely to need emergency medicine, which can be costly. If a patient maintains regular visits to a health care provider, receives any vital immunizations, and establishes a regimen for managing any chronic health conditions, that person should maintain overall better health. HMOs generally negotiate lower monthly rates and premiums than other types of plans, so long as the beneficiary goes to a physician that is part of the HMO provider network. If a patient with an HMO plan chooses to go to a provider who is not in the HMO network, the costs of those services would not be eligible for coverage or reimbursement by the insurance company or employer. So although a beneficiary may pay less into an HMO plan, there are fewer choices in terms of which providers a patient may choose.

PREFERRED PROVIDER ORGANIZATIONS

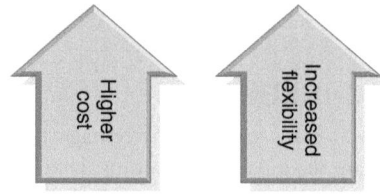

Although the preferred provider organization (PPO) also focuses on preventive care, this type of benefit plan allows patients more flexibility with the health care providers they choose to seek out for their health care needs. PPOs are generally more expensive in terms of monthly premiums, whereas plan deductibles tend to be lower than HMOs. PPO plan providers also work with an established network of approved providers. Beneficiaries pay lower co-pays when using in-network providers, and they have the freedom to pay more in order to see the out-of-network provider of their choice. Beneficiaries of PPOs do not need referrals to see specialists. Another advantage of the PPO plan—in light of the higher monthly premium—is that there is a limit to the out-of-pocket expense that a beneficiary will be subject to during a plan year. Once that out-of-pocket maximum has been reached, the PPO pays 100%. The beneficiary would only be responsible for co-pays for the remainder of the plan year.

Patients who seek out PPO plans must do so with the understanding that their PCP may not provide them with as comprehensive care as the HMO network provider; patients may see whomever they choose rather than managing all their preventive and specialized care through one PCP. However, most beneficiaries with PPOs generally do receive the majority of their preventive and general care from a PCP, while enjoying the flexibility of *seeking a second opinion* or specialized care whenever they choose.

How Pharmacy Technicians Use This Information

Patients with benefit plans that have a deductible may not always know when their entire deductible has been met. So it may be alarming for them to discover that a prescription for which they were expecting a lower fixed amount or co-pay has to be paid at full price until the plan deductible has been met. During the process of troubleshooting a pharmacy benefit issue, it is important for a pharmacy technician to verify if a plan requires a deductible and whether it has been met. If not, the technician should carefully explain this situation to the patient.

HIGH DEDUCTIBLE HEALTH PLANS

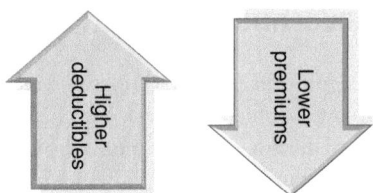

As the name suggests, a high deductible health plan (HDHP) is structured for a high initial out-of-pocket deductible that must be met, which proportionately lowers the monthly premium. The higher the deductible, the lower the monthly premium. Once the deductible has been met, the plan covers 100% of in-network expenses, so there would not be a co-pay (so long as the beneficiary goes to an in-network provider).

How Pharmacy Technicians Use This Information

Patients may occasionally receive services, including prescriptions, from an unapproved provider—for which their pharmacy benefits may not apply. Or prescriptions from a specialty provider may require a higher co-pay. When troubleshooting prescription benefit eligibility, a pharmacy technician should verify whether a health care provider is in or out of the insurer's network and communicate this information to the patient as a reason for the increased cost of the prescription.

HEALTH SAVINGS ACCOUNTS

Many employers are eligible to offer employees a health savings account (HSA)—also referred to as a flexible spending account. An employee may elect to have a percentage of his or her pretax salary (up to a maximum amount allowed by tax law) deposited into an account to be applied to that individual's eligible health care expenses. Using an HSA lowers the employee's taxable income and therefore his or her tax liability. However, the funds deposited must be used within that plan year or the employee will lose them and the tax benefit. HSAs are generally set up in one of two ways: either the beneficiary receives a debit account along with a debit card to use at the point of care, or the beneficiary pays for services out of pocket and submits claims to the HSA administrator for reimbursement. A claim is a paper or electronic invoice that details the medical/pharmaceutical care that was provided, the date on which that service was provided, and the payment required. Generally, claims for HSA reimbursement may be submitted by e-mail or fax to the claims administrator for processing. Although over-the-counter drugs were once eligible for HSA reimbursement, as of 2011 the ACA no longer allows for OTC drugs reimbursement. Additionally, in 2013, the amount that an individual may have deposited into an HSA to apply to medical expenses was reduced to a maximum of $2500 per plan year.

How Pharmacy Technicians Use This information

Patients may be unclear at times concerning what types of qualifying medications are covered by their HSA. For example, some plans cover certain types of over-the-counter medication and devices. Pharmacy technicians should verify with the benefit provider the types of items that are eligible for HSA debit or claim reimbursement and provide that information to the patient.

WHAT'S COMING IN 2014?

The Affordable Care Act will require each state to create, by 2014, more resources for individuals who are uninsured. Many individuals who remain underinsured or uninsured in the United States are those who are self-employed or those who work for small businesses that cannot afford to provide their employees with costly medical and pharmacy benefits. To close this gap, states will be required to create two new sources of health insurance coverage for these groups of individuals:

American Health Benefit Exchange. Quality, affordable plans for those who are employed (not low income) and uninsured.

Small Business Health Option Plan. Quality, affordable benefit packages that owners of small businesses (an average of 100 or fewer employees) may offer to their employees.

Government-Provided Benefits

A significant percentage of the American population is unable to afford health insurance because of low income or a permanent disability that prevents them from working. Because the accessibility of health care is a public health issue, the U.S. government has programs that will provide health care benefits to individuals who cannot afford to pay out of pocket because of unemployment, a permanent disability, or low income. As noted in Chapter 2, the federal government may intervene in a free market to avail public goods that a private market might otherwise not provide to the entire population because of inherent risks or limited profit margins. For such individuals, the state and federal governments provide health care benefits under Medicaid or Medicare. There are several key differences between these two programs; the most notable is that Medicaid is a state-governed plan, whereas Medicare is federally governed. Let's begin with Medicaid plan highlights.

MEDICAID

State Medicaid plans are administered by each state's welfare agency or Department of Health and Human Services. Medicaid provides both comprehensive and long-term care to low-income patients who meet any of the following qualifying criteria (Medicare.gov, 2008):

- Pregnant women
- Children under the age of 19
- People 65 and over
- People who are blind
- People who are disabled
- People who need nursing home care

More than 60 million low-income individuals in the United States receive Medicaid benefits. This accounted for $353.8 billion in 2010. It was estimated that Medicaid covers 36% of all births, 50% of all HIV patients, and 68% of all nursing home patients in the United States (MedicaidProgram.net, 2011). The costs for Medicaid are generally shared between federal and state funding sources, whereas local Medicaid services are exclusively managed by each state. Each state may have individual eligibility requirements as well as stipulations on the types of services that Medicaid programs may provide. Common examples include the following:

- Health care
  - Including home health care services to qualifying elderly patients residing in a state that offers a community first choice option (effective October 2011)
- Dental care
- Prescription drug coverage
- Annuities
  - Help to protect the assets of eligible individuals against the expected costs of nursing home care

The Affordable Care Act will expand Medicaid eligibility to a larger population of pregnant women—and individuals under the age of 65 who are adults with no children—whose incomes fall within an established percentage of the national poverty level average.

One of the greatest challenges associated with Medicaid costs is the accurate tracking of state expenditures for Medicaid claims. For example, audits of New York's Medicaid system by the state comptroller revealed that New York wasted at least $92 million in Medicaid funds because of billing errors, improper payments, and poor record keeping during a 5-year period.

How Pharmacy Technicians Use This Information

It is important that pharmacy technicians be knowledgeable concerning the eligibility requirements and Medicaid plan highlights within their state. Pharmacy technicians should verify plan information with representatives of the state agency that governs their state Medicaid plan, which may then be communicated to a patient.

MEDICARE

Medicare is a national health care plan that provides benefits to citizens age 65 and older, as well as many individuals with qualifying disabilities who are unable to work. A common example would be an individual with permanent kidney failure, which necessitates regular kidney dialysis or organ replacement. According to one web-based resource, there were 47,672,971 total Medicare beneficiaries across the United States in 2011 (The Henry J. Kaiser Family Foundation, 2011). Nearly all of those individuals qualified for Medicare Part D prescription drug coverage. This accounted for nearly $3.7 billion in prescription drug costs alone in 2009.

Anyone who pays federal taxes also pays into the federally funded Medicare plan; Medicare tax for 2011 was 1.45% for working individuals and their employers and was 2.9% for the self-employed.

Medicare benefits are divided into various parts, based on the type of benefit to which each is applied:

Medicare Part A. Provides benefits for inpatient hospital stays as well as long-term care in a skilled nursing facility, hospice, or home:
- Premiums are between $0 and $450/month depending on how long the enrollee or his or her spouse accrued Medicare-approved employment
- There is generally a deductible to be met before Part A pays for inpatient stays
- There are co-insurance payments for hospital stays longer than 60 days

Medicare Part B. Like traditional health care benefits, Part B covers preventive care as well as benefits for regular maintenance care in a physician's office. The plan covers provider services, hospital outpatient care, and home health care:
- The premium for Part B coverage was around $115 for enrollees in 2011

Medicare Part D. This portion covers prescription drug expenses and is managed by an approved private-party pharmacy benefit management company:
- Monthly premiums apply and vary depending on the plan; for most basic plans, the deductible was about $310 for 2011
- These are stand-alone plans that must be purchased in addition to Medicare Parts A and B
- Some plans may offer members customized options such as fixed co-payments with no deductibles
- Extensive generic drug coverage is available, particularly during coverage gap

WHAT IS THE PART D COVERAGE GAP?

Because of the cost of pharmacy benefits, most Medicare Part D plans have a maximum benefit dollar amount of coverage that is outlined in the plan. Once that maximum is reached, the beneficiary will be responsible for 100% of his or her prescription drug costs out of pocket, until a specified dollar amount has been reached. In 2011, the initial medication coverage limit was $2840 (Q1 Group, LLC, 2011). Beneficiaries must cover the out-of-pocket threshold of $4550. This "donut hole" is of great concern to Medicare beneficiaries, considering their often-limited sources of retirement income. This is of particular concern to individuals who take multiple prescription drugs as well as those who take costly drugs out of medical necessity in order to sustain their chronic conditions and quality of life.

As a result of the Affordable Care Act of 2010, individuals who have reached their prescription benefit threshold are now eligible to receive 50% off of Medicare-covered brand name drugs and a 7% discount off of generic drugs. Some Part D plans offer additional generic drug coverage during the coverage gap as well. Several provisions of the Affordable Care Act have been designed to gradually close the coverage gap by 2020.

MEDICARE ADVANTAGE PLANS

Also referred to as Part C Plans, Medicare Advantage Plans are provided by Medicare-approved private insurance companies. These plans are available for individuals who meet basic Medicare eligibility requirements, and they may enroll during the same enrollment periods for Medicare.

TECH NOTE!
Pharmacy technicians may stay current with industry rules and standards by periodically researching information related to pharmacy benefits. The U.S. Department of Health and Human Services provides excellent online resources on the Medicare.gov and Healthcare.gov websites.

They cover all the same services as Medicare, except for hospice care, which is still covered by Medicare Part A. Most include pharmacy benefits, so enrollment in a separate Part D plan is generally not necessary or allowed except for certain qualifying circumstances. Eligibility requirements include the following:

- Enrollment in Parts A and B (including premiums for Part B enrollment)
- All preexisting conditions are accepted, with the exception of end-stage renal disease (ESRD)

Pharmacy Benefit Managers (PBMs)

Whether a private or government-sponsored insurance plan, many pharmacy benefit plans are structured and managed by a pharmacy benefit management (PBM) company. Examples include the following:

- CVS/Caremark
- Wellpoint
- Express Scripts
- AdvancePCS

Just as with other forms of managed care, PBM companies form partnerships with health and pharmaceutical care organizations and negotiate competitive tiered pricing for prescription drug benefit plans. PBM companies negotiate plan structures with the following:

- Managed care organizations, such as Texas Health Resources or Humana
- Medicaid and Medicare
- Local government entities
- Pharmacy organizations, such as mail-order pharmacies

PBMs negotiate pricing based on several factors of key importance to their industry partners, such as:

- Drug/compound ingredient costs
- Dispensing fees
- Retail pharmacy networks
- Cost-sharing
- Prior authorization
- Step therapy
- Therapeutic substitution
- Formularies
- Medication therapy management (MTM) programs and services

Providers who work with PBM networks may prescribe within the parameters of an established drug formulary, whereas other products may be approved with prior authorization. They work to establish step therapy pricing, as well as other tiered pricing structures. An example of a tiered pricing structure includes the following:

Tier 1. Generic drugs: $5 to $10 co-pay for a 1-month supply

Tier 2. Brand name drugs that have no generic equivalent: $15 to $20 co-pay for a 1-month supply

Tier 3. Brand name drugs with generic or therapeutic equivalents available: $30 to $40 co-pay for a 1-month supply

Tier 4. Specialty drugs, such as biologics or gene therapy: a percentage of the cost of the drug as a co-payment

PBMs usually partner with mail-order pharmacies to offer 90-day supply programs for maintenance drugs as well as drugs for which patients are offered incentives for using the lower-cost generic versions. They also provide pharmacists and patients with clinical support by checking for drug interactions, appropriate dosing, excessive utilizations, and other patient-specific factors.

How Pharmacy Technicians Use This Information

Pharmacy technicians may need to conduct research with a PBM to determine a beneficiary's pricing for a particular medication. Technicians should seek out resources for staying current on the basic plan structures as well as benefit eligibility requirements that must be met for patients to use their benefits.

Insurance Terminology: The Language of Pharmacy Benefits Management for Pharmacy Technicians

There are a variety of industry-related terms that pharmacy technicians must be able to understand and actively apply when providing customer service to pharmacy patients. Reviewing these terms may help one to understand the structure of a pharmacy benefits plan. Table 12-1 details each of the terms that relate to pharmacy benefits, which are defined and described in greater detail in this section.

When a patient brings a prescription to a pharmacy to have it filled and processed for payment with his or her pharmacy benefits, a claim—or type of electronic bill—is generated in the pharmacy order management system. This claim contains—in condensed electronic code—details related to the patient, the drug benefit, the prescription information and drug cost, and other pharmacy pricing information that may be factored into the total cost being requested for payment. The following describes the electronic claim submission process:

1. When a claim is sent electronically—or *adjudicated*—the insurance company—or *payer*—will return an electronic response.
    - The response will generally reflect the amount that the insurance provider will pay for the prescription, as well as what the patient's portion will be, or the co-pay amount.
2. If plan criteria are not met, based on the type of drug benefits that the insurance company provides, then the claim may be rejected.
    - If a claim is rejected, a rejection code will be included with the electronic adjudication response from the insurance company.
3. A pharmacy staff member may need to conduct research with the benefit provider to find out additional details concerning the rejection code and to determine what needs to be added, removed, or modified in the claim in order for the insurance company to approve it.

This seeming back-and-forth troubleshooting process accounts for a large portion of what pharmacy staff members spend their time on during their working hours. Pharmacy technicians must become familiar with claim rejection codes—as well as strategies for correcting them—in order to communicate appropriately with pharmacy benefit providers. Often there is a relatively simple piece (or pieces) of information that must be added to the electronic claim in order to meet adjudication acceptance requirements. Table 12-2 provides a list of common claim rejection codes. As shown, a prescription may be rejected because of an incomplete patient profile, drug profile, or insurance plan setup. Entering the missing information and resending the claim often solves the problem.

Sometimes, however, a patient may need to return to his or her caregiver for a variety of reasons before a prescription order can be filled. For example, a patient may need to be examined by the caregiver or have laboratory testing done and submitted to the insurance company before medication therapy is initiated or continued. Pharmacists play a key role during the patient counseling session in informing patients of guidelines that must be followed during the course of their medication therapy. If a drug will require a medical examination before each refill, the pharmacist should advise patients of this condition so that they may complete that process prior to coming to the pharmacy to have the prescription filled.

Learning that their prescription cannot be filled and that they must return to their prescriber for further medical treatment is not happy news for patients. When communicating this information, pharmacy technicians must demonstrate a sense of empathy, in which they attempt to identify with the patient's difficult situation and communicate a genuine sense of caring and concern about the inconvenience.

STRUCTURED PRICING AND DRUG FORMULARIES

Whether through a private or publicly governed benefit plan, pharmacy benefits are typically defined by a listing of drugs for which a particular plan will provide special pricing or established co-pay rates, based on the type and cost of the drug. This listing is known as a formulary. Many companies further categorize drugs into therapy levels. Insurance companies generally set forth a list of products—usually lower-cost drugs—that a prescriber should use as the first line—or step—of therapy. If that drug achieves the desired therapeutic effect, then the patient should be encouraged to continue using that product. If the drug does not achieve the desired effect—or produces an

TABLE 12-1 **Pharmacy Benefits Terminology**

Insurance Terminology	Definition/Explanation
Appeal process	Steps that should be taken by a Medicare Part D beneficiary to request a reevaluation of a decision made about prescription coverage.
Appointed representative	A person designated by the Medicare beneficiary to act on his or her behalf in the prescription drug benefit coverage appeal process.
Brand name drug	A trademarked commercial name given to a generic drug product, often protected by drug patent.
Claim	A paper or electronic invoice that details medical/pharmaceutical care that was provided, the date on which that service was provided, and the payment required.
Contraindication	A category of drug information that indicates interactions among various drugs or classes of drugs that may result in serious complications if the drugs are taken during the same course of therapy.
Coverage determination	Sets forth the types of benefits that the plan may allow, based on the beneficiary's eligibility.
Coverage gap	The period in Medicare drug benefit coverage in which an established maximum is reached, at which point the beneficiary will be responsible for 100% of prescription drug costs out of pocket, until a specified dollar amount has been reached.
Covered drug	A prescription medication for which a beneficiary's prescription drug benefit pays at least part of the cost during the plan year.
Denial	Rejection on the part of the drug benefit provider to cover a particular medication, based on plan limitations or drug coverage restrictions.
Exception	A determining factor in a beneficiary's appeal of a prescription drug coverage denial. Beneficiaries may wish to establish a legitimate justification for gaining coverage of a particular drug, based on medical necessity. Also referred to as "coverage determination." An example would be appealing coverage for a drug that would not normally be covered under the plan's formulary, based on established and documented medical necessity, or a request to pay a lower-tier co-pay exception for a higher-tier medication because the beneficiary has no therapeutic options with the lower-tier drug products.
Formulary	A list of which medicines a benefit plan covers and at what level of co-payment.
Generic drug	A drug that does not have a trademarked name, and is the therapeutic equivalent of a brand name drug, while it has been manufactured at a much lower cost.
Out-of-pocket threshold	The maximum dollar amount that a patient may pay before the benefit plan will provide additional coverage. Future provisions of the ACA may lower these amounts for patients.
Over-the-counter (OTC) drugs	Drugs that can be purchased without a prescription and are not paid for by insurance or through a health care savings account unless prescribed by an eligible caregiver.
Pharmacy benefit management (PBM) company	A company that manages pharmacy benefits and may assist an insurer in providing a pharmacy benefit plan.
Prior authorization	A form of drug benefit coverage determination that requires a prescriber to obtain advance approval for a particular product before the patient will receive benefit coverage.
Step therapy	A provision of a prescription drug benefit in which the prescriber must initially try drugs from lower (cost) tiers before use of a higher tier (more expensive) drug is covered under the drug benefit.
Therapeutic substitution	The process of switching an existing prescription to another—usually less expensive— medicine that is chemically different (not a generic), but is used to treat the same clinical condition.
Tiered co-pay	Groups of medicines with the same co-payment. Prescription drug plans group drugs on their approved formulary into these tiers, for which there will be a different co-payment amount.

TABLE 12-2   **Insurance Rejection Codes and Resolutions**

Category	Rejection Code (M/I = Missing or Invalid)		Resolution
Insurance card information	M/I Group Number M/I Cardholder ID Number M/I Person Code		Verify patient's plan information as noted on benefits card, or call plan provider
Prescription information	M/I Date of Service M/I Prescription/Service Reference Number M/I Fill Number M/I Days Supply M/I Compound Code M/I Product/Service ID M/I Dispense as Written (DAW)/Product Selection Code M/I Ingredient Cost Submitted M/I Number Refills Authorized Prior Authorization Not Required M/I Prior Authorization Supporting Documentation	Active Prior Authorization Exists—Resubmit at Expiration of Prior Authorization Prior Authorization In Process Authorization Number Not Found Prior Authorization Denied Date Written Is After Date Filled Days Supply Limitation for Product/Service	Verify information entered in pharmacy database May need to contact prescriber for further information or approvals (such as prior-authorization requests)
Patient information	M/I Birth Date M/I Smoker/Non-Smoker Code M/I Prescriber Location Code M/I Patient Gender Code M/I Patient Relationship Code M/I Patient Location M/I Pregnancy Indicator		Verify information entered under patient profile and update
Prescriber information	M/I Primary Care Provider ID		Verify information entered under prescriber profile Verify provider eligibility with benefit provider
Electronic processing error	M/I Pharmacy Number M/I Bin Duplicate Paid/Captured Claim Claim Has Not Been Paid/Captured Claim Not Processed Submit Manual Reversal Reversal Not Processed	DUR Reject Error System Unavailable/Host Unavailable Time Out Scheduled Downtime Payer Unavailable Connection to Payer Is Down Host Processing Error	Verify information entered for electronic claims submission in the pharmacy system Resend electronic claim May need to seek technical support from the company the pharmacy management system provider
Eligibility issue	M/I Other Coverage Code M/I Eligibility Clarification Code M/I Coordination of Benefits/Other Payments Count Pharmacy Not Contracted With Plan on Date of Service Submit Bill to Other Processor or Primary Payer Patient Is Not Covered Patient Age Exceeds Maximum Age Filled Before Coverage Effective Filled After Coverage Expired	Filled After Coverage Terminated Product/Service Not Covered Prescriber Is Not Covered Primary Prescriber Is Not Covered Refills Are Not Covered Other Carrier Payment Meets or Exceeds Payable Prior Authorization Required Plan Limitations Exceeded Discontinued Product/Service ID Number Cost Exceeds Maximum Refill Too Soon	May need to refer to the benefit plan provider, may be information that could be provided related to verifying eligibility status May need to contact prescriber to obtain prior-authorization information Claim may need to be submitted to a different benefit provider

undesired effect when taken alone or in combination with other drugs that the patient may be actively taking—then the prescriber may seek other therapeutic options. This practice is known as **step therapy**.

How Pharmacy Technicians Use This Information

If a patient has difficulty gaining approval for benefits coverage on a particular drug, a pharmacy technician may wish to gain information on whether or not there is documentation on file related to whether step-therapy plan requirements have been met. If there is a lower-tiered drug that a patient must have tried (unless the prescriber has established a therapeutic basis for an exception), the patient needs to *first* try the lower-tier drug, then move up to a higher-tier drug if the first-step product does not achieve the intended therapeutic result. In this instance, the pharmacy technician would refer this matter to a pharmacist, who would then call the prescriber to make a therapeutic substitution to a lower-step drug.

Often a prescriber may already be aware that prescribing a particular drug may create issues for a patient in terms of his or her pharmacy benefit coverage. A prescriber may preemptively request approval based on medical necessity by submitting a prior-authorization request to the insurance company. If approved, the patient would then receive drug benefit coverage for that prior-authorized product. Some limitations for therapy often apply in this case. If a claim is rejected, prior authorization may be obtained after the fact. Either the patient will contact the prescriber and request that the prescriber contact the insurance company to submit a prior-authorization request, or a pharmacy staff member will call to inform the prescriber that a prior-authorization request is required for the patient to obtain the prescription using the prescription drug plan benefits.

There may be a formulary listing of drugs that are covered by a prescription benefit plan, whereas the patient's co-payment might increase based on the cost of the product. This is another type of tiered drug pricing. For example, the patient might obtain an inexpensive antihistamine at a co-pay of only $10, so long as the generic product is used. If the patient wished for a brand name version of that drug, however, the co-pay may increase to $20. If the patient wished to gain a prescription for a newer antihistamine product, one for which only a brand name version is available, the co-pay for that drug may increase to $40. This pricing structure is commonly referred to as the *tiered co-pay*.

Relax, Relate, Research, and Resolve: Working with Patients and Their Pharmacy Benefits Management

Often, frustrated patients may already be aware of issues concerning the successful processing of their prescriptions. But just vocalizing those frustrations to someone who will hear, understand, and express a desire to help can make all the difference in the world. When interacting with an angry or frustrated patient, it is a good idea to follow these four steps:

1. *Relax.* Maintain a steady, normal tone of voice and volume. Allow the patient to vent without redirecting blame or responding defensively. Remember that *these patients are not angry with you,* so try not to personalize or internalize their actions.
   a. If a patient is getting out of control or evidences signs that he or she could become a danger to him or herself, other patients, or pharmacy staff members, then a pharmacist should be notified immediately. Pharmacies are generally equipped with emergency "panic" buttons that will signal local law enforcement in the event that staff members or other patients are placed in a threatening or dangerous situation.
   b. Once a patient is allowed to release his or her frustration, make another attempt to calmly and clearly communicate, asking open-ended questions. The process of explaining the information may, in itself, create a diversion and diffuse a patient's emotional response.
2. *Relate.* Try to view the problem from the patient's perspective by imagining how you might feel if placed in that situation and the action that you would wish to be taken to assist you. Personalizing a patient's position often helps pharmacy staff members to better demonstrate empathy and express genuine concern for a patient's needs.

3. *Research.* Take another look at the types of rejection codes shown in Table 12-2. Many of these rejections are preventable! If the patient is effectively interviewed when the prescription is accepted, many common rejection errors can be prevented from occurring in the first place. Ask appropriate, probing questions, and ensure that you clarify patient's responses. Always ensure the following:
   a. The patient's information is verified and the patient has an active and updated profile.
   b. The prescriber's information is verified and the prescriber is eligible on the patient's insurance plan.
   c. The patient presents the most current insurance plan information, and all information, such as dependent codes, is verified for accuracy.
   d. All information on the prescription has been verified for validity and accuracy. Check the date to ensure that the prescription is still valid *before* the patient walks away.
   e. Be efficient and plan your work whenever possible. Do as much of the legwork as possible while the patient is waiting, or while the patient is gone, to minimize wait time. Write down information that you gain, using clear, concise documentation. This will eliminate the need to ask the patient to repeat any information unnecessarily.
4. *Resolve.* Take ownership of the patient's issue and assure the patient that you will take whatever steps are necessary and allowed within your scope of practice as a pharmacy technician in order to offer assistance. Then, follow through! If a claim was rejected because of a pharmacy-related issue such as an order-entry error or failure to gather vital information, apologize on behalf of the pharmacy, whether or not you were the individual directly involved with the error. Often a patient's anger and frustration are quickly diffused when a pharmacy staff member accepts accountability for an error.

Chapter Summary

- Health care benefits allow the population greater access to services that will allow them to stay healthy, treat minor illness or injury, and assess risk factors for certain types of diseases.
- The accessibility of health care and immunizations allows the health care community to control the spread of communicable diseases that would affect the health of the population at large.
- The goal of health care reform is to identify a strategy for ensuring that everyone has access to health care, regardless of social status.
- Medical benefit insurability is based on a patient's prior and current health and medical history of illness.
- As a result of the Affordable Care Act, signed into effect by President Obama in 2010, there are emerging federal and state-sponsored insurance coverage plans for individuals with preexisting conditions who have been uninsured for at least 6 months. These are referred to as preexisting condition insurance plans (PCIPs).
- Health and pharmacy benefits may be administered either through a private source or through a program funded by either the federal government or a state agency.
- A beneficiary is an individual who is eligible to receive health care benefits.
- There are a few key terms that may apply to both private and government benefit plans that pharmacy technicians need to be aware of: primary care provider (PCP), premium, co-pays, and co-insurance.
- Private health insurance may be provided by an individual's employer.
- Managed care is administered by organizations known as health maintenance organizations (or HMOs), preferred provider organizations (PPOs), or high-deductible health plans.
- Many employers are eligible to offer employees a health savings account—also referred to as a flexible spending account. Employees elect to have a percentage of their pretax salary (up to a maximum amount allowed by tax law) deposited into an account to be applied to their eligible health care expenses.
- The Affordable Care Act will require each state to create, by 2014, more resources for individuals who are uninsured.

- The state and federal governments provide health care benefits under Medicaid or Medicare. Medicaid is a state-governed plan, whereas Medicare is federally governed.
- Medicaid plans are administered by each state's welfare agency or Department of Health and Human Services.
- Medicare is a national health care plan that provides benefits to citizens age 65 and older, as well as many individuals with qualifying disabilities who are unable to work.
- Anyone who pays federal taxes also pays into the federally funded Medicare plan.
- Medicare tax for 2011 was 1.45% for working individuals and their employers, and it was 2.9% for the self-employed.
- Medicare benefits are divided into various parts, based on the type of benefit each applies to.
- Many pharmacy benefit plans are structured and managed by a pharmacy benefit management (PBM) company.
- PBMs usually partner with mail-order pharmacies to provide 90-day supply programs for maintenance drugs as well as those for which incentives may be offered for using the lower-cost generic products.
- Pharmacy benefits are typically defined by a listing, or formulary, of drugs for which a particular plan will provide special pricing or established co-pay rates.
- Insurance companies generally set forth a list of products—usually lower-cost drugs—that a prescriber should use as the first line—or step—of therapy.
- When a claim is sent electronically to the insurance company, the company will return an electronic response.
- If plan criteria are not met, based on the type of drug benefits that the patient's benefit plan specifies, then a claim may be rejected.
- A pharmacy staff member may need to conduct research to learn what must be corrected in an order before the insurance company will approve it.
- When interacting with an angry or frustrated patient concerning billing issues, a pharmacy technician may follow these four steps: relax, relate, research, and resolve.

REVIEW QUESTIONS

Multiple Choice

1. This may be either paper or electronic and details prescription information and what payment is required:
   a. Coverage determination
   b. Claim
   c. Denial
   d. Exception

2. What provision of a pharmacy benefit plan requires that a lower-level drug be prescribed first before a higher-level drug is prescribed?
   a. Step therapy
   b. Therapeutic substitution
   c. Coverage determination
   d. Tiered co-pay

3. What would a patient request of his or her prescriber in order to gain approval for a medication that the benefits company would normally not approve?
   a. Appeal
   b. Therapeutic substitution
   c. Prior authorization
   d. Step therapy

4. What is the list of drugs that a particular pharmacy benefit plan may cover?
   a. Coverage determination
   b. OTC drugs
   c. Formulary
   d. Coverage gap

5. This sets forth what types of services are not covered by a medical/pharmacy benefit plan:
   a. Coverage determination
   b. PBM
   c. Step therapy
   d. Formulary

6. At which point in Medicare Part D coverage does the patient pay 100% of the co-insurance?
   a. Coverage gap
   b. Appeal
   c. Exception
   d. Step therapy

7. What is the fixed amount that a beneficiary must pay for a particular service?
   a. Coinsurance
   b. Co-pay
   c. Premium
   d. Deductible

8. What type of private health benefit requires that beneficiaries gain most of their health care from one primary plan-approved provider?
   a. HMO
   b. PPO
   c. HDHP
   d. HAS

9. What type of private health benefit allows beneficiaries to see out-of-network providers?
   a. HMO
   b. PPO
   c. HDHP
   d. HAS

10. Which part of the Medicare benefit plan covers medication costs?
    a. Part A
    b. Part B
    c. Part C
    d. Part D

Short Answer

1. What is the sole nonqualifying preexisting condition that will disallow a person from enrolling in a Medicare Advantage Plan?

2. Give a short answer concerning how a pharmacy technician might resolve the following pharmacy claim rejections, based on information provided in the chapter:
   - Dependent's age exceeds the maximum age limit on record
   - Missing days' supply
   - Missing "Dispense As Written" (DAW) code
   - Invalid patient gender code
   - Patient is not covered

3. Describe the types of coverage determinations details that a pharmacy plan beneficiary may wish to clarify with the benefit plan provider.

Bibliography

Center for American Progress. (2011). *SHOPping Around: Setting Up State Healthcare Exchanges: A Roadmap.* Retrieved 7/6/2011, from Center for American Progress: www.americanprogress.org/issues/2011/07/shop_exchange.html

Healthcare.gov. (2010, September 23). *Understanding the Affordable Care Act: Provisions.* Retrieved 6/6/2011, from Healthcare.gov: www.healthcare.gov/law/provisions/choice_access/index.html

Henry J. Kaiser Family Foundation. (2011). *Implementation Timeline.* Retrieved 7/6/2011, from Health Reform Source: healthreform.kff.org/timeline.aspx

Henry J. Kaiser Family Foundation. (2011). *Total Number of Medicare Beneficiaries, 2011*. Retrieved 7/4/2011, from Statehealthfacts.org: www.statehealthfacts.org/comparemaptable.jsp?ind=290&cat=6&sort=a

Illinois Department of Healthcare and Family Services. (2011). *HIPAA Claim Rejection Codes*. Retrieved 7/6/2011, from HFS Illinois Department of Healthcare and Family Services: www.hfs.illinois.gov/hipaa/faq3.html

Richardson, J., The Health Strategies Consultancy, LLC. (2003, June 26). *PBMs: The Basics and an Industry Overview*. Retrieved 7/7/2011, from ftc.gov: www.ftc.gov/ogc/healthcarehearings/docs/030626richardson.pdf

MedicaidProgram.net. (2011). *1 Medicaid Program–Waste of Medicaid Funds*. Retrieved 7/4/2011, from MedicaidProgram.net: www.medicaidprogram.net/articles/137707/Medicaid-Program

MedicaidProgram.net. (2011). *Medicaid Program*. Retrieved 7/4/2011, from MedicaidProgram.net: www.medicaidprogram.net/articles/137707/Medicaid-Program

Medicare.gov. (2008, August 26). *Frequently Asked Questions About Medicare*. Retrieved 7/3/2011, from Medicare.gov–The Official U.S. Government Site for Medicare: questions.medicare.gov/app/answers/detail/a_id/2038/session/L3NpZC96eGh2MzZ5aw%3D%3D

Medicare.gov. (2011, last updated May 20). *How Advantage Medicare Plans Work*. Retrieved 7/5/2011, from Medicare.gov–The Official U.S. Government Site for Medicare: questions.medicare.gov/app/answers/detail/a_id/2254/c/3

Q1Group, LLC. (2011). *What Is the Outlook for Medicare Part D 2011?* Retrieved 7/5/2011, from Q1 Medicare.com: www.q1medicare.com/PartD-The-2011-Medicare-Part-D-Outlook.php

Wisconsin Physician Service Health Insurance. (2011). *Common Claim Codes Explained*. Retrieved 7/6/2011, from WPS Health Insurance: www.wpsic.com/customers/help_claims_codes.shtml

www.yourpharmacybenefit.org. (2011). *Private Insurance–Glossary*. Retrieved 6/30/2011, from Your Pharmacy Benefit.org: www.yourpharmacybenefit.org/medicare/glossary.asp

13

Cultural Competence: The Journey to Effective Communication in a Culturally Diverse Society

KEY TERMS

Active listening: The skill of focusing one's attention on what a person actually says and how he or she says it, rather than just hearing the person's voice.

Bias: A preference or an inclination, especially one that inhibits impartial judgment.

Cultural imperialism: The extensive infusion of one nation's culture into the culture of another nation.

Cultural norms: A set of behaviors that a particular cultural group commonly associates with itself.

Cultural relativism: The belief that the behaviors and customs of any culture must be viewed and analyzed by that culture's own standards.

Culture: Knowledge, language, values, customs, and material objects passed from person to person and from one generation to the next in a human group or society.

Ethnic pluralism: The coexistence of a variety of distinct racial and ethnic groups in one society.

Ethnocentrism: The assigning of a lesser value to cultures other than one's own; viewing one's own culture and way of life as superior to all others.

Media: The means through which communication is transmitted to the receiver as part of the communication model.

Message/feedback: Thought, idea, emotion, or information that is transmitted in the communication model.

Message incongruence: Instances in which the sender's direct and indirect communications transmit very different messages, from the receiver's perspective.

Prejudice: A negative attitude based on faulty generalizations about members of selected racial and ethnic groups.

Receiver: The person or group in the communication model that receives the message.

Sender: The person or group in the communication model that transmits the message.

What does culture mean to you? One definition of culture might be the knowledge, language, values, customs, and material objects passed from person to person and from one generation to the next in a human group or society.

The dictionary has several interesting definitions of culture that summarize the concepts presented in this chapter (Merriam-Webster Online, 2011):

- The integrated pattern of human knowledge, belief, and behavior that depends upon the capacity for learning and transmitting knowledge to succeeding generations
- The set of shared attitudes, values, goals, and practices that characterizes an institution or organization
- The customary beliefs, social forms, and material traits of a racial, religious, or social group; *also,* the characteristic features of everyday existence (as diversions or a way of life) shared by people in a place or time.

The first definition suggests that culture is defined by patterns established through the passing of knowledge, beliefs, and behaviors across generations. The second definition suggests that culture is an identity formed largely by the collective traits of an external group to which a person inherently belongs (e.g., ethnicity) or with which a person identifies (e.g., a social culture, such as the hippie culture of the 1960s). The third definition suggests that culture is a consummate set of established values that help define an institution or organization, the way the organization wants to be perceived, and the behaviors it expects from those who choose to be members.

In their interactions with a person of another culture, it is important that pharmacy technicians recognize the factors that have influenced the formation of the patient's culture or cultures. Also, within a culture, there may be subcultures or groups of people who share a distinctive set of cultural beliefs and behaviors that differ significantly from those of the larger society.

Generally, a set of behaviors is commonly associated with a particular cultural group *by that group;* these are called cultural norms. Some norms may be positive and others not. Often these norms are so integrated into a person's thought process that the individual may not be conscious of them and how they are displayed in his or her behavior.

The process of exploring another culture and its norms often allows each of us (or forces us, in some cases) to conduct a personal inventory of our own cultural norms and the ways they drive our interactions with others. Such an inventory may reveal attitudes, beliefs, and behaviors that others may find offensive or that may create a barrier to effective relationship building. There is great value in using self-discovery to identify behavioral modifications that create more openness to exploring and embracing the differences in others. It is important to recognize that a person does not have to agree or identify with the ideals and behaviors associated with a particular culture or subculture to communicate and interact positively with members of that group. Indeed, cultural identities tend to be concentric (overlapping), because we are all human beings. Bear in mind that a cultural norm should not be confused with a *stereotype,* which is a conventional, formulaic, and oversimplified conception, opinion, or image that has been widely used in a particular group of people, a culture, or a subculture. Stereotypes usually are based on outside individuals' perceptions and opinions, rather than on the viewpoint of the group.

Many commonalities can be identified and embraced as a foundation for establishing communication and relationships, whether personally or professionally. However, this requires a lifelong process of becoming *interculturally competent.* The journey begins here.

This chapter discusses various forms of communication and the degree to which cultural context influences how members of different cultures send and receive information. In this case, the term *context* refers to "implicit meaning" (in terms of culture). A basic model, or structure, applies to communication intended to transmit information from one source to another. This chapter discusses each of the key components of the communication model and the ways pharmacy technicians can demonstrate these behaviors in their healthcare role.

Communication Model

The communication model (Figures 13-1 and 13-2) comprises the following structural components:

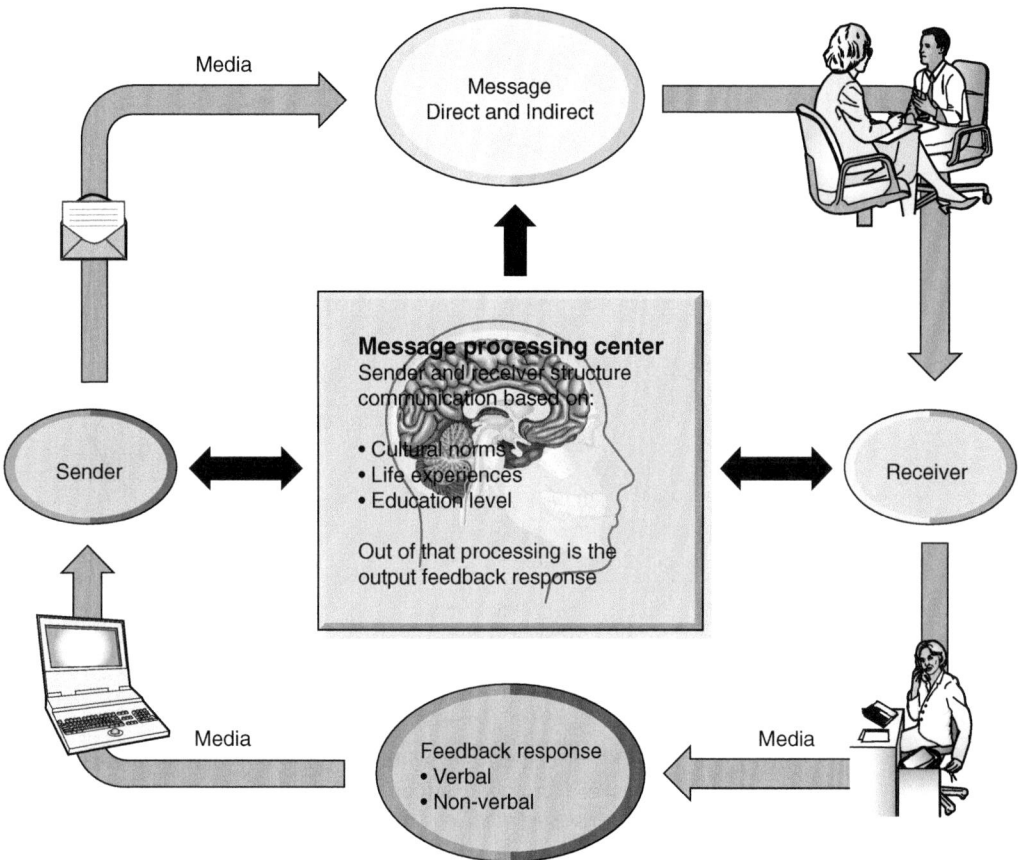

FIGURE 13-1 Communication model.

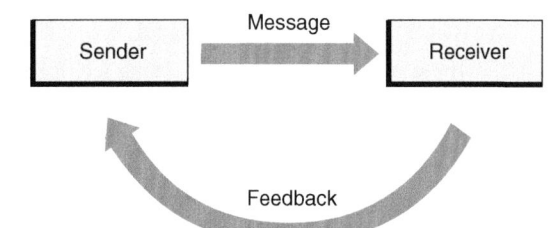

FIGURE 13-2 Communication is a two-way process. (From Perry A, Potter P: *Clinical nursing skills and techniques,* ed 7, St Louis, 2009, Mosby.)

- Sender: The person sending a message.
- Receiver: The person intended to receive the message.
- Message/feedback: The thought, idea, emotion, or information that is transmitted.

Media are generally the means through which the communication is transmitted to the receiver. The message may be sent to one or more people, directly or indirectly, by a variety of media.

- Directly
  - Speech
    - Face-to-face interaction
    - Telephone
  - Written communication
  - Electronic media (e.g., e-mail, text message, fax)
- Indirectly (nonverbal communication cues)
  - Gestures
  - Facial expressions

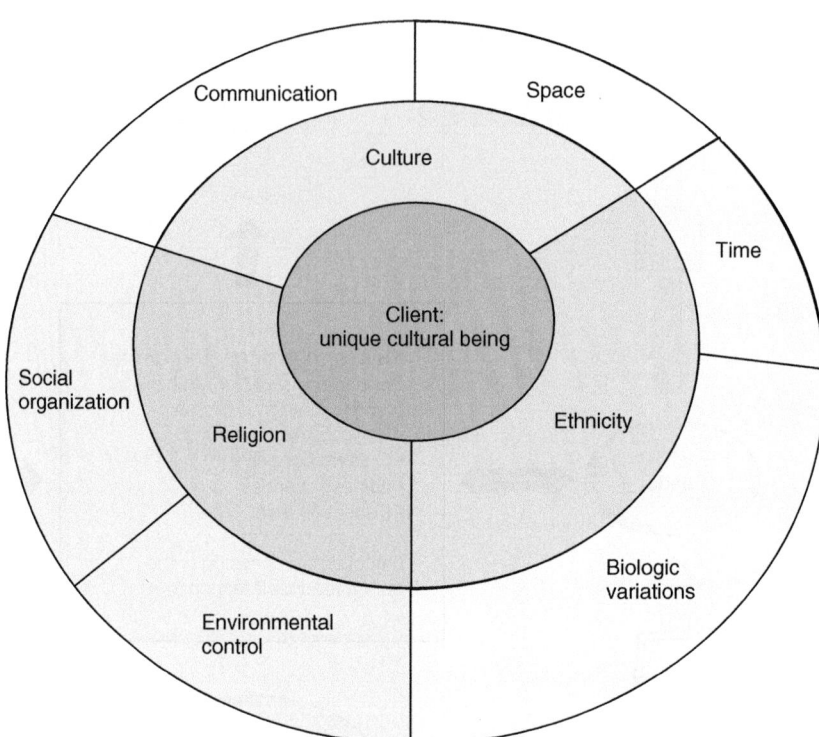

FIGURE 13-3 Model of the patient within a culturally unique heritage and the cultural phenomena that have a profound effect on nursing care. (From Giger J, Davidhizar RE: *Transcultural nursing: assessment and intervention,* ed 5, St Louis, 2008, Mosby.)

- Posture (body positioning)
- Eye contact

MESSAGE PROCESSING

The way a receiver processes a message may be influenced by:
- Personal experience
- Cultural context (Figure 13-3)
- Educational background
- Natural tendencies toward communication

Message processing may be filtered by a person's cultural norms, which can strongly influence the receiver's response to the sender. For example, a younger individual responding to a person who is older or in a position of authority may follow a cultural norm of showing respect for elders. Rather than speaking frankly, the younger person may choose to address the elder more formally, with a response that reflects the respect customarily extended to an elder.

The receiver of the message processes the information transmitted and responds with *feedback* that is based on the receiver's personal interpretation of the information. The extent to which the receiver processes the message in the context that the sender intended often varies widely. Because personal interpretation can be quite subjective, it is extremely important that the sender verify with the receiver that the message was received and interpreted as the sender intended. Otherwise, messages may be misinterpreted, creating conflict between sender and receiver.

MESSAGE INCONGRUENCE

Sometimes the sender's direct and indirect messages transmit very different meanings from the perspective of the receiver; this is called *incongruence.* Note the following examples of incongruent messages.
- A flustered, visibly agitated nurse comes to the main pharmacy, wags her finger at the technician who greets her, and loudly proclaims, "I'm not angry, I'm just here to ask about a medication fill error!"

TECH ALERT!
If the receiver seems confused, use the phrase, "What did you hear me say?" because sometimes what was intended and what was received are different.

- A disappointed pharmacist has tried, so far without success, to convince a physician to change an obviously inappropriate medication order. When asked how he is feeling, he meekly replies, "Oh, I'm just fine."
- A pharmacist hands an intravenous (IV) label to a technician, who bursts into tears. The pharmacist asks what is wrong, and the technician responds, "No, I'm okay, it's nothing at all."

Incongruence also may occur if cultural norms that drive communication are not recognized. In cases of message incongruence, it is important to ask a few simple, open-ended questions to help clarify what the person is truly trying to communicate. For example, "Although you said you were okay, you seem unhappy. How can I help?" or "What would make you feel better about this situation?"

RECEIVING AND GIVING FEEDBACK

Receiving Feedback

Once a message has been sent, the receiver processes the information and, based on his or her interpretation of it, sends feedback. The sender can receive the feedback in ways that allow him or her the best opportunity to understand it the way the receiver intends. The following are some positive characteristics to practice when receiving feedback.

- Openness: Listen without interrupting or arguing.
- Acceptance: Accept the feedback without devaluing it.
- Respect: Recognize the feedback's value and the value of the person who sent it.
- Engagement: Interact with the speaker and ask for clarification when appropriate.
- Active listening: Listen carefully and try to understand. It is okay to say, "I understand," which does not mean, "I agree," but allows both parties to feel the message had been sent and received.
- Thoughtfulness: Try to understand the personal behaviors and/or cultural norms that may influence the feedback.
- Interest: Show genuine interest in receiving feedback.
- Sincerity: Show a genuine desire to make personal changes if they are appropriate.

Conversely, certain behaviors should be avoided when receiving feedback.

- Defensiveness: Defending one's personal actions and objecting to the feedback.
- Attacking: Verbally attacking the person giving the feedback.
- Denial: Refuting the accuracy or fairness of the feedback.
- Disrespect: Devaluing the speaker and the feedback provided.
- Closed-mindedness: Ignoring the feedback and demonstrating no interest in receiving it.
- Inactive listening: Hearing words but not listening for their meaning and interpretation.
- Rationalizing: Finding explanations that remove personal responsibility.
- Patronizing: Listening and agreeing without intending to use the feedback to make any changes.

Giving Feedback

When a person receives a message, the information received is processed mentally, emotionally, and with a number of filters derived from the sources discussed earlier. Consider the following tips for giving feedback:

- Be clear and concise; do not pull unrelated information into the dialog.
- Have a positive emphasis; feedback is intended to uplift, not tear down.
- Be specific; avoid generalizations or extremes, such as "always" and "never."
- Focus; highlight the *behavior* observed, not the *person*.
- Be descriptive; give enough detail so that the receiver understands the feedback.
- Own your feedback; use "I" statements that demonstrate personal accountability.

Active Listening

Most people have experienced the frustration of attempting conversation with someone who was not actually *listening* to them. Active listening is the skill of not just *hearing* a person as he or she speaks, but of paying individual attention to what the person is actually saying and to *how* the person is saying it. Active listening is crucial to effective communication in the healthcare setting. In today's culture of multitasking, it can be very difficult to do. Pharmacy technicians must deal with numerous distractions; therefore, they must make a concerted effort to actively listen to each other and to patients so as to prevent a misunderstanding that could result in harm to a patient or pharmacy staff member. As a pharmacy technician, the following behaviors can help you make sure you are actively listening.

- Establish appropriate eye contact. This often requires some knowledge of cultural norms for eye contact. Limited eye contact, by itself, is not necessarily an indicator of inattention; some cultures consider steady eye contact offensive or inappropriate.
- Provide the communicator with an outward indicator of your attention, such as a nod or other facial or nonverbal cue.
- Allow the speaker to communicate without interruption.
- Concentrate on not mentally formulating a response while the speaker is still communicating.
- Once the speaker has finished and before you respond, ask questions, if necessary, to make sure you clearly understand what was communicated.

A commitment to active listening allows healthcare professionals to better understand and learn from each other. When cultural norms are a factor, asking open-ended questions about the individual's cultural preferences for communication—as well as behaviors that should be avoided—helps improve understanding. For example, in some cultures, a woman's husband speaks for her in certain official situations. A person who was not raised in that culture might find that difficult to understand. Again, you do not have to agree or identify with the ideals and behaviors associated with a particular culture or subculture to communicate and interact productively. Pharmacy technicians must acknowledge, respect, and adjust their patterns of communication whenever necessary to suit the needs of a widely diverse patient population.

Achieving Cultural Competence as a Pathway to Better Communication and Care of Patients

DEFINING CULTURAL EXPRESSION

The process of achieving cultural competence is an ongoing personal journey. Often the first place to begin exploring other cultures is to consider how an individual feels about his or her own culture. How people view their own ethnicity and cultural self may influence how they feel about and respond to individuals of other cultures. The field of sociology has defined several terms that best describe how individuals may view themselves and others from a cultural standpoint. These definitions apply to a variety of factors besides ethnicity.

- Cultural imperialism: The extensive infusion of one nation's culture into that of another nation.
- Cultural relativism: The belief that the behaviors and customs of any culture must be viewed and analyzed by the culture's own standards.
- Ethnic pluralism: The coexistence of a variety of distinct racial and ethnic groups in one society.
- Prejudice: A negative attitude based on faulty generalizations about members of selected racial and ethnic groups.

Many individuals confuse *cultural pride* with ethnocentrism. Cultural pride is pride in one's heritage and an active observance of traditions and ways of demonstrating and preserving a cultural heritage. In contrast, ethnocentrism means assigning less value to cultures other than one's own. Ethnocentrism can lead to offensive and destructive behavior; over time, negative attitudes may escalate to aggression against individuals of other cultures to which a person feels superior. Ethnic pluralism is the opposite of ethnocentrism; it acknowledges each culture as equal to others, all capable of coexisting peacefully. Pluralism allows each culture to maintain its own identity, while enabling people to learn and gain value and perspective from other cultures.

It is important to recognize that many nations, including the United States, are multicultural and have been for a long time. Avoiding acknowledging other cultures dismisses the tremendous value to be gained when people extend their perspective outside what they know and find comfortable.

So, How Does This Relate to Communication in Healthcare?

Most metropolitan areas in the United States are culturally diverse from the standpoint of ethnicity, social status, gender designations, and sexual orientation. Unless people do not travel outside their immediate residential area, they inevitably must interact with individuals of other cultures and social subcultures. The same is true in today's culturally diverse healthcare setting. Recognizing how we relate to our own cultural selves makes us more aware of how this affects our responses and ability to communicate effectively with individuals of other cultures, whether that culture is one of ethnicity or social or sexual orientation. Becoming more comfortable with our own definition of cultural awareness opens the door for personal growth and the ability to understand, rather than dismiss or avoid, other cultural groups.

The Only Thing to Fear Is Fear Itself

Often the underlying issue of a communications barrier is a fear of the unknown (e.g., whether a person of another culture understands you) or perhaps a fear of offending people as you try to gain an understanding of their cultural norms. To remove those barriers, you must be willing to open yourself to creating opportunities to learn, grow, and expand your appreciation of other cultures. A few strategies for increasing your own understanding might include any of the following as a starting point.

- Conduct your own research.
  - Find trusted sources of information about various cultures, particularly sources that describe cultural norms in a culture or subculture.
- Ask appropriate questions.
  - Ask someone of another culture, with whom you have a rapport and a professional relationship, to share his or her perspective on how you might better understand that culture and the types of behavior that should be avoided.
    - Asking people to provide perspective gives them the freedom to share what they choose and are comfortable with sharing, rather than limiting their responses to your questions.
    - Avoid asking questions that are derived from a stereotype.
  - Be careful not to ask personal questions or questions about sensitive subjects that an individual may find offensive (e.g., sexual orientation, politics, or religious affiliation). Simply ask, "What would you like me to know about your culture that will help me to better understand patients of that culture?"
  - If you do not understand what the person says, say so! No one wants to be patronized with an insincere nod and smile. Clarify what you did not understand and ask for additional information.
- Ask a professional.
  - Depending on the size of the community pharmacy facility, the human resources or training department is likely to have educational resources and may offer professional development workshops on cultural awareness and diversity training.
  - If a patient does not speak English or is a nonnative English speaker, obtain the professional services of an interpreter.
    - When speaking to patients, always speak to and maintain eye contact with the patient, not the interpreter.
- Experience another culture for yourself.
  - Try another culture's food, music, or other traditional forms of entertainment.
  - Volunteer for mission trips inside and outside the United States.
  - Travel to and tour countries with other cultures.

TECH NOTE!
Find opportunities to learn more about different cultures so that you are comfortable interacting professionally with individuals from many backgrounds.

SCIENCE OF INTERCULTURAL COMPETENCE

According to Professor Michael Bynam of the University of Durham in England, cultural competence has five key elements (Bynam, 2002):

- *Attitudes:* Curiosity and openness, readiness to suspend disbelief about other cultures and belief about one's own.

- *Knowledge:* Knowledge of social groups and their products and practices in one's own and in one's country and of the general processes of societal and individual interaction.
- *Skills of interpreting and relating:* The ability to interpret a document or event from another culture and to explain it and relate it to documents from one's own.
- *Skills of discovery and interaction:* The ability to acquire new knowledge of a culture and cultural practices and the ability to operate knowledge, attitudes, and skills under the constraints of real-time communication and interaction.
- *Critical cultural awareness/political education:* The ability to evaluate critically and on the basis of explicit criteria perspectives, practices, and products in one's own and other cultures and countries.

Attitudes

The first step to achieving cultural competence is to recognize and work toward changing attitudes that act as a barrier to engaging members of other cultures in our society. Attitudes are our feelings and emotions about something; other cultures, in this context. Frequent encounters with members of other cultures can help healthcare professionals gain knowledge that helps them better understand the other person's culture, clarify misconceptions, and begin to develop appreciation of and respect for other cultures. Also, an increased awareness of their attitudes toward and perspectives on other cultures can make pharmacy technicians more sensitive to how they treat patients who share their cultural backgrounds, in addition to those of different backgrounds. Our attitudes may be formed or altered by a number of influences, such as:

- Our life's experiences
- The shared experiences of friends and/or family
- News and social media
- Religious or political affiliation
- Peer pressure

Any of these influences may shade our perspective about a different culture, and it is important to recognize when one of these influences is interfering with our ability to embrace another culture without showing bias (i.e., a preference or an inclination, especially one that inhibits impartial judgment). It is important to recognize that as human beings, we harbor bias as a natural tendency or as a learned behavior based on personal preferences or the preferences of those close to us. Modifying our subconscious human reaction when we encounter another culture can be difficult; it is how we choose to respond that makes all the difference. Because an attitude is generally an emotional response, we can modify our attitude toward a subject if we are provided with information that alters our perspective.

Psychologists have long established a link between attitudes and behavior; harboring a negative attitude about something without some manifestation in behavior, however remote or covert, is difficult. Research in the area of behavioral and social psychology has reflected that, during our initial encounters with something new, our subconscious registers an immediate negative or positive attitude, regardless of whether we are aware of it.

External influences, often referred to as "peer pressure," may alter people's behavior in a way that may conflict with their own attitudes and beliefs so as to please the majority or preserve the status quo. Social marketing (e.g., antidrug and smoking cessation campaigns) has promoted a positive change in attitude and behavior with regard to those types of unhealthy behaviors. Frequent participation in exercises that increase cultural awareness in the workplace may help achieve a similar end over time.

Knowledge

One of the best ways to diffuse a misconception is to clarify it with facts. Resources that allow you to gain knowledge (e.g., libraries, newspapers, diversity training courses) can be used to increase your awareness and improve your ability to interact more effectively in a culturally diverse environment.

Skills of Interpreting and Relating

Once we have opened ourselves to a change in the attitudes that often prompt unhealthy responses to other cultures, the next step is to find common ground, based on the information gained in researching other cultures. We should seek ways to relate other cultures to our own, to find common threads that are universal to a variety of cultures. The art, food, and music of other cultures are a great place to start.

Patients' cultural background often strongly influences how they approach "modern" healthcare in terms of Western medical practice. Many people still practice traditional forms of medicine passed down for generations, either in place of or in addition to modern therapeutics. Healthcare professionals, including pharmacy technicians, must find ways to acknowledge patients' cultural practice of medicine when presenting them with prescription medications. Prescribers should learn about the traditional products used, including any ingredients that have medicinal properties that may interact with prescribed medication. Pharmacy technicians should further encourage patients to share that information when consulting with a pharmacist during patient counseling. Relating modern pharmaceuticals to traditional preparations may increase patients' overall comfort with using modern drugs and increase the likelihood that they will take the medication as prescribed. A pharmacist may need to clarify clinical information, which may require the services of an interpreter, if available.

Skills of Discovery and Interaction

The best way to reset an old or inaccurate perception about a particular culture is to have a positive cultural experience, from which new ideas and discoveries about various cultures can be made. Healthcare professionals can look for opportunities to talk with members of other cultures, to discover how each responds to different forms of communication and to build relationships with those from other cultures. To achieve this level of intercultural competence, a pharmacy technician can interact with other members of the pharmacy team, patients, and members of the healthcare community.

Critical Cultural Awareness/Political Education

Improved cultural competence should be a call to action in our local, state, and global communities, because it relates to cultural awareness, social justice, and passing the torch of learning cultural competence to another person or persons. In the healthcare setting, this may be achieved by modeling culturally sensitive behavior, treating all patients with respect, avoiding behaviors that those of other cultures may consider offensive, and taking a stand when one encounters behavior that is culturally insensitive or blatantly inappropriate.

Communicating to Your Audience

When a child asks you a question, you probably take a minute to ask yourself how best to answer the question in a way the child will understand. This simple adjustment is the act of *communicating to your audience*. You must frame your communication to suit the understanding, aptitude, education, and communication ability of your audience. Just as a concept is explained differently to an adult than to a child, the level of communication between a pharmacy technician and a patient is different from that between a pharmacy technician and the staff pharmacist, a physician, or other healthcare professional. For communication in the pharmacy setting, pharmacy technicians should consider the following:

- What type of communication is most appropriate (e.g., telephone, face to face, or written)? What is the level of technical expertise of the person with whom the technician is communicating?
- What does the target audience need? Information? Feedback? Troubleshooting? It is important to communicate in a clear, logical manner, based on your audience's needs.

TARGET AUDIENCE: HEALTHCARE PROFESSIONAL

When communicating with a provider, pharmacy technicians should address the individual formally and be prepared to obtain the information needed to serve the person. When communicating with a healthcare professional, technical language generally is appropriate, depending on the person's technical knowledge. Always make sure the individual's needs have been met. If the communication is in writing, state the purpose of the communication clearly and concisely and specify the information needed. Make sure all written forms of communication have been proofread for grammatical and typographical errors before they are sent.

TARGET AUDIENCE: COWORKER

When communicating with a peer, some level of professional rapport is likely to exist, so communication should be conducted in a way that builds and sustains that relationship. Communicate openly and honestly, making sure to use technical language only as necessary. When passing along information about a task, make sure the communication includes the details needed to perform the task and always ensure that your coworker has a clear understanding of what has been communicated.

TARGET AUDIENCE: PATIENT

Establish the Patient's Level of Communication

It is important to establish how best to communicate with patients based on their overall knowledge of their health status, their educational level (often indicated by a person's vocabulary or verbal articulation), and their emotional state. Communicating with patients who are in pain or upset can be difficult. If a patient is upset, first try to address the person's emotional state by attempting to empathize or by showing compassion and caring about the person's physical and emotional well-being. Often an angry or frustrated patient simply wants to be *heard and acknowledged*. Applying active listening skills may rapidly diffuse a tense situation and bring a patient to a place emotionally where the pharmacy staff member can communicate with the person productively.

Speakers of Other Languages

If a patient speaks English as a second language, using both verbal and nonverbal communication, in addition to illustrations and pictures, may help ensure that the patient receives the message you intended to send. Whenever possible, use the services of a professional interpreter. When a family member acts as the interpreter, the healthcare professional cannot be sure of the level of understanding of the person doing the interpreting, unless the family member is also a healthcare professional. If the interpreter does not truly understand the information being interpreted, the risk arises that inaccurate or incorrect information will be relayed to the patient. It also is important to gain a sense of the gestures to which a patient may respond well and also gestures that should be avoided because patients of certain cultures may find them offensive.

Gather as Much Information as Possible

When communicating with patients, it is important to gather as much pertinent information as possible to prevent patients from having to repeat themselves or return to the pharmacy unnecessarily because of incorrect or incomplete information. Pharmacy technicians should always have a pen and paper handy when communicating with patients to ensure that all necessary details are documented and verbally clarified for completeness and accuracy.

Avoid Using Technical Language

Generally, using common language whenever possible is the best course. Technical language can be misinterpreted or misunderstood, leading the patient to take a medication incorrectly. In every interaction with patients, it is *crucial* that pharmacy technicians make sure the patient has a clear understanding of the information he or she received.

Practice Cultural Competence

A patient's cultural designation may call for observance of a traditional value, such as speaking to a spouse or honoring a request to avoid products derived from certain plant and animal sources. These preferences should be acknowledged, respected, and honored whenever possible and when in the best interests of the patient's health and safety.

Observe Appropriate Spacial Awareness and Physical Contact

Various cultures view spacial distance between individuals quite differently. Therefore, pharmacy technicians should be alert to the patient's nonverbal cues about his or her comfort with the personal space they provide. Individuals who value a greater spacial separation usually keep a safe distance when communicating and may step back or move away if they feel a person has intruded on that space. As a pharmacy technician, you must adjust this distance based on the patient's comfort, not your own. Touching generally should be avoided; if it is necessary to assist the patient, always ask for permission before coming into physical contact with a patient or the person's children.

Consider Eye Contact

Various cultures view eye contact differently. In the United States, direct eye contact is considered an acknowledgement of attention and verbal engagement. However, many cultures may consider constant direct eye contact inappropriate, offensive, or even threatening. As with spacial awareness, pharmacy technicians should be observant of patients' nonverbal cues and adjust their level of eye contact accordingly.

Exploring Typology Assessment to Understand the Cultures Around You

Magazines frequently contain a variety of polls and surveys to help the reader better define the type of mate for which he or she is best suited, the type of career the person may enjoy, or the types of consumer products that may interest the individual. Such poll questions target basic underlying preferences that certain groups of people are likely to have in common.

Similar types of assessments can be used in the healthcare setting. Individuals' basic tendencies drive the types of roles in which they operate best (and worst). The credo for the journey to understanding those around you is, as *Hamlet*'s Polonius said, "To thine own self be true." Often the factor that most strongly drives miscommunication is a lack of knowledge (or acknowledgement) of underlying influences that affect how we decode messages. Our cultural contexts, life experiences, personal ideals, and many other influences weigh in on how we interpret information received. For example, a person who has a bad experience with a particular consumer product is not likely to communicate positively about that product. As human beings, our personal experiences often shape our perspective on several levels. Many underlying factors of which we may or may not be aware influence our response to various situations and to the messages we receive.

A variety of typology assessments are available that can help a person explore his or her inherent tendencies based on questions that identify preference patterns. The Myers-Briggs assessment and the Jung Typology assessment are just two examples. These instruments are available online, and students can fill out the questionnaires to help them determine their typology. Based on the results, the student may search for information on his or her type and on other types. These assessments can be valuable exercises in the healthcare setting, because they allow individuals to better learn the personalities of coworkers, to a degree that many individuals may have difficulty expressing on their own.

Chapter Summary

- Culture may be defined as:
  - Patterns established through the passing of knowledge, beliefs, and behaviors across generations.
  - An identity that is formed largely by the collective traits of an external group of which one is inherently a part (e.g., ethnicity) or with which one identifies.
  - A consummate set of established values that help to define an institution or organization, how that organization wants to be perceived, and the behaviors that it expects from those who choose to be members of the organization.
- A culture may also have subcultures, or groups of people who share a distinctive set of cultural beliefs and behaviors that differ in some significant way from those of the larger society.
- Cultural norms are behaviors commonly associated with a particular cultural group, by that group.
- A person does not have to agree or identify with the ideals and behaviors associated with a particular culture or subculture to communicate and interact positively with members of that group.

- Many commonalities can be accepted as a foundation for establishing communication and relationships, whether personally or professionally.
- The structural components of the communication model are sender, receiver, and message/feedback.
- Media are generally the means through which the communication is transmitted to the receiver. The message may be sent to one or more people, directly or indirectly, and by a variety of media.
- The receiver processes the message sent in light of personal experience, cultural context, educational background, and natural tendencies as they relate to communication.
- If the sender's direct and indirect messages transmit very different meanings from the perspective of the receiver, this is called incongruence.
- Feedback can be received in ways that allow the person receiving it the best opportunity to hear and understand the message the way the other person intended.
- Certain behaviors should be avoided when receiving feedback, including defensiveness, attacking, denial, disrespect, closed-mindedness, inactive listening, rationalizing, and patronizing.
- Important tips for giving feedback include: Be clear and concise; do not pull unrelated information into the dialog; have a positive emphasis; be specific; avoid generalizations or extremes (e.g., "always" and "never"); highlight the behavior observed, not the person; give enough detail for the receiver to understand; own your feedback, using "I" statements that demonstrate personal accountability.
- Active listening is defined as the skill of not just *hearing* a person as they are speaking, but of paying individual attention to what the person says and how he or she says it.
- Pharmacy technicians must acknowledge, respect, and adjust their patterns of communication whenever necessary to suit the needs of a widely diverse patient population.
- Often the place to begin exploring other cultures is to consider how one feels about his or her own culture.
- *Ethnocentrism* can lead to offensive and destructive behavior; negative attitudes may escalate over time into aggression against other cultures to which a person feels superior.
- The opposite of ethnocentrism is *ethnic pluralism*, which acknowledges all cultures as equal, capable of coexisting alongside one another peacefully.
- The process of becoming more comfortable with one's own definition of cultural awareness opens the door for personal growth and understanding of other cultural groups, rather than dismissing or avoiding them.
- Individuals can remove barriers created by fear or uncertainty about the traditions and values of other cultures by doing their own research, asking appropriate questions, asking a professional, and experiencing another culture for themselves.
- The five key elements of cultural competence are attitudes, knowledge, skills of interpreting and relating, skills of discovery and interaction, and critical cultural awareness/political education.
- A communicator must adjust the communication to suit the understanding, aptitude, education, and communication ability of the audience.
- When communicating with a patient care provider, address the individual formally and obtain only the information needed.
- When communicating with a peer, communicate in a way that builds and sustains the professional relationship.
- Establish how best to communicate with patients based on their knowledge of their health status, their educational level, and their emotional state.
- A variety of typology assessments can be used to explore an individual's inherent tendencies based on questions that identify preference patterns. These assessments can be valuable exercises in the healthcare setting, because they individuals to better understand the personalities of coworkers, to a degree that many individuals have difficulty expressing on their own.

REVIEW QUESTIONS

Multiple Choice

1. Listening to understand is a demonstration of:
   a. Bias
   b. Active listening
   c. Culture
   d. Incongruence

2. An inclination that inhibits impartial judgment is a:
   a. Bias
   b. Cultural norm
   c. Prejudice
   d. Stereotype

3. A pharmacy staff member inappropriately expresses a negative attitude about a patient that is based on faulty generalizations. This is an example of:
   a. Generalization
   b. Imperialism
   c. Prejudice
   d. Bias

4. A patient who explains how the preparation of a root extract has been passed down through family generations is attempting to express an element of her:
   a. Culture
   b. Norm
   c. Subculture
   d. Relativism

5. A set of behaviors typically self-assigned by a cultural group is known as:
   a. Cultural norm
   b. Cultural imperialism
   c. Ethnocentrism
   d. Stereotypes

6. The belief that the ideals of a particular culture should be viewed in light of that culture's own standards is also known as cultural:
   a. Ethnocentrism
   b. Pluralism
   c. Relativism
   d. Imperialism

7. A healthcare provider tries to indoctrinate a patient with the notion that the practice of medicine in the provider's country should be adopted in all countries. This is an example of cultural:
   a. Imperialism
   b. Pluralism
   c. Relativism
   d. Ethnocentrism

8. A pharmacist insists to a technician that her culture's traditions in pharmacy practice are primitive and inferior to those of the pharmacist's country. This is an example of:
   a. Ethnocentrism
   b. Incongruence
   c. Prejudice
   d. Bias

9. A pharmacy technician interacts with a patient and asks for clarification when receiving the patient's feedback. This is what type of feedback reception?
   a. Engaged
   b. Respectful
   c. Interested
   d. Sincere

10. A healthcare professional shows that he values a patient's perspective, regardless of whether he agrees with it. This is what type of feedback reception?
    a. Respectful
    b. Thoughtful
    c. Interest
    d. Sincere

TECHNICIAN'S CORNER

1. For what target audience might technical language be least appropriate?
2. Explain what is meant by spacial awareness.
3. How might certain cultures view prolonged eye contact? How should a healthcare provider determine the appropriate level of eye contact during communication with a patient?

Bibliography

Bynam, M. (2002, April 23). *Assessing Intercultural Competence in Language Teaching.* Retrieved 7/17/2011, from http://inet.dpb.dpu.dk/infodok/sprogforum/Espr18/byram.html

International Committee of the Red Cross. (2005). *International Humanitarian Law: Treaties and Documents.* Retrieved 7/14/2010, from www.icrc.org/ihl.nsf/full/470?opendocument#top

Kendall, D. *Definitions cited on web page derived from Sociology in Our Times: The Essentials, 2nd Edition.* Retrieved 7/18/2011, from www.sociology.ohio-state.edu/classes/Soc463/garoutte/glossary_of_terms_kendall.htm

Lasagna, L. (2010). *The Hippocratic Oath: Modern Version (Written in 1964).* Retrieved 7/14/2010, from www.pbs.org/wgbh/nova/doctors/oath_modern.html

Levine, C.N.D. (1993). *Building a New Consensus: Ethical Principles and Policies for Clinical Research on HIV/AIDS.* In T.A. Shannon, editor: *Bioethics: Basic Writings on the Key Ethical Questions That Surround the Major, Modern Biological Possibilities and Problems.* Mahwah, New Jersey: Paulist Press.

Lewis, M.A. (2002). *Medical Law, Ethics & Bioethics for the Health Professions,* 6th Edition. Philadelphia: FA Davis.

Loo, T. (2006). *How to Define Your Life Purpose.* Retrieved 7/11/2010, from http://ezinearticles.com/?How-to-Define-Your-Life-Purpose&id=331527

Merriam-Webster Online. *Culture.* Retrieved 7/13/2011, from www.merriam-webster.com/dictionary/culture

Santa Clara University, Markkula Center for Applied Ethics. (2009). *A Framework for Thinking Ethically.* Retrieved 7/14/2010, from www.scu.edu/ethics/practicing/decision/framework.html

The Free Dictionary. (2011). *Stereotype, Bias [Definitions].* Retrieved 11/18/2011, from www.thefreedictionary.com/stereotype

The Nuremberg Code. (1949). In A. Mitscherlich, F. Mielke, *Doctors of Infamy: The Story of the Nazi Medical Crimes.* New York: Schuman.

Vasquez, A.S. (1988). *Conscience and Authority.* Retrieved 7/14/2010, from www.scu.edu/ethics/practicing/decision/conscience.html

WordNet Search 3.0. (2010). *Code [Definition].* Retrieved 7/10/2010, from http://wordnetweb.princeton.edu/perl/webwn?s=code

World Medical Organization. (1996). *Declaration of Helsinki, British Medical Journal,* 313:1448.

14 Infection Control

LEARNING
OBJECTIVES

By the end of this chapter, students will be able to competently:

1. Relate the importance of maintaining infection control in both community and institutional practice settings.
2. Identify the three major components in the infection cycle.
3. Describe the modes of transmission for various diseases.
4. Identify the four factors that affect the survival of bacteria.
5. Describe key behaviors that prevent the spread of particulate and microbial contamination in the pharmacy environment.
6. Describe methods for performing proper hygienic and aseptic hand washing.
7. Describe various types of personal protective equipment that can be used to control infection in the pharmacy environment.
8. Explain the different types of isolation, risk, and precautions used to keep pharmacy personnel from being exposed to disease.
9. Review standards of the Occupational Safety and Health Administration (OSHA) related to infection control in the healthcare environment.

KEY TERMS

Infection: The successful invasion of the body by pathogenic organisms and the reaction of tissues to their presence and the toxins they generate.

Infection reservoir: A means through which a pathogen may be spread.

Mode of transmission: A vehicle or mechanism through which infection may be transmitted and spread.

Nonpathogenic: Describes an organism that normally resides in the body and requires special circumstances to cause a disease.

Nosocomial infection: Refers only and specifically to infections acquired in the hospital setting.

Pathogenic: Describes an organism that can cause a disease anywhere in the body.

Personal protective equipment (PPE): Items health care workers can wear to create a physical barrier that will help to prevent the spread of disease.

Susceptible host: Any person in the vicinity who is in the pathway of the reservoir in which an infecting agent is being carried or spread.

Introduction

It is ironic that the health care environment, where individuals go to treat disease and infection, is a hotbed for disease-spreading microorganisms. Because the health care environment is constantly exposed to disease-causing agents, controlling the spread of infection is a matter of public health. Organizations like the Centers for Disease Control (CDC) and the Occupational Safety and Health Administration (OSHA) have established standards and guidelines that detail measures that may prevent infections associated with air, water, and other elements in the health care environment. These organizations have conducted various studies which suggest that although the health care environment contains a variety of microorganisms, only a few are of significant concern to susceptible individuals. However, the *number* of susceptible individuals increases in the health care setting.

In 2007, the CDC's Healthcare Infection Control Practices Advisory Committee (HICPAC) reviewed its 1996 isolation precaution standards. Those original standards delineated sources of infection primarily in the hospital environment and set forth guidelines for how to create barriers to prevent the spread of infecting agents to other hospital areas. Because the face of health care delivery has extended past the acute care hospital setting into areas such as home health, ambulatory care, specialty sites, and long-term care, there was a need to revise these standards to reflect both the risks and the preventive measures that can be universally applied across multiple health care settings. These 2007 standards also address key revisions to isolation and protective equipment and environment guidelines that can be applied to more susceptible patient populations, such as those who have received hematopoietic stem cell transplants (HSCTs).

Today's infectious disease control measures have been impacted by the emergence of particularly virulent (strong and highly resistant to antimicrobial therapy) pathogens, such as severe acute respiratory syndrome (SARS), swine flu, and methicillin-resistant *Staphylococcus aureus* (MRSA). This has prompted a renewed focus on what must be done in the health care setting to better isolate these pathogens and prevent their spread to other health care areas and patients. In light of the risks involved in a variety of health care settings, the term nosocomial infection now refers only and specifically to infections acquired in the hospital setting. For all other settings, the term *health care–associated infection* (HAI) is now applied.

There are numerous opportunities for the introduction of contaminants into the health care setting, given the number of physical surfaces, equipment, and supplies that both patients and care providers may come into contact with. In the pharmacy environment specifically, there are also factors that increase the risk of contamination of the nonsterile and sterile products being prepared therein. From the standpoint of patient safety, there is always a degree of risk that a patient might acquire a health care–associated infection, and this continues to be a subject of great concern and interest to regulatory organizations as well as leaders across the health care industry. Care must be taken to ensure that all members of the health care team, as part of their daily processes, practice specific behaviors that will prevent the introduction and spread of infection in the patient care environment.

A primary goal of the pharmacist and pharmacy technician practice that is related to infection control is the preparation, dispensing, and distribution of pharmaceutical products that may be safely administered to and by patients. During the manufacturing or manual preparation process, these products must have been subject to controls that ensure their quality, purity, and efficacy. Members of the health care team must then ensure that the products administered, as well as the routes through which medication is administered, are not compromised by either microbial or foreign particulate contamination.

The term *infection control* implies that there will always be the possibility of infection—we must simply find ways to *control* the amount of infection and the extent to which it spreads. To accomplish this goal, one must have a clear understanding of where a disease-causing agent may originate and how it is sustained (thereby creating the risk of being spread beyond its source). This chapter examines how infection begins and is spread, which is commonly referred to as the "chain of infection" or the infection cycle (Figure 14-1). Based on the factors known about how infection is spread, there are controls that, when adhered to, significantly minimize the introduction and spread of infection. It is critical for pharmacy technicians to be knowledgeable about how infection is spread and the behaviors that must be adopted to minimize that risk. Adherence to policies and guidelines not only protects patients: these policies are also designed to protect members of the health care team from unnecessary exposure to and contraction of disease-causing agents.

The Chain of Infection

According to the new CDC standards, there are three critical links to the chain of infection.

AN APPROPRIATE RESERVOIR

There must be an infection reservoir, which is a means through which a pathogen can spread, such as the air or dust particles in the air, food that is infected with the agent, or a surface that has been

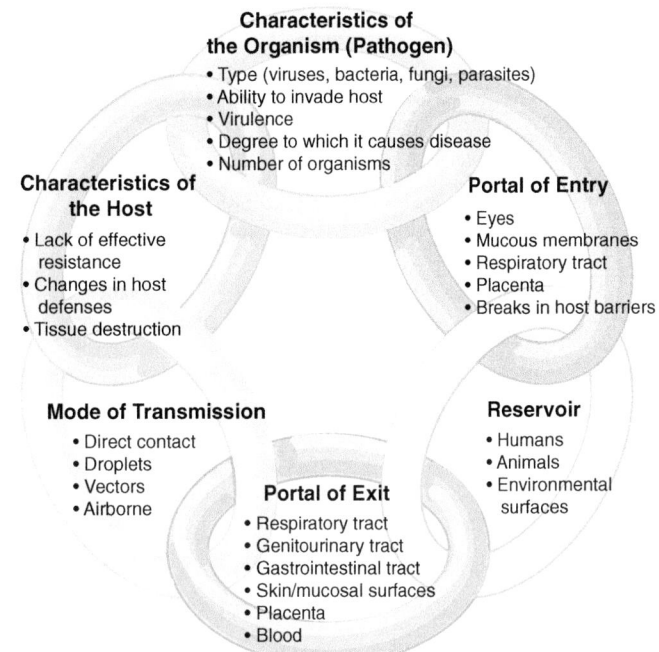

FIGURE 14-1 Chain of infection. (From Harkreader H, Hogan MA, Thobaben M: *Fundamentals of nursing: caring and clinical judgment,* ed 3, Philadelphia, 2007, Saunders.)

contaminated with the agent. There must be an adequate number of disease-causing agents, which can include the following:

* Bacteria, such as *H. pylori*
* Fungi, such as *Candida albicans and Aspergillus fumigatus*
* Viruses, such as hepatitis A or *H. influenzae*
* Parasites, such as lice or scabies
* Prions (similar to viruses, but without genetic material) responsible for degenerative diseases of the nervous system

Someone who is exposed to that reservoir may become a susceptible host to infection.

Human reservoir sources include patients, their household guests, and any facility employees. Any individual may be an active host of a pathogen, or an uninfected carrier. The endogenous bacterial flora of patients (those bacteria naturally residing in the gastrointestinal and respiratory tracts) may also serve as reservoir sources of HAIs.

A SUSCEPTIBLE HOST

Many organisms cannot survive for a very long time outside of a living organism. It is the host organism that creates an environment where the infecting agent can gain nourishment for growth and reproduction. Sometimes the reservoir supplies conditions for growth, sometimes it does not.

As noted in the pharmacology chapter, the body's lymphatic system supplies an innate immune response, which targets and seeks to destroy foreign substances that invade its environment. However, a patient whose immune response has been lowered because of his or her disease state is susceptible to developing an infection from an agent that the body would normally be able to fight. The condition of the person who is exposed to a significant reservoir of infecting agent will register a response based on the type of infecting agent, its virulence, the route of exposure, and the person's immune response.

A susceptible host may also be any person in the vicinity who is in the pathway of the reservoir through which the infecting agent is being carried or spread. Any patient or staff member may be a susceptible host, depending on the method through which the infecting agent is being transmitted as well as the transmission vehicle.

TABLE 14-1   **Transmission of Disease via Various Routes**

Disease	Infecting Agent	Form	Mode of Transmission
AIDS	HIV	Virus	Contact via mucous membrane or percutaneous exposure
Aspergillosis	*A. fumigatus*	Fungus	Airborne
Chicken pox	Varicella zoster	Virus	Airborne, direct contact
Flu	*H. influenzae*	Virus	Droplet contact
Herpes	HSV-1, HSV-2	Virus	Direct or indirect contact
Malaria	Plasmodium	Parasite	Vector borne by mosquito
Measles	Measles virus	Virus	Airborne
Pneumonia	*S. aureus*	Bacteria	Direct or indirect contact
SARS	SARS coronavirus	Virus	Droplet contact
Scabies	*S. scabiei*	Parasite	Direct contact
Strep Throat	*S. pyogenes*	Bacteria	Droplet contact
Tuberculosis	*M. tuberculosis*	Bacteria	Droplet contact
Whooping cough	*B. pertussis*	Bacteria	Droplet contact

A MODE OF TRANSMISSION

There must be a vehicle or mechanism through which infection can be transmitted and spread. The primary modes of transmission are as follows:
- Contact
- Vehicle
- Airborne
- Vector borne

Table 14-1 lists various diseases, the infecting agent that causes them, and the mode of transmission through which the disease can spread.

Contact Transmission

Contact transmission is the most common form of pathogen transmission and is divided into three categories: direct contact, indirect contact, and droplet (which may occur as a result of direct or indirect contact).

Direct contact transmission occurs when microorganisms are transferred from one infected person to another person without a contaminated intermediate object or person.[1] Direct contact transmission may occur under any of the following circumstances:
- Blood or blood-containing fluids entering the host's body after contact with the infected human reservoir source
- Transfer of a parasite from the patient's body to a caregiver's exposed skin

Indirect contact transmission occurs when microorganisms are transferred to a susceptible host following their transmission onto an intermediate object or person. This may occur in any of the following situations:
- Poor hand hygiene following the care of an infected patient, after which the caregiver comes into contact with other patients, devices, or equipment that other caregivers then come into contact with
- Use of contaminated devices with multiple patients
- Use of a contaminated device to prepare multiple doses of medication
- Introduction of microbial or particulate contamination because of poor aseptic technique during the process of intravenous (IV) admixture (such as coughing or sneezing in a laminar airflow hood environment, or touch contamination)

- Shared toys among infected pediatric patients
- Contaminated personal protective attire spreading contamination to other patient care areas after exposure to the infected blood or body fluids of an infected patient

Droplet contamination may occur as a result of an infected host coughing, sneezing, or talking during a clinical procedure or in the presence of individuals near enough to make contact with the droplets of infected body fluid. Based on epidemiological studies, a distance of approximately 3 feet in diameter around an infected host would allow for direct droplet contact transmission of a respiratory bacterial or viral agent. Generally, the droplet particle size is what defines it as contact—rather than airborne—contamination. Airborne contaminants may travel distances far greater than 3 feet.

Airborne Transmission

Airborne transmission generally results from the spread of either airborne droplets or small particles containing infectious agents that remain actively infective over time and distance traveled, can be transmitted via air currents, and can be inhaled by susceptible hosts. Generally, airborne transmission occurs without the susceptible host ever coming into contact with the human reservoir carrier.

Vector-borne Transmission

Vector-borne infection generally occurs when a susceptible host is bitten by an insect carrying a pathogen or by an intermediary animal (such as a rat) that was infected previously. The source vector is typically an arthropod such as a tick, mosquito, or flea. Although this is less common in the health care environment, there is certainly a chance that an infected vector could gain access to patient care areas and infect patients or staff members with the infecting agent.

Infecting Agent Survival Factors

Given the types of infecting agents that spread disease, one must consider if the health care environment creates an ideal atmosphere for the survival and flourishing of microbial contamination. Four key factors influence the survival of an infecting agent and its ability to spread disease:

- Type of organism
  - Pathogenic organisms are those that are generally not indigenous, or normal residents, or flora of the human body; pathogenic organisms are capable of causing disease through any portal of entry in the human body
  - Nonpathogenic organisms are normally found in the body and only cause infection in the case of overpopulation or if an organism migrates or is introduced into the body outside of its normal internal environment
- Number of organisms
  - When it comes to infection, there is strength in numbers; depending on the type of organism, some single-cell bacteria may replicate in as few as 15 minutes, whereas others typically take between 8 and 24 hours to replicate to a number that could cause and spread disease
- Resistance of host
  - The more susceptible the host, the greater the chance that the infecting agent will survive, because the body's defenses are compromised and unable to deploy either innate or cell-mediated immune responses to fight off disease
- Environmental factors
  - Aerobic microorganisms need air to survive, whereas anaerobic microorganisms may survive with or without air
  - Environmental temperatures such as room temperature are conducive to bacterial growth
  - The acidity or alkalinity of the host site is also a consideration
  - Presence of nutrients, such as dextrose in solution

The absence of any of these factors might interrupt the infection cycle and prevent the transmission of infecting agents to hosts. Members of the health care team must take all necessary measures to prevent the spread of HAIs in the patient care setting. The following section discusses several measures of infection control that can be deployed in a variety of health care settings.

Universal Precautions That Combat Transmission Portals of Entry

The type of reservoir in which the infecting agent has been transported often determines the mode of transmission. There must be a means of entry into the body, which may include the following:

Digestive system—if the product is ingested

Respiratory system—if the product is inhaled

Integumentary system—if there is a break in the skin or mucous membranes

Genitourinary tract—such as with a sexually transmitted disease or contact with a contaminated instrument such as a catheter or speculum

Circulatory system—an agent introduced into the bloodstream via a needle stick

Based on these transmission entry points, members of the health care team can employ measures to create physical barriers that will safeguard both them and patients against the transmission of disease through various portals of entry.

Preventing Particulate and Microbial Contamination in the Pharmacy Environment

There are a variety of ways in which health care workers can protect themselves, and the environment in which they provide patient care, from the introduction and spread of disease-causing agents. One of the most effective methods for preventing the spread of infection is proper hand washing. According to a *Morbidity and Mortality Weekly* report generated by the CDC, the self-reported reasons for poor adherence to proper hand washing techniques included the following:

- Irritation and dryness of hands following hand washing
- Inconvenient location of sinks or too few sinks
- Shortage of soap and paper towels
- Too busy/insufficient time for hand washing—"patient's needs take priority"
- Understaffing/overcrowding in the health care environment

Pharmacy staff members must recognize the importance of practicing good hand hygiene as a means to prevent the spread of infecting agents. Particularly as our hands come closest to the equipment and supplies that are used in the preparation of sterile pharmaceuticals, the practice of proper hand hygiene is critical and must never be compromised in favor of workflow processes.

In fact, the process of aseptic hand washing should take no more than 2 minutes from start to finish when properly performed. In a broad sense, the term *hand hygiene* includes hand washing with either plain or antiseptic-containing soap and water and the use of alcohol-based products (gels, rinses, foams) that do not require the use of water.[1] The following section gives a breakdown of each of the steps involved in proper aseptic hand washing.

HYGIENIC AND ASEPTIC HAND WASHING TECHNIQUES

The primary difference between hygienic and aseptic hand washing is that hygienic hand washing is designed to be performed in a general health care environment where particulate and microbial counts are not specifically monitored. Aseptic hand washing adds measures that allow individuals to reduce the amount of human particulate (like hair and dead skin cells) and infecting agents that may be on the surface of the skin and may spread contamination in an environment where particulate and microbial counts are strictly monitored and measured. Although pharmacy technicians are not required to perform aseptic hand washing outside of the controlled environment, these measures offer a highly effective way to help prevent the spread of infection.

STEPS FOR PERFORMING PROPER ASEPTIC HAND WASHING

Step 1: Remove *all* jewelry and roll sleeves *above* the elbow.

Step 2: Turn on water and adjust temperature to lukewarm.

- The stream of water should be adjusted to prevent unnecessary splashing (Figure 14-2).
- Rinse hands and forearms under the stream of water, using caution not to touch any fixtures on the sink.

TECH ALERT!
Studies have shown that artificial nails and nail extensions harbor a variety of disease-causing agents, such as yeasts and gram-negative bacilli. Many health care organizations disallow employees involved in direct patient care (including pharmacy employees) from wearing artificial nails in light of the risks of the spread of infection, particularly among highly susceptible patient populations.

Step 3: Apply a generous amount of the disinfecting solution to fingertips (Figure 14-3).

*   Use a fingernail pick to clean under the surface of each nail, then use a brush to scrub the surfaces of fingernails (if available and appropriate).

Step 4: Use a sponge to apply disinfecting solution to hands:

*   All four surfaces of each finger should be cleaned by placing each finger in the center of the palm and rotating in a circular motion. Be sure to include the surfaces of the palm, outer hand, and between each finger.
*   The antibacterial cleansing agent used should remain in contact with the skin for 15 seconds for hygienic hand washing and 30 seconds for aseptic hand washing in order for it to perform its bactericidal activity.

Step 5: Use a sponge to apply disinfecting solution to forearms *all the way up to the elbow.*

*   All four surfaces of the wrist and arms should be cleaned using a circular motion.

Step 6: Hands should be rinsed in an upright, vertical position beginning with the fingertips and rinsing down to the elbows (Figure 14-4).

*   This will rinse contaminants past the elbow region and away from the hands.
*   Make sure that all soap residue is removed.
*   Ensure that you do not touch any sink fixtures during the rinsing process.

Step 7: Water should be left running while all surfaces of the fingers, hands, and arms are dried with clean, dry paper towels.

*   Ensure that you do not touch any part of the towel dispenser during the drying process.

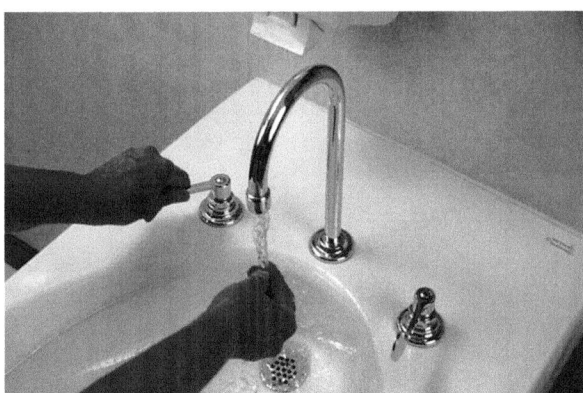

FIGURE 14-2 Turning on water. (From Potter P, Perry AG, Stockert P, Hall A: *Basic nursing,* ed 7, St. Louis, 2011, Mosby.)

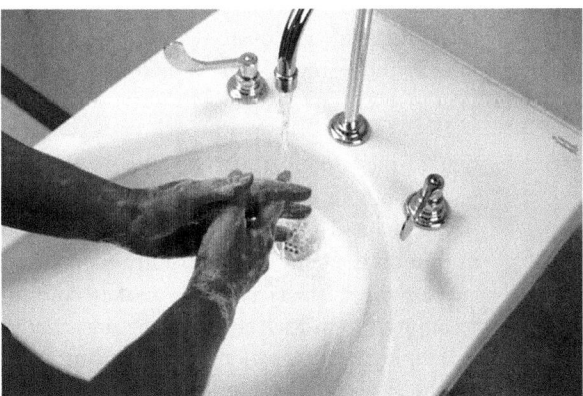

FIGURE 14-3 Lathering hands thoroughly. (From Potter P, Perry AG, Stockert P, Hall A: *Basic nursing,* ed 7, St. Louis, 2011, Mosby.)

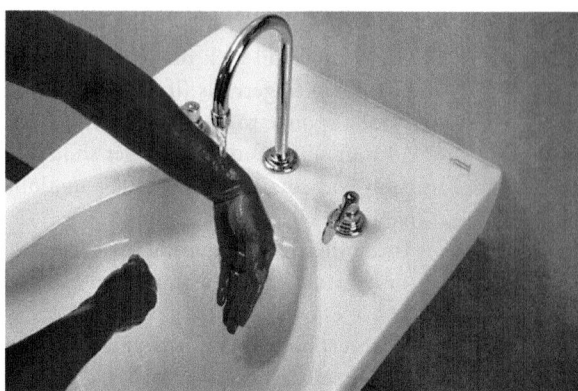

FIGURE 14-4 Rinsing hands. (From Potter P, Perry AG, Stockert P, Hall A: *Basic nursing,* ed 7, St. Louis, 2011, Mosby.)

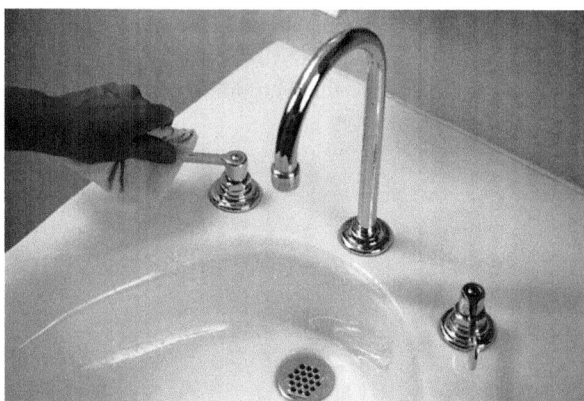

FIGURE 14-5 Turning off faucet with clean, dry paper towel. (From Potter P, Perry AG, Stockert P, Hall A: *Basic nursing,* ed 7, St. Louis, 2011, Mosby.)

Step 8: After all surfaces are dried, damp towels should be thrown away and new clean, dry paper towels should be used to shut off the water faucets.

- Be very careful to ensure that you do not touch any of the sink fixtures with bare hands (Figure 14-5).

In the absence of scrub sponges (such as in pharmacy environments where there is not a controlled area like a clean room), the cleansing steps may be performed using an approved antimicrobial cleansing agent.

Although a variety of cleansing agents are currently available, the most commonly used product is chlorhexidine gluconate (CHG), 4%. CHG not only kills bacterial flora on the skin, but it also inhibits the regrowth of bacteria for a period of time after hand washing.

MAINTAINING A HYGIENIC ENVIRONMENT

One of the best ways that a pharmacy technician can protect the products being prepared in the pharmacy is to create an environment that will not be conducive to various forms of pathogen transmission. The 2007 HICPAC guidelines state that the creation of a "safety culture" within an institution is among the best strategies to ensure that a hygienic health care environment is created and sustained. The elements of a safety culture include the following:

- Support from leaders within the organization
- Employee participation in safety planning
- The availability of appropriate protective equipment
- The creation of norms within the environment that set a standard for hygienic practice (for example, repeated emphasis on the use of alcohol hand rubs before entering patient care

areas or the performance of hygienic hand washing before and after providing care to the patient)
- New employee orientation training that communicates and reinforces infection control practices as an integral part of normal, accepted workplace behavior

PERSONAL PROTECTIVE EQUIPMENT

Every new pharmacy technician should enter a new pharmacy environment with the expectation of taking whatever measures necessary to prevent the spread of infection. The use of appropriate protective equipment must be practiced and incorporated into one's regular routine. Personal protective equipment (PPE) refers to items that health care workers can wear to create a physical barrier that will help to prevent the spread of disease among the patient, caregiver, and the health care environment (Figure 14-6). PPE items are selected based on the patient population being served and the types of disease transmission that are possible. PPE items may be worn individually or in combination, based on the risks involved. Examples of protective equipment used in the health care environment include the following:
- Shoe covers.
- Bouffant cap–style head coverings protect the environment from contamination that may originate in and on the scalp.
- Respirator, isolation, or surgical face masks. Protect against the spread of contamination via droplet or airborne transmission; may be worn by patients who may have infectious disease with airborne transmission or by health care workers to provide a barrier against contamination of the oral mucosa. Masks may be worn in combination with a face shield or goggles to further protect the eyes and skin from contact with infecting agents.
- Isolation gowns. Protect the arms and exposed body and clothing areas from contamination from blood, body fluids, and other potentially infectious materials in the health care environment. Gowns come in different varieties, based on the degree to which the gown needs to be resistant to exposure to contaminated bodily fluids.
- Gloves. Generally either latex or nitrile gloves are used in the health care environment to prevent the spread of infection resulting from touch contamination. Gloves may need to be changed frequently to prevent the spread of infection between wound sites on the same patient and among multiple patients and to prevent the creation of reservoirs on equipment and supplies in the health care environment.

PATIENT ISOLATION PRECAUTIONS

One of the best ways to prevent the spread of infecting agents in various health care environments is by identifying precautions that health care workers should adhere to. Two types of precautions should be observed: standard precautions and transmission-based precautions.

Standard precautions are behaviors that all health care workers should observe in order to prevent the introduction and spread of contaminants among health care workers, patients, and the health care environment. Elements of the standard precautions, as set forth in the 2007 HICPAC guidelines, include the following (Siegel, 2007):
- Hand hygiene
- Use of gloves, gown, mask, eye protection, or face shield, depending on the anticipated exposure
- Safe injection practices
  - Injuries caused by needles and other sharps have been associated with the transmission of HBV, HCV, and the human immunodeficiency virus (HIV) to health care personnel
  - Needle sticks and other sharps-related injuries may be prevented with the proper use of engineering controls such as needle-safe devices and the proper use of sharps containers
- Equipment or items in the patient environment likely to have been contaminated with infectious body fluids must be handled in a manner that prevents the transmission of infectious agents
  - Proper cleansing of patient care areas is critical, particularly when incontinence and exposure to urine and feces may be more common (such as among pediatric patients or elderly patients in long-term care facilities)
- For some interactions, only gloves may be needed; during other interactions, the use of gloves, gown, and face shield or mask and goggles is necessary

SEQUENCE FOR DONNING PERSONAL PROTECTIVE EQUIPMENT (PPE)

The type of PPE used will vary based on the level of precautions required; e.g., Standard and Contact, Droplet or Airborne Infection Isolation.

1. GOWN
- Fully cover torso from neck to knees, arms to end of wrists, and wrap around the back
- Fasten in back of neck and waist

2. MASK OR RESPIRATOR
- Secure ties or elastic bands at middle of head and neck
- Fit flexible band to nose bridge
- Fit snug to face and below chin
- Fit-check respirator

3. GOGGLES OR FACE SHIELD
- Place over face and eyes and adjust to fit

4. GLOVES
- Extend to cover wrist of isolation gown

SECUENCIA PARA PONERSE EL EQUIPO DE PROTECCIÓN PERSONAL (PPE)

El tipo de PPE que se debe utilizar depende del nivel de precaución que sea necesario; por ejemplo, equipo Estándar y de Contacto o de Aislamiento de infecciones transportadas por gotas o por aire.

1. BATA
- Cubra con la bata todo el torso desde el cuello hasta las rodillas, los brazos hasta la muñeca y dóblela alrededor de la espalda
- Átesela por detrás a la altura del cuello y la cintura

2. MÁSCARA O RESPIRADOR
- Asegúrese los cordones o la banda elástica en la mitad de la cabeza y en el cuello
- Ajústese la banda flexible en el puente de la nariz
- Acomódesela en la cara y por debajo del mentón
- Verifique el ajuste del respirador

3. GAFAS PROTECTORAS O CARETAS
- Colóquesela sobre la cara y los ojos y ajústela

4. GUANTES
- Extienda los guantes para que cubran la parte del puño en la bata de aislamiento

USE SAFE WORK PRACTICES TO PROTECT YOURSELF AND LIMIT THE SPREAD OF CONTAMINATION
- Keep hands away from face
- Limit surfaces touched
- Change gloves when torn or heavily contaminated
- Perform hand hygiene

UTILICE PRÁCTICAS DE TRABAJO SEGURAS PARA PROTEGERSE USTED MISMO Y LIMITAR LA PROPAGACIÓN DE LA CONTAMINACIÓN
- Mantenga las manos alejadas de la cara
- Limite el contacto con superficies
- Cambie los guantes si se rompen o están demasiado contaminados
- Realice la higiene de las manos

A

SEQUENCE FOR REMOVING PERSONAL PROTECTIVE EQUIPMENT (PPE)

Except for respirator, remove PPE at doorway or in anteroom. Remove respirator after leaving patient room and closing door.

1. GLOVES
- Outside of gloves is contaminated!
- Grasp outside of glove with opposite gloved hand; peel off
- Hold removed glove in gloved hand
- Slide fingers of ungloved hand under remaining glove at wrist
- Peel glove off over first glove
- Discard gloves in waste container

2. GOGGLES OR FACE SHIELD
- Outside of goggles or face shield is contaminated!
- To remove, handle by head band or ear pieces
- Place in designated receptacle for reprocessing or in waste container

3. GOWN
- Gown front and sleeves are contaminated!
- Unfasten ties
- Pull away from neck and shoulders, touching inside of gown only
- Turn gown inside out
- Fold or roll into a bundle and discard

4. MASK OR RESPIRATOR
- Front of mask/respirator is contaminated — DO NOT TOUCH!
- Grasp bottom, then top ties or elastics and remove
- Discard in waste container

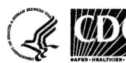

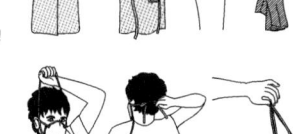

SECUENCIA PARA QUITARSE EL EQUIPO DE PROTECCIÓN PERSONAL (PPE)

Con la excepción del respirador, quítese el PPE en la entrada de la puerta o en la antesala. Quítese el respirador después de salir de la habitación del paciente y de cerrar la puerta.

1. GUANTES
- ¡El exterior de los guantes está contaminado!
- Agarre la parte exterior del guante con la mano opuesta en la que todavía tiene puesto el guante y quíteselo
- Sostenga el guante que se quitó con la mano enguantada
- Deslice los dedos de la mano sin guante por debajo del otro guante que no se ha quitado todavía a la altura de la muñeca
- Quítese el guante de manera que acabe cubriendo el primer guante
- Arroje los guantes en el recipiente de deshechos

2. GAFAS PROTECTORAS O CARETA
- ¡El exterior de las gafas protectoras o de la careta está contaminado!
- Para quitárselas, tómelas por la parte de la banda de la cabeza o de las piezas de las orejas
- Colóquelas en el recipiente designado para reprocesar materiales o de materiales de deshecho

3. BATA
- ¡La parte delantera de la bata y las mangas están contaminadas!
- Desate los cordones
- Tocando solamente el interior de la bata, pásela por encima del cuello y de los hombros
- Voltee la bata al revés
- Dóblela o enróllela y deséchela

4. MÁSCARA O RESPIRADOR
- La parte delantera de la máscara o respirador está contaminada — ¡NO LA TOQUE!
- Primero agarre la parte de abajo, luego los cordones o banda elástica de arriba y por último quítese la máscara o respirador
- Arrójela en el recipiente de deshechos

PERFORM HAND HYGIENE IMMEDIATELY AFTER REMOVING ALL PPE

EFECTÚE LA HIGIENE DE LAS MANOS INMEDIATAMENTE DESPUÉS DE QUITARSE CUALQUIER EQUIPO DE PROTECCIÓN PERSONAL

B

FIGURE 14-6 A, Donning personal protective equipment. **B,** Removing personal protective equipment. (From Centers for Disease Control and Prevention: *Guidelines for isolation precautions: preventing transmission of infectious agents in healthcare settings 2007,* Atlanta, Ga, June 2004, Centers for Disease Control and Prevention. In Sorrentino S, Gorek B: *Mosby's textbook for long-term care nursing assistants,* ed 6, St. Louis, 2011, Mosby.)

- Education and training on the principles and rationale for recommended practices are critical elements of standard precautions because they facilitate appropriate decision making and promote adherence when health care workers are faced with new circumstances

Transmission-based precautions are measures that must be taken based on exposure to patients with known or strongly suspected infectious disease. They include the following:

- Placement of patients in single rooms when transmission of an infecting agent is a concern; particularly when airborne transmission is possible, single-room placement would be prescribed
- Contact precaution: requires gown and gloves
- Droplet precaution: mask required, may need gown and gloves if within 3 feet of patient
- Airborne precaution: mask or respirator required; depending on the pathogen, gown and gloves may be appropriate
  - Precautions during aerosol-producing procedures (like intubation) require the protection of the eyes, nose, mouth, gown, and gloves; caregivers within the immediate environment may need to don a respirator mask

Avoiding Infectious Disease

One of the best ways to avoid exposure to infectious disease when transmission-based precautions are in place is to limit exposure to susceptible areas. Although pharmacy technicians' exposure to such high-risk areas may be limited to the delivery of medication to a drug storage area, it is important to be observant of signage that may indicate an isolation precaution based on a particular type of disease transmission. Generally, signs will be placed outside the door of a patient who has been located in a single-patient room as a transmission-based precaution. Pharmacy technicians *must* ensure that they observe all standard and special precautions, including the donning of PPE that is appropriate for the transmission type. When the risk of serious infectious disease is present, pharmacy technicians should avoid contact with the affected areas unless their presence is absolutely necessary to deliver essential care to the patient or service to a member of the nursing staff.

Proper hygienic hand washing before and after contact with an area for which there is a transmission-based precaution is one of the best ways to minimize the risk of spreading the infection to other health care workers, patients, and other environments in the health care setting.

Chapter Summary

- The health care environment is a breeding ground for disease-spreading microorganisms.
- Organizations like the Centers for Disease Control (CDC) and the Occupational Safety and Health Administration (OSHA) have established both standards and guidelines that detail measures to help prevent infections associated with air, water, and other elements in the health care environment.
- *Nosocomial infection* now refers only and specifically to infections acquired in the hospital setting. For all other settings, the term *health care–associated infection* (HAI) may now be applied.
- Every member of the health care team should practice daily behaviors that will prevent the introduction and spread of infection in the patient care environment.
- There are three critical links to the chain of infection: appropriate reservoir, susceptible host, and mode of transmission.
- One of the most effective methods for preventing the spread of infection is proper hand washing.
- *Hand hygiene* includes both hand washing, with either plain or antiseptic-containing soap and water, and the use of alcohol-based products that do not require the use of water.
- The primary difference between hygienic and aseptic hand washing is that hygienic hand washing is designed to be performed in a general health care environment where particulate and microbial counts are not specifically monitored.
- The most commonly used cleansing agent is chlorhexidine gluconate (CHG) 4%. CHG not only kills bacterial flora on the skin, but it also inhibits the regrowth of bacteria for a period of time after hand washing.

- Pharmacy technicians may protect the products being prepared in the pharmacy by creating an environment that will not be conducive to various forms of pathogen transmission.
- The elements of a safety culture include the following:
  - Support from leaders within the organization
  - Employee participation in safety planning
  - The availability of appropriate protective equipment
  - The creation of norms within the environment that set a standard for hygienic practice (for example, repeated emphasis on the use of alcohol hand rubs before entering patient care areas or the performance of hygienic hand washing before and after providing care to the patient)
  - New employee orientation training that communicates and reinforces infection control practices as a integral part of normal, accepted workplace behavior
- Examples of protective equipment that may be used in the health care environment include the following:
  - Shoe covers
  - Bouffant cap–style head coverings
  - Respirator, isolation or surgical face masks
  - Isolation gowns
  - Gloves
- Members of the health care team may prevent the spread of infecting agents in various health care environments by identifying precautions that health care workers should adhere to.
- Two types of precautions should be observed: standard precautions and transmission-based precautions.
- One of the best ways to avoid exposure to infectious disease when transmission-based precautions are in place is to limit exposure to susceptible areas.
- Technicians must ensure that they observe all standard and special precautions, including the donning of PPE that is appropriate for the transmission type.

REVIEW QUESTIONS

Multiple Choice

1. The invasion of an infecting agent and reaction of the tissues involved describes a(n):
   a. Pathogen
   b. Infection
   c. Susceptible host
   d. Nonpathogen

2. An organism that can cause a disease anywhere in the body is known as a(n):
   a. Pathogen
   b. Infection
   c. Susceptible host
   d. Nonpathogen

3. The means through which an infecting agent can be spread is referred to as a:
   a. Reservoir
   b. Susceptible host
   c. Mode of transmission
   d. Nosocomial infection

4. Any person to whom an infecting agent may be spread is a:
   a. Reservoir
   b. Susceptible host
   c. Mode of transmission
   d. Nosocomial infection

5. Human reservoir sources include:
   a. Patients
   b. Health care workers
   c. Guests of patients
   d. All of the above

6. A countertop that has been touch-contaminated with an infecting agent may serve as a:
   a. Reservoir
   b. Susceptible host
   c. Mode of transmission
   d. Nosocomial infection

7. Transmission by contact from one person to another constitutes this type of transmission:
   a. Indirect contact
   b. Direct contact
   c. Droplet
   d. Airborne transmission

8. Liquid particles that travel 3 feet or less carrying pathogens characterize this type of transmission:
   a. Vector borne
   b. Airborne
   c. Droplet
   d. Direct contact

9. This type of transmission occurs generally without the susceptible host ever coming into contact with the reservoir carrier:
   a. Indirect contact
   b. Airborne
   c. Droplet
   d. Both A and B

10. This type of transmission-based precaution would require the wearing of a respirator mask:
   a. Droplet
   b. Direct Contact
   c. Airborne
   d. All of the above

TECHNICIAN'S CORNER

1. List other health care environments, besides acute care settings, where isolation precaution standards may be applied.
2. Explain how disease can be introduced through the integumentary system portal of entry.
3. Why should health care workers avoid wearing false nails?

Bibliography

Biology Online. (2011). *Prion*. Retrieved 7/26/2011, from Biology: www.biology-online.org/dictionary/Prion

Ciesin Thematic Guides. (2011). *Changes in the Incidence of Vector-Borne Diseases Attributable to Climate Change [Summary of Key Vector-Borne Diseases]*. Retrieved 7/27/2011, from Ciesin Thematic Guides: search.yahoo.com/search?p=define+vector+borne

The Herb Doc. (2011). *A Systems Approach to Good Health and Nutrition*. Retrieved 7/26/2011, from The Herb Doc: www.theherbdoc.com/ConsumerEducation/_borders/Top-ConsumerEd.htm

Siegel, J.D. R. E. (2007). *2007 Guideline for Isolation Precautions: Preventing Transmission of Infectious Agents in Healthcare Settings*. Retrieved 7/26/2011, from www.cdc.gov/ncidod/dhqp/pdf/isolation2007.pdf

U.S. Army Medical Department Center and School—Academy of Health Sciences. (2011). *Lesson 1: Communicable Diseases*. Retrieved 7/27/2011, from tpub.com: www.tpub.com/content/armymedical/MD0540/MD05400005.htm

15 Pharmacy Materials Management

By the end of this chapter, students will be able to competently:

1. Describe the materials management process for both community and institutional pharmacy settings.
2. Explain how a formulary is used for determining items procured and maintained in pharmacy stock.
3. Discuss some of the factors that influence product selection.
4. Outline the roles and responsibilities of pharmacy technicians in the inventory management process.
5. Identify various storage requirements for pharmaceuticals.
6. Examine how technology has impacted the process of materials management.
7. Detail the process for the removal of products from inventory.
8. Describe the process for maintaining a record of controlled substances received, stored, and removed from inventory.
9. Explain the importance of deterring theft or medication diversion.
10. Describe the three types of voluntary manufacturer recall and the role of pharmacy technicians in gathering recalled pharmaceuticals.

KEY TERMS

Acquisition cost: The net price paid by a pharmacy for a product.

Basic stock: Amount of physical inventory maintained to meet an average demand level.

Carrying costs: Costs associated with carrying and maintaining inventory; includes outdates, product deterioration, storage, inventory taxes, and insurance.

Discontinued: Product that will no longer be produced or carried.

Expired product: Product that has exceeded its dating and may no longer be dispensed to a patient.

Order cycle time: The amount of time that elapses between the placement of an order and the receipt of the products via shipment.

Perpetual inventory management: The process whereby physical inventory counts are taken at the start of each shift, as well as before and after each medication fill.

Procurement: The process of obtaining goods and services.

Procurement costs: Costs associated with the ordering, shipping, and receiving of pharmaceuticals, including order transmission fees, receiving, and processing of the purchase order for payment.

Purchase order: Hard copy or electronic form on which drug orders are entered and sent to a drug supplier for processing.

Recalled product: Product that is subject to a voluntary process whereby the manufacturer requires that all distributed units of a particular item or items be returned to the manufacturer directly because of some degree of product defect.

Safety stock: The amount of inventory maintained to account for unexpected or anticipated fluctuations in demand and in order cycle times.

Introduction

The third principle of the Code of Ethics for Pharmacy Technicians states that a "pharmacy technician assists and supports the pharmacist in the safe, efficacious and cost effective distribution of health services and healthcare resources." One of the primary ways to accomplish this goal is by carrying out the pharmacy procurement process.

Procurement may be defined as the "process of obtaining goods and services from preparation and processing of a requisition through to receipt and approval of the invoice for payment. It commonly involves (1) purchase planning, (2) standards determination, (3) specifications development, (4) supplier research and selection, (5) value analysis, (6) financing, (7) price negotiation, (8) making the purchase, (9) supply contract administration, (10) inventory control and stores, and (11) disposals and other related functions" (BusinessDictionary.com, 2011).

Whether in the community or institutional pharmacy setting, inventory management processes impact a pharmacy's ability to provide needed products and services to patients. In the community setting, particularly the independent pharmacy, the effective management of inventory often determines the success or failure of the pharmacy as a business. In the hospital setting, management of inventory is critical to ensuring that both standard and emergency medication supplies are readily available to patients whose inpatient care needs are generally of a more critical nature than are the needs of patients in an ambulatory care (community) setting.

Figure 15-1 itemizes each of the key components of the pharmacy materials management process. This chapter examines each of those components and their application to community or hospital pharmacy practice.

WHAT IS THE ROLE OF THE PHARMACY TECHNICIAN?

Inventory management is one area of pharmacy practice in which a highly skilled pharmacy technician may have an opportunity to work independently and perform specialized tasks alongside the supervising pharmacist. In fact, key opportunities for advancement to the position of purchasing technician exist in both community and institutional pharmacy settings. This chapter describes the roles and responsibilities of pharmacy technicians at each level of the procurement process. Students should begin to see how pharmacy technicians use their acquired skills in the area of materials management to serve patients, pharmacists, and their pharmacy organization in a meaningful and impactful way.

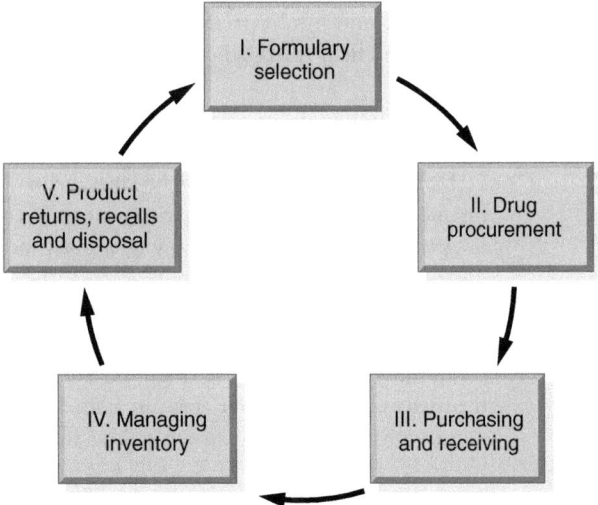

FIGURE 15-1 Pharmacy materials management process.

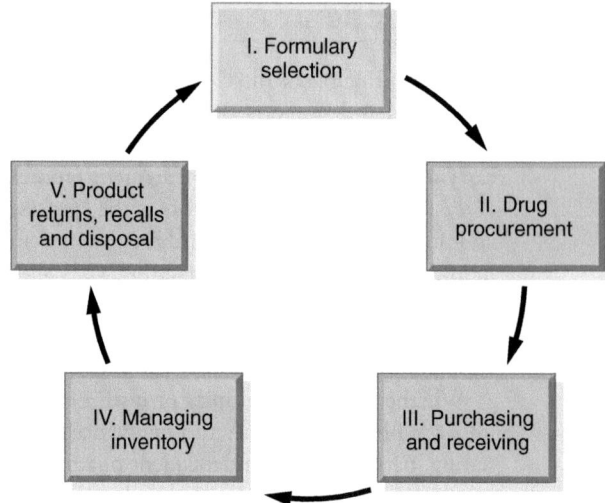

I. Formulary Selection

The *first* component of materials management is the establishment of inventory and what types of items will be stocked at a particular pharmacy location. A formulary is a list of drug products that are available for dispensing at a pharmacy. In general, formularies are established by a pharmacy and therapeutics—or P & T—committee that has been established within a community or institutional pharmacy organization. The P & T committee is composed of physicians and pharmacists within that organization who meet regularly to discuss the necessity of various types of medication on the formulary—or under consideration for addition to the formulary—in terms of how to optimize clinical outcomes for patients in a manner that also controls cost. This team of medical professionals establishes what drug products will be best utilized by the majority of the patient populations that they serve in a particular area.

In the institutional pharmacy setting, formulary selections standardize the management of various conditions, based on clinical data that support the efficacy of a particular product or products. In the end, the formulary determines which brand name and generic drugs will be made available for use by patients. Quite often, contractual supplier agreements such as group purchase organizations (GPOs) will identify many formulary selections in the hospital and health-system settings. GPO agreements will be discussed later in this chapter.

In community pharmacy practice, the types of medical benefits plan that a pharmacy accepts often determine the availability and cost of the drugs that will be made available to patients. Formularies help managed care organizations control costs by prescribing a range of drug products that are
- Cost-effective
- Most clinically appropriate for the patient

Managing prescription benefit costs helps keep the overall costs for those services affordable for most patients. One cost savings measure that affects materials management is the utilization of generic drug products. Many pharmacy benefit plans offer savings of 30% to 60% off the dispensing cost when a patient accepts the generic equivalent of a brand name drug when available.

Managing the cost of purchasing the drugs is a significant challenge for pharmacies in both the community and hospital settings. Pharmacies must consider the acquisition cost of the drugs themselves, to which other costs are added to arrive at the final dispensing price. In general, community pharmacy pricing structure is as follows:

Average Wholesaler Price (AWP) + Dispensing Fee
(on a scale that is based on the drug price) + Fixed % of the AWP

Example: Fee structure is AWP + 10% markup + $5 dispensing fee

$$\$10 \times \$1.10 = \$11$$
$$\$11 + \$5 = \$16$$

A drug with an AWP of $10 would be dispensed to the patient at a cost of $16.

There are additional costs that are not related to the drugs but still constitute major budgetary considerations: nonacquisition costs. According to a National Cost of Dispensing Survey conducted by the Coalition for Community Pharmacy Action in 2007, nonacquisition costs include the following:
- Prescription department salaries and benefits
  - May include licensure and continuing education for pharmacist/technician staff
- Other prescription department costs
  - Prescription dispensing materials (pill counters, bottles, compounding supplies)
  - Information/drug information technology
      Information technology (IT) support for pharmacy management software
      Drug information databases
      Facilities costs
  - Rent/mortgage
  - Utilities
- Other store/location costs
  - Marketing/advertising
  - Accounting, legal, and professional fees
  - Insurance, taxes, and licenses
  - Complying with federal and state regulations (e.g., the Health Insurance Portability and Accountability Act [HIPAA])
- Allocated corporate overhead, where applicable

Items that will be included in the physical inventory—that is, items that are available for purchase—must be selected based on their usage levels and anticipation of usage (such as seasonal products like cold and flu medication or vaccines). Pharmacies control purchasing costs by establishing relationships with reputable vendors that will offer them good pricing on drugs based on various usage criteria.

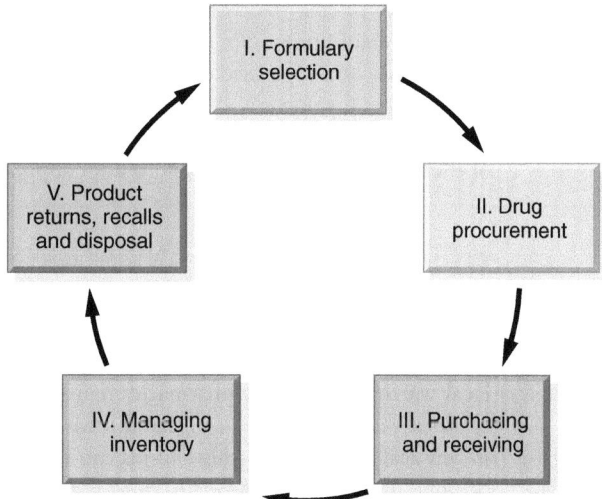

II. Drug Procurement

Pharmacies obtain their inventory by establishing relationships with companies that supply pharmaceutical products. The organization's pharmacy and therapeutics committee will have conducted cost analyses to compare pricing on various formulary drug products that are therapeutically equivalent; this process helps the committee to determine which products will be made available in the physical inventory. Pharmacies may then purchase products from any of the following sources:

- Drug wholesalers
- Group purchase organizations
- Prime vendor organizations
- Direct suppliers (pharmaceutical companies)

Drug manufacturers supply drug distributors—wholesalers—with the products that they have produced. This is one area in which there has been ongoing concern because of the number of disreputable secondary distributor sources that might potentially supply pharmacies with harmful or ineffective counterfeit drugs. Drug manufacturers must ensure that they demonstrate "supply chain integrity" by following ethical practices and conducting business only with reputable wholesaler sources, as well as establishing equitable pricing for both wholesalers and direct-buy pharmacies. The "fee for service" model that many manufacturers and wholesalers have adopted creates more transparency in the drug wholesaling industry and reduces the number of disreputable secondary distributor sources that may be closed or guarded concerning their pricing structures.

Pharmacies must carefully evaluate possible suppliers based on volume purchase discounts, discounts offered for drugs that are dispensed by private pay (cash), any special or promotional discounts offered, and the product return policies each supplier offers. Products may need to be returned for a variety of reasons; some suppliers may give pharmacies credit toward the purchase of new product in exchange for the return of an expired product.

DRUG WHOLESALERS

Pharmacies may purchase drugs from wholesalers. Wholesalers are businesses that sell to other businesses, not to the customer directly.

GROUP PURCHASE ORGANIZATIONS (GPOs)

Because of the sheer volume of drug products utilized in the hospital pharmacy environment, hospitals generally enter into a contractual agreement with an organization through which they may purchase the majority of their pharmaceutical products. Many hospitals procure their drug supplies through a group purchase organization (GPO). Multiple hospital organizations join a GPO to gain competitive pricing that is based on the volume of products being ordered by the entire group of member organizations. Not only may GPOs negotiate with drug wholesalers for competitive pricing, but they also track generic drug pricing on all the drugs that they cover. This allows them to bid for better pricing on individual items that they have identified as having the most competitive pricing through a particular source. Under a GPO agreement, hospitals generally procure 90% or greater of their products from one prime vendor supplier.

PRIME VENDOR ORGANIZATIONS

Much like—or in conjunction with—GPOs, prime vendor suppliers provide pharmaceutical products to pharmacies for highly competitive pricing. Pharmacies must generally agree to procure 90% or greater of their total supply from one sole source. Prime vendor suppliers usually have a local warehouse whereby pharmacies may gain supply on short notice, which reduces the amount of stock that must be kept on hand. This allows less of the pharmacy's free capital to be tied up in physical inventory, so those funds can be allocated to other areas of the budget. The advantage of same-day ordering and delivery is that it helps pharmacies advance patient care through the timely provision of pharmaceutical products that would take 24 hours or longer to procure through other sources.

DIRECT SUPPLIERS

Purchasing products directly from drug manufacturers is generally the most costly option for pharmacies. This is typically done only in emergency situations when a product is unavailable through any other approved source. Direct purchase may require more space for inventory storage as well, which is another disadvantage of this purchasing option.

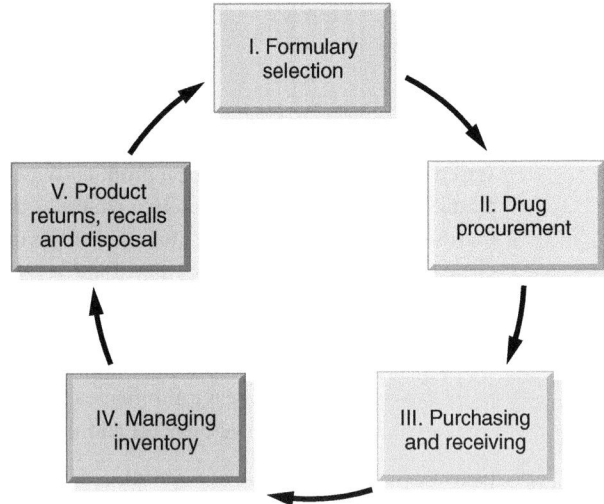

III. Purchasing and Receiving

GENERATING A PURCHASE ORDER

A pharmacy supply order, or purchase order, may be generated via computer and Internet-based technology provided by the drug supplier or with the use of other types of purchasing software. Software provided by the supplier, particularly a prime vendor or GPO supplier, allows pharmacies to accurately maintain an appropriate amount of inventory on hand based on the needs of current patients. Many pharmacy inventory management systems provide a formulary listing of products that the pharmacy stocks; products are generally listed by their National Drug Code (NDC) numbers. Pharmacies generate electronic purchase orders that are sent directly to the supplier for processing. Box 15-1 lists each of the line items typically included on a purchase order.

A computerized inventory management system may be designed to provide points at which stock is automatically ordered when it falls below a target quantity on hand (QOH). Additionally, pharmacies have manual means for staff members to write down items that are low in stock or have been dispensed at an unusually high volume and will run low sooner than usual. Line items on a purchase order may be entered in several ways:

- Manually
- Using a bar code scanner
- Through automated order generation based on stock levels

Electronic orders generally return confirmation of the receipt of the order, along with an estimated date and time of delivery. Same-day ordering and delivery may be accomplished through a

BOX 15-1 **Items Included on a Pharmacy Purchase Order**

- Shipping address
- Date order was placed
- Purchase order number
- Ordering department name/location
- Expected date/time delivery
- Shipping terms
- Account number or billing designation
- Quantity of items ordered
- Unit price/extended price
- Total price of the order
- Buyer's name and phone number

prime vendor supplier, so long as the order is generated and transmitted by an established cutoff time (such as 9 a.m.).

RECEIVING A SHIPMENT

Once an order has been shipped to the pharmacy, the supplier will generally deliver it within an agreed time frame. Pharmaceutical products may be shipped in boxes, cartons, refrigerated containers, plastic bins, or even on large wooden pallets in the case of very large orders. When shipments arrive, they must be signed for in order to confirm receipt. Every shipping container should include a listing of the items enclosed, such as a packing list or shipping invoice that indicates items shipped and billed to the pharmacy. Every item in the shipment must then be verified to ensure the following:

- The correct item was sent
- The correct quantity of ordered items was sent
- All products received are within their expiration date, intact, and shipped in the most appropriate containers to protect the physical and chemical integrity of the products contained within

Pharmacy shipments must never be placed on inventory shelves until all products have been properly received.

Pharmacies that use a bar coding system allow for more efficient receiving of drug shipments. A bar code scanning device is used to scan each product and enter the number of units received. Once scanned, that product is then entered into the pharmacy's system as quantity on hand. Failure to scan in new items received will result in inaccurate QOH in the inventory system. Inaccurate inventory management causes a variety of problems, including the pharmacy's ordering products before it is necessary, which results in excess inventory, diminished inventory space, and poor management of the pharmacy's drug purchasing budget. Because drug products are the single greatest investment for a pharmacy organization (generally accounting for 60% to 70% of the total budget allocation), it is extremely important that accurate stock levels be maintained.

STOCKING SHIPMENT

Incorporating new stock into a pharmacy's physical inventory is an important step in the receiving process, as pharmacy staff members must rely on stock being placed in the designated locations. Items that require special storage, such as refrigeration or protection from light, must be stored appropriately to maintain the physical and chemical stability of the drug. Box 15-2 indicates temperature ranges for various stock storage requirements. Failure to stock products properly increases costs because of the human resources needed to collect damaged products or relocate products stocked incorrectly, shipping charges for returns, and potential health risks to the patient in the event that a degraded product was mistakenly dispensed.

Stock that may be considered hazardous (such as chemotherapeutic drugs) or corrosive (such as acids, bases, or compounding materials that are flammable, like alcohol) must be stored appropriately. In the hospital pharmacy setting, cytotoxic and other hazardous types of drugs are stored separately, whether they are stored on shelves or in refrigerated compartments. Products that are corrosive or flammable must be stored in a fire-resistant locker or cabinet.

Pharmacy shelves or bins must be labeled with product NDC bar codes in addition to product names. Pharmacy technicians involved in stocking drugs should pay particular attention to shelf/bin labels to ensure that products have been placed in the correct storage locations. Stock may be separated by active or backup storage designation, and it is important that pharmacy technicians are aware of which designation the shipment item falls into. Internal and external products must always be separated. Also, products that have look-alike or sound-alike names should be physically

TECH NOTE!
Check product packaging for storage information. Pharmacy technicians must be aware of temperature gradients so that they will know the appropriate temperature range at which various drug products must be stored to preserve the product's physical and chemical stability.

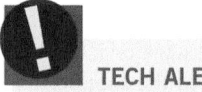

TECH ALERT!
The best way to manage a medication fill error is to prevent it from happening in the first place.

BOX 15-2   **Pharmacy Inventory Storage Temperatures**

Cold: 36° to 46° F
Cool: 46° to 59° F
Room temperature: 59° to 86° F
Warm: 86° to 104° F
Excessive heat: above 104° F (for drugs requiring warming)

separated to minimize the risk of incorrect product selection during the fill process. The best way to manage a medication fill error is to prevent it from happening in the first place. Proper stock placement is the first step.

When a new product is placed in stock, it will likely have a longer manufacturer stability date than products already in stock. The newest products should be moved to the rear, and older products that will expire sooner should be brought to the front. Products that are short-fills should be marked with a brightly colored label or sticker placed on the packaging, or the expiration date should be highlighted so that pharmacy staff members know that those products need to be used first. This process is known as stock rotation.

TECH ALERT!
Internal and external products are absorbed and utilized differently by the body and contain different delivery systems. They must be stocked in separate locations to avoid a medication fill error caused by the wrong route of administration!

TECH NOTE!
Vaccinations are an example of a range of products for which safety stock may be maintained.

TECH NOTE!
In the event of drug shortages, back orders, or the discontinuation of drug products, it is important that both prescribers and patients are made aware of these inventory challenges. Communicate unavailability while suggesting alternatives. Refer the patient or prescriber to the pharmacist to discuss therapeutic alternatives.

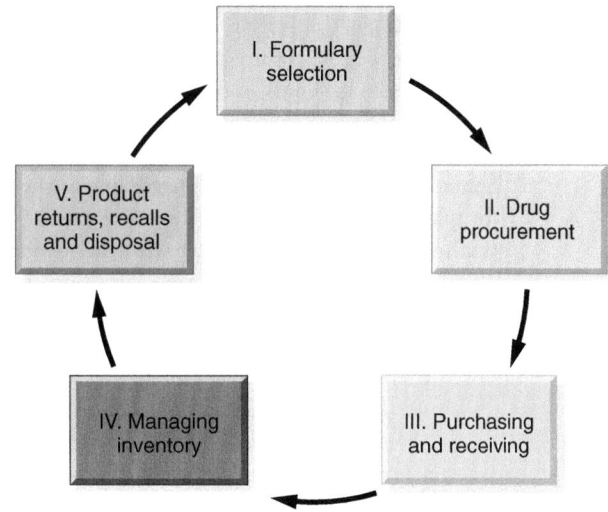

IV. Managing Inventory

As noted throughout this chapter, proper management of pharmacy inventory is critical for delivering patient care and optimizing a pharmacy's most expensive asset: its drug supply. Physical inventory must be evaluated regularly to ensure that products used the most frequently are kept in stock and those for which an average demand has been established are always available. Order cycle time—which is the turnaround time from when products are ordered to when the shipment arrives—must also be taken into consideration.

Inventory management requires maintaining a balance between what items should always be kept in stock, in light of local demands and actual storage space for physical inventory. In a community setting, failure to have the appropriate products in stock may result in the loss of a customer to another pharmacy, not only for that first fill but for future prescription fills. Pharmacy managers must carefully consider the cost of maintaining stock levels in light of the items that are dispensed most frequently.

Physical inventory may be divided into various categories, based on several key criteria:
- High-cost items
- High/low dispensing trends
- Products in which external factors influence usage

Basic stocks include those items of physical inventory that must be maintained based on established average demand. Safety stocks include inventory stores that are maintained in anticipation of fluctuations in use. Vaccinations are an example of products for which safety stock may be maintained. Products are often designated in terms of their frequency of use or stability: the terms *fast movers* and *slow movers* are often used when evaluating the frequency of dispensing turnover. Product expiration is another key factor. If a product that is a slow mover also has a short expiration date, it might be ordered infrequently or only when a patient needs it. Some pharmacies may ask regular patients to inform them a day or two ahead of time when a short-dated or extremely expensive product is needed, so that the item does not have to be stocked on a daily basis.

Because basic stock items must be kept in physical inventory at all times in order to meet the average demand, a minimum number of units of these items should be maintained in the physical inventory. That minimum QOH is known as the par level. For example, if 10 patients are regularly dispensed 30 capsules of drug X, the par level would be set at no less than 300 capsules. An additional safety stock of 300 capsules may be added to that number if drug X was a product for which usage could reasonably increase. Using an automated inventory system, minimum and maximum order stock quantities may be entered. If the physical inventory count on that drug falls below the par level, then the inventory system would automatically place that drug in a queue to be ordered when the next purchase order is generated. It is vital to recognize how important the pharmacy technician's role is during the receiving process: this automated ordering feature will work only if receiving processes are conducted properly so that QOH numbers are accurate.

An automated inventory system may also indicate the cycle order time; based on the criticality of keeping a particular product in stock, that item may need to be ordered more frequently or further in advance in anticipation of an extended cycle order time.

LOANING AND BORROWING

Sometimes a product may be unavailable or the order may be on its way, and a temporary measure for making the product available to the patient may be necessary. Pharmacies have a long-standing tradition of assisting each other with the loaning of products, pending replacement following the receipt of an incoming purchase order. Both hospital and community pharmacies generally have a loan/borrow form on which items to be loaned or borrowed are noted. One may even designate certain portions of the supply order to be shipped to another location in order to replace borrowed items. The only exception to this rule is with Schedule II narcotics. When a Schedule II narcotic is borrowed, a Drug Enforcement Administration (DEA) form 222 is completed, which basically transfers that stock from one pharmacy to another as a purchase. This transaction transfers accountability for the maintenance of that narcotic inventory from the source location to the receiving location. Each pharmacy location must ensure that the transfer of Schedule II narcotic inventory is properly documented and that items are immediately counted for accurate quantities.

LOCAL AND NATIONAL SHORTAGES

Sometimes there may be a local or national shortage of a particular drug for various reasons:
- Manufacturer recall
- Unavailability/shortage of raw materials needed to manufacture the drug product
- Shipping challenges resulting from a natural disaster, disease outbreak, or terrorist attack

When these events occur, pharmacies need to carefully monitor the dispensing of products that are in short supply. If there is a public health concern, pharmacies may be required to surrender supplies for equal distribution across regional areas. Dispensing may be limited to patient populations with the greatest risk of health problems if they don't receive the medication. This has been a common practice during national shortages of flu vaccine, particularly the recent H1N1 flu vaccine. During the national shortages, supplies were limited for distribution to children, elderly patients, and individuals who were highly susceptible to disease because of conditions that lowered their immune response.

INVENTORY CYCLE COUNTS

Physical inventory is divided into sections based on frequency of use. Each section is inventoried on a fixed regular schedule. This allows the entire inventory of products to be counted on a weekly or monthly basis. An average inventory turnover rate—the average rate at which products are dispensed—may then be measured over a year's time to help pharmacy managers better assess what items should remain in physical inventory. Fast movers, short-dated products, and expensive items are counted more frequently, whereas slow movers are counted less frequently. Reports are generated during each cycle count so that product usage trends can be established. Based on those trends, the frequency with which certain products are cycle-counted may be increased. Deviations in the counts are counted as *losses,* or shrink. Losses may be due to product receiving or restocking errors, product damage/disposal, or theft. Pharmacy managers must ensure that losses are carefully monitored, particularly when theft may be an issue.

Aside from verifying the number of units of each product in stock, cycle counting also allows pharmacy staff to verify that products are of the highest level of quality possible. Recall that principle 8 of the Code of Ethics for Pharmacy Technicians states that "A pharmacy technician never assists in the dispensing, promoting or distribution of medications or medical devices that are not of good quality or do not meet the standards required by law." True, cycle counts are tedious and time consuming, but they are critical to the inventory management process. While they are verifying stock levels, pharmacy technicians should also verify the following:

- Product packaging checks to ensure that each has not been compromised.
- Product expiration dates:
  - Products that are due to expire within 60 to 90 days of the date of the cycle count should be marked with a brightly colored sticker or have the expiration date emphasized using a highlighter marker.
  - Short-dated items should be rotated to the front to ensure that they are dispensed first. Of course, any items that have expired should be removed from stock and processed for either return or proper disposal.
- Products that have been discontinued—will no longer be manufactured or carried by that pharmacy—should be identified and either marked for immediate dispensing or removed from physical inventory for return or proper disposal.

USE OF PHARMACY AUTOMATION AND TECHNOLOGY IN INVENTORY MANAGEMENT

Many pharmacies use a computerized pharmacy management system that is furnished either by their drug supplier or by one that interfaces electronically with the supplier's ordering system. Computerized supply management systems allow for more efficient tracking of inventory product-dispensing trends and allows for broader formulary availability.

In a retail pharmacy setting, computerized or web-based inventory management systems offer valuable resources to community pharmacies, both independent and chain stores, such as the following:

- Detailed product information for product selection for ordering
- User-friendly technology
- Order status tracking
- Real-time inventory QOH reporting
- Back order alerts
- Daily updates on drug pricing
- Purchase/account history

Bar Code Scanning

The use of bar code scanning technology (Figure 15-2) continues to advance in many industries, including the community and hospital pharmacy practice. Bar code scanners not only allow for

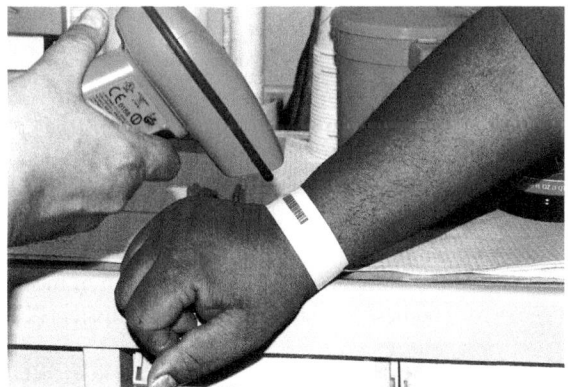

FIGURE 15-2 Bar code reader used to scan the client's wristband. (From Kee JL, Hayes E, McCuistion L: *Pharmacology: A nursing process approach*, ed 6, Philadelphia, 2009, Saunders.)

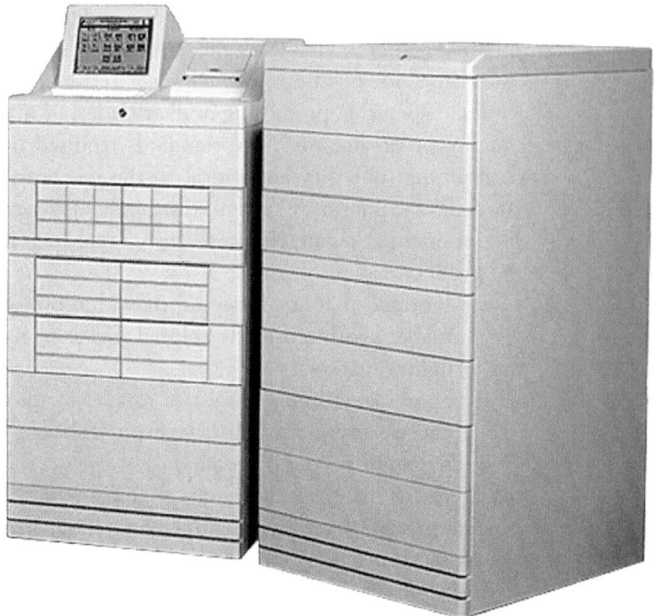

FIGURE 15-3 Computerized medication management system. (From Kee JL, Hayes E, McCuistion L: *Pharmacology: a nursing process approach*, ed 6, Philadelphia, 2009, Saunders. Courtesy Pyxis Corp., San Diego, California.)

better tracking of inventory, but they also permit more accurate product selection during the prescription order and fill process. Bar code scanners that are used specifically for inventory management allow for real-time adjustment of inventory QOH stock levels during the fill and dispensing process and may also include keypads that allow quantities to be entered and adjusted during the receiving and cycle count processes.

In a hospital pharmacy setting, tracking inventory is a greater challenge because medication storage areas are located all over the hospital, not just in the central pharmacy. Pharmacy stock may be located in areas such as the following:

• Central pharmacy
• IV room
• Refrigerated cases
• Satellite pharmacies
• Medication storage areas for nursing unit floor stock or patient-specific dispensing
• Pharmacy automated storage devices, such as a carousel shelving
• Remote drug storage devices, such as a Pyxis (Figure 15-3) or Omnicell automated medication and supply dispensing machine/cabinet

Use of a computerized inventory and workflow management system allows for the following measures of efficiency:

• Allows staff that would otherwise be needed for inventory counting to be reallocated to other pharmacy workflow tasks
• Recaptures the amount of time spent by inventory staff during the processing of ordering and receiving
• Allows for better tracking of product end dates
• Prime vendor software allows for submission of orders for same-day or next-day delivery
• Allows for better physical security by controlling access to medication supplies
• Provides necessary documentation of medication usage data for reporting to hospital accrediting bodies, such as The Joint Commission (TJC)

ANTICIPATING COMMUNITY NEEDS

Formulary selection may be based on established demographic data gathered on the residential areas and communities surrounding a pharmacy. Pharmacies with a large retirement community may offer products and services that would be in greater demand for that patient population. Pharmacies with single-family home communities may require more medication for pediatric patients. Additionally, during cold, flu, and allergy seasons, there will be an increase in the volume of products that are dispensed for these conditions, so ordering trends would increase during those periods.

Inventory Management and Disaster Preparedness

Hospital pharmacies must stock enough emergency medicine to meet the needs of the area population in the event of a mass casualty situation that could be due to a natural disaster, disease outbreak, or chemical/biological terrorist attack. Pharmacies are required to keep safety stock on hand so that area hospitals can respond appropriately in a mass casualty situation. The disaster-preparedness of a hospital could strongly impact the survival rates of citizens in that area in the event of a mass casualty situation, such as a hurricane, tornado, or terrorist attack.

Inventory Management of Narcotic and Controlled Medication Stock

Narcotic and controlled medication is generally kept in a secure location, such as a vault or locked cabinet. Because of the theft and abuse potential of these products, the stock levels must be closely monitored. Perpetual inventory management is a process whereby physical inventory counts are taken at the start of each shift, as well as before and after each medication fill. Additionally, products that are Schedule II narcotics must be ordered and tracked on DEA form 222. Discrepancies caused by manufacturer shortages or waste (product spillage or disposal after falling on the floor) must be carefully documented to ensure the accountability of controlled products. Pharmacy technicians involved in the dispensing and inventory management processes for narcotic and controlled medication must not only display ethical behavior, but they should do so with an added sense of accountability for maintaining accurate perpetual inventory. Any observed or suspected theft of narcotics or controlled medication should be reported to the pharmacist in charge or appropriate authority. Failure to report theft may place the observer at risk of professional discipline or prosecution, along with the offending party or parties.

LOSS, FRAUD, WASTE, AND ABUSE

Recall that principle nine of the Code of Ethics for Pharmacy Technicians states that a "pharmacy technician does not engage in any activity that will discredit the profession, and will expose, without fear or favor, illegal or unethical conduct in the profession."

TECH ALERT!
Failure to report theft may place the observer at risk of professional discipline or prosecution, along with the offending party.

As noted earlier, losses may be due to product receiving or restocking errors, product damage/disposal, or theft. Unfortunately, the theft of drugs is a major problem that costs pharmacies thousands of dollars a year. Although theft for personal use has not been as great a concern for pharmacy technicians, theft of products for private sale has been a major issue among an alarming number of pharmacy technicians. Each year, some pharmacy technicians are professionally disciplined for the misappropriation of pharmaceutical products. State boards of pharmacy have inspectors and code enforcement officers who investigate claims involving theft. Theft of controlled and narcotic substances may also be subject to investigation by the Drug Enforcement Administration, as well as local law enforcement. Pharmacy technicians must carefully consider the severe consequences of theft in the pharmacy and avoid this behavior at all costs.

In the event that a pharmacy technician suspects another pharmacy staff member of theft or observes this behavior, there are anonymous methods through which that information can be disclosed for investigation by the appropriate authorities. Inappropriate waste, fraudulent sales practices, and signs of physical dependence on controlled substances are all issues that pharmacy technicians must not involve themselves in and must report immediately. Pharmacies generally have a fraud, waste, and abuse hotline to which anonymous reporting may be made. In rare instances, a person's identity may have to be revealed if live testimony is necessary in a criminal trial. Although testifying in court may be uncomfortable, the risk of having to give legal testimony should not serve as a deterrent to a pharmacy technician making the right decision to report unethical and illegal activity.

Pharmacy managers may take some security measures to discourage the theft and other forms of misappropriation of pharmacy stock, including the following:
- Adjusting the locations of security cameras
- Close monitoring of high-risk items
- Random drug testing

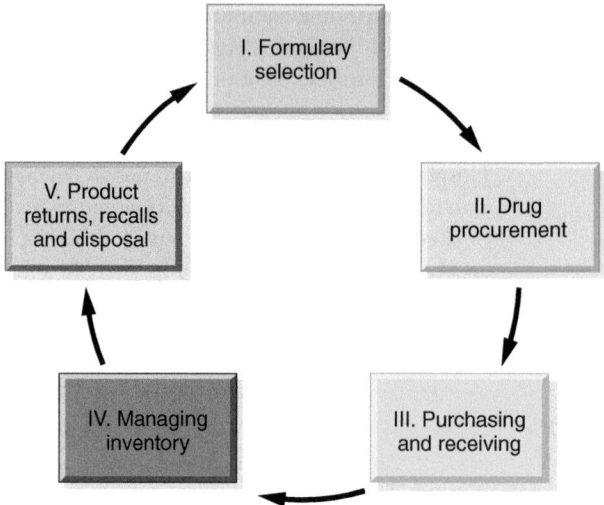

V. Product Returns, Recalls, and Disposal

The most common reason for drugs to be returned is expiration. Products that reach their beyond-use dating must be removed from stock immediately. They may then be processed for:
• Partial or full credit by the manufacturer
• Preparation for proper disposal

Each drug manufacturer or supplier has a return policy, as well as documentation that must be completed as part of the credit return process. Also, some manufacturers allow products to be returned for proper disposal whether or not credit is extended, as other packaging materials may be recycled.

In the community pharmacy setting, products that are identified as expired (or about to expire) during cycle counts are manually removed from stock.

In a hospital pharmacy setting, packaging often allows unused drugs to be returned to stock for reuse. Because of unit dose packaging, there can be thousands of individual doses that must be checked for expiration dating. Drug expiration dates are checked on a monthly basis both in the central pharmacy areas and wherever else medications are stored. This is part of the medication or nursing unit inspection. Following the unit inspection, pharmacy staff members document products found to be expired and gather them for return to the manufacturer or for proper disposal. Additionally, pharmacy technicians check returned medication from floors to verify product dating and package integrity prior to returning those individual doses back into pharmacy's physical inventory.

Because of the sheer volume of credit returns of drug doses in a pharmacy, many hospital pharmacies and a growing number of community pharmacies enlist the services of an outsource company to sort and document products for return or disposal.

PROPER DRUG DISPOSAL

Properly disposing of expired or damaged pharmaceutical products is critical to protecting the local and global environment. The Resource Conservation and Recovery Act (RCRA) gives the Environmental Protection Agency (EPA) the authority to control the generation, transportation, treatment, storage, and disposal of hazardous waste.[2] The U.S. Geological Survey conducted research in 1999 that indicated the extent to which there are traces of antibiotics and other pharmaceuticals in groundwater supplies that are fed by lakes and rivers. Although many of these deposits are the result of drug metabolites excreted by the human body, flushing drugs into sewer systems can be very harmful, because universal standards are in place for identifying and filtering out various pharmaceutical compounds from water supplies. Pharmacy technicians should always consult with a

BOX 15-3   **Voluntary Drug Recalls**

Type 1. Products with incorrect labeling or products that have microbial contamination, for which use could lead to serious health consequences up to and including death.
Type 2. Products for which use may lead to a temporary health problem or serious (but not life-threatening) health complications.
Type 3. Products that do not present a health risk but may violate packaging or labeling restrictions.

pharmacist before pouring a liquid down the sink or flushing medication down the toilet. Every pharmacy should have an established standard operating procedure related to the proper disposal of pharmaceutical products.

VOLUNTARY DRUG RECALL

The Food and Drug Administration, under the Federal Food, Drug and Cosmetic Act of 1938, may request that a product be recalled, based on concerns about the product's efficacy, purity, or functionality. Most drug recalls are done voluntarily by the drug or product manufacturer. Drug recalls are classified according to severity and risk to public health. Box 15-3 details each of the types of drug recalls.

In the event of a voluntary drug recall, a drug manufacturer notifies all individuals who have purchased the product subject to the recall. If individual batches (lots) are affected, the recall notice will detail the specific lots that need to be checked.

Pharmacy staff members place an immediate priority on the collection of all recalled products, including any compounded medication in which the recalled drug may be an ingredient. Any product within the specified lots is immediately returned to the drug manufacturer. Credit toward new product is extended to any pharmacy that returns recalled products, or units recalled are replaced with product unaffected by the recall when possible.

The Future of Inventory Management: RFID Technology

What is RFID? If you live in an area with a toll road that uses, for automated billing purposes, a remote toll tag to track the number of times you cross, then you are already aware of how radio frequency identification (RFID) can be utilized. Although this technology is not new, it is generally very costly and is not yet available for mainstream application in today's modern health care setting. The establishment and utilization of an RFID system requires the application of expensive radio-frequency tags, readers, network interfaces, and cables in order for the system to have widespread utilization in a community or hospital pharmacy setting. The most common current health care application of RFID is patient identification bands, in which an RFID reader (like a bar code scanner) is used to positively verify individual patient identifiers prior to the administration of medication or other medical treatment. The advantage of RFID over the standard analog bar code scanner is that the radio frequency tags can be read through various types of materials (a patient's tag could be scanned and the reader would pick up the ID tag without the patient having to be repositioned, as the wristband need not be visible for scanning).

Future applications of RFID extend to every aspect of the pharmacy supply chain and include the following:
• Use in mail-order pharmacies to ensure proper product identification during the order fill and shipping process
• Tracking of patient shipments, as well as pharmacy purchase order shipments and contents of shipping containers
• Tracking of inventory in the pharmacy, as well as tracking of inventory as it leaves the pharmacy and is distributed to various areas of a hospital
• Tracking of durable medical equipment and supplies that are distributed to patients in the retail pharmacy setting or to patient care areas in the hospital pharmacy setting

Chapter Summary

- Whether in the community or hospital pharmacy setting, inventory management processes impact a pharmacy's ability to provide needed products and services to patients.
- Procurement may be defined as the process of obtaining goods and services.
- Key opportunities for advancement to the position of purchasing technician exist in both community and hospital pharmacy settings.
- The key components of the pharmacy materials management process include formulary product selection, purchase order and receiving, managing inventory, and product recalls and returns.
- A formulary is a list of drug products that are available for dispensing at a pharmacy.
- Vendor relationships exist with drug wholesalers, group purchase organizations, prime vendor organizations, and direct suppliers.
- Pharmacies evaluate possible suppliers for purchase advantages, such as volume purchase discounts and credit toward the purchase of new product in exchange for the return of expired products.
- Pharmacies generate electronic purchase orders that are sent directly to the supplier for processing and may be generated via manual entry, use of a bar code scanner, or automated order generation based on stock levels.
- Pharmaceutical products may be shipped in boxes, cartons, refrigerated containers, plastic bins, or large wooden pallets.
- Every item in the shipment must be verified to ensure that the correct item was sent, the correct quantity of ordered items was sent, and all products received are within their expiration date, intact, and shipped in the most appropriate shipping containers.
- Incorporating new stock into a pharmacy's physical inventory is an important step in the receiving process.
- Inventory management requires maintaining a balance between what items should always be kept in stock in light of actual storage space for physical inventory.
- *Order cycle time*—which is the turnaround time from when products are ordered until the shipment arrives—must also be taken into consideration.
- *Basic stocks* include those items of physical inventory that must be maintained based on established average demand.
- *Safety stocks* include inventory stores that are maintained in anticipation of fluctuations in use. Both hospital and community pharmacies generally have a loan/borrow form on which items may be loaned or borrowed in emergency short-fill situations.
- In a retail pharmacy setting, computerized or web-based inventory management systems offer valuable resources to community pharmacies.
- Bar code scanners that are used specifically for inventory management allow for real-time adjustment of inventory QOH stock levels during the fill and dispensing process.
- In a hospital pharmacy setting, tracking inventory is a greater challenge because medication storage areas are located all over the hospital.
- Stock may be managed in automated storage devices, such as carousel shelving or automated dispensing machines. The use of a computerized inventory and a workflow management system allows for various measures of efficiency.
- Key issues that affect pharmacy inventory management include anticipating community needs, disaster and mass-casualty preparedness, narcotic and controlled medication storage, and loss/fraud/waste/abuse.
- Each drug manufacturer or supplier has a return policy, as well as documentation that must be completed as part of the credit return process.
- Some manufacturers may also allow products to be returned for proper disposal.
- Drug expiration dates are checked monthly, both in the central pharmacy areas and wherever else medications are stored.
- The proper disposal of expired or damaged pharmaceutical products is critical to protecting the local and global environment.
- The Food and Drug Administration, under the Federal Food, Drug and Cosmetic Act of 1938, may request that a product be recalled based on concerns about the product's efficacy, purity, or functionality.

- In the event of a voluntary drug recall, a drug manufacturer notifies all individuals who have purchased the product subject to the recall.
- Pharmacy staff members place an immediate priority on the collection of all recalled products.

Multiple Choice

1. The net price that a pharmacy pays for a particular product is referred to as the:
   a. Acquisition cost
   b. Procurement cost
   c. Carrying cost
   d. Dispensing cost

2. Basic stock is composed of items for which:
   a. There is no need to maintain stock
   b. There is an established average demand
   c. There are special order needs
   d. There are additional costs

3. A particular cream that will no longer be produced by a drug manufacturer should be considered:
   a. Out of stock
   b. Unavailable
   c. Discontinued
   d. Unsafe for dispensing

4. The period of time between when an order is placed and when the shipment arrives at the pharmacy is referred to as the:
   a. Order cycle time
   b. Order fluctuation time
   c. Shipping time
   d. Receiving time

5. Pharmacy physical inventory that is maintained to account for unexpected or anticipated fluctuations in demand is known as:
   a. Emergency stock
   b. Fluctuation stock
   c. Basic stock
   d. Safety stock

6. The following types of drugs need to be stored in a flame-resistant cabinet:
   a. Acids
   b. Corrosive compounding materials
   c. Isopropyl alcohol
   d. All of the above

7. Moving older products to the front of the shelf describes the inventory process of:
   a. Stock rotation
   b. Restocking
   c. Motion inventory
   d. Stock replacement

8. A Schedule II narcotic may:
   a. Be borrowed using a DEA schedule 222 form and returned once the borrowing pharmacy has received more stock
   b. Be borrowed using a DEA schedule 222 form and considered to be a nontransferable purchase
   c. Not be borrowed, as this is against the law

9. When a drug product expires, it may be:
   a. Returned for partial or full credit by the manufacturer
   b. Thrown in the garbage
   c. Prepared for proper disposal
   d. Both A and C

10. A product in which there is microbial contamination that could pose a risk to patients' health may be subject to a type ___ recall.
    a. 1
    b. 2
    c. 3
    d. 4

TECHNICIAN'S CORNER

1. How do formularies help managed care organizations?
2. What types of storage requirements would affect the physical and chemical stability of a drug product?
3. How should products with look-alike or sound-alike names be stored in a pharmacy?

Bibliography

American Pharmacy Alliance. (2002). *Information*. Retrieved 8/15/2011, from http://www.ameripharm.com/apa_info.html

Bacheldor, B. (2006, November 7). *RFID Brings Further Automation to Mail Order Pharmacy*. Retrieved 8/15/2011, from RFID Journal: http://www.rfidjournal.com/article/view/2801

BusinessDictionary.com. (2011). *[Definition of] Procurement*. Retrieved 8/8/2011, from BusinessDictionary.com: http://www.businessdictionary.com/definition/procurement.html

Coalition for Community Pharmacy Action. (2007, January 26). *Executive Summary of the National Cost of Dispensing (COD) Study Final Report*. Retrieved 8/10/2011, from Coalition for Community Pharmacy Action: http://www.rxaction.org/publications/National_COD_Study_Executive_Summary.pdf

Groundwater Foundation. (2011). *Pharmaceuticals and Personal Care Products (PPCPs): An Emerging Issue*. Retrieved 8/15/2011, from http://www.groundwater.org/gi/docs_pack/fa13.pdf

Hunt, M. (2007, April 16). *Squaring Off: Should Every Hospital Join a GPO?* Retrieved 8/9/2011, from Drug Topics: Voice of the Pharmacist: http://drugtopics.modernmedicine.com/drugtopics/Pharmacy/Squaring-off-Should-every-hospital-join-a-GPO/ArticleStandard/Article/detail/417486

National Association of Chain Drug Stores (NACDS). (2004, October). *Issue Brief: Elements of a Pharmacy Dispensing Fee*. Retrieved 8/9/2011, from http://ovha.vermont.gov/budget-legislative/appendix3b.pdf

National Community Pharmacists Association (NCPA). (2008). *Managing the Pharmacy Inventory*. Retrieved 8/10/2011, from http://www.ncpanet.org/members/pdf/ownership-managinginventory.pdf

Regulatory Affairs Associates. (2010, December 5). *The FDA Recall Process: How It Works*. Retrieved 8/15/2011, from http://www.regaffairs.net/top-news/33

United States Environmental Protection Agency (EPA). (2011, August 11). *Summary of the Resource Conservation and Recovery Act of 1976*. Retrieved 8/15/2011, from United States Environmental Protection Agency (EPA): http://www.epa.gov/lawsregs/laws/rcra.html

16 Medication Safety and Error Prevention

KEY TERMS

Adverse drug event (ADE): A severe, unexpected patient reaction to medication administration.

Medication error: Any preventable event that may cause or lead to inappropriate medication use or patient harm.

Medication misadventure: An event in which a patient suffers harm after administration of medication for which a fill error occurred.

As is emphasized repeatedly throughout pharmacy technician course work, the primary goal of pharmacy technician practice is to support the pharmacist in the safe, efficacious dispensing of quality pharmaceutical products and services. Protecting the health, welfare, and safety of patients is the first priority of every pharmacist and pharmacy technician. Although relatively few medication errors occur, compared with the number of prescriptions filled each year, each of those errors represents a human life that was negatively affected, or maybe even ended, by a medication dispensing error.

Every member of the pharmacy profession and the healthcare team must take extra care to practice behaviors that minimize the risk of a medication error. Unfortunately, errors do occur, and the number continues to rise. When an error occurs, pharmacy and other healthcare personnel have an ethical and a legal obligation to report it. This is not just a measure of accountability for the individuals involved in the error; it is also a way to educate the rest of the pharmacy profession across the United States. Sharing cases of medication dispensing errors and resulting medication misadventures with other pharmacists and pharmacy technicians is helpful, because dispensing errors occur much more easily than one might think. Information sharing helps prevent that error in pharmacies in other cities or towns.

This chapter also discusses how medication errors can be prevented in five key areas:
- Order entry
- Fill process
- Pharmacy processes
- Storage practices
- Communication

Pharmacy technicians must consider the five rights of safe medication administration during the order entry, fill process, nonsterile pharmaceutical compounding process, unit-dose packaging process, medication unit inspection, cycle count, and sterile intravenous (IV) admixture, all of which they will perform in the course of their careers. Remember, the five rights are:
- Right patient
- Right drug
- Right dose
- Right route
- Right time

This chapter first presents some basic definitions that apply to medication safety and errors. It then examines how medication errors and misadventures can occur when one or more of the five rights go wrong. Resources provided by national organizations (e.g., the Institute for Safe Medication Practices [ISMP]) for investigating, reporting, and preventing medication errors are also discussed.

Defining Medication Errors and How They Occur

The National Coordinating Council for Medication Error Reporting and Prevention (NCCMERP) has encouraged the healthcare professions to use the following standard definition of a medication error (NCCMERP, 2011):

> "A medication error is any preventable event that may cause or lead to inappropriate medication use or patient harm while the medication is in the control of the health care professional, patient, or consumer. Such events may be related to professional practice, health care products, procedures, and systems, including prescribing; order communication; product labeling, packaging, and nomenclature; compounding; dispensing; distribution; administration; education; monitoring; and use."

A medication error is an event that occurs because a prescription was filled incorrectly, at any point in the order entry, fill, compounding or dispensing process. A medication error becomes a medication misadventure *when a patient is affected by that error*. A medication misadventure caused by the pharmacy may be an event in which a patient suffers harm after administration of medication for which a fill error occurred. A medication misadventure caused by a patient or patient caregiver occurs when the medication is given or self-administered incorrectly.

Medication errors occur for a variety of reasons. In a survey done in 2006, 80% of the 150 pharmacists surveyed reported that difficulty with product identification is probably the main reason patients and caregivers make medication errors.

In 1996 and 1997, the Massachusetts Board of Registration in Pharmacy conducted a comprehensive study on the causes of medication errors. Survey responses indicated that the pressure of both internal and external stimuli or stressors contributed to or created ideal conditions for errors. Pharmacists who contributed to the study data gave the following as reasons for medication errors:
- Internal stressors
  - Too many telephone calls
  - No time to counsel

- External stressors
  - Overload/unusually busy day
  - Too many customers
  - Lack of concentration
  - No one available to double-check
  - Staff shortage
  - Similar drug names
  - Illegible prescription
  - Misinterpreted prescription

Medication errors that occur as a result of staffing issues are common in both institutional and community pharmacies, particularly when the workflow is regularly heavy and stressful. Some common ways in which inadequate staffing creates dangerous opportunities for medication errors are:

- Increased workload, which often can result in a compromise in quality in favor of production
- Inadequate pharmacist availability for questions and assistance
- Short cuts that result in fewer multiple checks
- Overwork, which adversely affects staff members' morale and general sense of commitment and accountability to job tasks

Realistically, in a busy workplace, a heavy customer load results in profitability, so no business wants to eliminate its customer flow. Therefore, the workflow must be managed properly to ensure that quality is not compromised or abandoned in the pursuit of meeting workflow demands. Although good customer service in a retail industry generally is characterized by the provision of products and services in a timely manner, pharmacists and pharmacy technicians face the particular challenge of filling prescriptions as quickly as possible while ensuring that all necessary steps in the order entry and fill process are performed.

PROCESS BREAKDOWN

Regardless of whether internal or external stressors are present, all pharmacy technicians must recognize that every task associated with pharmacy practice should be well documented as a process in the pharmacy's standard operating procedures. A process is effective only when it is followed consistently; processes create a control in which an expected final product is produced when steps are followed in the same manner on a consistent basis. Deviation from the process, or process breakdown, can have serious workflow consequences, particularly in healthcare. In fact, an important way to research a medication error is to determine the point or points where a process breakdown led to the error.

No simple solutions exist for easing or coping with the internal and external stressors of pharmacy practice. All pharmacy technicians must strive to perform their tasks with accuracy and safety as the first priority, and timeliness as a valuable second priority.

Some additional common causes of medication errors, particularly in institutional pharmacies, include:

- Communication breakdown
  - Incorrect transcription during a verbal order
  - Illegible handwriting that is not verified for clarification
  - Improper pass-down of information when multiple individuals process a particular order
- Inventory storage practices
  - Internal and external products stored together
  - Oral and injectable products stored together
  - Difficult to read storage labeling
  - Incorrect storage labeling
  - Incorrect product locations
  - Look-alike or sound-alike products stored close together
  - Poor or inadequate lighting in drug storage areas
- Repetition/acquired blindness
  - Short cuts or poor technique develop over time
  - Recognizing the product shape and pulling the drug, without actually reading the label

BOX 16-1   Medication Errors Resulting from Breakdown in Adherence to the Five Rights
of Medication Administration

RIGHT PATIENT
- Similar or multiple names in a database without distinguishing patient identifiers
- Wrong patient's refill number selected

RIGHT DRUG
- Wrong product with a similar name selected
- Wrong form of the right drug selected
- Wrong product selected because of illegible handwriting and misinterpretation
- Wrong product selected during the fill process
- Wrong information entered on the dispensing label

RIGHT DOSE
- Wrong strength of an oral solid drug selected
- Wrong concentration strength of a liquid drug
- Wrong release rate of a product selected
- Use of an unapproved abbreviation that results in order entry error in drug dosing

RIGHT ROUTE
- Wrong formulation of a drug selected (e.g., adult rather than pediatric formulation)
- Intravenous (IV) administration of an oral drug
- Oral administration of an IV drug
- Incorrect otic or ophthalmic product selected

RIGHT TIME
- Wrong dosing frequency entered into pharmacy system and printed on dispensing label
- Wrong administration interval entered on an IV solution label
- Wrong IV drip flow rate entered and noted on an IV solution label
- STAT or one-time dose sent multiple times and administered multiple times by patient caregiver
- Scheduled dose not delivered at the right time, which may result in patient response to late dose, or patient caregiver may miss a scheduled dose as a result of delayed delivery

RIGHT DOCUMENTATION
- Incorrect labeling of medication and/or products
- Improper pharmacy records

- Spelling and order entry errors result from lack of attention
- Overconfidence develops as a result of mastering a routine

RELATING MEDICATION ERRORS TO THE SIX RIGHTS OF MEDICATION ADMINISTRATION

Recall each of the six rights of medication administration that should be observed during the processes of medication order acceptance, review, entry, fill, and dispensing, administration, and distribution. Box 16-1 lists possible errors that can occur that relate to these six rights.

How Medication Misadventures Occur

Medication misadventures may or may not result from a medication error. Recall that a medication misadventure caused by the pharmacy may be an event in which a patient suffers harm after administration of medication for which a fill error occurred. A medication misadventure caused by a patient or patient caregiver occurs when the medication is given or self-administered incorrectly. The U.S. Agency for Healthcare Research and Quality (AHRQ) noted the following types of medication errors that result in an adverse drug event (ADE) (AHRQ, 2011):

- Missed dose
- Wrong technique
- Illegible order

- Duplicate therapy
- Drug-drug interaction
- Equipment failure
- Inadequate monitoring
- Preparation error

Many misadventures occur as the result of a pharmacodynamic action of the drug, indicated by an ADE (a severe and unexpected patient reaction to medication administration). Because of the pharmacodynamics of drugs, the onset of an adverse reaction may be delayed or may occur within a short time after administration; it depends on the drug's onset of action. Examples of medication misadventures that occur as the result of a severe, unexpected reaction include:

- Adverse drug reactions: Unexpected; more serious than a side effect
- Allergic drug reactions: Caused by known or unknown drug, food, or environmental allergy
- Drug-drug interactions: Often result from the use of drugs from multiple therapeutic classes; over-the-counter (OTC) drugs that affect prescription drugs; or poor drug therapy monitoring by the pharmacist or other healthcare providers

Medication misadventures may also occur as a result of a patient's lack of knowledge and understanding of the medication. Some patient-related causes of medication misadventures are:

- Noncompliance with the prescribed regimen
- Limited health literacy
- Lack of necessary patient education and drug therapy monitoring

One of the best ways to prevent misadventures that occur as a result of misunderstanding is to ensure that patients receive medication counseling from a pharmacist.

Strategies for Ensuring Medication Dispensing Safety and Error Prevention

At this point you have studied a variety of scenarios that create opportunities for medication fill errors. By now you may realize that even when a pharmacy technician is well trained, competent, and has a good understanding of workflow processes, a breakdown of those processes can occur as a result of internal or external stressors (or both). However, you can get these processes back on track. Preventing medication errors requires commitment and focus. Let's examine strategies for preventing medication errors in the following key areas:

- Order entry
- Fill process
- Pharmacy processes
- Storage practices
- Communication

ORDER ENTRY

- Eliminate errors caused by poor handwriting by using a computerized order entry system, rather than handwritten order entry.
- Pharmacists can practice read-backs during telephone verbal order transcription for confirmation and clarification.
- Pharmacists can discourage the use of high-risk abbreviations by prescribers (Table 16-1). Ask the prescriber to spell it out instead.
- Verify the original order during transcription; if necessary, call back the prescriber for clarification.
- Verify the accuracy of labels before filling the prescription.

FILL PROCESS

- Gather materials first.
- Read the label twice.
- Double-check ingredients before filling the prescription (Figure 16-1).
- Check the product by name, strength, and National Drug Code (NDC) number during the fill process.
- Avoid distractions and complete a fill before moving to another task.

TABLE 16-1   **Dangerous Medication Abbreviations***

Abbreviation	Intended meaning	Common error
U	Units	Mistaken as a zero or a four (4), resulting in overdose. Also mistaken for "cc" (cubic centimeters) when poorly written.
μg	Micrograms	Mistaken for "mg" (milligrams), resulting in an overdose.
Q.D.	Latin abbreviation for "every day"	The period after the "Q" has sometimes been mistaken for an " I," and the drug has been given "QID" (four times daily) rather than daily.
Q.O.D.	Latin abbreviation for "every other day"	Misinterpreted as "QD" (daily) or "QID" (four times daily). If the "O" is poorly written, it looks like a period or an "I."
SC or SQ	Subcutaneous	Mistaken as "SL" (sublingual) when poorly written.
T I W	Three times a week	Misinterpreted as "three times a day" or "twice a week."
D/C	Discharge; also discontinue	Patient's medications have been prematurely discontinued when D/C (intended to mean "discharge") was misinterpreted as "discontinue," because it was followed by a list of drugs.
HS	Half strength	Misinterpreted as the Latin abbreviation "HS" (hour of sleep).
cc	Cubic centimeters	Mistaken as "U" (units) when poorly written.
AU, AS, AD	Latin abbreviation for "both ears," "left ear," and "right ear," respectively	Misinterpreted as the Latin abbreviation "OU" (both eyes); "OS" (left eye); "OD" (right eye)
IU	International Unit	Mistaken as IV (intravenous) or 10 (ten)
MS, MSO_4, $MgSO_4$	Confused for one another	Can mean morphine sulfate or magnesium sulfate

*As designated by the National Coordinating Council for Medication Error Reporting and Prevention (NCCMERP).

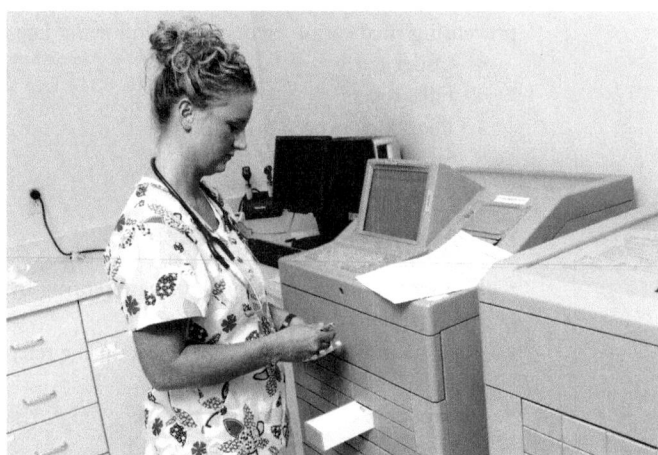

FIGURE 16-1 Double-check the ingredients of all prescriptions before they are filled. (From Hopper T: *Mosby's pharmacy technician: principles and practice,* ed 3, Philadelphia, 2011, Saunders.)

- Attach the appropriate auxiliary labels.
- Use charts and reference materials; do not work from memory.

PHARMACY PROCESSES

- Staffing shortages are a reality; pharmacists and pharmacy technicians must learn to establish good workflow processes to compensate for understaffing.

- Never compromise good filling practices for production; work that must be done twice because of fill errors is inefficient and unproductive.
- Do not allow bad habits or poor attitudes to take root; be responsible for your own work.

STORAGE PRACTICES
- Notify a pharmacist if poor lighting is an issue; you are probably not the first person to notice.
- Use TALLman LeTTering: In tall man lettering, key letters or syllables are noted in upper case, which helps distinguish between drugs with similarly spelled names.
- Store look-alike/sound-alike products in separate areas and post signs or labels to alert and warn staff members.

COMMUNICATION
Pharmacists and pharmacy technicians can help prevent medication errors and misadventures by learning from their mistakes. The profession of pharmacy cannot treat medication errors and misadventures as dirty little secrets; they must be openly and honestly shared with the rest of the healthcare community. The goal is to prevent another member of the profession from committing that same or a similar error and perhaps harming a patient. Not only is medication error reporting the right ethical decision, it also helps protect the health, welfare, and safety of patients across the pharmacy profession.

The following publications carry information on medication errors and misadventures and how to report them:
- *ISMP Medication Safety Alert!* (newsletters)
- *FDA Drug Safety Newsletter*

AHRQ has established the following measures to help prevent medication errors that result in ADEs:
- Use the U.S. Food and Drug Administration's (FDA's) Medwatch program to report serious ADEs.
- Improve incident reporting systems.
- Create a better (less punitive or discipline-driven) atmosphere to encourage more consistent ADE reporting.
- Rely more on pharmacists to advise physicians on medication therapy.
- Put increased emphasis on promoting healthcare provider education on medication use.
- Improve nursing medication administration and monitoring systems.

Institute for Safe Medication Practices: A Resource for Error Reporting and Information and Resource Sharing

The ISMP is a not-for-profit organization dedicated to educating the healthcare community, providers and patients alike, in safe medication practices and ways to prevent and protect themselves from medication errors.

Several publications are available to practitioners that highlight errors that occur in specific areas of patient care, such as acute care (for the cardiac and general intensive care units) and ambulatory care (for community pharmacies).

A nursing publication, *Nurse Advise-ERR*, is specifically designed to provide information about medication administration and ways to prevent errors during administration.

The publication *Safe Medicine* is designed for consumers and provides information on ways patients can help prevent medication errors and misadventures through communication with their caregivers and pharmacists and through sources of healthcare education.

ERROR REPORTING
Pharmacy Reporting
When an error occurs, the pharmacy files a detailed report with the U.S. Pharmacopeia/Institute for Safe Medication Practices (USP-ISMP) Medication Errors Reporting Program (MERP). Depending on the nature of the error, ISMP follows up when appropriate.

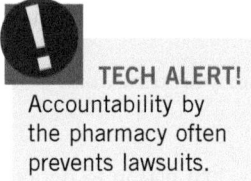

Individual Reporting

When an error occurs, time is often a critical factor in reporting, particularly for contacting the patient to prevent the individual from administering the incorrect prescription fill. Personal accountability is a must, regardless of the implications for disciplinary action. When a pharmacy technician discovers an error, he or she must notify the pharmacist in charge or a staff pharmacist immediately. The pharmacist then contacts the patient to inform the person of the error and takes steps to retrieve the misfilled product and/or provide the patient with medical advice if he or she has already administered the wrong medication. All individuals involved in the medication error should complete any necessary internal documentation, providing as much detail as possible.

Chapter Summary

- Medication errors are part of the reason healthcare costs continue to rise.
- All members of the pharmacy profession must consistently practice behaviors that minimize the risk of a medication error.
- A medication error is any preventable event that may cause or lead to inappropriate medication use or patient harm while the medication is in the control of the healthcare professional, patient, or consumer.
- Medication misadventures may be caused by a pharmacy or by a patient.
- Medication errors that occur as a result of staffing issues are common to both hospital and community pharmacies, particularly when the workflow is regularly heavy and stressful.
- Common causes of medication errors, particularly in hospital pharmacies, may include communication breakdown, poor inventory storage practices, and repetition/acquired blindness.
- Inventory storage practices may create opportunities for medication selection or fill errors, or both.
- Acquired blindness occurs when a person relies on the color or size of packaging they are accustomed to seeing, rather than *actually reading* the package labeling.
- Errors caused by handwriting can be eliminated through the use of computerized order entry systems instead of handwritten order entry.
- Pharmacy technicians should review their habits and practice improvements that help prevent medication errors.
- Publications concerned with the reporting of medication errors and misadventures include *Pharmacy Today, U.S. Pharmacist, ISMP Medication Safety Alert!* newsletters (and other newsletters), and the *FDA Drug Safety* newsletter.
- The Institute for Safe Medication Practices (ISMP) is a not-for-profit organization dedicated to educating the healthcare community, providers and patients alike, in safe medication practices and ways to prevent and protect themselves from medication errors.
- When an error occurs, the pharmacy files a detailed report with the USP-ISMP Medication Errors Reporting Program (MERP). Depending on the nature of the error, ISMP follows up when appropriate.
- When a pharmacy technician discovers an error, he or she must notify the pharmacist in charge or a staff pharmacist immediately. The pharmacist contacts the patient to inform the person of the error and takes steps to retrieve the misfiled product and/or provide the patient with medical advice if he or she has already administered the wrong medication.
- All individuals involved in the medication error should complete the necessary internal documentation, providing as much detail as possible.

1. How does process breakdown increase the risk of a medication error?
2. Give an example of an error that may occur as a result of poor adherence to verifying the right patient.
3. What steps should a pharmacy technician take when he or she discovers that a medication error has occurred?

Bibliography

Agency for Healthcare Research and Quality (AHRQ). (2001, March). *Reducing and Preventing Adverse Drug Events to Decrease Hospital Costs*. Retrieved 8/17/2011, from www.ahrq.gov/qual/aderia/aderia.htm# MedicationErrors

Gianutsos, G. (2008, December 1). *Identifying Factors That Cause Pharmacy Errors*. Retrieved 8/15/2011, from www.uspharmacist.com/continuing_education/ceviewtest/lessonid/105916/

Institute for Safe Medication Practices. (2011). *ISMP Medication Safety Alert! Newsletters*. Retrieved 8/16/2011, from http://ismp.org/newsletters/default.asp.

Massachusetts Office of Health and Human Services. (2011). *Reasons for Prescription Errors: Medication Error Study Results*. Retrieved 8/15/2011, from www.mass.gov/?pageID=eohhs2terminal&L=8&L0=Home&L1= Provider&L2=Certification%2c+Licensure%2c+and+Registration&L3=Occupational+and+Professional&L 4=Pharmacy&L5=Medication+Error+Prevention&L6=Medication+Error+Study&L7=Results+of+the+ Medication+Error+S

National Coordinating Council for Medication Error Reporting and Prevention (NCCMERP). (2011). *About Medication Errors*. Retrieved 8/17/2011, from www.nccmerp.org/aboutMedErrors.html

Pharmacy Times. (2006, August 1). *Study Looks into Rx Drug Errors* Retrieved 8/17/2011, from www. pharmacytimes.com/publications/issue/2006/2006-08/2006-08-5742/

USA Today. (2009). *A Prescription's Path through a Pharmacy*. Retrieved 8/16/2011, from www.usatoday.com/ money/graphics/rx_error/flash.htm

17 The Structure and Organization of Institutional Pharmacy Practice

LEARNING
OBJECTIVES

By the end of this chapter, students will be able to competently:

1. Explain the organizational structure, functions, responsibilities, and operation of hospitals and health systems, central pharmacies, and decentralized (satellite) pharmacies.
2. Define various types of organizations classified as institutional pharmacies.
3. Briefly describe regulatory standards for hospital and health system practice, including The Joint Commission (TJC) Accreditation and Medication Management Standards and TJC's National Patient Safety Goals.
4. List the roles and responsibilities of pharmacy technicians in various types of institutional pharmacies.
5. Identify key components of the medication order.
6. Explain how medication orders are processed in an institutional pharmacy.

KEY TERMS

Decentralized service: Any pharmacy service located outside the central pharmacy service area; also referred to as a "satellite."

Health system: An incorporated group of hospitals comprising a complex of facilities, organizations, and skilled personnel who provide healthcare within a geographic area.

Medication reconciliation (Med Rec): Creating a written or electronic list of any medications the patient currently is taking, including prescription medications, over-the-counter (OTC) medications, and herbal and nutritional supplements.

Triage: The process of prioritizing the order in which patient care is administered based on the severity of patients' injuries or disease.

This third unit of the text discusses one of the most challenging and interactive environments for pharmacy technicians: hospital and health system pharmacy practice. In the first two units, you learned about the pharmacy profession in general, in addition to the organizational structure and workflow processes of community pharmacies. Community pharmacies focus on dispensing medication and patient counseling as their chief tasks. Information collected from the patient during the dispensing process enables the pharmacist to provide continuing medication management, particularly for patients who seek such consultation.

In contrast, the institutional pharmacy focuses primarily on the scheduled distribution of pharmaceutical products and clinical services. Hospital patients generally have more serious illness and conditions. In the hospital, nurses, physicians, and other healthcare practitioners continually review, assess, and apply clinical data to determine the appropriate medications for a patient. In the community pharmacy, the patient is the staff's primary "customer"; however, in the institutional pharmacy, other members of the healthcare team, primarily nurses and physicians, are the primary customers.

The communication and workplace skills required of pharmacy technicians in an institutional pharmacy are notably more complex than those required for a community pharmacy. Individuals who provide pharmaceutical products in an institutional pharmacy not only serve patients, but also strongly affect the capability of *other* members of the healthcare team to serve patients. Although pharmacists may interact with patients along with other healthcare providers, pharmacy technicians' interaction with patients is comparatively limited in this environment, although that may vary, depending on the size of the organization.

Hospital pharmacy practice falls under the umbrella of institutional practice, which generally includes the following settings:

- Hospitals and health systems
- Nursing homes
- Hospice facilities

Unlike hospitals, nursing homes and hospice facilities typically do not have on-site pharmacies; they must rely on an institutional pharmacy to provide medication therapy management.

This chapter gives you, as a student, the opportunity to gain additional perspective on the type of pharmacy practice that would best suit you and your lifestyle, career goals, and workplace strengths. Each hospital and healthcare system has a unique culture. Based on the types of patients served, hospitals have varied clinical focuses, specialties, mission statements, and organizational ideals. Recall Chapter 3, in which you were challenged to identify and affirm your own ideals; in doing so, you may recognize how those ideals will guide the way you provide patient care. While exploring the institutional pharmacy career path, you may want to research area hospitals and health systems to learn their ideals and then evaluate how those ideals align with your own. Aligning yourself with an organization with similar ideals or with ideals into which you might want to grow may be an excellent career move.

Because of the scope of the workflow processes that are typically performed in institutional pharmacies, the topic has been divided into two chapters. This chapter focuses on the following foundational principles of institutional practice:

- Organizational structure
- The various roles and responsibilities of pharmacy technicians
- The types of information that must be reviewed and verified on the physician/medication order

Chapter 18 builds on those topics and approaches the specific workflow processes performed in various institutional settings as they relate to the distribution of pharmaceutical products and services.

To develop a broad perspective on how pharmacy practice affects healthcare in the institutional practice setting, you must first understand the organizational structure of the hospital and health system.

The Hospital and Health System Settings

A hospital may be considered an establishment that offers services to help maintain the health and vitality of a local community or demographic region. A health system is an incorporated group of hospitals comprising a complex of facilities, organizations, and skilled personnel who provide healthcare within a geographic area. The health system allows for an individual hospital to benefit from operating within the system rather than on its own. The services provided by a hospital and/or health system allow citizens to maintain health, address chronic disease, and use life-saving emergency, trauma, and critical care services. Depending on the location, such as a rural area, the services a hospital provides may be critical for a community. In addition, a regional hospital creates jobs for the citizens in that area. In many ways a hospital is an organic entity, much like a tree, in that it extends many branches of healthcare services to a community, and draws from community resources, in part, to sustain itself.

The World Health Organization (WHO) described the primary components of a well-functioning health system, which is committed to performing the following key community services (World Health Organization, 2010):

- Improving the health status of individuals, families, and communities
- Defending the population against whatever threatens its health

- Protecting people against the financial consequences of ill health
- Providing equitable access to people-centered care
- Making it possible for people to participate in decisions affecting their health and health system

The hospital organization involves a variety of services that support patient care, employees, and the physical hospital environment. Together these services establish a *continuum of care. Continuity of care* is the tracking of patients through their clinical experience at a hospital; it includes every service used in the patient's care (e.g., administrative functions, such as admissions and billing).

The organizational structure of a hospital outlines the management and leadership for each of the service areas. The size and range of a hospital's clinical services influence the complexity of its organizational structure. For the purposes of this chapter, visualize the organizational structure of a hospital as taking the form of a pyramid (Figure 17-1). Keep in mind that the hierarchy of each service may vary based on the organization.

In general, the members of the hospital's healthcare team may be classified into one of three primary functional groups:

- Governing body
- Medical staff
- Hospital staff

The governing body generally consists of the Board of Directors or Trustees and the hospital administrators. The medical staff generally consists of professional clinicians who have been granted the appropriate prescribing or clinical practice authority at that facility, such as:

- Physicians
- Psychologists
- Podiatrists
- Dentists
- Clinical pharmacists

Members of the medical staff may serve on committees that provide direction for the clinical services provided by a hospital or health system. Such committees may include:

- Review of pharmacy and therapeutics (P&T)
- Credentialing

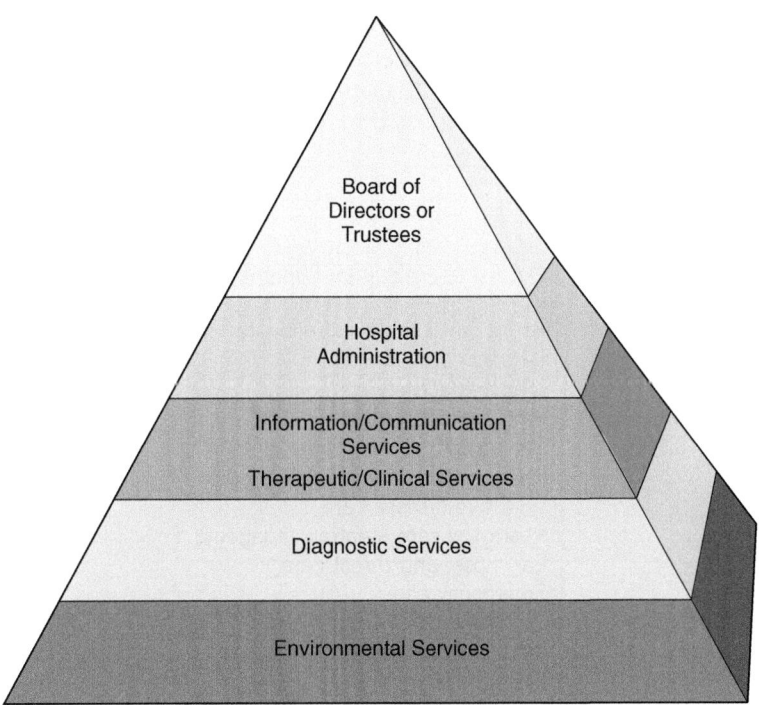

FIGURE 17-1 General hospital organizational structure.

- Quality assurance
- Drug and clinical service utilization review

BOARD OF DIRECTORS OR TRUSTEES

Members of the Board of Directors or Board of Trustees generally are unpaid volunteers who collaborate to make strategic recommendations for a hospital or health system based on local and regional community needs. The board represents the needs of the local and regional community leaders and the interests of groups that provide financial support to the hospital, particularly not-for-profit groups.

HOSPITAL ADMINISTRATORS

Hospital administrators are the principal leaders and generally the primary decision makers. They follow the recommendations of the Board of Directors and determine how each of the services may best promote the hospital's mission, values, strategic planning priorities, and goals. Administrators are responsible for the following:

- Hospital budgeting and finance
- Establishment of the hospital's standard operating policies and procedures
- Marketing and public relations

CLINICAL SERVICES

A hospital provides a variety of clinical services that are based on the healthcare needs of the people in its demographic area (Box 17-1).

The medical staff generally provides leadership in each of the primary clinical areas. Services such as pharmacy, pathology, and radiology generally are considered support services. Support services provide data that the medical staff uses to make decisions on a patient's care. Other types of professional clinical support services include:

- Physical or occupational therapy (or both)
- Medication therapy reconciliation
- Pastoral care
- Guest services (including interpreters for patients and families who speak languages other than English)
- Dietary and nutrition services

DIAGNOSTIC SERVICES

Diagnostic services assist the medical staff members in the diagnosis of a patient's condition. The following are diagnostic services.

BOX 17-1   **Hospital Clinical Services**

Acute care (adult and neonatal)	General surgery
Cardiac care	Social work/social services
Diabetes and endocrinology	Men's health
Pain management	Speech and language pathology
Pediatrics	Metabolic disease care
Physical and occupational therapy	Spine care
Digestive disease care	Neuroscience
Pharmacy care (central, inpatient)	Tissue/organ transplantation services
Ear, nose, and throat care	Nutritional/dietary services
Emergency care	Urology
Psychiatric/behavioral care	Oncology/cancer care
Respiratory therapy	Orthopedics
General internal medicine	Wellness and fitness
Senior care	Women's health

- *Radiology* (imaging services). Many imaging machines are now mobile devices, so patients often do not need to leave their rooms. Magnetic resonance imaging (MRI) must still be performed in the imaging department.
- *Pathology* (clinical laboratory services). The clinical laboratory provides diagnostic services to establish the origin of disease, in addition to laboratory values that reflect the functionality of body systems. The medical staff members analyze the results of the clinical laboratory tests to help them make decisions on patient care.
- *Emergency department.* The emergency department (ED) staff plays a critical role in providing both diagnostic services and acute care for patients whose conditions vary in severity. A vital function of the emergency department is to prioritize the order in which patient care is administered, based on the severity of a patient's injury or disease; this process is known as triage. Triage ensures that patients whose conditions require immediate treatment receive care before those with less serious conditions. After diagnosis and initial basic treatment have been performed, the ED staff determines whether a patient may be discharged for follow-up outpatient care or requires a hospital stay.

    From a cost-containment standpoint, every effort should be made to ensure that the most appropriate clinical decisions are made in the emergency department. Failure to admit a patient may result in worsening of the person's condition and the need for further clinical services on either an outpatient or inpatient basis. Unwarranted admission results in the unnecessary provision of expensive services, which drives up healthcare costs for patients and healthcare organizations.

Medication Reconciliation

As part of the patient intake process in the emergency department, an ED staff member (e.g., nurse or medical assistant) interviews the patient and creates a written account of any medications he or she currently takes, including prescription medications, OTC medications, and herbal and nutritional supplements. This process is referred to as medication reconciliation. It is an extremely important part of establishing a patient's medical history. If a patient is admitted for inpatient treatment, prescribers and clinical pharmacists need to know about any conditions for which a patient has been previously treated and any medication the person takes or to which he or she may be allergic. Some in the pharmacy profession have suggested that medication reconciliation be performed by a hospital pharmacy technician. They point out that a pharmacy technician who previously worked in a community pharmacy already is familiar with the types of information collected to establish a patient's medical history.

Communication and Information Services

Information services is a nonclinical service that provides crucial support to patients, medical staff, and other members of the hospital team. It is responsible for:

- Admissions
- Billing and collection
- Medical records
- Information technology
- Education and training
- Human resources/employee services

The information collected by this department allows for tracking of patients and the clinical services they receive and facilitates billing and processing of medical benefits. Information services also provides support for the technologic devices used in various areas of a hospital. In fact, in the field of health information technology, new roles are emerging for managing the stream of clinical information that must be available to all members of the healthcare team. Support services specific to the management of hospital employees include education and training and human resources.

ENVIRONMENTAL SERVICES

Members of the environmental services staff provide maintenance for the hospital's physical environment. Their work includes infection control procedures, which are crucial. Note the following examples:

- Housekeeping and laundry staff members play a crucial role in preventing the spread of infectious agents that may be present on contaminated linens and on surfaces in treatment areas, examination rooms, and inpatient areas.
- Engineering services staff members maintain the general environmental controls, such as heating and cooling, ventilation, and air filtration.
- Biomedical engineering services staff members provide technical support by monitoring, repairing, and performing preventive maintenance on medical equipment and supplies.
- Central supply staff members provide support services ranging from sterilizing surgical instruments to assembling medical supplies and distributing them to various areas of the hospital.

Environmental services functions may be provided by hospital staff or may be outsourced to contracted employees.

Continuity of Care

In healthcare, quality care generally is measured by patient treatment outcomes that are also cost-effective. In hospitals and health systems, many individuals collectively contribute to that outcome, because caregivers draw from the expertise of other members of the healthcare team. Continuity of patient care has been defined as "care over time by a single individual or team of health care professionals and the effective and timely communication of health information" (Cabana and Jee, 2004). To be highly effective, continuity of care in a hospital must involve both medical and hospital staff members. Members of the medical staff (e.g., prescribers and pharmacists), along with diagnostic teams (e.g., radiology and laboratory services), establish a clinical pathway to:

- Determine the cause or causes of a patient's medical condition based on the medical history and diagnostic data collected (e.g., laboratory tests and imaging results)
- Determine treatment options, including medical and pharmaceutical care
- Complete a regimen of medical and pharmaceutical treatment on an inpatient basis as necessary
- Stabilize the patient's health condition to the extent that the person may be discharged
- Perform discharge planning, including a course of treatment to be followed on an outpatient basis

A variety of administrative functions performed by hospital staff ensure that the stream of health information is made available to all healthcare team members. The processing of patients through various areas of the hospital and documentation of the treatment received must be accurate in both medical records and billing/accounting records.

The Institutional Pharmacy Practice Setting

By now you should have an idea of the structure and functions of the different branches of the hospital. Now, let's turn our attention specifically to the hospital pharmacy. The types of pharmacy support services provided in a hospital may include:

- Central pharmacy services
- Decentralized pharmacy services
- Outpatient pharmacy services (may be part of the hospital or may be privately owned and operated)

CENTRAL PHARMACY

The central pharmacy is the main source of pharmaceutical products, services, and clinical support for the hospital; this support is available 24 hours a day, 7 days a week, 365 days a year. Clinical pharmacists review all written or electronically generated medication orders and verify the clinical appropriateness of all medications prescribed, taking into account patient-specific information. Medication orders may be entered manually or electronically or transmitted by fax. Once an order has been formally verified (approved), the medication is made available for administration to the patient by a caregiver. The means by which a caregiver obtains medication depends on the type of medication and the type of preparation required. Recall that the primary outcome of pharmaceutical services in the institutional setting is distribution. In the central pharmacy, staff members prepare verified doses of medication that will be administered by caregivers in patient care areas. Medication generally is distributed to the following areas:

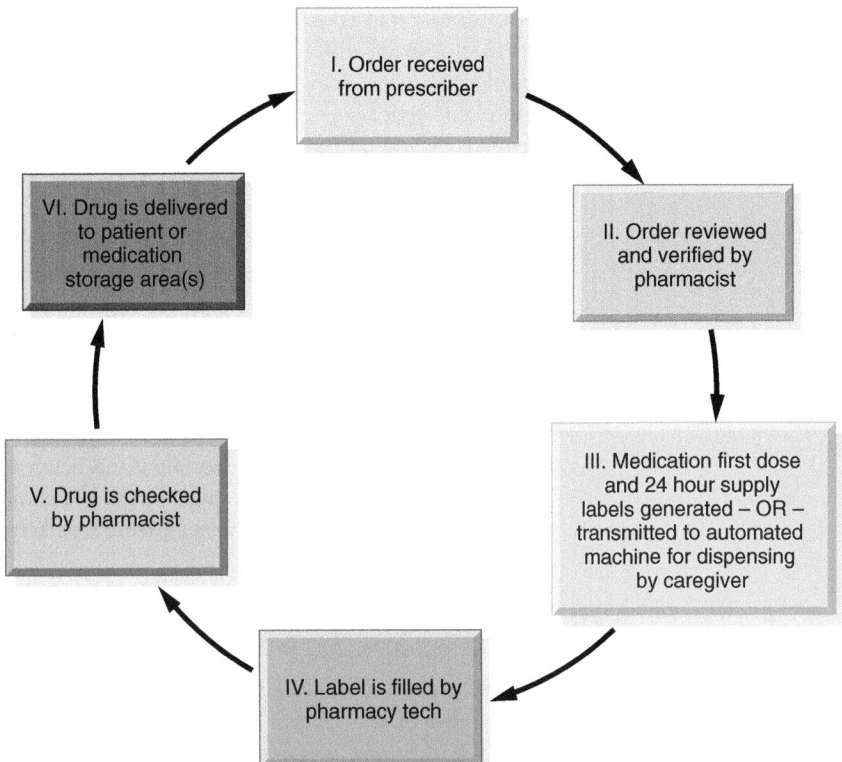

FIGURE 17-2 Basic order entry and fill workflow for processing a medication order.

- Patient's bedside
- Restricted-access medication storage room or area
- Automated dispensing machine or cabinet

The Joint Commission, a national organization that accredits hospital and health organizations, has established rules for preparing medications. For all medications that require preparation, such as reconstitution or the addition of multiple ingredients, the procedure must be performed by pharmacy staff members who have been appropriately trained in the proper aseptic technique. Because injectable solutions must remain sterile, they must be prepared *aseptically;* that is, using techniques that prevent contamination of sterile solutions with solid particulate matter or microbial disease-causing organisms.

BASIC WORKFLOW PROCESSES OF CENTRAL PHARMACY

Figure 17-2 shows the basic workflow started when an order is received from the prescriber. Once the pharmacist verifies the order, the dose or doses are either transmitted electronically to a patient profile on a computerized medication dispensing machine for removal and administration by a caregiver, or labels are generated and the medication is filled by a central pharmacy technician. Once the medication has been filled and packaged in its final dispensing container, a pharmacist must check the dose for accuracy. Once checked, the dose may be delivered to the patient care area or to the patient's bedside if the medication is needed urgently.

Decentralized Pharmacy Services

Any pharmacy service outside the central pharmacy service area is considered a decentralized service. Some patient care areas serve a specific patient population or patients that need a narrow range of products and services. These care areas require dedicated pharmacy services, which may be provided by a decentralized *satellite pharmacy.* A satellite pharmacy is a scaled-down version of the central pharmacy. Satellite pharmacies typically are equipped with technology, equipment, and supplies that enable them to provide point-of-care pharmaceutical products and consultative services to such clinical areas as the following:

- Intensive care unit (ICU)
- Pediatric/neonatal (PICU)
- Oncology
- Transplant services
- Preoperative and postoperative treatment areas
- Same-day surgery
- Emergency department

Satellite pharmacies generally are staffed with at least one pharmacist and a technician, although in some cases a pharmacy technician may perform tasks independently and set work aside to be checked and verified by a pharmacist or checking technician.

The workflow process of a satellite pharmacy is very similar to that of the central pharmacy; however, fewer doses are prepared, and the hours of operation are specified rather than round the clock. Often the pharmacist and pharmacy technician in a satellite pharmacy come to know the clinical staff working in their area, and they may seek opportunities to build relationships with staff members that result in more efficient workflow and better patient care. Pharmacists and pharmacy technicians may better serve their customers' needs in a clinical area by performing rounds to gather information about preparing medications patients are likely to require, particularly during periods the satellite pharmacy may be closed.

OUTPATIENT PHARMACY SERVICES

On discharge from the hospital, the patient may be given a treatment plan that includes taking short-term medications or continuing drug therapy as an outpatient. The size of the hospital determines the number of pharmacists and technicians that staff the outpatient pharmacy service. The structure and workflow processes of the outpatient pharmacy are very similar to those of a community pharmacy (Figure 17-3). Discharge medication orders are processed in the same way as outpatient prescriptions, with a few exceptions. For example, discharge planning includes an expectation that the patient will follow up with his or her primary caregiver; therefore, refills typically are not authorized on discharge prescriptions.

The Regulatory and Governing Bodies of Hospital and Health System Pharmacy Practice

Regulatory standards in pharmacy practice, as in any other strictly related industry, have been created for the protection of its stakeholders and to ensure the highest level of quality for the products and

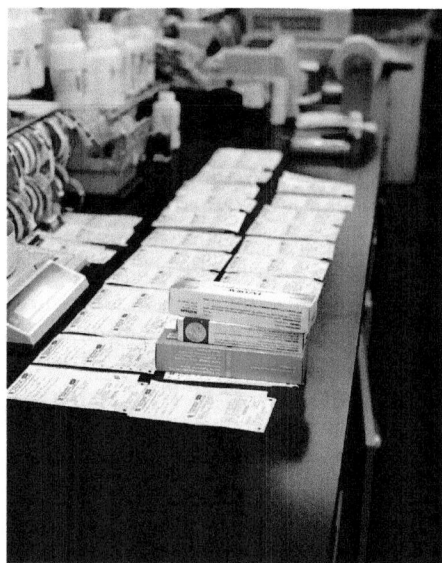

FIGURE 17-3 Station for filling outpatient medication orders. (From Hopper T: *Mosby's pharmacy technician: principles and practice,* ed 3, Philadelphia, 2011, Saunders.)

BOX 17-2   Benefits of Accreditation by The Joint Commission

- Helps organize and strengthen patient safety efforts
- Strengthens community confidence in the quality and safety of care, treatment, and services
- Provides a competitive edge in the marketplace
- Improves risk management and risk reduction
- May reduce liability insurance costs
- Provides education on good practices to improve business operations
- Provides professional advice and counsel, enhancing staff education
- Provides a customized, intensive review
- Enhances staff recruitment and development
- Provides deeming authority for Medicare certification
- Recognized by insurers and other third-party payers
- Provides a framework for organizational structure and management
- May fulfill regulatory requirements in some states

clinical services offered. Hospitals generally seek The Joint Commission accreditation, because this has a variety of benefits (Box 17-2). TJC sets forth standards of practice for many clinical services, including pharmacy. These standards, based on data contributed by expert members of the healthcare community, establish expectations for hospital performance. The standards pertain specifically to the way each organization creates an ideal environment for patient care, and measures of patient safety are included. Medication Management (MM) is the specific standard that addresses the responsibilities of a hospital's department of pharmacy. For example, standard MM.01.02.01, EP 1, which applies to look-alike/sound-alike drugs, states, "The hospital develops a list of look-alike/sound-alike medications it stores, dispenses, or administers" (The Joint Commission, 2011).

A TJC surveyor (inspector) may visit an accredited facility at any time to verify that a hospital's organizational structure and processes are consistent with the established standards. For pharmacy technicians, it is important to be aware of key compliance issues, such as:

- How frequently training is conducted.
- Instances in which a pharmacist needs to check their work.
- How often quality assurance processes (e.g., expiration date checks and cleaning) are conducted.
- How errors are handled, documented, and corrected.

TJC surveyors may make inquiries of any hospital staff member, so it is important that every staff member know the hospital's standard operating procedures and those that apply directly to pharmacy technician practice.

NATIONAL PATIENT SAFETY GOALS

The Joint Commission established National Patient Safety Goals (NPSGs) in 2002 to address areas of key concern in patient safety across healthcare systems. A panel of healthcare practitioners and other experts form an advisory group that consults with TJC about annual revision of the NPSGs. Based on issues relevant to current practice, NPSGs may be changed or revised, or new goals may be added. The NPSGs for 2011 concerned:

- Identifying patients correctly
- Improving staff communication
- Safe medication use
- Infection prevention
- Identifying patient safety risks
- Preventing mistakes in surgery

The measures for safe medication use included proper labeling of medication, exercising caution with patients taking anticoagulant medication, and proper procedure for medication reconciliation. Pharmacy technicians should stay current on the NPSGs and the way those measures should be observed by pharmacy personnel.

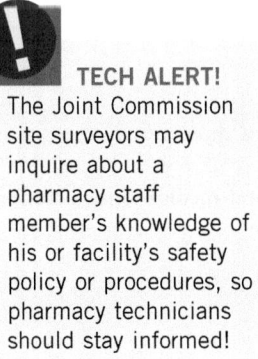

TECH ALERT!
The Joint Commission site surveyors may inquire about a pharmacy staff member's knowledge of his or facility's safety policy or procedures, so pharmacy technicians should stay informed!

TABLE 17-1   **Duties Pharmacy Technicians May or May Not Legally Perform**

May perform	Example	May not perform
• Dispensing, record keeping, pricing, performing administrative functions • Preparing doses or precompounded medications • Preparing doses of extemporaneously compounded, nonsterile medications • Transporting medication to and from floors or units • Replenishing floor stocks	• Receiving written prescriptions • Answering and directing phone calls • Preparing patient records • Keeping workspaces clean • Retrieving medication from supply shelves • Preparing labels • Counting and pouring medication • Reconstituting premade medication powders • Weighing and measuring bulk materials • Compounding • Selecting containers • Maintaining and filing compounding records • Aseptically mixing parenteral products • Selecting equipment for compounding procedures • Packaging products • Preparing drug carts or trays • Delivering controlled drugs • Retrieving, reconciling, and recording credit for unadministered medications • Returning unadministered medications to unit-dose bins and injectables to stock • Checking for expiration dates • Removing overstocks	• Taking verbal prescription orders over the phone (except in some states) • Delivering a product without the final check by a pharmacist • Modifying a compounding formula in any way without the expressed consent or direction of a pharmacist • Recommending a dosage adjustment based on the patient's weight or condition • Advising a patient to continue taking a medication after discharge • Speaking to a nurse about a patient's medical condition and suggesting which medications should be discontinued

Role and Duties of a Pharmacy Technician in an Institutional Pharmacy

A hospital pharmacy has several workstations at which a pharmacy technician may perform a variety of tasks. Legally, pharmacy technicians may perform some tasks but not others (Table 17-1). Individual state boards of pharmacy may allow or disallow certain tasks, so it is important for pharmacy technicians to know what legally falls within their scope of practice in their state.

In general, a pharmacy technician may work in any of the following central pharmacy work areas:
- USP <797>–compliant controlled clean room
- Supply and purchasing
- Compounding areas
- Telephone/order entry area
- Picking/restocking area
- Narcotic vault
- Central supply/floor stock
- Investigational drug service
- Accounting/purchasing
- IS support
- General medication delivery/other miscellaneous tasks

Let's examine the tasks a pharmacy technician may perform in each of those areas.
- USP <797>–compliant controlled clean room
    - Mix intravenous (IV) sterile enteral and parenteral solutions and medications, including chemotherapy and cytotoxic/hazardous drugs
    - Restock drugs, equipment, and supplies
    - Label premixed solutions
    - Clean and disinfect prescribed areas
    - Deliver medication, as needed

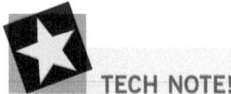

TECH NOTE!
The *continuum of care* includes any hospital service that influences the care a patient receives during an outpatient or inpatient stay. *Effective continuity of care* ensures that patients have a quality experience throughout the various hospital services provided. The continuum of care symbol indicates that a service is on the continuum of care.

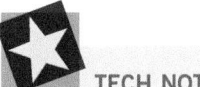

- Supply and purchasing
  - Inventory pharmacy stock
  - Process drug returns
  - Order and requisition inventory items
  - Receive and restock shipped inventory items
  - Process loan/borrow requests
- Compounding areas
  - Complete batch logs and use approved compounding formulations
  - Perform extemporaneous and bulk compounding
  - Label final product
- Telephone/order entry area
  - Place outbound phone calls to nursing floors and decentralized pharmacy areas as directed
  - Appropriately route inbound phone calls to various areas of the pharmacy, including triaging calls about order verification and clinical consultation that must be forwarded to pharmacists
  - Process medications returned from nursing floors to credit patient accounts
  - Process order sets to charge to patient accounts
- Picking/restocking area (manual or using automation/robotics)
  - Package solid and liquid dose medication in unit-dose packaging
  - Select patient-specific unit doses for first, STAT, and refill doses to be delivered to nursing areas
  - Complete restocking, including new inventory and credit returns
- Narcotic vault
  - Process patient-specific doses of narcotics and controlled medication
  - Process returns of narcotics and controlled medications
  - Inventory and reconcile all products dispensed, including completed drug administration records returned from nursing floors
- Central supply/floor stock
  - Process bulk orders from nursing floors for IV solutions and tubing
  - Deliver bulk orders to decentralized storage areas and/or automated medication dispensing machines
- Investigational drug service
  - Help with regular training on new drug study protocols
  - Help with training hospital staff in new drug study protocols
  - Prepare oral, topical, and parenteral study drugs per protocols established by study sponsor organizations
  - Manage inventory of investigational drugs
  - Label products
- Information Systems support
  - Provide support to pharmacy IS team for hardware and software
  - Investigate issues and troubleshoot
- Accounting and purchasing
  - Perform accounting functions related to patient billing and procurement of nondrug supplies (e.g., office supplies and forms)
  - Process staff travel reimbursements
  - Maintain vendor relationships
- General medication delivery and other miscellaneous tasks
  - Hand-deliver medication to various areas of the hospital
  - Refill automated medication dispensing machines in nursing areas, if applicable
  - Deliver medication via pneumatic tube system (Figure 17-4)
  - Perform monthly inspection of nursing unit drug stocks for expired and damaged drugs
  - Log medication refrigerator temperatures daily
  - Perform monthly inspection of drugs in all central pharmacy drug storage areas for expired or damaged drugs
  - Report and gather drugs in the event of a drug recall

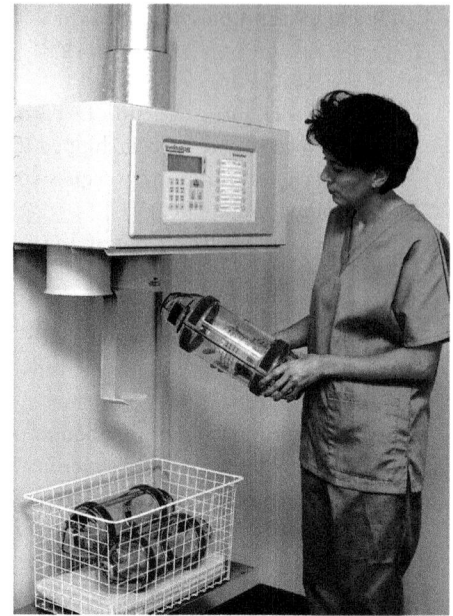

FIGURE 17-4 Pneumatic tube system. A pneumatic tube system is used to transport orders to the pharmacy and medications to hospital floors. (From Hopper T: *Mosby's pharmacy technician: principles and practice,* ed 3, Philadelphia, 2011, Saunders.)

DECENTRALIZED (SATELLITE) PHARMACY AREAS

Similar to central pharmacy operations, a pharmacy technician may perform any of the following tasks in the satellite pharmacy:

- IV admixture
- Perform rounding to verify that a daily 24-hour supply is maintained in nursing areas
- Calculate drip rates as necessary
- Prepackage specialty surgical procedure kits, such as for anesthesia, organ transplantation, or cardiac procedures
- Count narcotics
- Deliver medications
- Restock satellite pharmacy areas
- Perform monthly inventory and unit inspection of all medication stored in satellite area
- Perform medication order entry and label processing, as prescribed by satellite staff pharmacists

Processing Medication Orders

In the central pharmacy, orders most often are transmitted electronically or by fax. The physician order contains a variety of clinical information, including medication orders. Although most physician orders are filed directly into the patient's record, copies of the medication orders are forwarded to the pharmacy for verification, processing, and filling. Pharmacists generally perform order entry in hospital pharmacies; however, some hospitals allow pharmacy technicians to perform this task. A key step in medication order entry is identifying items on the physician order that apply to pharmacy order entry. Pharmacists and technicians must be able to determine which items on the physician order must be entered. The same types of medical and sig code abbreviations seen in a community pharmacy may be noted on a physician order, and these must be interpreted accurately for transcription.

Medication may be distributed only on the written order of a:

- Licensed physician
- Physician assistant
- Nurse practitioner
- Pharmacists per verbal order (must be countersigned by a physician within 48 hours)

TECH NOTE!
Calculation of drip rates allows a satellite pharmacy technician to better plan workflow processes. For example, suppose a liter of an IV drip is running at 75 ml/hour. Based on that rate, the patient will need a bag every 13 hours. Two bags would be needed to provide a 24-hour supply.

TECH NOTE!
Pharmacy rounding allows a pharmacy technician to obtain information about a medication fill that an order may not provide. For example, if a patient is due for discharge or an order is expected to change, a satellite technician may learn that information from the nursing staff before an order is written; this additional information may prevent the preparation of unnecessary doses.

In addition, the prescriber must be certified by the institution as having order writing privileges in that facility.

Just as with an outpatient prescription, key pieces of patient and drug information must be provided on the physician order:

- Patient information
  - Name
  - Room number
  - Hospital number (if applicable)
  - Age, weight, height, allergies, and gender (may be included)
- Drug information
  - Name
  - Strength
  - Dosage written in metric measurements
  - IV solutions orders
    - Name and strength of each additive
    - Name and volume of base solution
    - Flow rate or frequency
    - Routes of administration
    - Frequency of administration

COMPUTERIZED MEDICATION MANAGEMENT SYSTEMS

Most hospitals use a medication management system that allows pharmacists to consult a volume of clinical information; this enables them to make informed decisions on the therapeutic appropriateness of medication orders. Various medication management systems offer features that provide pharmacists with vital information, such as:

- Automatic dosage calculation
- Standardized order sets that have been established by the P&T committee of that institution
- Alerts related to the formulary status of drugs ordered
- Allergy screening
- Multiple therapeutic class screening
- Drug-drug interaction screening
- Laboratory values and other useful diagnostic data
- Nursing procedures, which may help determine when medication needs to be prepared and/or delivered
- Full medication administration history (Figure 17-5)
  - All orders, even those that were discontinued, are noted in a patient's profile to provide a complete medication use history
  - Medication reconciliation list compiled when the patient was admitted

MEDICATION ORDER PROCESSING AND DISTRIBUTION

Once medication orders have been entered and verified by a pharmacist, a few fill or distribution options may be carried out by a pharmacy technician.

- If the order is for *bulk* solutions that a caregiver may self-dispense using an automated dispensing cabinet, the order may be activated electronically and made available for dispensing from the automated cabinet in the patient care area.
- If the order is for a *new* medication that will be administered at a regular interval and the dose must come from the pharmacy initially, a label is generated in the central pharmacy. A pharmacist fills and labels the container and checks the product. The dose then may be delivered to the floor. The average expected turnaround in most hospitals is 2 hours from the time the order is received.
- If the order is for a *STAT* medication, the drug must be administered within 30 minutes or less from the time the order was written. Once the label has been generated, the dose should be filled by a pharmacy technician, checked by a pharmacist, and delivered immediately to the patient's bedside or to the medication storage area.

Patient ID stamp John Douglas 523469 Room 569-A	MEDICATION ADMINISTRATION RECORD GENERAL HOSPITAL	ALLERGIES: **NKDA**

DATE START STOP	MEDICATION DOSAGE, ROUTE ADMINISTRATION TIME	First Shift 07:00 to 14:59	Second Shift 15:00 to 22:59	Third Shift 23:00 to 06:59
	Ord. 08-01-11 5% Lactated Ringer's Sol. 1000 mL IV TKO at 20 mL/hour continuous			
	Ord. 08-01-11 losartan (Cozaar) tablet 50 mg once daily AM and HS Hold for systolic BP less than 130. Call MD.			
	Ord. 08-01-11 Insulin glargine (Lantus) 20 units subcut. daily at 8 AM Give on time. Record on insulin MAR. Do not mix with other insulins or medications.			
	Ord. 08-02-11 norfloxacin (Noroxin) 400 mg q12h × 3 days STOP 8-05-11 after 6 doses Take with glass water 1 hr before or 2 hr after meals		·	

This type of a 24-hour printed MAR for routine scheduled medications can be computer or pharmacy generated. It mentions some administration priorities and includes both the generic and the trade name to reduce chance of error. Separate MARs may be used for one-time-only and prn orders (refer to p 138) and certain drugs such as heparin and insulin, which require coagulation or blood glucose assessment prior to administration.

SIGNATURES (FIRST & LAST NAME)	INITIALS	SIGNATURES (FIRST & LAST NAME)	INITIALS	SITE CODES	MEDICATIONS NOT GIVEN
				LU - L Gluteus RU - R Gluteus LT - L Thigh RT - R Thigh LA - L Abdomen RA - R Abdomen LV - L Ventrogluteal RV - R Ventrogluteal LM - L Arm RM - R Arm LD - L Deltoid RD - R Deltoid	NPO - NPO RF - Refused WH - Withheld

FIGURE 17-5 Example of a computer-generated medication administration record for as needed (PRN) medications. (*Example of an unclear order that must be clarified with the prescriber or pharmacy or both.) (From Mulholland J: *The nurse, the math, the meds: drug calculations using dimensional analysis,* ed 2, St Louis, 2011, Mosby.)

Checking the Five Rights of Medication Administration

Pharmacists are required to check the work of pharmacy technicians, because technicians work under the licenses of the pharmacists to whom they are responsible. Therefore, every dose of medication prepared by a pharmacy technician must be verified by a pharmacist for accuracy and correctness. A dose of medication must *never* be dispensed or distributed for administration to a patient without a pharmacist's check. Pharmacists must verify:

- Generated pharmacy labels for accuracy
- Orders entered for correctness and therapeutic appropriateness
- Unit-dose cassettes, drawers, or envelopes, checking them against a printed medication profile fill list to verify that all drugs dispensed are active, correct, and properly labeled

Tech-Check-Tech

A new opportunity for advancement in hospital pharmacy practice is the position of checking technician. When a new standing order is written for a patient, the order is entered in the patient's profile. If the order is not changed, it is printed along with other medication orders scheduled to be filled for a 24-hour supply delivered to medication storage areas once or twice daily (the medication distribution process is discussed in detail in Chapter 18). Such orders that have been previously verified for clinical appropriateness may be filled by a technician, whose work may be verified by a checking technician. Only a few U.S. pharmacies currently have a Tech-Check-Tech program. Individuals who want to be considered for the job of checking technician must undergo extensive training that includes subjects such as:

- Medication therapy management
- Pharmacology
- Techniques for preventing medication errors
- Pharmaceutical mathematics

When they have completed their training, these technicians typically must demonstrate their skill in checking filled medication doses (usually more than 500 doses) by achieving an accuracy rate of 99.7% or better. A checking technician is evaluated for skill and accuracy biannually or annually. The use of checking technicians helps to enhance the role of the hospital pharmacy in patient care, because it allows pharmacists to spend more time providing consultation services to the healthcare teams in patient care areas. The use of pharmacy technicians in these challenging roles that do not require clinical decision making is good for the profession, because it improves pharmacists' ability to serve patients and creates an excellent opportunity for career advancement for technicians.

Chapter Summary

- Institutional pharmacy practice includes the following settings: hospitals and health systems, nursing homes, and hospice facilities.
- Hospitals establish a continuum of care, in which a variety of services support patient care, employees, and the physical hospital environment.
- The three primary groups in a hospital are the governing body, the medical staff, and the hospital staff.
- The governing body includes the Board of Directors or Trustees and the hospital administrators.
- Diagnostic services include radiology and pathology.
- Medication reconciliation is an important part of the emergency department intake process; some suggest that this task be performed by a pharmacy technician.
- Pharmacy support services provided in a hospital may include central pharmacy services, decentralized pharmacy services, and outpatient pharmacy services.
- The central pharmacy is the main source of pharmaceutical products, services, and clinical support for the hospital; it operates 24 hours a day, 7 days a week, 365 days a year.
- In the central pharmacy, technicians review all medication orders and verify the clinical appropriateness of all prescribed medication.
- Injectable solutions must be prepared aseptically, using techniques that prevent contamination of sterile solutions with solid particulate matter or microbial disease-causing organisms.
- Decentralized pharmacy (satellite) services are provided outside the central pharmacy and meet the needs of patient care areas that require dedicated pharmacy services because they have a specific patient population or one that requires a narrow range of products.
- Outpatient pharmacy services dispense medication for self-administration or use on an outpatient basis.
- The Joint Commission established National Patient Safety Goals (NPSGs) to address key areas of concern regarding patient safety in health systems. The measures for safe medication use include proper labeling of medications, exercising caution with patients taking anticoagulant medications, and using proper procedure for medication reconciliation.
- The pharmacy technician may work in the following areas:
  - USP <797>–compliant controlled clean room
  - Supply and purchasing
  - Compounding areas
  - Telephone/order entry area

- Picking/restocking area
- Narcotic vault
- Central supply/floor stock
- Investigational drug service
- Accounting/purchasing
- IS support
- General medication delivery/other miscellaneous tasks
- Some hospitals allow pharmacy technicians to perform order entry. A key task in medication order entry is to identify items on the physician's order that apply to pharmacy order entry.
- Medication management systems give pharmacists access to clinical information that enables them to make informed decisions on the therapeutic appropriateness of medication orders.
- A pharmacy technician may have several fill or distribution options, depending on whether the order is for a bulk, new, or STAT medication.

REVIEW QUESTIONS

Multiple Choice

1. These members of a healthcare organization represent the interests of a hospital's local community:
   a. Medical staff
   b. Hospital staff
   c. Hospital administrators
   d. Board of directors

2. These members of a healthcare organization generally are the lead decision makers on how the organization may achieve its clinical mission:
   a. Medical staff
   b. Hospital staff
   c. Hospital administrators
   d. Board of directors

3. Pastoral care is provided by a hospital's:
   a. Support staff
   b. Medical staff
   c. Engineering services
   d. Central supply

4. A pharmacy technician may legally perform all of the following tasks *except:*
   a. Modify a compounding formula
   b. Replenish floor stock
   c. Prepare medication labels
   d. Deliver controlled medications

5. A pharmacist may generate a medication order as long as it is countersigned by a physician within ____ hour(s)?
   a. 1
   b. 8
   c. 24
   d. 48

6. The institutional practice setting may include which of the following?
   a. Hospital
   b. Nursing home
   c. Hospice
   d. All of the above

7. A patient's continuum of care at a hospital includes:
   a. The medical treatment history with that hospital
   b. The medication use history at that hospital
   c. Tracking of the patient's entire clinical experience at that hospital
   d. Tracking of a patient's daily self-maintenance of his or her health condition

8. At a hospital, who must be granted prescribing or clinical practice authority at that facility to see patients?
   a. Clinical pharmacists
   b. Psychiatrists
   c. Physicians
   d. All of the above

9. This group at a hospital or in a health system represents the interests of the surrounding community:
   a. Physicians
   b. Board of trustees
   c. Facility administrators
   d. Hospital staff members

10. This part of a hospital's governing body determines how best the services provided by a hospital will serve the needs of the surrounding community.
    a. Board of directors
    b. Facility administrators
    c. Medical staff
    d. Hospital staff members

TECHNICIAN'S CORNER

1. Explain how rounding is useful to pharmacy technicians in terms of workflow and fill processes.
2. What types of information must be included on an order for an IV solution?
3. Explain how a health system affects its surrounding community.

Bibliography

Baylor Healthcare System. (2011). *Specialties and Services*. Retrieved 8/19/2011, from www.baylorhealth.com/SpecialtiesServices/Pages/Default.aspx

BusinessDictionary.com. (2011). *Healthcare System*. Retrieved 8/18/2011, from www.businessdictionary.com/definition/health-care-system.html

Cabana, M., Jee, S. (2004, December). *Does Continuity of Care Improve Patient Outcomes?* Retrieved 8/24/2011, from www.jfponline.com/pages.asp?aid=1830

Cedars-Sinai Medical Center. (2007, January 4). *Tech-Check-Tech: New California Regulation Will Help Prevent Medication Errors, Free Pharmacists for More Direct Patient Care*. Retrieved 8/28/2011, from www.cedars-sinai.edu/About-Us/News/News-Releases-2007/Tech-Check-Tech-New-California-Regulation-Will-Help-Prevent-Medication-Errors-Free-Pharmacists-For-More-Direct-Patient-Care.aspx

Community Hospital Corporation (CHC). (2009). *Organizational Structure*. Retrieved 8/19/2011, from www.communityhospitalcorp.com/content/default/?id=17

Memorial Medical Center. (2011). *Board of Directors*. Retrieved 8/19/2011, from www.mmcwm.com/board.

The Joint Commission. (2011). *Facts about the National Patient Safety Goals*. Retrieved 8/23/2011, from www.jointcommission.org/facts_about_the_national_patient_safety_goals/

The Joint Commission. (2011, January). *Facts about Hospital Accreditation*. Retrieved 8/26/2011, from www.jointcommission.org/assets/1/18/HospitalAccreditation_1_31_11.pdf

The Joint Commission. (2011, June 10). *2011 Hospital National Patient Safety Goals*. Retrieved 8/28/2011, from www.jointcommission.org/assets/1/6/HAP_NPSG_6-10-11.pdf

World Health Organization. (2007). *Everybody's Business: Strengthening Health Systems to Improve Health Outcomes*. Retrieved 8/19/2011, from www.who.int/healthsystems/strategy/everybodys_business.pdf

World Health Organization. (2010, May). *Key Components of a Well Functioning Health System*. Retrieved 8/18/2011, from www.who.int/healthsystems/EN_HSSkeycomponents.pdf

18

Institutional Pharmacy Practice II: Drug Distribution Systems

LEARNING OBJECTIVES

By the end of this chapter, students will be able to competently:

1. Explain how drug distribution drives workflow processes in a hospital pharmacy.
2. Describe the pharmacy technician's role in the use and management of various types of automated drug dispensing systems.
3. Outline the unit-dose batch process.
4. Describe the technician's role in the medication cart fill process.

KEY TERMS

Automation: The use of computer-based systems, as part of a workflow process, to perform functions that otherwise would be performed manually.

Drug distribution system: The process by which drugs are distributed to various storage areas; also, a machine or an automated system used to distribute drugs in both the pharmacy and patient care areas.

Prepackage: The process in which drugs in bulk containers are placed in unit-dose packaging, either manually or by automation.

Repackage: The process in which drugs retained in the manufacturer's packaging are enclosed in overwrap packaging for inventory management and to establish per-unit dosing.

Unit dose: An individual single-use package of drug product.

Unit-dose cart fill: A process in which patient-specific doses are prepared in individual packaging and distributed to patient-specific storage areas.

Chapter 17 presented an overview of the duties of pharmacy technicians in hospital pharmacies. Remember, the outcome of community pharmacy workflow is drug *dispensing;* the outcome of hospital pharmacy workflow is drug *distribution*. A variety of factors determine the types of technology a pharmacy uses to distribute medication doses to patient care areas, including:

- The size of the hospital (i.e., number of beds)
- The scope of clinical services provided
- The average patient load

A small hospital may be able to manage the distribution of drugs with a small staff and more manual processing. For example, the pharmacist may electronically verify doses in the medication management system and generate labels. The pharmacy technician fills those orders, has them checked by the pharmacist, and hand-delivers them to the patient care areas. In a medium to large hospital, however, thousands of doses may have to be prepared and distributed over a 24-hour period. The process in which patient-specific doses are prepared in individual packaging and distributed to patient-specific storage areas is called a unit-dose cart fill, or cart fill for short. Pharmacies use automation to increase the efficiency of time-consuming cart fill processes so that patients' doses are delivered before the scheduled administration times. Pharmacy technicians contribute to the hospital's continuity of care by delivering 24-hour cart fills in a timely manner.

Automation can be defined as the use of computer-based systems, as part of a workflow process, to perform functions that otherwise would be performed manually. Automated pharmacy systems can perform tasks such as drug packaging, intravenous (IV) admixture, product selection, and inventory management. For *continuity of care,* automation plays a critical role in patient-specific dose dispensing, because doses are more readily available for administration by a patient caregiver. Automation has improved three key areas of pharmacy practice:

- Patient safety
- Inventory control
- Workflow efficiency

Individual patient profiling improves accountability for each scheduled dose and reduces the number of doses dispensed incorrectly. Remote inventory management is better accomplished when distributed inventory can be tracked from a central location. Workflow is more efficient, because more doses may be dispensed at once, eliminating the need for multiple fills and deliveries. Staff members who otherwise would have to make drug deliveries can be assigned to other pharmacy functions.

A number of automated processes are used to distribute drugs to various hospital areas. Drug distribution system may refer to (1) a process in which drugs are distributed to various storage areas or (2) a machine or an automated system used to distribute drugs within the pharmacy and to patient care areas.

This chapter discusses the common applications of automation in hospital pharmacies, including:

- Medication packaging and repackaging
- Medication preparation
- Patient-specific dosage dispensing
- Medication delivery
- Medication order entry
- Inventory management
- Working with other healthcare services

Preparing for Distribution: Unit-Dose Medication Packaging and Repackaging

Each state's Board of Pharmacy establishes standards of practice for the use of technology in pharmacy processes; always, patient safety is expected to be the primary goal, not simple convenience or efficiency. One safeguard of patient safety is making sure the pharmacist checks every prescribed dose of medication before it is administered; this ensures the drug's clinical appropriateness, given patient-specific factors. Once the pharmacist check has been performed, the verified doses can be distributed to patient care areas.

Unlike the customers of community pharmacies, hospital patients are administered medication one dose at a time. Because prescribers' orders may change frequently, patients typically are dispensed no more than a 24-hour supply at one time. Although pharmacies order medications in bulk quantities, the drug must be prepackaged into individual doses before distribution to patient care areas. Solid dosage forms may be packaged into small blister containers; semisolid and liquid dosage forms may be packaged in unit dose cups or oral syringes. Prepackaging may be performed manually or an automated fill process.

Unit-dose packaging must contain all necessary medication information so that the pharmacist can verify each dose for accuracy. The packaging also may include a bar code that can be scanned during the stocking and filling processes.

Medication provided in the manufacturer's packaging (e.g., a syringe or a blister pack) may have to be repackaged in an overwrap plastic container that allows for bar code scanning and that also can be more easily picked out of an automated or robotic drug storage and distribution system. This type of automation is based on a computer database that contains product information and allows reporting of the unit-dose cart fill, usage history, and other administrative information.

Some vendors of automated systems may provide support services, such as staff members who specifically perform unit-dose prepackaging and repackaging. However, unit-dose packaging generally is done by the hospital pharmacy staff.

TECH NOTE!
A delay in crediting medications can result in a significant amount of untracked Inventory. Many hospitals try to ensure that final billing of a patient's charges is completed within a few days of the discharge date. Timely crediting of unused medications helps streamline pharmacy inventory and hospital billing processes.

Unit-dose packaging can be customized to accommodate a variety of product sizes. A unit-dose packaging machine is designed to place individual units of a drug (except for liquids) in partly transparent packaging; this allows the contents to be identified easily but also protects the product from damage or contamination. Unit-dose packaging also preserves the physical and chemical integrity of the product. When kept in airtight packaging, unused medications can be recycled and redistributed to other patients.

For accurate inventory management, it is very important to carefully account for unit-packaged medications. Unused doses must be returned to the central pharmacy from patient care areas; there, the price of the medication is credited to the patient's account, and the drug is recaptured in the pharmacy's physical inventory.

Unit-dose packaging systems are now able to perform automated filling of syringes with sterile solutions. A variety of products must be dispensed in a syringe, and previously these were prepared manually in batches by the pharmacy staff. With an automated syringe-filling device, several syringes can be filled in a short time.

The process of drug packaging includes the following steps:

- Proper cleaning, calibration, and setup of packaging equipment and supplies
- Hygienic hand washing and donning of gloves
- Proper product selection using multiple product identifiers (e.g., bar code scanning and verification of the product name, strength, dosage form, and dispensing unit) (Figure 18-1)
- Proper packaging selection (based on the product size or storage requirements, such as protecting the contents from light)
- Documentation of the product packaging (packaging log) (Figure 18-2)
- Verification and checking by a pharmacist (may be performed before or after drug packaging)

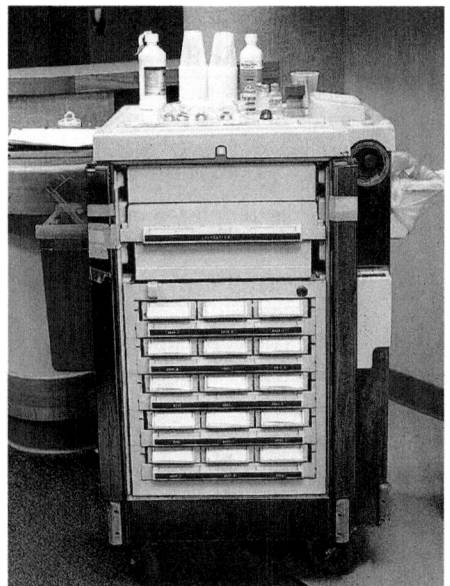

FIGURE 18-1 Unit-dose cabinet. Unit-dose drug distribution systems use single-unit packages of drugs, which are dispensed to fill each dose requirement as it is ordered. Each package is labeled with the drug's generic and brand name, manufacturer, lot number, and expiration date. When dispensed by the pharmacy, the individual packages are placed in labeled drawers assigned to individual patients. The drawers are kept in a large unit-dose cabinet at the nurses' station; in some institutions, individualized containers or envelopes may be locked in a cabinet in the patient's room. The pharmacist typically refills the drawers every 24 hours. In long-term care facilities, they are usually exchanged on 3- or 7-day schedules. (From Clayton B, Stock Y, Cooper S: *Basic pharmacology for nurses,* ed 15, St Louis, 2010, Mosby.)

	Date	Drug (generic)	Strength	Dosage form	Amount	MFG	MFG lot#	MFG exp date	Pharmacy expiration date	Pharmacy lot #	Tech	RPH
1	2/11/2011	aspirin	81mg	tab	100	Bayer	JGH405	7/15/2012	Jun-11	A1001	LP	TG
2	2/12/2011	perphenazine	2mg	tab	100	Schering	XYZ124	12/1/2012	Jul-11	A1002	TK	DS
3												
4												
5												
6												
7												
8												
9												

FIGURE 18-2 Example of a unit-dose log record. (From Hopper T: *Mosby's pharmacy technician: principles and practice,* ed 3, Philadelphia, 2011, Saunders.)

Automation in Drug Storage: The Unit-Dose Medication Carousel and Robotics Systems

MEDICATION CAROUSELS

Proper drug storage systems allow for better inventory management and ensure that drugs are kept under conditions that maintain their stability. In addition, drug storage must be planned carefully to minimize medication selection errors. As mentioned earlier, medium and large hospitals may distribute thousands of individual doses for administration in various patient care areas. Pharmacies do not have unlimited medication storage space; automated dispensing systems offer an excellent solution to this problem. With an automated drug carousel, a few shelves of medication are accessible at a time; the rest of the shelving extends unseen into spaces above the ceiling. Shelves rotate down, like a carousel, when a product is selected, and the shelf on which the product is stored then rests in the picking location.

A carousel system generally uses the following components:
- Label printing system (generally laser or thermal printer)
- Bar code scanner for product identification
- Main carousel unit and product staging surface
- Mechanism for identifying correct product location
- Bins for storage of individual products on carousel shelves

The selected products generally are placed in small reclosable baggies and labeled with the product information or the patient-specific label information, or both. Packaged and labeled products are set aside for checking by a pharmacist. After they have been checked, the doses are sorted by patient or drug storage area (or both) and delivered to the various drug storage areas.

The pharmacy technician's duties when working with a medication carousel include:
- Performing inventory management processes (e.g., stocking, checking expiration dates, and verifying product inventory counts).
- Picking doses for distribution.
- Checking doses (if applicable): A trained checking technician may check the doses picked by another technician as long as the doses are part of a batch fill previously verified by a pharmacist and they do not include any new orders.

ROBOTICS SYSTEMS

Robotics systems also can streamline medication pick and fill processes significantly (Figure 18-3). A batch fill that normally may take 3 to 4 hours can be completed in 45 minutes. From a patient safety standpoint, a robotics system can select hundreds of products within minutes with few or no errors. This significantly reduces the turnaround time for medication delivery to storage in

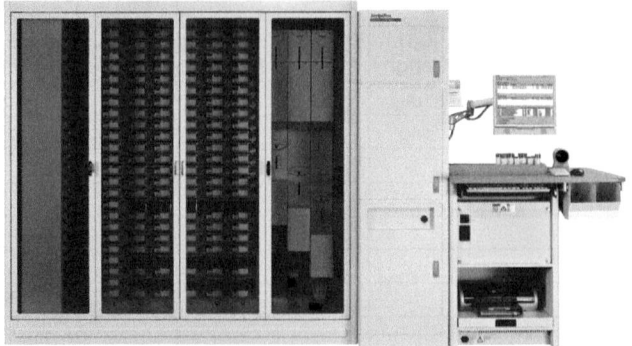

FIGURE 18-3 SP 200 robotic prescription dispensing system (ScriptPro), a fully automated, robotic prescription dispensing system. It accepts prescription dispensing instructions from pharmacy computers and delivers filled and labeled vials at a rate of up to 100 prescriptions per hour. (From Hopper T: *Mosby's pharmacy technician: principles and practice,* ed 3, Philadelphia, 2011, Saunders.)

patient care areas. It also allows pharmacy staff members to be better used for other pharmacy tasks.

Automated IV admixture is a recent addition to pharmacy technology. Some robotics systems perform IV admixture of both standard and cytotoxic drugs. This type of technology is very useful for mixing hazardous products and significantly reduces the time required for each fill process. These enclosed, controlled-environment systems also eliminate the risk of introduction of contaminants into the sterile solutions.

Pharmacy robotics systems generally are set up with unit-dose packages that have been staged in rows around a robotic arm–type mechanism. When dose pick requests are sent to the robotics system electronic queue, the robotic mechanism moves on a hydraulic rail or track to the appropriate location. After the product's bar code has been scanned, the dose is removed from its location and placed in a dispensing bin or envelope. If the wrong drug has been placed in a particular location or if the product is out of date, the pick is placed in a reject bin for manual processing.

Pharmacy technicians generally are responsible for maintenance work on robotics systems, including:

- Calibrating packaging sizes for various products to be stocked in the robot picking area
- Filling "bins" of drug supply in the robot picking area
- Stocking IV admixture robots with aseptic compounding equipment (e.g., needles, syringes, and sterile vials of diluents and IV drugs)
- Cleaning up the robot picking area, because doses may fall during the picking process

A variety of products, because of their packaging or size, may not be ideal for a unit-dose batch fill. Pharmacies often stock the robotics system with 200 to 300 of their most used drugs; less frequently used drugs and those that cannot be used with the robotics system are processed manually by pharmacy technicians or may be picked using another automated system, such as a carousel.

Patient Caregiver Dispensing: The Use and Management of Automated Drug Dispensing Systems

Automated dispensing machines improve continuity of care by giving caregivers better access to medications that must be administered to patients (Figures 18-4 and 18-5). The hospital's pharmacy department ultimately is responsible for setting up, positioning, filling, and maintaining these machines and for training hospital staff in their use. Also, it cannot be overemphasized: pharmacy staff members must help ensure patient safety by making sure that doses have been verified for accuracy by a pharmacist before they are placed in an automated device. It is equally important that

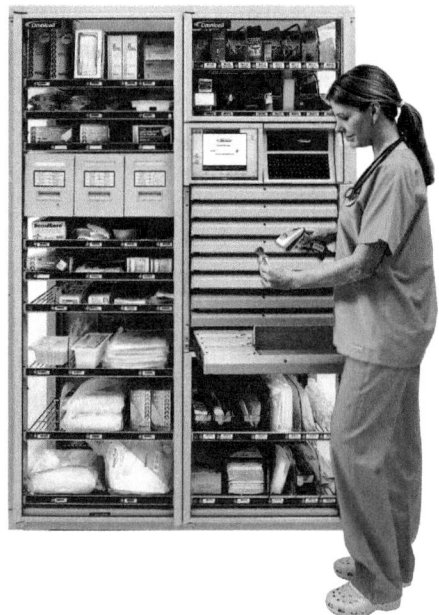

FIGURE 18-4 OmniRx is an example of an automated dispensing system used in hospital units. (From Hopper T: *Mosby's pharmacy technician: principles and practice,* ed 3, Philadelphia, 2011, Saunders.)

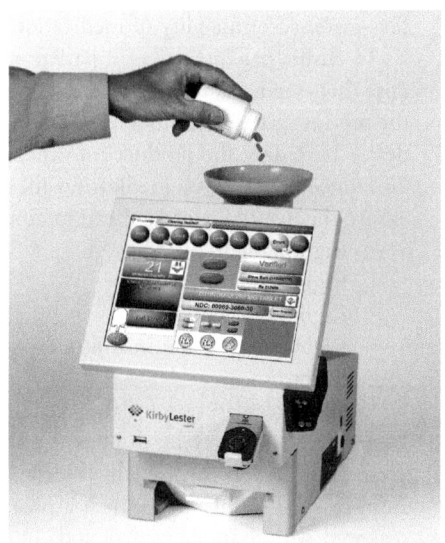

FIGURE 18-5 The KL20 is a full-featured counting and verification device for medication dispensing. It includes accurate counting, multiple checks and balances, visual images, barcode scanning, workflow software — all these functions in one tabletop-sized system to ensure that every order is being dispensed correctly. Photo courtesy of Kirby Lester.

drugs stocked in a dispensing device be placed in the proper locations, so that caregivers can be confident that the correct medication is in that location. Caregivers, in turn, must exercise great caution by making sure that the correct medication is removed from the dispensing machine and in the appropriate quantity. Every dose *must* be verified one final time before it is administered to the patient.

A variety of drug dispensing systems currently are available, and many more are likely to reach the market as this technology continues to advance. The following are examples of dispensing systems:

- AutoPharm (Talys)
- MedDispense (Metro)
- MedSelect (Amerisource Bergen)
- AcuDose (McKesson)
- MTS MedLocker (MTS)
- Serve Rx (MDG Medical)
- Pyxis MedStation 3500 (Cardinal Health)

USING ELECTRONIC PATIENT PROFILING FOR CAREGIVER DISPENSING

Medication can be removed from an automated dispensing machine by patient name or, in an emergency, by individual product. Under normal circumstances, medication orders are entered electronically by authorized caregivers and transmitted electronically to a pharmacist (in some the orders may be handwritten and transcribed into a computer-based system by a nurse or other caregiver). The pharmacist in the central or satellite pharmacy reviews the patient's clinical data to determine the therapeutic appropriateness of the prescribed medication. When an order has been cleared for filling, the pharmacist "verifies" the medication in the system, which activates the machine for dispensing.

The pharmacy's medication management system often is designed to interact with a variety of other computer-based systems inside and outside the pharmacy department. Dispensing labels may be generated in the pharmacy or sent up to label-printing devices in satellite pharmacies, or the product may be made available under the patient's medication profile in an automated dispensing machine in the patient care area. These automated cabinets generally provide room-temperature storage for medications. Refrigerator devices that have been customized for restricted access allow for greater accountability of medication doses that must be stored under refrigerated conditions.

To ensure patients' safety, a patient-specific label is generated and affixed to any patient-specific dose that originates in the pharmacy. This label also is verified and checked by a pharmacist before the product is delivered to a medication storage area. However, doses dispensed from an automated device have only the product information; they are not labeled with patient-specific information. To reduce the risk of a medication fill error, it is very important that proper steps be followed to ensure the five rights of medication administration:

- Right patient
- Right dose
- Right medication
- Right route of administration
- Right time

Hospital regulatory standards require that doses be verified by a pharmacist before dispensing. Unverified doses may be dispensed only in a documented emergency in which the patient's survival would be jeopardized by a delay in the dispensing and administration of the medication. Also, in rural hospitals in which a pharmacist may not be on-site for order review, orders may be reviewed within an allowed period. In such cases the prescriber may obtain the medication from the automated machine or drug locker and must personally witness complete administration of the dose.

Hospital pharmacy and therapeutics (P&T) committees generally establish a list of drugs used in acute care or that may be appropriate in emergencies (these are commonly referred to as *override drugs*). The Joint Commission recognizes that the use of override drugs may be required in some cases, but it urges facilities to keep the list of such drugs to a minimum so that as many medication doses as possible are verified by a pharmacist before administration to a patient.

RESTRICTED ACCESS TO AUTOMATION

Access to automated dispensing machines must be limited to pharmacy staff members and authorized individuals who have been trained and are directly involved in patient care and medication administration. The pharmacy must provide a user identification (ID) and password to authorized medical and hospital staff members and must keep these identifiers on file. Some automated devices

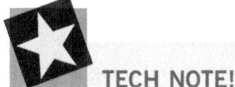

have bioscan devices that identify authorized users by fingerprint in addition to user name. A device usage history is recorded and kept on file for every person who accesses the automated device. This history may include:

- The identity of the person who accessed the device
- The patient profile or profiles that were accessed
- The name, strength, dose, and quantity of drug removed
- The name, strength, dose, and quantity of drug returned to the machine unused
- Documentation of the process for the dispensing and/or wasting of narcotic medications (dispensing individual must dispose of unused product in the presence of a witness)
- Log-in timeouts: The amount of time an authorized user has to perform functions in the automated device is limited to ensure that the system is not left unattended or accessible to unauthorized individuals. Dispensing devices can be formatted to time out automatically after a short period of inactivity and to allow access to the device for a maximum amount of time per log-in.

Organization of Drug Supplies in an Automated Device

Generally, drugs are stored in drawers that contain any of the following, based on the type of medication:

- Individual medication doses
- Multiple strengths of individual doses
- Multiple doses of several legend drugs
- Multiple doses of several nonlegend drugs

Drugs for which quantities must be strictly monitored, such as high-cost medications and controlled substances, typically are stored in individual pockets that dispense one dose at a time.

At least monthly, pharmacists and pharmacy technicians must inventory all the drug pockets and drawers of each dispensing machine and inspect the contents to verify:

- Placement of products in their correct location
- Inventory quantities (discrepancies must be documented and reconciled)
- Product expiration dates, so that short-fill medications can be removed and returned to the pharmacy
- Product packaging, to make sure it is not compromised or damaged
- The drug return bin, which must be emptied and its contents returned to the pharmacy

Each of these items may be verified *whenever* a pharmacy technician enters an automated device to add or remove inventory.

Chapter Summary

- Automated devices help large organizations manage significant workload, allow for better use of staff pharmacy technicians, and facilitate more efficient and accurate inventory management. Most important, automation improves patients' safety. Automated devices, such as robotics systems, significantly reduce the risk and incidence of human fill errors.
- Staff pharmacy technicians provide most of the maintenance support of automated devices, such as upkeep and cleaning, filling and loading, troubleshooting, and generation of a variety of usage and batch fill process reports.
- Unit-dose cart fill processes enable pharmacy staff to prepare a 24-hour supply of pharmacist-verified doses for distribution to various areas of the hospital. Cart fills may include the preparation of doses labeled for individual patients or doses that will be removed from an automated dispensing device by a caregiver in a patient care area.
- Medication orders should be filled only after a pharmacist has verified each dose to be the most clinically appropriate, given patient-specific factors. Only in emergency situations may medication be dispensed from nursing floor stock or automated dispensing machines. Other limited exceptions may exist, such as policies for rural hospitals or in other situations as set forth by an individual state's Board of Pharmacy.
- Pharmacy technicians may serve key roles related to various forms of automation. Technicians may perform any of the following tasks:

- Unit-dose prepackaging and/or repackaging of medications
- Proper cleaning, calibration, and setup of packaging equipment and supplies
- Picking of unit-dose medication for the patient-specific cart fill using automated drug storage carousels
  - Properly trained checking technicians may check the doses picked by another technician provided the doses are part of a batch fill previously verified by a pharmacist and no new orders have been included.
- Inventory management processes, such as stocking, checking expiration dates, and verifying product inventory counts
- Calibrating of packaging sizes for various products to be stocked in the robot picking area
- Filling "bins" of drug supply in the robot picking area
- Stocking IV admixture robots with aseptic compounding equipment (e.g., needles, syringes, and sterile vials of diluents and IV drugs)
- Cleanup of the robot picking area, because doses may fall during the picking process
- Tasks required for maintenance of automated drug dispensing devices, including:
  - Verifying correct product locations in the device
  - Verifying inventory counts
  - Checking product expiration dates so that short-fill medications can be removed and returned to the pharmacy
  - Ensuring that product packaging is not compromised or damaged
  - Checking the drug return bin, which must be emptied and the contents returned to the pharmacy
  - Maintenance of devices and troubleshooting of technical problems
  - Training of hospital staff in the use of automated devices

REVIEW QUESTIONS

Multiple Choice

1. The process in which drugs retained in the manufacturer's packaging are enclosed in an overwrap packaging is referred to as:
   a. Prepackaging
   b. Repackaging
   c. Automation
   d. None of the above

2. An individual, single-use package of drug product is also known as an:
   a. Unit dose
   b. Single dose
   c. Individual dose
   d. Sole dose

3. Standards that apply to the use of automation technology are defined by:
   a. The Joint Commission
   b. Each state's Board of Pharmacy
   c. Each facility's Board of Trustees
   d. Each facility's Chief Nursing Officer

4. Unlike customers in a community pharmacy, hospital patients:
   a. Receive their medication therapy all at once
   b. Are administered one dose at a time
   c. May only receive up to a 24-hour supply
   d. b and c

5. Pharmacy inventory stock may be more efficiently managed using:
   a. Carousel shelving
   b. Automated dispensing machines
   c. Robotics systems
   d. a and c

6. The process in which drugs in bulk containers are placed in unit-dose packaging is referred to as:
   a. Prepackaging
   b. Repackaging
   c. Automation
   d. a and b

7. The process in which patient-specific doses are prepared in individual packaging and distributed to patient-specific storage areas is known as:
   a. Unit-dose packaging
   b. Cart fill
   c. Drug distribution
   d. Drug picking process

8. A manufactured unit-dose cup of a liquid medication may need to be _____ before it is placed in a robot staging area.
   a. Emptied into a bulk container
   b. Repackaged
   c. Prepackaged
   d. None of the above

9. A storage carousel system often has which form of technology to assist the user with product identification?
   a. Bar code scanning
   b. Thermal printers
   c. Product staging areas
   d. Storage bins

10. Robotics systems are ideal for dispensing:
    a. Less frequently used drugs
    b. More frequently dispensed drugs
    c. Bulky supplies that otherwise would take up considerable space
    d. Expensive drugs

TECHNICIAN'S CORNER

1. How does unit dosing of medication assist in the recycling of unused doses?
2. What types of medication fills may a properly trained checking technician check?
3. Name the five tasks involved in the monthly inspection of an automated dispensing system.

Bibliography

Shack & Tulloch. (2008). *A "Stacked" Medication Supply Chain Rollout Leads to Rapid Safety, Efficiency, and Cost Benefits.* Retrieved 9/1/2011, from www.mckesson.com/static_files/McKesson.com/MPT/Documents/MAIFiles/CaseStudy_Comanche.pdf

State of Minnesota Pharmacy Board. (2001, March 1). *Automated Medication Storage and Distribution System Guidelines.* Retrieved 8/30/2011, from www.phcybrd.state.mn.us/forms/autohosp.pdf

Texas Administrative Code. (2011). *Subchapter D Institutional Pharmacy, Rule 291.72, Definitions (2001).* Retrieved 8/31/2011, from http://info.sos.state.tx.us/pls/pub/readtac$ext.TacPage?sl=R&app=9&p_dir=&p_rloc=&p_tloc=&p_ploc=&pg=1&p_tac=&ti=22&pt=15&ch=291&rl=72

Washington State Legislature. (2006, November 13). *Chapter 246-872 WAC: Automated Drug Distribution Devices.* Retrieved 8/30/2011, from http://apps.leg.wa.gov/WAC/default.aspx?cite=246-872&full=true

19 Aseptic Admixture and Compounding of Sterile Preparations

LEARNING OBJECTIVES

By the end of this chapter, students will be able to competently:

1. Explain the rationale for creating a controlled environment.
2. Explain the regulatory standards of practice for aseptic intravenous (IV) admixture.
3. Recognize key components of a USP <797>–compliant clean room.
4. Describe the proper use and maintenance of products and equipment in preparing compounded sterile products.
5. State the storage, labeling, and documentation requirements for various types of injectable drugs.
6. Describe proper aseptic technique for preparing sterile vials and ampules.
7. Describe each of the types of sterile supplies that are used during the aseptic admixture process.
8. Compare and contrast the types of glass and solution containers into which drug additives may be injected.
9. Describe proper aseptic technique for the preparation and handling of hazardous drugs in ampules, vials, and other containers.
10. Discuss various methods for solution and container sterilization.
11. List types of parenteral drugs commonly prepared in a controlled environment.
12. Describe each of the quality assurance processes that must be performed daily, weekly, and/or monthly in the controlled environment.
13. Perform various mathematical calculations to solve compounding problems.

KEY TERMS

Ante-area: The designated location in a controlled environment where labels are prepared and hand washing and garbing are performed. The ante-area must be maintained under ISO Class 8 conditions.

Aseptic admixture: The skill of preparing intravenous (IV) solutions in a manner that prevents the introduction of contaminants, so that the final product remains or becomes sterile.

Aseptic hand washing: The process of washing the skin surfaces of the hands and forearms, using an antimicrobial skin cleanser, to remove particulates and contaminants from the fingertips to the elbows without recontamination during the hand washing process.

Aspirate: The release of air and/or drug particles from a vial.

Bactericidal: A term used to describe a cleanser that kills bacteria.

Bacteriostatic: A term used to describe a cleanser that inhibits the growth of bacteria; also referred to as persistent activity.

Barrel: The part of a syringe used to accurately measure the amount of a sterile drug.

Bevel: The sharp, pointed tip of a needle.

Buffer area: The area of a controlled environment where sterile pharmaceuticals are prepared. The buffer area must be maintained under ISO Class 7 conditions at all times.

Chemical stability: The ability of a drug's active ingredients to maintain their chemical integrity and potency.

Controlled environment: A designated area in a pharmacy where environmental factors, such as continuous airflow, temperature, humidity, and air quality, are maintained consistently and measured regularly.

Gauge: The diameter of the interior of a needle's lumen.

Heel: The flat, rounded end of a needle, opposite the bevel at the needle's tip.

HEPA filter: A high-efficiency particulate air filter; it removes particulates but not vapors or gases.

Hub: A transparent, plastic casing used to attach a needle to the tip of a syringe.

Hypertonicity: A term used to describe a solution that has a higher concentration of dissolved ingredients; it draws fluid out of red blood cells (RBCs), causing them to shrink, and increasing the plasma fluid volume.

Hypotonicity: A term used to describe a solution that has a lower concentration of dissolved ingredients; it causes fluid to flow across the red blood cell (RBC) membranes, resulting in swelling and bursting of RBCs.

Isotonicity: A term used to describe a solution that has a tonicity similar to that of blood; therefore, it causes no movement of fluid across the membranes of RBCs.

IV admixture: The process in which one or more active drug ingredients are introduced into a solution that will be injected or infused into a patient by a parenteral route.

Lumen: The hollow space inside the shaft of a needle.

Microbiologic stability: A drug's ability to resist microbial growth and maintain sterility.

Multiple-dose containers: Per U.S. Pharmacopeia (USP) requirements, a container that has a preservative and an antibacterial agent, as well as a maximum volume of 30 ml, to limit the number of punctures to the container's closure.

Needles: Sharp, bevel-pointed instruments used to transfer liquid drawn into a syringe.

Open system: A drug container that, once broken, provides no physical barrier between the sterile contents of the container and the external hood environment.

Pass-throughs: Hatches used to pass products between the clean room and the outside environment.

Pharmacy engineering control (PEC) devices: Specialized equipment primarily used to create ideal controlled environments for the preparation of compounded sterile preparations.

Physical stability: A drug's ability to maintain its appearance, taste, suspension, and/or dissolution.

Plunger: The part of a syringe that slides into and out of the barrel to manipulate the sterile substance.

Quality assurance (QA): Measures used to evaluate the effectiveness of quality control procedures.

Quality control (QC): The process established in a controlled environment to ensure that all regulations and procedures are followed in the preparation of compound sterile preparations (CSPs).

Response time: The time required for an antiseptic cleanser to kill microorganisms.

Single-dose containers: An IV drug container that is not reusable and does not contain a preservative.

Sterile: The state of being free of microbial or solid particulate contamination.

Syringe: A cylindrical, sterile container used to measure the amount of drug needed.

Therapeutic stability: A drug's ability to maintain its expected therapeutic effect.

Toxicologic stability: A drug that maintains no significant increase in toxicity.

For a pharmacy technician, the ability to perform aseptic admixture of sterile intravenous (IV) products is one of the most sought-after and marketable hands-on skills. Often, pharmacy technicians who have worked in a community pharmacy and who want to transition to hospital pharmacy practice first obtain training in the preparation of sterile products. Students who develop this capability in their formal education courses have the advantage of beginning entry-level careers with a very important skill set already established.

IV admixture is the process in which one or more active drug ingredients is introduced into a parenteral solution that will be injected or infused into a patient by a parenteral route. Aseptic admixture is the preparation of IV solutions in a manner that prevents the introduction of contaminants, so that the final product remains or becomes sterile. In pharmacy practice, the word sterile means without microbial or solid particulate contamination. When injectable drugs are prepared, distributed, dispensed, and administered, sterility of the final product is critical. Introduction of contaminants into a prepared solution may have serious consequences for a patient's health. A solid particulate contaminant may cause a traveling clot in the patient's vascular system, which may block a major blood vessel or lead to a heart attack, or both. Microbial contamination may cause mild to severe systemic infections that could lead to death if left untreated.

Extreme care and specialized training are necessary for all who prepare compounded sterile preparations (CSPs). To maintain compliance and protect patients' health, pharmacy technicians involved in the production of CSPs must be knowledgeable about the legally enforceable professional standards that regulate the preparation of sterile pharmaceuticals.

WHY ARE COMPOUNDING STANDARDS NECESSARY?

Standards are important primarily because they protect the health, welfare, and safety of patients receiving parenteral drugs prepared by pharmacists and pharmacy technicians in a hospital, for home infusion, or in a nursing home. The best way to protect patients is to minimize the chances of healthcare-acquired infections (HAIs), which occur as a result of contamination of medication prepared by pharmacy staff members. Contamination of IV solutions during preparation is a well-documented public health issue, a problem that has generated a great deal of discussion and critical assessment over the past 40 years.

In the 1970s a surge of thousands of HAIs resulted in serious illness and death; these infections were found to have originated in IV solutions that had been contaminated during preparation. The medical and pharmacy professions began to examine the overwhelming need to review the procedures for preparing IV solutions and identify risk factors for contamination. During the 1980s and 1990s, organizations such as the U.S. Food and Drug Administration (FDA), U.S. Pharmacopeia (USP), and American Society of Health-System Pharmacists (ASHP) conducted various quality surveys and published materials that established practice guidelines related to the preparation of sterile pharmaceuticals. These guidelines made practice recommendations centered on the pharmacist's responsibility for ensuring proper preparation, labeling, storage, dispensing, and delivery of CSPs. A particularly important publication was the *1992 ASHP Technical Assistance Bulletin*. Contamination of IV admixtures continued to raise concern in the next decade, particularly in light of high-profile cases of patient injury or death. One such case, in 2006, involved 11 patients who had had cardiac surgery. The patients developed serious infections as a result of administration of a contaminated admixture, and three died. These deaths highlighted the importance of the *1992 ASHP Technical Assistance Bulletin*.

The first legally enforceable standard that applied across the profession of pharmacy was established by the USP in January, 2004; that standard is USP Chapter <797>. Among pharmacy professionals, this standard raised widespread concern about the drastic changes—and potential cost—involved in modifying IV preparation areas to achieve full compliance. From 2005 through 2007, various modifications to the original standard were discussed among leaders in the industry. The final draft of revisions to USP <797> became official on June 1, 2008.

OTHER SOURCES OF STERILE PRODUCT COMPOUNDING STANDARDS

In addition to the ASHP and USP, the following organizations have contributed to the establishment of standards for the preparation, storage, handling, and administration of CSPs.
American Society for Parenteral and Enteral Nutrition (ASPEN); set forth standards for:
- Labeling of parenteral nutrition formulations
- Standard nutrient ranges and sample formulations
- Extemporaneous compounding of parenteral nutrition formulations
- Stability and compatibility of parenteral nutrition formulations
- In-line filtration of parenteral nutrient admixtures

TABLE 19-1   **ISO and U.S. Standards for Clean Room Classification**

Class name		Particle Count	
ISO class	U.S. FS 209E	ISO, (m³)	F2 209E, ft³
3	Class 1	35.2	1
4	Class 10	352	10
5	Class 100	3,520	100
6	Class 1,000	35,200	1,000
7	Class 10,000	352,000	10,000
8	Class 100,000	3,520,000	100,000

Adapted from former Federal Standard No. 209E, General Services Administration, Washington, DC, 20407 (September 11, 1992) and ISO 14644-1:1999, Cleanrooms and associated controlled environ ments—Part 1: Classification of air cleanliness. For example, 3,520 particles of 0.5 µm per m³ or larger (ISO Class 5) is equivalent to 100 particles per ft³ (Class 100) (1 m³ = 35.2 ft³).

Occupational Safety and Health Administration (OSHA); set forth standards for:
- Use of personal protective equipment (PPE)

National Institute for Occupational Safety and Health (NIOSH)
- As an agency of the Centers for Disease Control and Prevention (CDC), alerts healthcare organizations to help reduce healthcare workers' occupational exposure to hazardous drugs
- Specifies that hazardous drug compounding should be performed in a biologic safety cabinet (BSC) that is vented 100 percent to the outside

International Organization for Standardization (ISO)
- Regulates clean room standards for a variety of industries
- Publishes standards for clean rooms and associated controlled environments
- Presents classes on evaluating clean room environments based on airborne particle counts

In Table 19-1, the U.S. standards for clean room classification are noted according to U.S. units of measurement. By law, Federal Standard 209E can be superseded by new international standards. It is expected that 209E will be used in some industries over the next 5 years, but that eventually it will be replaced internationally by ISO 14644-1. Because the ISO is an international organization, the current standards are expressed in metric units. ISO Class 5 is the standard level of airborne particulate that must be sustained in pharmacy engineering control (PEC) devices, such as a laminar airflow hood. ISO Class 7 is the standard for the controlled environment buffer room, and ISO Class 8 is the standard for the controlled environment ante-area.

A contaminated solution is a *reservoir* that supplies the *infecting agent* through an injectable *route of administration* to the *susceptible host* patient. Preparers of sterile IV solutions must be trained in how to prevent the introduction of infecting agents that may create ideal conditions for an HAI.

This chapter discusses the key elements of USP <797> and how these standards directly affect pharmacy technician practice. A good way to start is to examine the practice standards themselves. The next section provides an overview of the current revised standards. and following sections explain how those standards are applied to the environment, equipment, supplies, and procedures involved in aseptic admixture of sterile solutions.

USP Chapter <797>

USP <797> provides guidelines and standards for pharmacy technician practice in five key areas:
- The environment in which sterile preparations are prepared
- The PPE used in that environment
- The procedures performed for admixture of various types of sterile preparations
- Quality assurance (QA) guidelines that help to regulate controlled environments and those who prepare CSPs
- QA measures to assess the amount of airborne and surface contaminants in the controlled environment despite the preventive procedures and controls in place

BOX 19-1   Compounded Sterile Preparations Regulated by USP <797> Standards

• Biologic	• Nutrient
• Diagnostic	• Radiopharmaceutical
• Drug	

USP, U.S. Pharmacopeia.

BOX 19-2   Types of Sterile Manufactured Preparations Regulated by USP <797> Standards

• Aqueous bronchial inhalations	• Irrigations for wounds and body cavities
• Aqueous nasal inhalations	• Ophthalmic preparations
• Baths and soaks for live organs and tissues	• Tissue implants
• Injections of any type	

USP, U.S. Pharmacopeia.

USP <797> regulates certain CSPs (Box 19-1) and manufactured compounded preparations (Box 19-2).

In 2004 The Joint Commission (TJC) announced that it would survey facilities to ensure compliance; however, that position changed in 2006. Currently, TJC considers USP <797> "a valuable set of guidelines—contemporary consensus-based safe practices—that describes a best practice for establishing safe processes in compounding sterile medications"; however, it no longer requires organizations to implement the guidelines as a condition of accreditation. It is important to note that many of the TJC Medication Management standards are similar to those of USP <797>, and that TJC "will expect to see structures and processes that ensure safe practices for compounding sterile medication." Therefore, pharmacy technicians must know how their state interprets the guidelines and uses them to assess their hospital environments and those who prepare sterile pharmaceuticals.

As noted earlier, the purpose of compounding standards is to prevent the introduction and spread of contaminants into CSPs. The environment in which CSPs are prepared must be designed, constructed, and maintained so as to minimize contamination risks.

Controlled Environment

ISO standards cover air quality in the controlled environment. An effective means of preventing the spread of contaminants into CSPs in the preparation areas is to limit the number of airborne particles, which could be acting as reservoirs for disease-causing microorganisms.

CLEAN ROOM

The space in which sterile medications are prepared may be referred to as an *IV room* or *lab,* a *clean room,* or a *controlled environment.*

This text uses terminology consistent with USP <797>; therefore, *controlled environment* is used primarily. A controlled environment is a designated area in a pharmacy in which environmental factors such as continuous airflow, temperature, humidity, and air quality are maintained consistently and measured regularly. Controls for airflow and air pressure are created, sustained, and monitored in the controlled environment. To protect the stability of products prepared there, clean room environments are maintained in the standard room temperature range (59° to 86° F). Humidity must also be kept low, because high humidity can affect the integrity of products and the packaging of supplies stored in the controlled environment.

From ceiling to floor, the controlled environment must be constructed in a way that prevents the collection, growth, and spread of contaminants through various modes of transmission. A controlled environment must be constructed of material that is:
  • Nonporous
  • Nonshedding (does not give off any residue)
  • Able to undergo regular cleaning without degrading

Ceilings must be constructed of nonshedding light fixtures, and all corners must be smoothed, or coved. Fan-powered high-efficiency particulate air (HEPA) filtration allows capture of airborne particulates. The filtered air blowing down on a continuous vertical plane also creates positive pressure in the clean room area; that is, the air pressure is higher in the clean room space than outside it. This allows the inside air to be forced out whenever the clean room door is opened, thus creating an "air barrier" that minimizes the amount of potentially contaminated outside room air that enters the controlled environment.

A clean room may be constructed with two main areas, an ante-area and a buffer area. The ante-area is where label preparation takes place, as well as the hand washing and garbing (covered later in the chapter). The ante-area must be maintained under ISO Class 8 conditions at all times. The buffer area is where the sterile pharmaceuticals are actually prepared, so the requirements for air quality are more stringent; the buffer area must be maintained under ISO Class 7 conditions at all times.

Pass-throughs are hatches that are used to pass products between the clean room and the outside environment without the clean room staff having to leave the area and disturb the positive pressure airflow. This reduces the frequency of staff exiting the controlled area and potentially introducing airborne contaminants into it. Only one side of the pass-through opens at a time, so little or no air exchange takes place. Some pass-throughs are designed to HEPA filter air during each pass to ensure that potentially contaminated outside air does not enter the buffer room. New clean technology will include automated features. This allows safe passage of supplies into the clean room, transfer of products out of the clean room after preparation, and better inventory management.

CLEAN ROOM EQUIPMENT

Any item allowed into the clean room must have the same nonporous, nonshedding composition that can sustain frequent cleaning (Figure 19-1). Storage, equipment, and supplies should be minimized in the buffer area to reduce contamination risks.

Commonly Used Clean Room Furniture

- Stainless steel wire shelving units are ideal, particularly if they have wheels so they can be moved for cleaning.
- Stainless steel tables are best, because they do not generate particles and surfaces are easy to clean.
- Chairs may be padded with a nonporous material, such as vinyl.
- Stainless steel is recommended for supply carts, which should be mounted on wheels and castors.

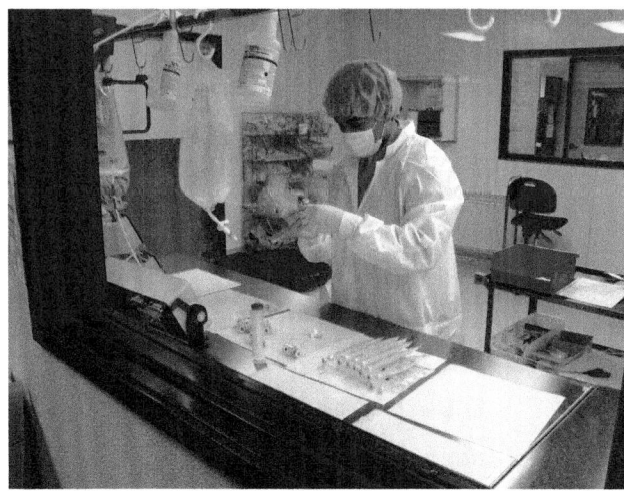

FIGURE 19-1 Clean room. (From Hopper T: *Mosby's pharmacy technician: principles and practice*, ed 3, Philadelphia, 2011, Saunders.)

- For USP <797> compliance, any carts used for product transport in the clean room must remain in the controlled areas at all times. Products must be removed from outer boxes and packaging, sprayed with isopropyl alcohol (IPA), and wiped down before they are transferred to a clean room cart and taken into the clean room.

Other Equipment and Supplies Commonly Used in a Clean Room

Tacky mats are multiple sheets of plastic film coated with adhesives that must be used on the floor in the clean environment to trap particulates from the soles of IV preparers' shoes. Because they quickly become dirty, the topmost sheet should be peeled off frequently so that a fresh tacky surface is always uppermost.

Repeater pumps are used for batch preparation. Tubing connects a large-volume source to smaller volume bags or syringes. The pump may be operated manually or programmed to draw a defined volume at timed intervals.

Total parenteral nutrition (TPN) compounding machines are used to mix large volumes of TPN formula. Compounding machines are programmed to draw defined volumes of IV solutions and various drugs into a central collection IV bag.

Electronic balances may be used to measure the quantity of drug to be added to an IV or irrigation solution.

PERSONNEL GARB AND ATTIRE

Pharmacy professionals involved in the preparation of sterile pharmaceuticals in the controlled environment must wear PPE to ensure that no surface contaminants are introduced into the clean room and that no contaminant from the controlled environment (e.g., residue from a hazardous drug preparation) is transferred into other areas of the pharmacy. PPE is also commonly referred to as *clean room garb* and *attire*.

Clean room PPE also shields the controlled environment from the thousands of particles shed by the human body (Table 19-2).

Various types of PPE must be worn, and the items must be put on in a particular order (Box 19-3). The point of the order of garbing is to cover first the "dirtiest" parts of the body (i.e., those that shed the most particulates). After proper hand washing the remaining items are put on, and this should provide total coverage of exposed skin and outer scrubs.

Artificial nails are more likely to harbor gram-negative pathogens than natural nails, both before and after hand washing; for this reason, they are not allowed in the controlled environment. Cosmetics, also, are not allowed, because they shed particulates during motion.

PHARMACY ENGINEERING CONTROLS

As mentioned earlier, PECs are specialized pieces of equipment primarily used to create ideal controlled environments for the preparation of CSPs. They include the laminar airflow workbench (LAFW), commonly referred to as the *IV hood* (Figure 19-2). The types of devices used are

TABLE 19-2   **Number of Airborne Particles Generated by the Human Body in 1 Minute***

Activity	Number of particles
Motionless/sitting/standing	100,000
Head, arm, neck, leg motion	500,000
All of the above with foot motion	1 million
Standing to sitting position and vice-versa	2.5 million
Walking at 2 miles per hour	5 million
Walking at 3.5 miles per hour	7.5 million
Walking at 5 miles per hour	10 million

*Particles are 3 microns or larger in size.

BOX 19-3 **Personnel Cleansing and Garbing Order**

- Remove all personal outer garments.
- Remove cosmetics.
- Remove jewelry from hands, wrists, or any other visible body parts.
- Remove artificial fingernails (if wearing them).
- Put on personal protective equipment (PPE) and perform procedures in the following order:
  1. Put on dedicated shoes or shoe covers.
  2. Put on head and facial hair covers.
  3. Put on face masks and eye shields.
  4. Perform hand cleansing procedures.
  5. Put on nonshedding gown.
  6. Put on sterile, powder-free gloves.
     - Apply isopropyl alcohol (IPA) to gloves before beginning compounding and intermittently during the compounding process.

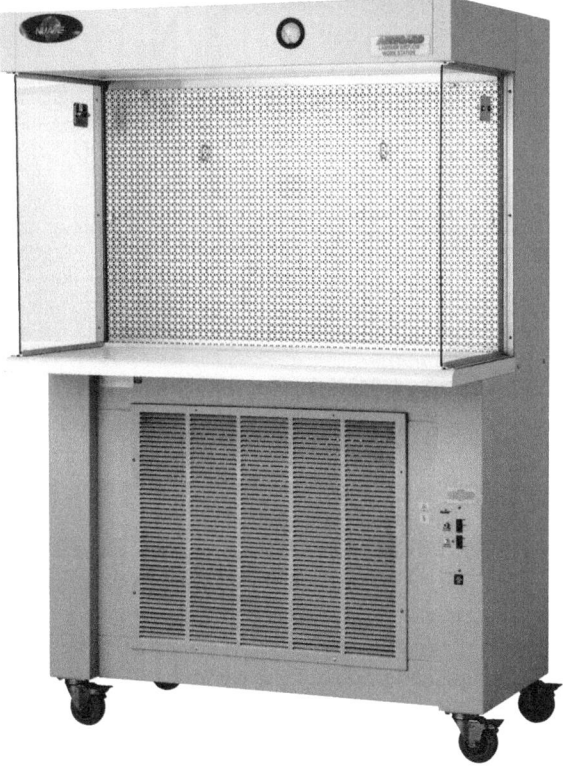

FIGURE 19-2 Airegard 301 (horizontal laminar flow hood clean bench). (Courtesy of NuAire, Inc., 2011.)

determined by the types of drugs prepared within them and the environment in which the device is stored.

PECs in the clean room have three primary functions:
- To provide clean air in the clean zone
- To provide a constant airflow, preventing unclean room air from entering the clean zone
- To remove and prevent any particulate matter 0.3 micron or larger from entering the clean zone

The LAFW has three main components:
- A *prefilter,* which traps dust, lint, and other large contaminants and must be cleaned or changed at least monthly and documented

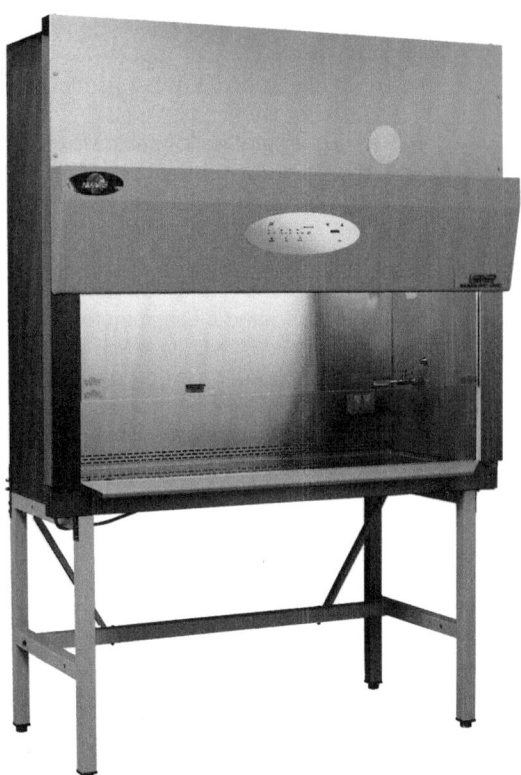

FIGURE 19-3 Vertical flow hood. (Courtesy of NuAire, Inc., 2011.)

- A HEPA filter, which removes particulates (microorganisms), but not vapors or gases and must be checked every 6 months
- A *work surface,* which is the clean zone where aseptic compounding takes place. Work must be performed 3 to 6 inches from the outer edge (depending on whether the hood has an air intake grill).

To create ISO Class 5 air quality, the LAFW must run continuously for at least 30 minutes before use. Work surfaces must be prerinsed with sterile water, if necessary, then disinfected with 70% IPA, and allowed to dry before use.

A vertical LAFW also is used in the aseptic preparation of sterile pharmaceuticals; its airflow design creates a safer environment for the mixing of cytotoxic and other hazardous drugs (Figure 19-3). A vertical LAFW specifically designed for the preparation of hazardous drugs is called a biologic safety cabinet. A BSC is also referred to as a *glove box* (Figure 19-4). BSCs are classified according to the amount of air exhausted from the work area and the amount of air that is filtered and recycled back into the contained work area (Table 19-3).

The five main components of an LAFW are:

- A *glass shield:* This must be kept closed, except for an 8-inch opening to maintain airflow.
- *Air intake grills:* These are located at the front and back of the hood; they create negative pressure to suck in contaminants and prevent them from exiting the containment area within the hood.
- A *recirculation exhaust blower:* This pulls air from the containment center back through a plenum into the unit to be refiltered and exhausted. Depending on the BSC class, air may be exhausted directly back into the room after filtration or exhausted into a separate duct system to prevent air contamination.
- *Clearance:* The hood must have at least 14 inches of ceiling clearance and 12 inches of clearance on all sides for reliable measurement of airflow.
- A *HEPA filter:* This removes particulates and microorganisms; a vertical LAFW has a filter that supplies filtered air to the work surface, and a filter to filter air before it is exhausted from the top of the cabinet.

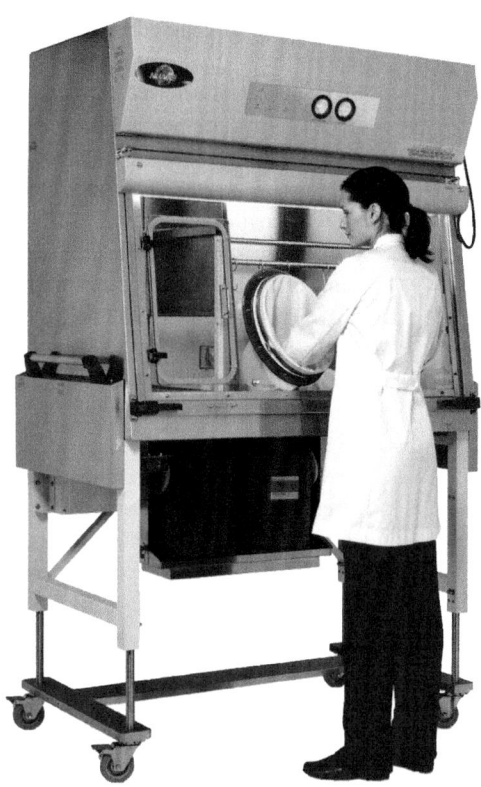

FIGURE 19-4 Labgard 437: Glove box (also called a biological safety cabinet) for IV admixture. (Courtesy of NuAire, Inc., 2011.)

TABLE 19-3   **HEPA Filtering System Standards**

Class	Risk levels	Safety level	Filtering system
I	Low- to moderate-risk biologicals	Biosafety level I	HEPA system filters air before it is exhausted.
II	Low- to moderate-risk biologicals	Biosafety level II	HEPA system filters exhaust air to room or to a facility exhaust system.
III	High-risk biologicals	Biosafety level III	Containment of hazardous materials.

From Hopper T: *Mosby's pharmacy technician: principles and practice*, ed 3, Philadelphia, 2011, Saunders.
HEPA, High-efficiency particulate air [filter].

- A *work surface:* This is the clean zone, where all aseptic manipulations of sterile pharmaceuticals are performed. These procedures must be performed at least 3 inches from each air intake grill.
  - Drapes and mats must not block the intake grills.
  - To prevent interruption of airflow, items should not be hung on an IV pole directly above items on the work surface.
  - Because of the vertical airflow, manipulations should be performed 3 inches or more above the work surface.
- The air of the containment area should be purged for at least 3 minutes between preparations to remove any airborne contaminants.
- Some LAFWs may have an alarm/alert system that indicates when the glass shield is not at the appropriate height.

The barrier isolator is a PEC with the same components as an LAFW; however, all the components are contained. Minimum standards for preventing microbial contamination must be met when using the barrier isolator:

* It must be constructed of durable material that is easy to clean inside and out.
* It must have a pass-through system that isolates the interior of the unit from the room when materials are transferred into and out of the unit.
* It should include height adjusters for users.
* It must maintain positive air pressure to keep external airborne particles out.
* It must use a double-glove system to prevent leaks and tears that would compromise the interior environment.
* It must use a unidirectional or turbulent airflow that sweeps or mixes with airborne contaminants and flushes them from the containment area through an exhaust system.

The barrier isolator has five primary components.

Main chamber
* All interior surfaces are continuous (no sharp corners or edges) and easy to clean; sterile water is used as a prerinse, and then 70% IPA is used for cleaning.

Glove ports
* Workers can change gloves without exposing the interior of the cabinet to the outside environment.
* Gloves are available in various sizes and diameters.

Transfer hatches
* Internal surfaces are continuous and easy to clean.
* Hatches are angled to allow products to be passed easily into the main chamber.
* Test point allows QA air sampling.
* Hatch doors apply a vacuum that prevents outside air from entering the interior chamber.
* When the outside hatch is closed, an automatic factory interlock seals the door for 2 minutes to allow air to be flushed and exhausted.

Base frame
* The frame allows for height adjustment so that the operator can work standing or seated.
* Many are equipped with an adjustable foot rest.
* Many have electrical or pneumatic operation for height adjustment.

Monitoring and alarm system
* Airflow and the status of transfer hatch doors are continuously monitored.
* Control system logs power failures and other events.
* System gives an audible error message when readings deviate from the preset conditions.
* The device's integrity is demonstrated by a pressure hold test, which takes 10 minutes, and is monitored by the control system.
* A leak test may also be performed.

Performing Tasks in the Controlled Environment

The tasks performed in a controlled environment are determined by the risk of contamination. The ASHP and USP have established risk levels based on the potential for contamination of a CSP during preparation (Box 19-4).

Each risk level specifies:
1. Conditions dictating what may be compounded, based on the risk of contamination
2. Maximum storage limitations and requirements
3. QA measures that must be followed in the preparation of CSPs
4. QA standards that must be met to qualify a pharmacy professional to prepare CSPs per risk level (media fill challenge)

IMMEDIATE-USE COMPOUNDED STERILE PRODUCTS

Immediate-use CSPs are defined as low-risk preparations that are used only for emergencies or immediate patient administration. This classification is not intended for any product that needs extended storage or batch compounding. Six criteria must be met for a drug to be included in the immediate-use risk classification:
1. Compounding process must not exceed 1 hour.
2. Aseptic techniques must be followed.

BOX 19-4   **Risk Levels Based on the Potential for Contamination**

IMMEDIATE USE
- For emergent use or situations in which low-risk compounding would add risk because of delays
- No storage or batch compounding
- Continuous compounding process lasting less than 1 hour
- Use of aseptic technique
- Drug to be administered less than 1 hour after preparation begins or otherwise discarded
- Simple transfer of sterile nonhazardous drugs or diagnostic radiopharmaceuticals

LOW RISK
- Simple admixtures compounded using closed system transfer methods
- Prepared in International Organization for Standardization (ISO) Class 5 laminar airflow workbench (LAFW) located in an ISO Class 7 buffer area with an ISO Class 8 ante-area
- Examples include reconstitution of single-dose vials of antibiotics or other small-volume parenterals, or preparation of hydration solutions

LOW-RISK; LESS THAN 12 HOURS BEYOND USE DATE
- Simple admixtures compounded using closed system transfer methods
- Prepared in ISO Class 5 pharmacy engineering control (PEC) devices
- Compounding area segregated from noncompounding areas
- Administration starts no later than 12 hours after preparation

MEDIUM RISK
- Admixtures compounded using multiple additives and/or small volumes
- Batch preparations (e.g., syringes)
- Complex manipulations (e.g., total parenteral nutrition [TPN])
- Preparation for use over several days
- Prepared in ISO Class 5 LAFW located in ISO Class 7 buffer area with ISO Class 8 ante-area
- Examples include pooled admixtures, parenteral nutrition solutions using automated compounders, batch-compounded preparations that do not contain bacteriostatic components

HIGH RISK
- Nonsterile (bulk powder) ingredients
- Open system transfers
- Prepared in ISO Class 5 LAFW located in ISO Class 7 buffer area with separate ISO Class 8 ante-area
- Examples include compounded sterile preparations (CSPs) prepared from bulk, nonsterile components or final containers that are nonsterile and must be terminally sterilized

3. Compounding must involve three or fewer simple product transfers into the final dispensing container.
4. Preparer (if the pharmacist) must immediately witness complete administration of an unlabeled preparation, *or* the preparation must have a label that indicates:
   a. Patient information
   b. Names and amounts of all ingredients
   c. Name/initials of the preparer
   d. The exact 1 hour beyond-use date (BUD)/time, whether stored at room temperature or under refrigerated conditions.
5. Administration must begin within 1 hour from the exact time the preparer began preparing the product.
6. If administration has not begun within 1 hour, the product must be promptly, properly, and safely discarded.

LOW RISK

The following conditions must be met in order for a CSP to be considered low risk.
- All ingredients and equipment used are sterile.
- Basic or standard manipulations are performed.

- Single transfers and three or fewer products are used in the preparation.
- Storage for:
  - 48 hours at room temperature
  - 14 days at refrigerated temperatures
  - 45 days at frozen temperatures
- A relatively simple media fill challenge is performed annually.

A provisional low-risk level also may be assigned for some products given a BUD of 12 hours or less. These higher risk conditions, to which the provisional low-risk level would apply, include:

- All QA garbing, aseptic technique, and environmental testing are followed.
- Procedures are the same as for low-risk CSPs, except that the PEC is not located in an ISO Class 7 buffer area.
- Preparations are patient-specific and requested by a medication order.
- The product BUD is 12 hours or less, so administration must be started less than 12 hours after preparation, whether the product is stored at room temperature or refrigerated temperatures.
- The compounding area is segregated from other areas, including (but not limited to) unsealed windows, high traffic areas, food service, or construction, to reduce the risk of contamination.

MEDIUM RISK

CSPs considered medium risk involve more opportunities for the introduction of contaminants, or additional time for the growth of bacteria. Medium-risk CSPs meet the following conditions:

- All ingredients and equipment used during preparation are sterile.
- Multiple individual or small doses for multiple patients or multiple doses for a single patient are prepared.
- Mixing is prolonged.
- Multiple transfers involving multiple ingredients are performed.
- Storage for:
  - 30 hours at room temperature
  - 9 days at refrigerated temperatures
  - 45 days at frozen temperatures
- A more challenging media fill test must be performed at least annually, but may be required more frequently by some institutions or whenever the controlled room supervisor determines that additional competency assessment is appropriate.

HIGH RISK

High-risk compounding generally is discouraged from a patient safety standpoint unless preparation of the formulation is critical to the patient's health and all steps may be safely and properly performed. High-risk CSPs meet the following conditions and descriptions:

- Nonsterile ingredients and/or equipment are used during transfer to final dispensing containers.
- Ingredients, devices, and mixtures are exposed to air quality at or below ISO Class 5.
- Nonsterile water is exposed for at least 6 hours before sterilization.
- Storage for:
  - 24 hours at room temp erature
  - 3 days at refrigerated temp eratures
  - 45 days at frozen temp eratures
- The most complicated media fill challenge is required at least biannually,

Aseptic Clean Room Processes

TOOLS OF ADMIXTURE: COMPOUNDING SUPPLIES

Let's take a look at several types of equipment used to prepare sterile products and learn how to use them to prepare these products aseptically.

Sterile drugs, which usually are stored in vials and ampules, must be removed aseptically before use. A syringe and needle are required for this manipulation. Needles are sharp, bevel-pointed instruments used to transfer liquid drawn into a syringe. They have six major components, all of which come in contact with the sterile drug and must be kept sterile:

- The bevel is the sharp pointed tip of the needle; the bevel is angled to prevent coring when it is inserted into a vial or ampule to withdraw a substance.
- The lumen is the hollow space inside the shaft of the needle.
- The heel is the flat, rounded end, opposite the bevel at the tip of the needle.
- The gauge is the diameter of the interior of the lumen; the larger the gauge, the smaller the opening.
- The hub is the transparent plastic casing used to attach the needle to the tip of the syringe.
- *Length* identifies how long the needle is from the tip to the hub and is used to determine the depth of the injection.

A standard needle allows free transfer of a sterile solution into a syringe. Needles may also be double ended with a plastic centerpiece; these are used to transfer drugs from one vial to another. Double-ended "transfer" needles may be handled only by the plastic centerpiece to prevent contamination of either end.

A vented needle contains air chambers that allow air to be released when inserted into a vacuum-packed sterile vial or large-volume glass container.

A needle known as a *spike* may be used as a stand-alone transfer device or may be found at the end of a solution transfer set or fluid administration set (spikes may be vented or nonvented).

A filter needle contains a microfilter that captures any particulates, preventing contamination of the syringe or bag to be injected. A filter needle's filter pores must be no longer than 5 microns to prevent the transfer of particulate matter. Filter needles are used to draw up solution from a glass ampule, and they must be used in only one direction (either to withdraw or to inject).

The syringe is the sterile container used to measure the amount of drug needed. Syringes come in many sizes, because IV preparers may be required to draw up different volumes of sterile drug. The syringe has three major components.

- The *tip* is used to attach the needle and is available in both Luer-Lok and slip tip forms. A Luer-Lok has threads for screwing and locking the needle into place. The slip-tip is just slipped onto the needle. The tip must be kept sterile.
- The barrel is used to measure the amount of sterile drug accurately. It is marked with *graduations* (lines), which indicate units of measurement, usually cc's (cubic centimeters) or ml's (milliliters).
- The plunger slides into and out of the barrel to manipulate the sterile substance. The inner core of the plunger must remain sterile.

Before drawing from or injecting into a sterile container, consider the following questions:

- Does the drug need to be filtered?
- Does the drug need to be protected from light?
- Will the drug be affected by glass or plastic?

The answers to these questions help determine the type of container into which the sterile drug will be injected and the equipment the IV preparer must gather before performing IV admixture. IV drugs that will be administered parenterally may be dispensed in a syringe or in a volume of IV solution. Small-volume IV solutions are available in 50- to 250-ml containers; large-volume solution containers may be 500 to 3,000 ml in volume. Sterile containers may be made from plastic or glass. The most appropriate dispensing container may depend on drug additive sorption (the drug attaches itself to the solution container), light sensitivity, or sensitivity to leaching (plastic bag molecules detach and disperse in the IV solution).

Plastic containers are the most widely used type; they are easier to handle, lighter in weight, less likely to break, and do not require air exchange. Most containers have an add port for adding medication to the container, and all containers have an administration port for connecting tubing for administration to the patient.

Glass containers are vacuum systems that require a vent to facilitate air exchange. They are less permeable than plastic and must have a source for air exchange, such as an internal vent straw, an external vented needle, or a vented administration set. They may be amber colored to protect the contents from light while still being transparent enough to allow inspection of the contents for particulates.

Solution and vial container closures may be made of latex rubber and must provide enough elasticity to be snug, yet spring back to close the needle hole after penetration.

Sterile vials and ampules may be colorless or amber colored, glass or plastic, and may contain either liquid or dry powder for reconstitution. Vials may be single-dose or multiple-dose containers.

- Single-dose containers: These are not reusable and do not contain a preservative. They are limited in size by the USP to 1,000 ml. All ampules are considered single-dose containers, because they cannot be resealed once opened.
- Multiple-dose containers: Per the USP requirements, these contain a preservative and an antibacterial agent. They are limited in size to 30 ml to limit the number of punctures to the container's closure.

Vials that contain preservatives and large concentrations of alcohol are considered multiple-dose containers, because they do not provide an environment that supports germs and bacteria.

Miscellaneous Devices

The IV preparer may use a variety of sterile devices during the admixture process.

- A tamper-resistant IV port seal is placed over the additive port of an IV bag or glass bottle to which sterile products have been added. The seal creates a protective barrier from external contaminants.
- Syringe caps are used to secure a drug that is dispensed in a syringe. The cap may be pushed on for slip-tip syringes or twisted on for Luer-Lok–tipped syringes.
- Syringe connectors are used to transfer sterile preparations aseptically from one syringe to another.
- Amber bags are used to protect a finished product from light during delivery and administration.
- Fluid dispensing systems are used to transfer fluid from large-volume containers to smaller containers for reconstitution or batch IV preparation.
- Recapping devices are used to safely recap a needle for reuse.
- Syringe filters, which are 0.2 micron, attach to the Luer-Lok tip of a syringe. They filter either solutions pulled into the syringe or those pushed out of the syringe into a sterile solution.
- Sharps containers are used to dispose of used IV needles, syringes, or any devices used in the preparation of sterile products that may pose a risk of injury or exposure to drug products if discarded in the standard garbage. Sharps containers must be stored on a stand or rolling cart and must be replaced when they are three-fourths full, to prevent needle sticks.

CODE OF CONDUCT IN LAFW AREAS

Pharmacy professionals who prepare CSPs in the clean room have 14 primary responsibilities (Table 19-4). Each of these responsibilities must be met through adherence to established practice standards before, during, and after aseptic admixture and during drug delivery. Behaviors in the controlled environment are all process-driven; processes create a standardized control that, when followed consistently, provides the same desired outcome. The following behaviors involve a specific process, in which the steps must be performed in a particular order:

- Aseptic hand washing
- Cleaning of the horizontal or vertical LAFW
- Cleaning of the BSC
- Aseptic preparation of drug vials
- Aseptic preparation of drug ampules

A general set of best practices must be followed before, during, and after the process of aseptic admixture. These key behaviors may be considered a code of conduct in the LAFW environment. These behaviors help IV preparers to best protect the integrity of the ISO Class 5 air quality within the hood and to minimize the risk of contaminants being introduced into the sterile preparations. The following practices should be observed at all times:

- Perform all manipulations within 6 inches of the edge of the work surface and no closer than 6 inches in front of the HEPA filter.
- Avoid actions such as coughing, laughing, and excessive talking in critical areas.
  - Avoid unnecessary motion to reduce air turbulence.
  - The LAFW should run continuously. If it is turned off, it must be run for at least 30 minutes to purge particles from the air in the hood's critical areas.

TABLE 19-4   **Key Responsibilities for Those Who Prepare CSPs**

1. Personnel are adequately skilled, educated, instructed, and trained to perform and document their functions.
2. Ingredients have their correct identity, quality, and purity.
3. Open or partially used containers are properly stored.
4. Water-containing non-sterile CSPs are sterilized within 6 hours.
5. Proper and adequate sterilization is used.
6. Components are clean, accurate, and appropriate.
7. Potential harm from added substances is evaluated prior to dispensing.
8. Appropriate packaging is selected for sterility and stability.
9. Compounding environment maintains the sterility or purity of items.
10. Labels are appropriate and complete.
11. Beyond-use dates are appropriate and based on valid scientific criteria.
12. Correct compounding procedures are used.
13. Deficiencies in compounding can be rapidly identified and corrected.
14. Compounding is separate from quality evaluations.

- Assemble all necessary supplies before beginning the compounding (e.g., vials, ampules, syringes, needles, filters, and IV bags).
- Once sterile manipulations have begun, every effort should be made not to exit the critical area until all admixtures have been completed.
- Only objects that are essential to the compounding of sterile preparations should be placed in the LAFW. (Do not use pens, highlighters, labels, bins, or calculators in the hood.)
- No food or drink is allowed in any area of the pharmacy where sterile products are mixed or stored.

ASEPTIC HAND WASHING

Aseptic hand washing is the process of washing skin surfaces of the hands and forearms, using an antimicrobial skin cleanser, in such a way that particulates and contaminants are removed from fingertip to elbow without recontamination during the hand washing process.

The following are three examples of effective antimicrobial solutions, along with their (1) range of activity; (2) response time (the time required to kill microorganisms); (3) bactericidal action (i.e., kills bacteria); and (4) bacteriostatic action (i.e., inhibits the growth of bacteria).

- 70% isopropyl alcohol
  - Excellent activity against gram-positive and gram-negative bacteria, including those that are multidrug resistant (e.g., methicillin-resistant *Staphylococcus aureus* [MRSA] and vancomycin-resistant *Enterococcus* spp. [VRE])
  - Requires a 1-minute scrub
  - Immediate response (denatures proteins)
  - Persistent (residual) activity: None
- *Iodine and iodophors*
  - 7.5% to 10% concentration preferred
  - Excellent activity against gram-positive, gram-negative, and spore-forming bacteria and also mycobacteria, viruses, and fungi
  - Must allow hands to air dry 2 to 3 minutes for optimal response
  - Persistent activity: 30 minutes to 6 hours
  - Can cause some skin irritation and/or discoloration, depending on the concentration of iodine. The combination of povidone (Betadine) and iodine promotes sustained release of iodine on the skin and reduces irritation.

- *Chlorhexidine gluconate* (CHG)
  - Excellent activity against gram-positive bacteria and enveloped viruses (e.g., herpes simplex virus [HSV], human immunodeficiency virus [HIV], cytomegalovirus [CMV], influenza, and respiratory syncytial virus [RSV])
  - Affinity for binding to the skin, resulting in bacteriostatic activity
  - Response time: 30 seconds
  - Persistent activity: Up to 48 hours
  - Concentrations of 4% or higher can cause skin irritation after frequent use
  - Because of its bactericidal and bacteriostatic properties, CHG (e.g., Hibiclens) is the product of choice and is used in most hospital pharmacies. CHG is packaged in bulk bottles or individual packages. The individual packages include a nail pick and a scrub pad or sponge soaked in the chlorhexidine solution. Many facilities use the individual packages, which are more hygienic and allow for the scrubbing action that must take place for proper aseptic hand washing.

Eight essential steps *must* be followed for proper aseptic hand washing.

Step 1: Remove ALL jewelry and roll up the sleeves *above* the elbow.
  - Acrylic or other forms of false fingernails and nail polish cannot be worn in the hood, because polish may easily chip off, and false nails may harbor bacteria, fungi, and other harmful contaminants.

Step 2: Turn on the water and adjust the temperature to lukewarm.
  - Adjust the stream of water to prevent unnecessary splashing.
  - Rinse the hands and forearms under the stream of water, taking care not to touch any sink fixtures.

Step 3: Using a sponge, apply a generous amount of the disinfecting solution to the fingertips. Use a fingernail pick to clean under the surface of each nail; then use a brush to scrub the surfaces of the fingernails.

Step 4: Use a sponge to apply disinfecting solution to the hands. All four surfaces of each finger should be cleaned by placing each finger in the center of the scrub brush and rotating in a circular motion. Be sure to include the surfaces of the palm and outer hand and between all the fingers.

Step 5: Use a sponge to apply disinfecting solution to the forearms, all the way up to the elbows. All four surfaces of the wrists and arms should be cleaned with the sponge, using a *circular motion*. A circular motion detaches and removes surface contaminants and particulates, such as hair and dead skin cells, from the textured surfaces of the skin. Because the goal is to remove contaminants up to the elbow region, *do not* rub the hands up and down between the elbow and wrist. Instead, begin at the wrist and work your way to the elbow.

Step 6: The hands should be rinsed in a vertical position, beginning with the fingertips and rinsing down to the elbows. This rinses contaminants past the elbow region and away from the hands. Make sure all soap residue is removed. It is important to take care not to touch any sink surfaces during the rinsing process, because this would recontaminate the skin.

Step 7: Leave the water running while drying all surfaces of the fingers, hands, and arms with clean, dry paper towels. Take care not to touch any part of the towel dispenser during the drying process.

Step 8: After all surfaces have been dried, discard the damp towels and use new, clean, dry paper towels to shut off the water faucets. Take care not to touch any of the sink fixtures with bare hands.

Final tips:
  - If an IV preparer has a cut or open wound on the hands or arms, the hands should be washed and dried, and then an adhesive bandage should be placed over the area. Gloves should be worn and washed.
  - Only CHG-compatible lotions may be used on the hands so that the residual bacteriostatic properties of the CHG are not neutralized.

CLEANING THE HORIZONTAL LAMINAR AIRFLOW HOOD

Once the hands have been cleaned and gloved, the horizontal or vertical LAFW must be properly cleaned. This reduces the risk of contaminants in the critical areas being introduced into sterile products. The following steps must be performed in order:

Step 1: Clear all items from the workspace. Assemble cleaning materials, such as gauze and isopropyl alcohol. Sterile water for irrigation may also be used to preclean surfaces to remove dried substances that are less alcohol-soluble (e.g., potassium or dextrose). Apply an ample amount of alcohol to the gauze, taking care not to splash it onto the back cover of the HEPA filter.

Step 2: Using the fresh gauze soaked with alcohol, clean the IV pole, using one motion to sweep the entire pole, left to right. Do not double back on any areas, which may recontaminate those surfaces. Discard the gauze upon completion.

Step 3: Using a fresh gauze and alcohol, clean the sides of the hood in a vertical motion, using overlapping strokes to cover the entire surface area. Discard the gauze after use.

Step 4: Using a fresh gauze and alcohol, clean the entire work surface, using overlapping horizontal strokes to cover the entire work surface area. Discard the gauze after use.

When cleaning of the aseptic hood is finished, the staff member should sign the hood cleaning log. The log must be initialed once per shift for initial cleaning. However, IV preparers should perform aseptic hood cleaning *any time* the surfaces of the LAFW have been contaminated and after prolonged batch fills. Also, splashes and spills should be cleaned immediately after aseptic admixture has been completed.

CLEANING THE VERTICAL LAMINAR AIRFLOW HOOD (BIOLOGIC SAFETY CABINET)

Four steps *must* be followed to clean a vertical LAFW (BSC) aseptically.

Step 1: Clear all items from the workspace. Assemble cleaning materials, such as gauze and isopropyl alcohol. Sterile water for irrigation may also be used to preclean surfaces to remove dried substances that are less alcohol-soluble (e.g., potassium and dextrose).

Step 2: Using clean, sterile gauze and 70% IPA, clean the IV pole first so that any contaminants fall to the bottom of the hood, to be cleaned last. Discard the gauze after use. The glass cover may need to be raised slightly so that all surfaces can be reached, but it should be lowered as soon as possible to prevent contaminants from entering.

Step 3: Using clean, sterile gauze and 70% IPA, clean the two sides, back wall, and inside of the glass shield from top to bottom, using overlapping strokes. Always remember to stop at the bottom of the hood, remove your hand from the surface, and start back at the top of the hood to avoid bringing contaminants back up to the HEPA filter. Discard the gauze after use.

Step 4: Using fresh gauze and 70% IPA, clean the bottom surface of the hood, starting from the back wall and working toward the front glass in a side-to-side motion with overlapping strokes. Be sure not to double back over strokes, which may recontaminate surfaces.

PREPARING FOR ADMIXTURE EXERCISES

Awareness of personal behavior in the clean room and following proper aseptic processes are among the best ways IV lab staff can minimize the risk of introducing contaminants into the controlled environment and the sterile products mixed in it.

A few preparatory steps are required before IV admixture is started. IV preparers must:

- Make sure that the LAFW has been properly cleaned.
- Verify that all information on the label is correct and perform any necessary dosage calculations.
- Gather all drugs to be compounded.
- Gather all equipment and supplies to be used in that IV admixture process.

Next, the IV preparer must verify that all information on the sterile solution label is correct. (Remember the five rights: right patient, right drug, right strength, right route, and right dose.)

Perform all necessary dosage calculations, label documentation, and auxiliary labeling. After all, there is no point to using proper aseptic technique if an incorrect product is selected or if the incorrect dose is injected into the IV solution. Verifying dosing first is necessary to determine how much drug must be gathered and prepared for mixing.

Completing label documentation helps the IV preparer assess what products may need to be prepared before others, based on stability, handling, or special preparation requirements.

The next step is to gather all sterile drugs and IV solutions that will be mixed and then to gather all the supplies needed to prepare the products. Essential items include:

- Alcohol swabs
- Needles (including filter needles if you will be opening ampules or preparing a drug that must be filtered)

- Syringes (gather the appropriate sizes based on the volume of solutions to be drawn)
- Vented needles/spikes
- IV piggyback bags or bottles or large-volume IV solutions

Once all items have been gathered, inspect each one individually.

- Make sure the packaging of the needles, syringes, and so on is not damaged.
- Inspect IV solutions for expiration date, clarity, leaks, or physical deformity. Verify a second time that the correct solution has been selected. Any damaged or expired items should be discarded and replaced.
- Inspect ampules and vials; check expiration dates and verify a second time that the correct product and strength have been selected.

ASEPTIC PREPARATION OF STERILE VIALS

Sterile vials typically are vacuum-sealed containers with some volume of either positive or negative air pressure. When preparing drugs from sterile vials, it is very important not to aspirate the vial (i.e., release air or drug particles or both).

Aspiration may result in:

- Loss of active drug during the release, which will affect the final concentration
- Contamination of the preparer (which could be dangerous if a cytotoxic or hazardous drug is being compounded)
- Damage to the HEPA filter

Several steps must be performed, in the proper order, to prepare a drug from a sterile vial.

Step 1: Remove the colored dust cover from the top of the vial.

Step 2: Swab the rubber diaphragm a few times in the same direction with a sterile alcohol swab and set it aside. Wait a few seconds for the alcohol to dry before entering the vial.

Step 3: Draw back the plunger of the needle to the volume of liquid to be withdrawn from the vial.

- Place the needle, bevel up, on the top of the rubber diaphragm to prevent coring. Keeping the needle at a 45-degree angle, apply enough pressure to enter the vial. Insert the needle all the way to the hub.

Step 4: Invert the vial, making sure the laminar airflow is not blocked.

- Use a milking technique to withdraw fluid: first draw fluid, then inject air into the vial. Repeat this process until air has been removed from the syringe and the appropriate volume of solution has been added.

Step 5: Before removing the needle from the vial, tap the syringe to remove air bubbles, then inject them back into the vial. Make sure the needle is kept below the level of the liquid so that air is not reintroduced into the syringe. Recheck the contents of the syringe before withdrawing it from the vial.

Step 6: To prevent spills, place the vial upright on the work surface before withdrawing the needle. This also helps prevent solution from being aspirated into the preparer's eyes.

Step 7: Use a scooping motion or an approved recapping device to replace the needle cap.

Step 8: For a powder vial: Remove the dust cover from the vial and swab the rubber diaphragm with a sterile alcohol swab.

Step 9: Uncap the needle and insert it properly into the vial to prevent coring. Use the milking process to add the diluent liquid to the powder vial, making sure the needle does not come in contact with the powder. To prevent aspiration, withdraw the same volume of air as liquid that was added to the vial. Aspiration can be detected by the hissing sound produced by air escaping when the needle is removed and by the spattering of liquid.

Step 10: Make sure the powder vial is flat on the work surface before removing the needle.

Step 11: Use a scooping technique or an approved recapping device to replace the needle cap. As long as no parts of the needle, syringe tip, or plunger have been contaminated, the syringe may be reused to withdraw the reconstituted liquid.

Step 12: Roll the powder vial between the palms of the hands and gently invert it up and down to dissolve the powder. Rolling creates friction and heat and usually dissolves the drug more quickly. *Never* shake the vial, because it generates bubbles or foam, which prevent detection of incompatibilities and withdrawal of reconstituted drug. In addition, certain drugs may break down during the action of shaking, another reason to avoid this practice altogether.

TECH ALERT!
Multiple-dose containers, although convenient, pose an increased risk of contamination as a result of multiple transfers. IV preparers must take meticulous care to ensure that they do not introduce contaminants into multiple-dose vials (MDVs) and that they store the prepared medications under the correct conditions to maintain the product's physical, chemical, and antimicrobial stability.

Step 13: Inspect the reconstituted fluid for particulate matter (e.g., coring), precipitates, or any other particulates that may form as a result of incompatibility.

Step 14: Swab the rubber diaphragm and allow the alcohol to dry.

ASEPTIC PREPARATION OF STERILE AMPULES

Sterile ampules must be opened carefully, in such a way as to minimize the risk of glass particles entering the ampule. Even tiny glass fragments could be very harmful if injected into a patient. Once an ampule has been broken open, it becomes an open system, which means that no physical barrier exists between the sterile contents of the container and the external hood environment. The contents should be drawn immediately, using proper aseptic technique, to minimize the risk of contaminants entering the ampule. Any unused portion must be discarded immediately after injection of the volume required for the admixture.

Some ampules may have a colored ring or a dot marking a point on the neck of the ampule that has been weakened or scored to allow for easier breakage.

Thirteen important steps must be performed for aseptic entry of and withdrawal from a sterile ampule.

Step 1: Tap the contents of the ampule out of the neck and hub.

Step 2: Clean the ampule's neck with a sterile alcohol swab.

Step 3: Depending on the size of the ampule, wrap a piece of sterile gauze or a fresh alcohol swab around the neck. An ampule breaking device, if available, may be used instead of gauze.

Step 4: Breaking the ampule:
- Hold the ampule below the neck with one hand (or position the ampule breaking device near the neck of the ampule) and place the thumb of the opposite hand above the neck.
- Applying pressure to the neck, use a quick, firm snapping motion to break the ampule neck at a 20-degree angle; this prevents glass from falling back into the ampule.
- During the snapping motion, aim the ampule toward the side of the hood, away from the yourself and the HEPA filter. Be sure to hold on to the ampule neck after breaking it to prevent it from falling from your hands.

Step 5: Assemble the syringe and filter needle or filter straw, making sure that neither the syringe tip nor the hub of the filter needle is contaminated. Have a regular needle set aside.

Step 6: Hold the ampule or position it on the work surface. Draw a little more than the desired quantity of fluid from the ampule.

Step 7: Carefully use a scooping technique or an approved recapping device to replace the needle cap.

Step 8: Remove the filter needle or straw and replace it with a standard needle. Glass may be trapped inside the outer needle filter and will not enter the syringe; fluid must be drawn in only one direction using the filter needle; therefore, the needle must be replaced with a standard needle after the medication solution is drawn from the ampule.

Step 9: Remove any air bubbles by lightly tapping and inverting the syringe. Pull down the plunger slightly before expelling bubbles to avoid spilling liquid onto the work surface or into the HEPA filter.

Step 10: Measure the desired volume of fluid and then shoot excess fluid back into the ampule. Be careful not to touch the top or side of the ampule with the needle.

Step 11: The additive port of the final container should be swabbed with a sterile alcohol swab before the contents of the syringe are injected into the container.

Step 12: Mix the contents of the container by squeezing the additive port and inverting the solution a few times. *Never* shake the solution, because this creates bubbles. Inspect the solution for signs of incompatibilities (e.g., particulate matter, cloudiness, discoloration, bubble formation).

Step 13: All glass fragments, needles, and sharps should be placed in a sharps container and all other waste disposed of appropriately.

An experienced, proficient IV technician may want to advance to the specialized processes for admixture of hazardous drugs. However, it is important that the IV preparer understand the risks involved in the admixture of such drugs.

Preparation, Storage, and Handling of Cytotoxic and Hazardous Drugs

WHAT ARE HAZARDOUS DRUGS?

Hazardous drugs are pharmaceutical products that have one or more of the following six characteristics:

- Carcinogenicity (causes cancer)
- Teratogenicity (damages a developing fetus)
- Mutagenicity (reproductive toxicity, impairs fertility)
- Organ toxicity at low doses
- Genotoxicity (damages deoxyribonucleic acid [DNA])
- Similarity in structure or toxicity to other hazardous drugs

WHAT IS CHEMOTHERAPY?

Chemotherapy is drug therapy used to destroy or control the growth of cancer cells. Chemotherapeutic drugs are among several products classified as hazardous drugs.

- Many chemotherapeutic drugs are cytotoxic (i.e., they kill the cells).
- These drugs stop cell division by interfering with DNA, ribonucleic acid (RNA), and protein synthesis and by inhibiting mitosis.

TYPES OF CHEMOTHERAPEUTIC DRUGS

- Drugs that interfere with DNA synthesis (cell cycle S-phase agents)
- Drugs that interfere with mitosis (cell cycle M-phase agents)
- Non-cycle-specific drug, including:
  - Antibiotics
  - Alkylating agents
  - Hormones
- For S-phase or M-phase drugs to work:
  - The tumor cell must be in the cell phase the drug is targeting.
  - The drug must reach the cancer cell.
  - The cell must not be resistant to the drug.

WHAT ARE THE RISKS ASSOCIATED WITH HAZARDOUS DRUG ADMIXTURE?

The risk of exposure is constant *whenever* chemotherapeutic drugs are handled, primarily because these drugs kill both cancer cells (cytotoxicity) and some healthy cells. Some chemotherapeutic drugs are *mutagenic,* causing changes in the reproductive material of a cell. These cell changes may result in cancer, miscarriage, and birth defects redundant.

Studies conducted on nurses who had handled chemotherapeutic drugs over a prolonged period revealed traces of a particular drug in their urine. Some chemotherapeutic drugs may be absorbed through the skin and possibly through the lungs. In general, exposure to chemotherapeutic drugs may occur through any of the following modes of transmission:

- Inhalation
- Absorption
- Ingestion
- Accidental injection

The possible side effects of exposure to hazardous drugs may include the following:

- Acute side effects from skin exposure to the drug, which may include skin irritation (rash), blistering, and/or discoloration
- Long-term side effects, which may include:
  - Cancer
  - Birth defects
  - Miscarriage

Measures for protecting preparers of hazardous drugs against exposure include:

- Good preparation and handling techniques
- Using a BSC for all preparation

- Using barrier protection to prevent exposure through inhalation, absorption, ingestion, or injection

Most pharmacies do not allow IV preparers to perform admixture of hazardous drugs until they have sufficient experience with standard admixture and have been properly trained. Female IV preparers who are pregnant, may become pregnant, or are breast-feeding are not allowed to perform admixture of chemotherapeutic drugs because of the exposure risks involved.

Once an IV technician has demonstrated proficiency and confidence with the admixture of standard sterile products, he or she may progress to the specialized processes required for admixture of dangerous drugs, such as chemotherapeutic drugs. Many of the steps in the admixture of hazardous drugs are very similar to those of standard IV admixture; however, a few key differences exist, all of which are directed at protecting the preparer against contamination with a hazardous drug.

- All processes must be performed in a negative-pressure BSC environment.
- IV preparers first must put on hazardous IV preparation PPE, which includes a thicker impervious gown; a respirator mask; and the thicker, sterile, extended-cuff hazardous drug preparation gloves. When putting on gloves, the preparer first puts on a pair that is tucked under the cuff of the gown; a second pair is put on over the first, with the cuff extending over the gown. This second pair provides added protection.
- Luer-Lok syringes are used in the mixing of chemotherapeutic drugs, because they are much less likely to separate than are friction (slip tip) fittings; this reduces the risk of leakage or spills.
- All surfaces inside the BSC should be considered contaminated, so care must be taken to avoid contact with any surface during the admixture process.
- The BSC should be disinfected as explained earlier in the chapter. In addition, the hood should be decontaminated at least once a week to deactivate any cytotoxic drug residue that may remain in the BSC workspace.
- All admixture processes must be performed on an absorbent mat, which captures any particles of hazardous drug released. Upon completion of the admixture process, the absorbent pad must be disposed of properly.
- Waste disposed of during the admixture process must remain contained.
  - A small sharps container should be kept inside the BSC for disposal of sharps during the admixture process.
  - A plastic hazardous drug waste bag must be placed inside the BSC area for disposal of all nonsharps waste during the admixture process.
- When the admixture process is complete, hazardous drug PPE must be removed and properly disposed of in a chemotherapy disposal container.
- A chemotherapy spill kit must be kept handy so that any spills of hazardous drugs may be contained. Spill kits include the following items:
  - Eye protection
  - Respirator mask
  - Protective gown
  - Protective gloves
  - Absorbent spill pillows
  - Absorbent cloths
  - Hand broom and dust pan
  - Warning sign to indicate a hazardous drug spill
  - Incident report form

A spill of less than 5 ml may be considered a small spill and may be cleaned up using a spill kit. The National Institute for Occupational Safety and Health (NIOSH) considers any spill greater than 5 ml to be a large spill, which must be handled by an appropriate team of professionals trained in the containment of large, hazardous material spills. The hospital's environmental services department must have a process in place for handling the containment, cleanup, and decontamination of areas and individuals involved in a hazardous materials drug spill.

ASEPTIC PREPARATION OF HAZARDOUS VIALS AND AMPULES

Each of the steps listed in the following sections must be performed as part of the process of hazardous drug preparation. More detailed information is provided during training courses for the admixture of chemotherapeutic drugs. The purpose of these sections is to present an overview of the process as performed in a BSC.

Hazardous Vial Preparation

Step1: Set up the BSC work surface after it has been properly cleaned. Place a plastic-lined absorbent pad on the work surface and then place items for admixture on the pad. Have a hazardous materials waste bag accessible in the BSC work area for discarding nonsharps waste during the compounding process. The IV solution bag should have been spiked with IV tubing and the tubing should have been primed before the start of the admixture process. Spiking the bag before adding the hazardous drug ensures that if the tubing leaks, it will only contain solution.

Step 2: Remove the dust cover from the top of the vial.

Step 3: Swab the rubber diaphragm a few times in the same direction with a sterile alcohol swab and set it aside. Wait a few seconds for the alcohol to dry before penetrating the vial.

Step 4: Draw back the plunger of the needle to the volume of liquid to be withdrawn from the diluent vial.

- Place the needle, bevel up, on the top of the rubber diaphragm, to prevent coring. Keeping the needle at a 45-degree angle, apply enough pressure to enter the vial. Insert the needle all the way to the hub.

Step 5: Invert the vial, making sure that your hand positions allow for free vertical airflow passage.

- Use a milking technique to withdraw fluid: first, draw fluid, then inject air into the vial. Repeat this process until air has been removed from the syringe and the appropriate volume of solution has been added. *This is the only step in hazardous drug preparation that involves milking, because no hazardous drug ingredients are involved.*

Step 6: Before removing the needle from the vial, tap the syringe to remove any air bubbles, then inject them back into the vial. Make sure the needle is kept below the level of the liquid so that air is not reintroduced into the syringe. Recheck the contents of the syringe before withdrawing it from the vial.

Step 7: Place the vial upright on the work surface before withdrawing the needle to prevent spills. This also helps prevent solution from being aspirated into the preparer's eyes.

Step 8: Use a scooping motion or an approved recapping device to replace the needle cap.

Step 9: Remove the dust cover from the powder vial and swab the rubber diaphragm with a sterile alcohol swab. Allow the alcohol to dry.

Step 10: Spike the hazardous drug vial with a chemotherapy dispensing pin, which vents the vial and eliminates the need for milking during the remainder of the admixture process. Remove the needle from the syringe containing the diluent and use a Luer-Lok to attach the syringe to the dispensing pin. Invert the vial, making sure not to block vertical airflow.

Step 11: Inject diluent into the vial; because the dispensing pin provides contained venting, the milking technique is not required. Carefully swirl the drug with the syringe attached to the dispensing pin until the drug has completely dissolved.

Step 12: Inspect the reconstituted fluid for particulate matter (e.g., coring), precipitates or any other particulates that may form as a result of incompatibility.

Step 13: Draw the reconstituted liquid and inject air back into the vial. Remove all air bubbles and recheck the final amount of fluid.

Step 14: Before removing the syringe from the dispensing pin, pull back on the plunger to evacuate any fluid from the syringe tip.

Step 15: Properly affix a needle to the syringe. Once the additive port of the IV solution container has been swabbed with a sterile alcohol swab, the drug may be injected into the container.

Step 16: Carefully inject the drug into the solution. Raise the needle so that it is above the fluid level and pull back on the plunger to evacuate the syringe tip before removing the needle. Place the needle and syringe in a sharps container without recapping.

Step 17: Use an alcohol prep pad to wipe the external surface of the additive port to remove any hazardous drug residue.

Step 18: Affix a foil seal over the additive port and affix a hazardous drug label to the solution bag. Clean the outer surfaces of the bag with IPA and sterile gauze.

TECH NOTE!
Do not use the same puncture point in a vial, because air and fluid may leak when the vial is inverted.

Step 19: Mix the contents of the solution by inverting the bag a few times. *Never shake the bag.* Inspect the bag for signs of incompatibilities (e.g., particulates, cloudiness, fluid discoloration, bubble formation).

Step 20: Place the admixture solution and attached tubing in a hazardous drug delivery bag and seal the bag.

Step 21: Place all materials used during the admixture process in the hazardous waste disposal bag in the BSC. Seal the bag and then place it in the external, larger chemotherapy waste bin.

Step 22: Remove the hazardous drug preparation PPE in the following order: outer gloves, gown, mask, bouffant cap, inner gloves. Perform aseptic hand washing.

HAZARDOUS AMPULE PREPARATION

Hazardous ampule preparation begins with the same setup process as for vials: place the materials on a plastic-lined absorbent pad, along with IV solution that has been spiked with tubing, which has been primed. The following steps are then performed.

Step 1: Tap the contents of the ampule out of the neck and hub.

Step 2: Clean the ampule neck with a sterile alcohol swab.

Step 3: Depending on the size of the ampule, wrap a piece of sterile gauze or a fresh alcohol swab around the neck. An ampule breaking device also can be used.

Step 4: Breaking the ampule:
- Hold the ampule below the neck with one hand (or position the ampule breaking device near the neck of the ampule) and place the thumb of the opposite hand above the neck.
- Applying pressure to the ampule neck, use a quick, firm snapping motion to break the neck at a 20-degree angle; this prevents glass from falling back into the ampule.
- During the snapping motion, aim the ampule toward the side of the hood, away from yourself. Discard the top in the sharps container.

Step 5: Assemble a syringe and filter needle or filter straw, making sure that neither the syringe tip nor the hub of the filter needle is contaminated. Have a regular needle set aside.

Step 6: Hold the ampule or position it on the work surface. Draw a little more than the desired quantity of fluid from the ampule, taking care not to block vertical airflow.

Step 7: Carefully use a scooping motion or an approved recapping device to replace the needle cap.

Step 8: Remove the filter needle or straw and replace it with a standard needle.

Step 9: Measure the desired volume of fluid.

Step 10: Because hazardous drugs must be kept contained at all times, excess drug and air must be injected into a sterile empty vial. After removing the dust cover from a sterile empty vial, clean the rubber diaphragm and allow the alcohol to dry.

Step 11: Insert the needle into the vial and invert. Inject excess air bubbles and fluid into the sterile empty vial. Check for proper drug measurement, then pull back on the plunger slightly to clear the needle hub before removing the needle from the vial. Use the proper scooping method to recap the needle.

Step 12: Wipe the additive port of the final container with a sterile alcohol swab before injecting the contents of the syringe. After injecting the hazardous drug, pull back on the plunger to clear the needle hub of solution before removing the needle.

Step 13: Mix the contents of the container by squeezing the additive port and inverting the solution a few times. Cover the additive port with a foil seal. *Never* shake the solution, because this creates bubbles. Inspect the solution for signs of incompatibilities (e.g., particulate matter, cloudiness, discoloration, bubble formation).

Step 14: Discard all glass fragments, needles, and sharps in the contained sharps container and dispose of all other waste in the chemotherapy waste bag. Dispose of the waste bag, along with the outer gloves, in an external chemotherapy waste bin.

Step 15: Remove your chemotherapy PPE in proper order, ending with the inner gloves, and discard it in the chemotherapy waste bin. Perform proper aseptic hand washing.

Sterilization Techniques

A product is sterile when it is free of foreign particulates and microbial contaminants. The process of sterilization is performed either to destroy microorganisms or to remove foreign particulates.

According to The Joint Commission, the safest and lowest risk methods of admixture are performed when containers, devices, and admixture ingredients are sterile from the beginning. However, if a container or an admixture ingredient is not sterile, the IV preparer can sterilize it. The three main forms of sterilization are:

- Filtration sterilization
- Chemical sterilization
- Heat sterilization, including depyrogenation

Filtration sterilization is the most commonly used form of sterilization in hospital pharmacies. Filters may range from 0.22 micron to 0.1 micron. Special filter needles, filter straws, or filter attachments are affixed to a sterile syringe, and the admixture solution is drawn through the filter into the syringe. As fluid passes through the filter, any microorganism 0.22 micron or larger is trapped in the filter. The filter is then removed, and the filter-sterilized solution may be injected into the final dispensing container.

The following steps should be performed for filtration sterilization:

1. Gather the necessary supplies (e.g., needle, syringes, alcohol swabs, filter devices).
2. Withdraw the fluid into a syringe, passing the fluid through the filter device.
3. Remove and discard the filter device.
4. Switch to a standard needle and inject or transfer the filtered solution into the IV solution bag or bottle or into the final storage container; place a cap or seal (or both) on the dispensing container as necessary.

Chemical, or *cold*, sterilization generally is performed in manufacturing and industry, when containers or products may not withstand moist or dry heat sterilization.

In some cases a solution in an appropriate glass container may be sterilized using either dry or moist heat. Heat sterilization generally is used to sterilize glass containers, including glassware used in the preparation of sterile pharmaceuticals, or glass dispensing containers (e.g., dropper bottles for sterile ophthalmic solutions).

Dry heat sterilization may be used to perform depyrogenation. Pyrogens must be destroyed at a much higher temperature than moist heat can supply. The industry standard for dry heat sterilization is 300°C for 3 to 4 minutes.

Moist heat sterilization, as is done in an autoclave, may be performed using the following steps:

1. Wrap glassware and other devices for sterilization in autoclave-safe paper or sleeves that can be sealed and secured.
2. Place the items in an autoclave and sterilize at 121°C with 15 psi of steam pressure for 15 minutes.
3. Wait until the steam exhaust valve registers zero before opening the autoclave door.

Sterilization packaging should allow for full penetration of the sterilizing agent and should prevent exposure of contents to particulate or microbial contamination after the sterilization process. Contents must be easily identifiable, and packages should be stored in an area where humidity and temperature are controlled (e.g., a clean room ante-area) to protect the sterility of the contents.

Parenteral Drug Stability and Storage Requirements

IV drugs may remain stable as long as they are stored and handled under the appropriate conditions. Drug stability can be defined in terms of any of five key factors:

- Chemical stability: The ability of the drug's active ingredients to maintain their chemical integrity and potency.
- Physical stability: The drug's ability to maintain its appearance, taste, and suspension or dissolution.
- Microbiologic stability: The drug's ability to resist microbial growth and maintain sterility.
- Therapeutic stability: The drug's ability to maintain its expected therapeutic effect.
- Toxicologic stability: The drug's ability to maintain its original nontoxic state.

A significant change in the 2008 revisions of USP <797> is the increase in the stability window for medium-risk, refrigerated CSPs, from 7 days to 9 days. For home health and home infusion pharmacy practices, this allows IV preparers more time for shipment of a week's supply of drug to a facility or a patient's home. Once received, the patient has a full 7-day supply of IV drugs that may be safely stored under refrigerated conditions.

The revisions also limit the use of single-dose vials (SDVs), because the contamination risks for these containers have been a long-standing industry issue. The new guidelines allow for only 6 hours of BUD on a SDV that has been entered with a needle or other transfer device.

Depending on the type of injectable drug, special requirements may be a factor. Pharmaceutical drug references provide descriptions of the physical and chemical properties of injectable drugs, the ways they should be handled and prepared, and compatibility and stability information. Such references include:

- *Trissel's Handbook on Injectable Drugs*
- *Remington's Guide to Pharmaceutical Sciences*
- *King's Guide to Parenteral Admixtures*

These drug references provide key information about the types of products that may be mixed together, the types of IV solutions in which various drugs remain sterile when mixed, and drug-drug and drug-solution incompatibilities. The following types of drug storage and/or administration conditions may be necessary to preserve the physical, chemical, microbiologic, and therapeutic stability of CSPs while minimizing the risk of toxicity:

- Filter before administration
  - Some drugs may be stored in containers for which filtration may be necessary (e.g., ampules) or in which crystallization is an issue and filtration is necessary to ensure the patient's safety.
- Refrigeration
- Warming
  - Some drugs (e.g., mannitol) may revert to a partially crystallized form at room temperature and must be stored under warm conditions to maintain dissolution.
- No refrigeration
  - Some drugs become unstable and precipitate when refrigerated and must be stored at room temperature.
- Normal saline (NS) or dextrose 5% in sterile water (D_5W) for injection only
  - Some drugs may be incompatible with certain solutions or diluents, or the manufacturer may recommend a specific solution.
- Glass dispensing container
  - Some drugs may bind to the plasticizers in polyvinyl chloride containers, so they must be dispensed in glass containers to preserve the therapeutic stability of the CSP.
- Protection from light
  - Some drugs may physically or chemically degrade after prolonged exposure to light, particularly fluorescent lighting. Such products must be stored in dark- (often amber) colored containers or dispensed in a dark-colored bag that must remain in place during IV administration.
- Storage in the original container
  - Some products (e.g., oral nitroglycerin) may degrade or become unstable when removed from their original containers.

Care must be taken to follow the proper storage requirements to protect the integrity of CSPs. Most pharmacies post compound storage and stability charts for IV preparers to use, and that information should be kept current by the area supervisor or manager. It is important that IV preparers *never* work from memory in drug preparation; they must always consult the necessary references for the most current product stability information.

Creating and Assuring Quality in the Controlled Environment

QUALITY CONTROL

Quality control (QC) is the process established in a controlled environment to ensure that all regulations and procedures are followed in the preparation of CSPs. Quality assurance (QA) measures the effectiveness of the QC process.

- QC requires that all personnel complete prescribed training and competency assessments before they are approved to prepare patient doses
- QC also requires that all drug ingredients, compounding supplies, and equipment be verified for identity, sterility, and beyond-use date and have certificates of analysis or safety inspections.

The structure of the controlled environment and standard operating procedures (SOPs) for IV drug preparers should minimize the risk of contaminants being introduced into CSPs. To determine that environmental controls, such as HEPA filtration, are performing as expected, air sampling in the controlled environment must be conducted continually, based on the risk levels of the compounding performed in that environment.

All equipment must be capable of operating correctly. A written SOP must detail:

- An outline of the required equipment calibration
- Annual maintenance
- Monitoring for proper function
- Controlled procedures for use
- Time frames for usual activities
- Routine maintenance and frequency

Equipment calibration and maintenance reports must be kept on file for the lifetime of the equipment.

HIGH-RISK COMPOUNDING INGREDIENTS

Because of the risky nature of nonsterile ingredients, each nonsterile ingredient must be inspected for the following:

- Breaks in the container
- Loose-fitting cap or closure
- Deviation from the expected physical appearance
- Deviation from the expected aroma
- Deviation from the expected physical texture
- Evidence of physical or chemical deterioration

All ingredients must be stored under the most appropriate temperature, humidity, and lighting conditions.

- The beyond-use date is *1 year* from the date opened unless the manufacturer indicates otherwise.
- *All* high-risk CSPs are subject to sterility and pyrogen testing.

QUALITY CONTROL FOR VERIFICATION OF COMPOUNDED STERILE PRODUCTS

The following must be verified by a pharmacist before a CSP is dispensed or delivered:

- Prescription order
- Compounding procedure (written)
- Preparation records
- Expended materials used to make the CSP
- Aseptic mixing and sterilization techniques
- Accuracy and correct identities and amounts of ingredients
- Proper packaging and labeling
- Inspection of physical appearance against white/black surface for particulate contamination
- Checking of container and closure integrity
- Checking for leaks

DETERMINING ENVIRONMENTAL MONITORING PLAN IN THE CONTROLLED ENVIRONMENT

Any facility involved in the preparation of CSPs must have a plan for the types of environmental sampling and monitoring to be done. This is based largely on the risk level or levels of the compounding done at that facility.

The following list presents each of the key requirements of the environmental monitoring plan in terms of *what*, *when*, and *how*—that is, what the monitoring plan is; how often monitoring must be performed (by risk level); and how the monitoring is accomplished, including the types of materials or testing supplies required.

- What
  - Includes barrier isolators, hoods, clean room, and anteroom areas
- When
  - Monthly for low and medium risk
  - Weekly for high risk
- How
  - Electric air samplers (instead of passive agar plates), which actively measure established volumes of air; 48 hour incubation of samples
  - Hoods and isolators checked every 6 months and recertified (recertification is required if hoods are moved)

BUFFER/CLEAN ROOM MONITORING (ALSO KNOWN AS RECERTIFICATION OF THE CLEAN ROOM)

- What
  - Verify the approved structure, equipment, and supplies
    - No sinks or drains
    - No removal of equipment except for maintenance or repair
    - Verify structural integrity of clean room areas
- When
  - Annually
- How
  - Generally performed by an outside or contracted bioengineering company or laboratory

CLEANING/SANITIZING

- What
  - Cleansing of all surfaces within the clean room and ante-areas
- When
  - Daily
    - Remove all items and apply sanitizing agent
  - Weekly
    - Clean and sanitize ante-areas
  - Monthly
    - Clean areas attached to and adjacent to clean room areas, including shelving, walls, and ceilings, using approved cleansing agents
- How
  - Using approved sponges, mops, and wipers that are nonshedding and designated for exclusive use in buffer/clean room areas

AIR SAMPLING

- What
  - Test ISO Class 5, 7 and 8 areas according to established testing plan
  - Must include doorways or areas with significant air turbulence or that present opportunities for contamination
- When
  - Every 6 months
- How
  - Generally using growth medium to test for bacterial contamination
    - May use devices such as Bio-Culture, BACTair, airIDEAL, or Sampl'air
    - Incubate samples for 5 to 7 days
  - Test for the following acceptable colony-forming unit (CFU) levels/m^3 of air:
    - ISO 5 >1
    - ISO 7 >10
    - ISO 8 >100

SURFACE SAMPLING
- What
  - Surfaces in ISO Class 5, 7 and 8 environments
- When
  - Monthly for low and medium risk
  - Weekly for high risk
- How
  - Using agar plates or swabs

FINGERTIP SAMPLING
- What
  - 10% of fingertips of staff gloves
- When
  - Weekly for low and medium risk
  - Daily for high risk
- How
  - Using agar plates

EDUCATION AND TRAINING FOR CONTROLLED AREA STAFF MEMBERS

All personnel involved in the compounding of CSPs must prove their competence, as evidenced by the production of products free of contaminants (infecting agents or particulates). This begins with proper training, after which a hands-on skill demonstration must be performed.

Even if IV technicians complete an IV certification course, they must comply with each hospital pharmacy organization's process for validating competence before they are allowed to prepare doses for patients.

Gowning and gloving are among the most important measures for staff assessment, because direct touch contamination is the most common method of introducing infectious agents into CSPs by IV lab personnel.

How Is Proper Gowning and Gloving Assessed?

- At least three gloved fingertip samplings are performed before CSP compounding is allowed for "live" doses.
- Sterile agar touch plates are used *after* personnel have completed a media fill challenge appropriate for the type of compounding performed at their facility.
- Frequent and repeated disinfection of gloves with sterile 70% isopropyl alcohol during compounding processes should be encouraged.
- The preparer's competence must be assessed for each admixture procedure, including:
  - LAFW cleaning and behavior in the ISO Class 5 environment
  - Sterile vial preparation
  - Sterile ampule preparation
  - Sterile hazardous vial preparation
  - Sterile hazardous ampule preparation

The media fill challenge is designed to simulate the most challenging and stressful conditions encountered by IV admixture personnel.

ASSESSMENT RESULTS

Mistakes, complacency, and poorly structured processes occur. When they do, action must be taken by controlled area management or supervisors to correct them in a timely manner. If sampling results reflect an increase in air, surface, or glove contamination levels, the pharmacy facility must take corrective action, such as:
- Reevaluation of the adequacy of personnel work practices
- Reevaluation of cleaning procedures
- Reevaluation of operational procedures

- Evaluation of HEPA filtration in ISO Class 5, 7, and 8 areas
- Investigation into the type and source of contamination
- Determination of whether the sources of problems have been eliminated
- Cleaning of the affected area or areas
- Resampling
- Review of hand hygiene and garbing competence (may require more staff training)

IV Admixture Calculations

A crucial part of the admixture process is accurate dosage calculation. For proper dosage calculation, the IV preparer must:
- Read the label several times and verify the accuracy of the information
- Verify that the dosage is correct. (Through their work, IV technicians gain a sense of the normal therapeutic dosage ranges, so they can alert a pharmacist if a dosage is well above or below the common range.)
- Determine how much drug must be pulled from stock for the preparation, depending on package size
- Better prioritize tasks by beginning work on doses that require more admixture and that may be prepared sooner than those that require few manipulations

An IV preparer must determine two important facts before beginning the admixture process:
- The strength of the active ingredient (or ingredients) that must be measured
- The volume of the active ingredient (or ingredients) that must be measured and injected into the final container

The primary mathematical equation for IV admixtures is the ratio/proportion calculation. Calculation problems should be set up with the same units of measurement in the same positions on both sides of the equation to ensure that the dose is calculated correctly.

POWDER DRUG CALCULATION

With a lyophilized powder drug, a sterile diluent (e.g., sterile water) must be added to the powder to produce the additive solution. The IV preparer should check the package size to determine how much fluid may be added to the vial for proper reconstitution. The most common size for drug additive vials is 10 ml; some may be 20 ml, and 30 ml is the maximum volume. Some powder vials also are supplied in multiple-dose sizes (e.g., 100 ml or 200 ml). This allows for a larger volume of drug, which may be used to compound multiple doses of the drug. A liquid IV drug is expressed in terms of weight over volume.

Example: Many antibiotics are dosed in grams. If an IV preparer prepares a 1-g vial of cefazolin that is packaged in a 10-ml vial, the content of the reconstituted vial would be expressed as 1 g/10 ml or

$$\frac{1\ g}{10\ ml}$$

If the entire gram is to be dispensed, it should be expressed in the next smaller unit, which is milligrams. Because 1 g has 1,000 mg, the content of the reconstituted vial is expressed as

$$\frac{1,000\ mg}{10\ ml}$$

If the dose to be dispensed is 800 mg, the following ratio/proportion calculation is performed:

$$\frac{1,000\ mg}{10\ ml} = \frac{800\ mg}{x\ ml}$$

Perform cross-multiplication:

$$(x\ ml)\ (1000\ mg) = (800\ mg)\ (10\ ml)$$

$$x\ ml = (800\ mg)\ (10\ ml)\ /\ (1000\ mg)$$

$$x\ ml = 8$$

Isolate the unknown *(x)* by dividing each side of the problem by 1,000:

$$8 = x$$

Then, check to make sure the proportion is balanced:

$$\frac{1,000 \text{ mg}}{10 \text{ ml}} = \frac{800 \text{ mg}}{8 \text{ ml}}$$

The preparer should draw 8 ml aseptically from the vial and inject it into the dispensing container.

Drugs manufactured as liquids do not have to be reconstituted; ratio and proportion calculation is used to determine the volume of liquid to be injected into the dispensing container.

Example: An IV preparer receives a label for clindamycin, 180 mg in NS100. Clindamycin is dispensed in vials of 30 mg/ml; therefore, ratio and proportion calculation can be used to determine the volume of solution to be drawn.

$$\frac{30 \text{ mg}}{1 \text{ ml}} = \frac{180 \text{ mg}}{x \text{ ml}}$$

Perform cross-multiplication:

$$180 = 30x$$

Isolate the unknown *(x)* by dividing each side of the problem by 30.

$$6 = x$$

Then, check to make sure the proportion is balanced:

$$\frac{30 \text{ mg}}{1 \text{ ml}} = \frac{180 \text{ mg}}{6 \text{ ml}}$$

The preparer should draw 6 ml aseptically from the vial and inject it into the dispensing container.

PERCENTAGE STRENGTH CALCULATION

A medication order may require admixture of a particular percentage strength of a solution, or an IV preparer may need to know how much active drug is contained in a solution based on its percentage strength. Those who compound CSPs must know that any percentage strength is an expression of the number of grams per 100 ml of solution. Therefore, a drug with a percentage strength of 5% may be expressed as 5 g per 100 ml of solution.

Percentage strengths also may be expressed as decimals, by moving the decimal point two positions to the left to indicate that the percentage is an expression of hundredths. Therefore, 5% may be expressed as 0.05 g/ml.

Example

An IV preparer receives an order for dextrose 2.5% in water. This dose may be expressed in fraction form as:

$$\frac{2.5 \text{ g}}{100 \text{ ml}}$$

If the total solution volume is known, the amount of active ingredient needed can be calculated by using a ratio/proportion calculation.

MIXING STANDARD AND NONSTANDARD INTRAVENOUS SOLUTIONS

Active drugs can be added to a variety of parenteral solutions. Solutions are categorized, stocked, and labeled according to the percentage strength of their ingredients. IV solutions generally are concentrations of sodium chloride, dextrose, or lactated Ringer's solution. Standard solutions have been determined to have a pH and tonicity (balance of dissolved particles in a solution) similar to those of human blood plasma. Red blood cells (RBCs) and other blood constituents are suspended in plasma, and the RBCs themselves contain fluid. Introduction of a solution into the bloodstream can have one of three effects:

- Isotonicity: The solution has a pH and tonicity similar to those of blood; therefore, no movement of fluid occurs across the membranes of the RBCs.
- Hypertonicity: The solution has a higher concentration of dissolved ingredients than does blood; therefore, fluid is drawn out of the RBCs, causing them to shrink and increasing the plasma fluid volume.
- Hypotonicity: The solution has a lower concentration of dissolved ingredients than does blood; therefore, fluid flows across the RBC membranes, resulting in swelling and bursting of the RBCs.

Either hypotonicity or hypertonicity can pose a health risk to a patient; therefore, it is important that solutions be maintained as isotonic as possible so that little or no movement of water into or out of the RBCs occurs.

The standard isotonic solution of sodium chloride is 0.9%. This concentration strength is also known as *normal saline,* because it is equivalent to the "normal" tonicity and pH of blood plasma. The standard isotonic dextrose solution is 5%. Dextrose is mixed with sterile water in IV solutions, so IV solutions of dextrose generally are expressed as D_5W, or dextrose 5% in sterile water for injection. In terms of percentage concentration, D_5W contains 5 g of dextrose per 100 ml of solution. NS contains 0.9 g of sodium chloride per 100 ml of solution.

In certain cases a nonstandard hypotonic solution of sodium chloride or dextrose may be required. Often a patient may need one half or one fourth of the standard concentration. In such cases, the IV preparer adds concentrated dextrose or sodium chloride to a volume of sterile water for injection. Because of the risk of damage to RBCs, extreme care must be taken in preparing hypotonic or hypertonic solutions.

Chapter Summary

- Pharmacy IV preparation is strictly controlled by the regulations established by USP Chapter <797>.
- Pharmacy technicians who prepare IV solutions must know the five key areas of regulation in USP <797>:
  - The environment in which sterile preparations are prepared
  - The personal protective equipment that is used in that environment
  - The procedures for admixture of various types of sterile preparations
  - Quality assurance provisions that help regulate controlled environments and those who prepare CSPs
  - Quality assurance measures for assessing the amount of airborne and surface contaminants in the controlled environment despite the preventive procedures and controls in place.
- Pharmacy technicians who work in a controlled environment must make sure they perform the proper processes and follow the guidelines that maintain the integrity of the controlled environment. The fewer the airborne and surface contaminants, the lower the risk of those contaminants entering an IV solution.
- An effective means of controlling airborne contamination in the clean room is the use of PPE by IV preparers.
- CSP preparers should apply IPA to their gloves before beginning the compounding process and intermittently during the process.
- Aseptic hand washing must be performed after head and shoe covers have been put on. When hand washing is finished, the gown and gloves may be put on.
- PEC equipment must be run continuously and must be cleaned frequently to minimize contamination risks.
- Pharmacy technicians who are IV preparers must be knowledgeable about the handling of products at each of the three risk levels.
- Needles and syringes are the primary tools used during IV admixture. However, IV preparers should be knowledgeable about the many varieties of equipment and supplies used during the compounding process.

- Factors such as filtration, light sensitivity, and chemical properties influence the types of materials a preparer may gather before beginning the process of IV admixture.
- Quality assurance in the controlled environment consists of a variety of policies and procedures that constitute the best practices to ensure maintenance of the controlled environment and the absence of contamination of products prepared in it.
- Environmental monitoring allows those responsible for clean room areas to ensure that clean room controls are being maintained appropriately and that those who prepare CSPs do so only after proper training and periodic assessment of their skill level.
- A crucial step in IV admixture is accurate dosage calculation. Proper dosage calculation is critical to the patient's health when solutions of a nonstandard concentration must be compounded.
- The most important reason for USP <797> standards, in light of multiple contamination risks, is to protect the health, welfare, and safety of patients receiving parenteral drugs prepared by pharmacists and pharmacy technicians in a hospital, for home infusion, or in a nursing home.

REVIEW QUESTIONS

Multiple Choice

1. The skill of preparing IV solutions in a manner that prevents introduction of contaminants is referred to as:
   a. Sterile compounding
   b. Aseptic admixture
   c. Pharmaceutical compounding
   d. Sterile mixing

2. The component of a syringe that is used to measure accurately the amount of the sterile drug is the:
   a. Plunger
   b. Syringe tip
   c. Barrel
   d. Flange

3. The area in a controlled environment where sterile pharmaceuticals are prepared must be maintained under the conditions of ISO Class:
   a. 5
   b. 6
   c. 7
   d. 8

4. A term used for the ability of a product to maintain its expected medicinal effect is:
   a. Therapeutic
   b. Toxicologic
   c. Microbiologic
   d. Physical

5. Multiple-dose containers are limited to a maximum volume capacity of:
   a. 10 ml
   b. 30 ml
   c. 50 ml
   d. 100 ml

6. The agency that alerts health organizations to risks related to the handling of hazardous drugs is:
   a. NIOSH
   b. OSHA
   c. USP
   d. ISO

7. Low-risk compounds with a short BUD may be stored at room temperature for:
   a. 1 hour
   b. 8 hours
   c. 12 hours
   d. 24 hours

8. The air in the containment area should be purged, at least between preparations to remove any airborne contaminants, for:
   a. 1 minute
   b. 3 minutes
   c. 5 minutes
   d. 10 minutes

9. Concentrations of 4% or higher can cause skin irritation with frequent use of this cleanser:
   a. IPA
   b. Chloroxine
   c. Iodine
   d. CHG

10. The part of the LAFW that must be cleaned first is the:
    a. IV pole
    b. Sides
    c. HEPA filter
    d. Work surface

TECHNICIAN'S CORNER

1. Name the types of objects that are not allowed in the ISO Class 5 environment.
2. How is airflow controlled in the clean room environment?
3. Explain why compounding ingredients, devices, and supplies should be gathered before beginning aseptic admixture in an ISO Class 5 environment.

Bibliography

American Society of Health-System Pharmacists. (2007). *The ASHP Discussion Guide on USP <797> for Preparing Sterile Preparations*. Baltimore: The ASHP.

Ansel, H., Allen, L., Popavich, N. (1999). *Pharmaceutical Dosage Forms and Drug Delivery Systems*, 7th Edition. Philadelphia: Lippincott Williams & Wilkins.

Baxa Corporation. (2007). *Overview of USP General Chapter 797: Pharmaceutical Compounding—Sterile Preparations*. Retrieved 9/12/2011, from www.baxa.com/resources/docs/technicalPapers/USP797Overview.pdf

Grifols, U.S.A. (2011, March). *New and Noteworthy: Pass-Through Clean Room Carousel*. Retrieved 9/11/2011, from www.pppmag.com/new_noteworthy/?noteid=292

Hurst, M. (2008). *USP Chapter <797>: Understanding the Revisions—Technical Paper*. Retrieved 9/12/2011, from www.baxa.com/resources/docs/technicalPapers/USP797Revisions.pdf

Lasco Services. (2011). *USP 797 Compliant Clean Rooms: Why a Pharmaceutical Clean Room*. Retrieved 9/13/2011, from www.lascoservices.com/usp-797-cleanroom.html

PathCon Laboratories. (2009). *The Microbial Bioburden of USP 797 Compliance: Simplifying Environmental Quality and control Practices*. Retrieved 9/12/2011, from www.pathcon.com/documents/MB_USP_797.pdf

20 Green Pharmacy Practice

LiAnne Webster and Mark Floyd

LEARNING OBJECTIVES

By the end of this chapter, students will be able to competently:

1. Define sustainable healthcare culture.
2. Explain the risks of pharmaceuticals in the environment (PIE).
3. Describe green pharmacy practice within both the community and hospital pharmacy practice settings.
4. Briefly describe key components of green certification in the pharmacy practice.
5. Provide examples for energy conservation in the pharmacy and health care environments.
6. Describe how industry impacts PIE and how drug manufacturers can drive positive change.

KEY TERMS

Green pharmacy practice: Focuses on the utilization of resources that allow for the proper handling and processing of expired pharmaceuticals.

Sustainable health care culture: A healthcare environment in which production and processes optimize opportunities for the reduction of consumables that end up in landfills, the reuse of products when therapeutically appropriate and allowable by law, and the recycling of consumable materials whenever possible.

Introduction

Among the key goals of many health care organizations is the implementation of processes that optimize patient care while controlling costs. Additionally, the health care industry has taken strides toward creating a culture of environmental sustainability. Everything that we as human beings need is dependent—whether directly or indirectly—upon our natural environment. As defined by the Environmental Protection Agency (EPA), sustainability creates and maintains the conditions under which humans and nature can exist in productive harmony, that permit fulfilling the social, economical, and other requirements of present and future generations...[and] is important to making sure that we have and will continue to have, the water, materials, and resources to protect human health and our environment.

A sustainable health care culture is one that emphasizes the reduction of consumables that end up in landfills, the reuse of products when therapeutically appropriate and allowable by law, and the recycling of consumable materials whenever possible. Specifically, green pharmacy practice focuses on the utilization of resources that allow for the proper handling and processing of expired pharmaceuticals. The EPA has set forth a variety of guidelines pertaining to the disposal of both hazardous and nonhazardous waste materials in the health care environment. Additionally, it is important that members of the health care and pharmacy team practice behaviors that reduce the pharmaceutical waste that pollutes our local environment and the groundwater supplies that are fed by area lakes, rivers, and streams. This goal can be accomplished by educating and training staff on the proper handling and disposal of pharmaceuticals in patient care areas.

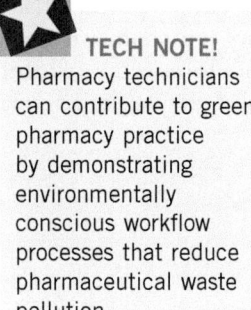

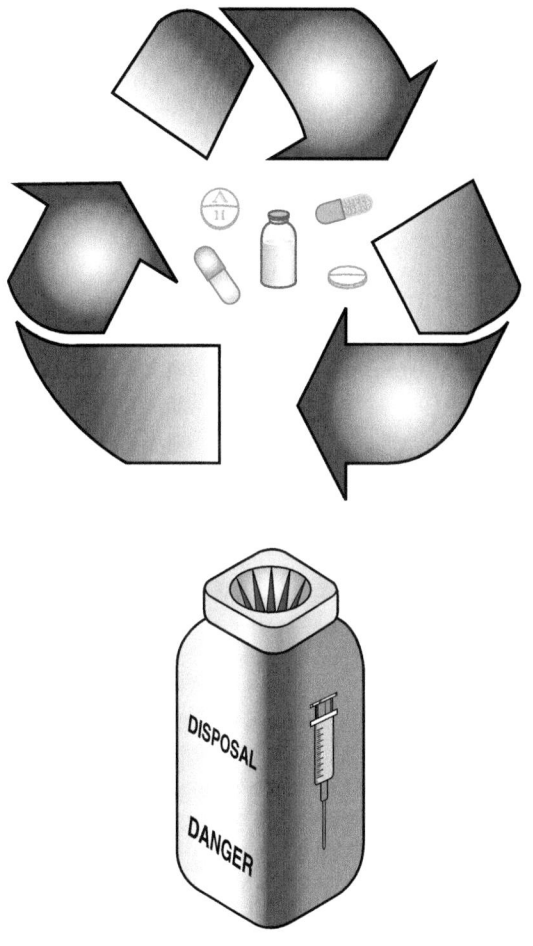

Pharmaceuticals in the Environment (PIE)

The overprescribing and overuse of pharmaceuticals by humans is a global problem that is challenging, particularly when pharmaceuticals are among the most cost-effective forms of preventive medicine. The human body excretes drug metabolites that are flushed through sewage systems and may leach contaminants into groundwater supplies via rivers, lakes, and streams. The improper disposal of expired or unused medication remains an ongoing consumer issue. This local and global concern is sometimes referred to as PIE, or pharmaceuticals in the environment. Prescription and over-the-counter (OTC) medication is left over in the medicine cabinets of almost every home in the United States. Consumers who do not know how to properly dispose of expired or unused pharmaceuticals may end up flushing them down the toilet or throwing them in the trash—thus creating a significant environmental impact over time. One of the gravest social concerns of unused or expired drugs is the risk of access and abuse by children and young adults. The abuse of OTC and prescription drugs by youth in America has both social and economic implications in the local and regional economies, particularly in the case of overdose that leads to the untimely death of a child. This chapter examines how green pharmacy practices can be established in both community and hospital pharmacy practice settings and how pharmacists and pharmacy technicians can better inform the public on the prevention of waste and pollution that occurs as a result of the improper disposal of pharmaceuticals.

Green Pharmacy in Community and Hospital Practice Settings

Green pharmacy practice in a community setting is measured by the ability of both independent and corporate pharmacy organizations to reduce pharmaceutical waste, educate consumers on the importance of proper disposal of medications, and provide them a solution by setting up medication take-back programs. This involves in-house training of pharmacy staff on the behaviors that encompass green pharmacy practice, as well as information that should be communicated to patients. There are many opportunities for incorporating green practices into a pharmacy organization that are largely underutilized and far from mainstream practice. The profession of pharmacy may further advance its organizations' sustainability by partnering with vendors that utilize green manufacturing processes, as well as:

* Recyclable printer paper/labels
* Recyclable drug storage containers
* Energy-efficient lighting
* Use of technology in a way that conserves energy
* Construction of pharmacies using globally sustainable materials

Green pharmacy in a hospital setting is measured by the ability of the department of pharmacy to become a more sustainable operation through education and training of green pharmacy practices such as:

* Purchasing of more green products
* Setting up recycling programs for glass, plastic, and paper products
* Ordering supplies from manufacturers that provide these types of products and are geared more toward sustainability

Although sustainability within the hospital environment is generally approached at the organizational—rather than departmental—level, each department may certainly do its part in increasing green awareness and integrating sustainable processes into daily operations.

What Is Green Certification?

Community pharmacies may obtain green certification through certifying agencies such as Eco-Path Texas, Leadership in Energy and Environmental Design (LEED), or Green Globe, to name a few. A green pharmacy certification focuses primarily on the reduction of pharmaceutical waste through medication take-back programs. Of course, there are a multitude of opportunities to expand an organization's overall culture of sustainability while maintaining compliance with state laws and regulations. This process often involves appointing a qualified expert or consultant who will spearhead an ongoing project and be responsible for its implementation. A green consultant would perform a baseline assessment of a pharmacy organization's operations and from that assessment identify potential cost savings, recommend green practices that could be reasonably implemented across the organization, and provide recommendations on how that organization can obtain certification through a third party. According to Mark Floyd, current regional president of the Lone Star chapter of the U.S. Green Chamber of Commerce, "a more effective and profitable process would focus on the triple bottom line of People, Profit and Planet." This requires both leaders and staff within an organization to approach the operations and daily practice of pharmacy through an *environmental lens*. Opportunities to expand an organization's culture of sustainability include the following:

* Optimizing energy efficiency
* Utilizing green cleaning and other environmental services
* Establishing green inventory management processes
* Offering ongoing staff *green awareness* training
* Instituting robust recycling programs
* Transitioning to paperless processes whenever possible
* Using alternative energy sources, such as sunlight or wind power

ACHIEVING GREEN THROUGH ENERGY CONSERVATION

Energy conservation is one measure that may reduce the overall carbon footprint of an organization and can be accomplished through any of the following measures:

* Proper maintenance of heating, ventilation, and air conditioning (HVAC) and pharmaceutical equipment
* Use of power strips to reduce phantom load (excess energy used to power up)
* Use of water-conserving fixtures and commodes
* Use of motion sensors for lighting fixtures and sinks

- Use of energy-efficient fluorescent or LED lighting
- Use of programmable thermostats
- Purchase of ENERGY STAR approved appliances and equipment
- Development of the practice of powering off desktop computers at the end of the work day or utilizing an energy-saving mode
- Reduction of unnecessary printing by using electronic fax, double-sided printing, and so on

Seeking Solutions to the Impact of PIE

TECH NOTE!
Pharmacy technicians can educate patients concerning programs such as medication take-backs that allow for the recapture of unused and expired medication and encourage consumer recycling of paper, plastic, and glass.

The environmental impact of pharmaceutical care continues to be monitored and measured as innovation progresses. The true impact may not be known for years, as with most of the environmental pollution that we encounter. Environmental data collection is necessary to quantify/measure all of the pharmaceuticals (i.e., medications, personal care products, residuals from humans and animals) that enter our lakes, rivers, and streams and is processed by local and regional waste water treatment facilities and municipalities. However, there has been progress in measuring some medications in our drinking water. There has been increasing concern among health officials that pharmaceuticals detected in surface waters could cause adverse environmental effects, including endocrine disruption in aquatic life and increased antibiotic resistance in humans. Two of the largest contributors to pharmaceutical metabolite waste entering the sewer system are believed to be hospitals and residential neighborhoods. This occurs as a result of the elimination of partially metabolized medications and expired unused drugs being flushed down the drain or the toilet.

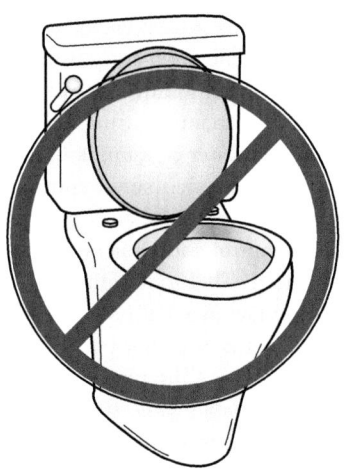

DRIVING CHANGE IN INDUSTRY

The agricultural and livestock industries inadvertently contribute PIE through the practice of injecting antibiotics to increase livestock production. Traces of antibiotic metabolites are excreted in livestock waste that may end up in the sewer system and even in local community wastewater treatment facilities. The EPA has established laws and regulations that control the use of pharmaceuticals in the farming industry. The use of antibiotics in the livestock industry is a major contributor to antibiotic resistance in humans because of the trace residue of those products in the meat that is produced. Global populations were projected to increase from more than 6.9 billion in 2011 to a predicted 8 billion by 2023 and a whopping 9 billion by 2050, according to the May 2011 United Nations projection. These projections emphasize the tremendous need for increased awareness and workable solutions by industries that are major contributors of waste and pollution (Box 20-1).

Several governmental and nongovernmental agencies and organizations have set forth laws, regulations, and guidelines that create a framework for environmentally conscious practices that reduce pollution and the contamination of natural resources. These organizations include the following:

- Food and Drug Administration (FDA)
- Environmental Protection Agency (EPA)
- Drug Enforcement Administration (DEA)
- U.S. Department of Agriculture (USDA)
- U.S. Fish and Wildlife Service (USFS)
- American Pharmacists Association (APhA)
- Teleosis Institute
- M&M Consultants of Dallas, Texas

BOX 20-1   Companies Leading in Green Manufacturing Practices

According to the *Newsweek* 2010 rankings of U.S. companies, the following are the top 10 green manufacturers:

1. Johnson & Johnson	6. Eli Lilly
2. Bristol-Myers Squibb	7. Merck
3. Allergan	8. Hospira
4. Pfizer	9. Biogen Idec
5. Abbott Laboratories	10. Life Technologies

There are a variety of companies that advance environmental initiatives through the secure handling and transportation of drugs that are recaptured as part of a medication take-back program, or as a means to manage expired medication generated by a pharmacy organization. These outsource companies perform the inventory of expired drugs and form partnerships with pharmaceutical companies that offer replacement inventory or purchase credit for the return of expired medication. Some drug manufacturers may also partner with companies such as Covanta Energy Systems, which utilizes co-generation and waste-to-energy technologies. More information may be gained through the Guaranteed Returns website at www.guaranteedreturns.com.

The drug manufacturing industry plays a large role in seeking opportunities to reduce pollution and groundwater contamination that occurs as a result of human sewage products. This is an area in which there are many opportunities for green chemistry, use of water-based solvents and more organic raw materials, and "pharmacovigilance" during the manufacturing process, which increases quality control and reduces drug recalls as a result of compromised drug efficacy or product contamination. The utilization of green manufacturing practices as a means to conserve energy and optimize raw material processing often equates to cost savings in a relatively short period of time. However, it is often not possible to both streamline manufacturing processes and incorporate more green practices. The pharmaceutical industry will continue to examine opportunities to become more sustainable while still producing the products and services needed by health care providers and patients across the United States.

Going Green for Good

Green practices must be incorporated into daily life. They should not be implemented as a socially fashionable cause, but rather integrated into the identity of an organization's culture and daily processes. Green health care practices may be incorporated into the inventory management system through the establishment of relationships with vendors that utilize green manufacturing processes. They may be incorporated into the health education of patients concerning the proper use, handling, and disposal of both prescription and over the counter medications. Prescription take-back programs may be implemented on a larger scale to encourage consumers to practice safe disposal of unused and expired pharmaceuticals on a regular basis. They can be advanced through the reuse of health care resources, as well as widespread recycling of paper, plastic, and glass materials. There are also many practical ways to conserve energy while organizations pursue future opportunities for seeking alternative sources of sustainable energy.

Entire pharmacy organizations should be familiar with the green pharmacy practices that are set forth by their hospital or health system. These practices may be further integrated into the education and training of pharmacists and pharmacy technicians within institutions of higher education across the United States and the health care community abroad.

Chapter Summary

- A sustainable health care culture emphasizes the reduction of consumables that end up in landfills, the reuse of products when therapeutically appropriate and allowable by law, and the recycling of consumable materials whenever possible
- Green pharmacy practice focuses on the utilization of resources that allow for the proper handling and processing of expired pharmaceuticals.
- The Environmental Protection Agency has established guidelines for the disposal of both hazardous and nonhazardous waste materials in the health care environment.
- The term *pharmaceuticals in the environment* refers to pharmaceutical contaminants seeping into groundwater supplies via rivers, lakes, and streams.
- Green pharmacy practice in a community setting is measured by the ability of both independent and corporate pharmacy organizations to reduce pharmaceutical waste, educate consumers on the importance of the proper disposal of medications, and provide solutions for reducing pharmaceutical contamination.
- Green pharmacy in a hospital setting is measured by the ability of the department of pharmacy to become a more sustainable operation through education and training of green pharmacy practices.
- The pharmacy profession can strengthen green practices through partnerships with vendors implementing green manufacturing processes.
- Green pharmacy certification primarily focuses on the reduction of pharmaceutical waste through medication take-back programs.
- Energy conservation is another way health care organizations can be "green."
- Several governmental and nongovernmental agencies and organizations have set forth laws, regulations, and guidelines for environmentally conscious practices that will reduce pollution and the contamination of natural resources.

REVIEW QUESTIONS

Multiple Choice

1. Green pharmacy practice in a community setting is measured by the ability of both independent and corporate pharmacy organizations to:
   a. Establish medication take-back programs
   b. Educate patients on the importance of proper drug disposal
   c. Reduce pharmaceutical waste
   d. All of the above

2. Which of the following are believed to be among the largest contributors to pharmaceutical metabolite waste entering the sewer system?
   a. Grocery stores
   b. Hospitals
   c. Residential areas
   d. Both b and c

3. The practice of pharmacovigilance may result in the _____ of drug recalls.
   a. Increase
   b. Decrease
   c. Elimination
   d. No effect on the incidence of drug recalls

4. This federal agency has established laws and regulations that control the use of pharmaceuticals in the farming industry:
   a. FDA
   b. EPA
   c. USDA
   d. USFS

5. A major contributor to antibiotic resistance is:
   a. Traces in fish raised in contaminated water
   b. Excessive drugs being stored in consumers' homes
   c. Trace residue in the meat of livestock raised using those products
   d. The lowered effectiveness of antibiotic drugs

6. Outsource companies assist pharmacies in inventory recycling by:
   a. Partnering with manufacturers that offer replacement inventory
   b. Identifying sources that offer purchase credit for the return of expired drugs
   c. Partnering with a company that uses waste-to-energy technology
   d. All of above

7. Drug manufacturing companies may seek out more sustainable manufacturing practices that utilize:
   a. Use of "green" chemistry in the bioengineering of synthetic drug products
   b. Use of water-based solvents
   c. Use of more organic raw materials
   d. All of the above

8. Green pharmacy practice in the hospital industry can be measured by the following policies:
   a. Purchasing of green products
   b. Setting up recycling programs for glass, plastic, and paper products
   c. Ordering supplies from manufacturers that provide these types of products and are geared more toward sustainability
   d. All of the above

9. Sustainability within the hospital environment is generally approached at the _____ level.
   a. Global
   b. Organizational
   c. Departmental
   d. Employee

10. Departmental sustainability may be increased through the use of:
    a. Recyclable drug storage containers
    b. Energy-efficient lighting
    c. Computers that may run continuously
    d. a and b

TECHNICIAN'S CORNER

1. What are the chief causes of pharmaceuticals in the environment?
2. How may pharmacy employees use technology in a way that conserves energy?
3. Aside from drugs being improperly disposed of, what is another social problem that has been created by the overage of expired/excess medications being stored in homes across the United States?

Bibliography

International Quality and Productivity Center. (2011). *Managing, Mitigating and Minimizing Risk to Ensure Global Compliance.* Retrieved 10/15/2011, from Pharmacovigilance North America 2011: http://www.pharmacovigilanceconference.com/Event.aspx?id=540540

Pfizer. (2007). *Pharmaceuticals in the Environment.* Retrieved 10/14/2011, from http://www.pfizer.com/files/Pfizer_PIE_Overview.pdf

PharmaTurns Solutions. (2008). *Eco-Friendly.* Retrieved 10/15/2011, from Greener Earth Initiative: http://greenerearthinitiative.org/green.html

Teleosis Institute. (2008). *Green Pharmacy Program: Helping Communities Safely Dispose of Unused Medications.* Retrieved 10/15/2011, from http://www.teleosis.org/pdf/GreenPharmacy_FullPreliminaryReport.pdf

Thomas, P. (n.d.). *Green Processes: PAT and QbD Take Root.* Retrieved 10/15/2011, from PharmaManufacturing: http://www.pharmamanufacturing.com/articles/2010/071.html?page=full

United States Environmental Protection Agency. (2011). *What Is Sustainability? What Is EPA Doing? How Can I Help?* Retrieved 10/15/2011, from http://epa.gov/sustainability/basicinfo.htm

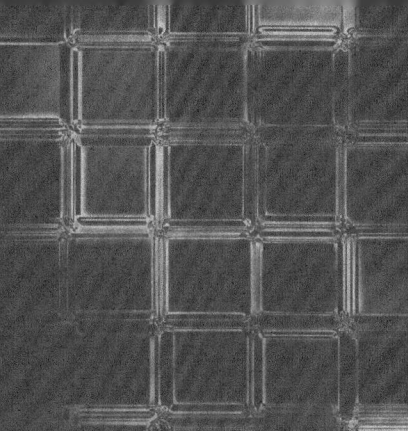

21

Preparing for What Lies Ahead: The Technician Career Path Overview

By the end of this chapter, students will be able to competently:

1. Explain the need for remote technician monitoring in various pharmacy settings.
2. Describe pharmacy settings that may utilize telepharmacy or remote pharmacy technician monitoring.
3. Describe the benefits of utilizing a remote monitoring system for the advancement of patient care and staffing challenges.
4. Describe key components of electronic supervision, detailing the various tasks that a pharmacist can monitor remotely.
5. Describe various states' laws and practice models related to remote technician monitoring.
6. Describe the framework for the managed care pharmacy practice, and explain the roles for pharmacy technicians at pharmacy benefit management (PBM) organizations.
7. Describe the nuclear pharmacy practice.
8. Describe the knowledge and skill training requirements of pharmacy technicians in the nuclear pharmacy practice.
9. Describe opportunities for pharmacy technicians in pharmaceutical sales and marketing.
10. Describe opportunities for pharmacy technicians in higher education.
11. Discuss future roles for pharmacy technicians, as identified by individuals across the profession of pharmacy and in industry settings.
12. Describe key elements of a well-written résumé.
13. Approach suggestions for how best to approach live and online job searches.
14. Describe behaviors that will prepare an applicant for a telephone interview.
15. Describe behaviors that will prepare an individual for a successful live interview, as well as the behaviors that one should avoid.
16. Define various types of interview questions.
17. Describe how best to approach behavior-based interview questions.

KEY TERMS

Radiopharmaceuticals: Agents used to diagnose certain medical problems or treat certain diseases and may be given by mouth, given by injection, or placed into the eye or into the bladder.

Telepharmacy: A system that uses an electronic method to monitor the dispensing of prescription drugs, review related drug use, and provide patient counseling services; the system uses technology such as audio, video, and still image capture.

Introduction

Now that students have had a chance to examine each of the areas of knowledge, skill, and attitudes that define the entry-level pharmacy technician practice, they should consider the opportunities that extend beyond the entry level. There are a variety of specialty practice areas that utilize pharmacy technicians. Based on the requirements, students may wish to consider them in the future. Those who began their practice with formal education are postured to be the most competitive, given projected changes to the face of the technician practice (as proposed by the National Association of Boards of Pharmacy):

- Clarify the terms *licensure, registration,* and *certification*
- License or register pharmacy technicians
- Accept certification from the Pharmacy Technician Certification Board (PTCB)
- Report pharmacy technician disciplinary information to a central clearinghouse
- Require pharmacy technician education that meets standardized guidelines
- By 2015, require pharmacy technicians to have completed an accredited education and training program as a condition of certification

According to the 2010-2011 Bureau of Labor Statistics, "employers favor those who have completed formal training and certification." Employment of pharmacy technicians is projected to increase by 31%, and that will only increase as qualified, well-trained pharmacy technicians elevate their careers to more innovative and specialized roles in the health care and pharmacy practice settings.

Examining Emerging, Specialty, and Prospective Areas of Technician Practice

The role of the pharmacist continues to evolve, creating more opportunities for the advancement of the pharmacy technician career path. The following subsections detail areas of the pharmacy technician practice that are up and coming, as well as some established *specialty* areas. Leading industry periodicals have also cited predictions about future roles and the utilization of pharmacy technicians in both community and health-system practices.

TELEPHARMACY AND REMOTE TECHNICIAN MONITORING

An online news report for WNDU in Indiana posted the following on September 5, 2009: "Did you know that more people die in hospitals on the weekends than on weekdays?" (McFadden, 2009). This article cited staffing shortages on weekends—and the inability of caregivers to be physically present while monitoring multiple patients at once—as a major contributor to mortality in the hospital setting. Specific to the acute care setting, intensive care specialists may now remotely monitor patients via cameras in patient rooms and alert onsite staff when issues arise. This is just one of several applications of this emerging technology. As many health care settings are looking for opportunities to further advance patient care and patient safety and minimize adverse events, they are seeking out technology to help them better manage staffing and workflow processes through remotely captured digital images or streaming video.

Telepharmacy is an area of the pharmacy practice that has been in use since the early 2000s, while ongoing advancements in technology have increased its visibility. The National Association of Boards of Pharmacy (NABP) modified its Model Pharmacy Act to include telepharmacy in its definition of pharmacy practice. Further, the American Society of Health-System Pharmacists House of Delegates adopted a policy position in 2007 that encourages state boards of pharmacy to "adopt regulations that enable the use of United States–based telepharmacy services for all practice settings." The Texas State Board of Pharmacy defines telepharmacy as a "system that monitors the dispensing of prescription drugs and provides for related drug use review and patient counseling services by an electronic method, including the use of the following types of technology: audio and video; still image capture; and store and forward."

The terms *electronic supervision* and *remote technician monitoring* are essentially synonymous. Either may be defined as a means by which the fill activities of pharmacy technician staff can be monitored and checked by a registered pharmacist offsite, using audio and/or visual technology. It is important to note that remote monitoring should not be used as a substitute for the adequate staffing of pharmacists in a hospital setting; rather, when the pharmacist is physically absent, remote monitoring allows onsite technicians to perform various job tasks, have their work checked remotely by a pharmacist, and then deliver those checked doses to medication storage areas as necessary. The result should be better provision of patient care, as well as increased patient safety because each dose will have been verified and checked by a pharmacist prior to dispensing.

Although telepharmacy would be appropriate in various practice settings, it is still a largely underused resource because of limited documentation concerning the overall positive outcomes on patient care as well as the hesitancy of individual states to adopt the corresponding legislation. The rural hospital practice setting is one area where there are wide applications for electronic monitoring because of the overwhelming need for pharmacy staffing.

What Is the Need for Remote Monitoring?

The primary need for a remote monitoring system is to allow a hospital or health system where there is a critical pharmacist staffing issue to still provide patient care and safety. This particularly applies to North Dakota. Of the 47 general acute care hospitals in the state, 39 are small, rural hospitals that staff one full-time pharmacist during the week or contract with a local community pharmacy for pharmacist support. Pharmacist support during weekends, evenings, and for vacation and emergency coverage is generally sparse. Additionally, because of The Joint Commission standards that require a 100% pharmacist order review, critical staffing shortages may threaten a hospital's accreditation compliance. Because most hospitals in the region are rural, graduates from area schools of pharmacy often choose to relocate to large markets; thus, the area experiences an ongoing shortage of pharmacists to cover these rural hospitals. In the early 2000s, this shortage contributed to the closure of several community pharmacies and threatened the survival of the region's hospitals as well. In an effort to revitalize the pharmacy services in the region and increase patient safety through pharmacist support, several area pharmacies participated in a pilot project to introduce remote monitoring services.

In a 2006 study, all 50 state offices of rural health were surveyed regarding rural hospital telepharmacy initiatives in their state. Box 21-1 notes each of the six states that had regulations in place related to telepharmacy as of July 2010. Table 21-1 notes other states that were involved in the study, as well as activity toward the utilization of telepharmacy within that state. About half of the hospitals cited in the study reported using federal grants to offset startup expenses. Other hospitals indicated that lack of funding was a barrier to purchasing updated medication dispensing equipment.

Study conclusions cited the need for additional research into how telepharmacy models affect medication safety in rural hospitals and how this technology may best be utilized. Other issues for consideration by state boards of pharmacy include the following:

BOX 21-1   **States That Have Implemented Telepharmacy Regulations**

North Dakota	Texas
Montana	Idaho
South Dakota	Utah

TABLE 21-1   **States That Have Implemented Limited Telepharmacy**

Utah	State board–approved telepharmacy pilot projects
Washington	State board–approved telepharmacy pilot projects
Arkansas	Offsite order entry allowed with documentation of improved patient care outcomes
Oklahoma	SBOP reviews requests on a case-by-case basis, has allowed remote order review by a pharmacist from one hospital in the area to another; pharmacist must have access to adequate clinical data in order to make informed clinical decisions
Minnesota	SBOP adopted guidelines for dispensing via telepharmacy; pharmacy sites must apply for variance to a specific regulation and gain board approval

- Physical location of pharmacists providing telepharmacy services
- Types of technology to be used
- Minimum amount of time a pharmacist must be onsite at a hospital
- Roles of pharmacists, pharmacy technicians, and nurses in medication distribution systems

MANAGED CARE PHARMACY

When many health maintenance organizations (HMOs) were established in the 1970s, prescription drug costs only accounted for about 5% of total health care expenses. With the steady increase of prescription drugs since the 1970s, the need to manage prescription drug utilization as both preventive and maintenance care continues to increase. Pharmacy benefit management (PBM) companies have been created specifically to develop and manage comprehensive and cost-efficient prescription drug benefits for a broad scope of patient populations. Roles that pharmacists play in the PBM organization include the following:

- Developing frameworks for the processing and the administration of drug benefit claims in a way that optimizes both clinical outcomes and cost containment
- Designing individual drug benefit plans
- Negotiating contract relationships between community pharmacies and PBM organizations
- Offering clinical consultive support and drug therapy analyses
- Providing clinical writers who develop drug utilization reviews, prior authorization guidelines, and disease management programs

The pharmacy technician's role in the PBM setting is primarily to provide information to a broad client base, determine the proper utilization of patient benefits, and collect and enter clinical data. Strong communication as well as organizational and clerical skills are essential in this practice setting. Specific job duties may include the following:

- Providing pharmacy benefit plan information to physicians, pharmaceutical companies, distributors, and plan members
- Assisting members with benefits claims processing
- Troubleshooting rejected claims
- Processing mail-order prescriptions

Specifically in the mail-order setting, medication filling, labeling, and packaging are tasks that would be performed by pharmacy technician staff.

NUCLEAR PHARMACY

What Is Nuclear Pharmacy Practice?

The Mayo Clinic defines radiopharmaceuticals as "agents used to diagnose certain medical problems or treat certain diseases [and] may be given by mouth, given by injection, or placed into the eye or into the bladder." Radiopharmaceuticals contain radioactive isotopes that help to identify the presence of disease in the human body and to diagnose diseases that affect every major human body system, including organs, vessels, and cellular structures. In the presence of disease, radioactivity is captured utilizing special imaging equipment. Some other radiopharmaceuticals are prepared in higher doses that have activity against cancer cells themselves or their replication. There are inherent risks involved with the handling and preparation of radiopharmaceuticals, and highly specialized training is required for both pharmacists and technicians working in this specialty area of practice.

A few colleges and universities, such as Purdue University and the University of Arkansas offer nuclear pharmacy training programs for both pharmacists and pharmacy technicians. Many nuclear pharmacies send new employees to the university setting to complete their education and training, as training guidelines are extensive and strictly regulated. According to guidelines set forth by the Nuclear Medicine program at University of Arkansas College of Pharmacy, "the nuclear Pharmacy Technician should demonstrate appropriate knowledge and understanding of the specific nuclear pharmacy site with emphasis on the technician duties and responsibilities, including standards of ethics governing pharmacy practice."

Key knowledge-based competencies for nuclear pharmacy technicians include an understanding of the following:

- Radiopharmaceutical terms, abbreviations, and symbols commonly used in prescribing, compounding, and dispensing radiopharmaceuticals
- Drug dosages by imaging procedure, routes of administration, and dosage forms, and the ability to distinguish therapeutic from diagnostic radiopharmaceutical utilization
- Procedures and operations related to the reconstitution, packaging, and labeling of radiopharmaceuticals
- Procedures and techniques related to aseptic compounding and parenteral admixture operations

  Key laboratory skill competencies include performance of the following:
- Mathematical calculations required for the usual dosage determinations and solution preparations in the compounding and dispensing of radiopharmaceuticals
- Usual technician functions associated with a specific radiopharmacy entity
- The essential functions related to drug purchasing and inventory control
- Manipulative and record-keeping functions associated with the compounding and dispensing of radiopharmaceuticals, as well as those associated with quality control testing

Because of the risks involved, entry-level pay is generally higher in this area of practice. However, because of the highly specialized nature of the nuclear pharmacy practice, there are few practice settings and a limited number of available positions.

PHARMACEUTICAL SALES, MARKETING, AND RESEARCH

Sales and marketing of pharmaceuticals offer a variety of well-paying career opportunities for pharmacy technicians who possess a 4-year undergraduate degree. Degrees in the areas of biology, chemistry, business, or marketing would be beneficial and provide a strong educational foundation. As in other areas of business, sales positions in this industry are best suited for individuals with strong communication skills. This career path is also suited for those who display self-confidence and are highly self-motivated. Those who wish to engage in this highly competitive industry must have experience in business-to-business processes and customer relations and have a proven performance record.

PHARMACY TECHNICIAN EDUCATION

The area of education and training presents unique career opportunities for pharmacy technicians, in both community and hospital pharmacy settings. Although a person may possess strong job skills and ability, specialized skills are required to communicate and demonstrate job tasks effectively as part of education and training. Education and training in the industry setting differs from that in the more traditional classroom setting, although both require a structure designed to meet established training goals and objectives. Training must be constructed in a manner that will allow learners to gain a foundational set of knowledge, skills, and attitudes that embody a particular profession. At the conclusion of training, written and hands-on skill assessments will provide documented proof that training was effective.

Modern education and training practices utilize a great deal of technology and are structured in a manner that best meets the needs of the target training audience. Adult learners tend to gain knowledge through visual, auditory, or hands-on demonstration (usually a combination of all three learning methods), and a balance of training methodologies will help them to meet a variety of learning styles.

The availability of quality resources for pharmacy technician training programs has significantly improved. As mentioned previously, the American Society of Health-System Pharmacists (ASHP) is currently the only professional organization that accredits pharmacy technician training programs. ASHP is also the primary organization that has established the best practices that have shaped the pharmacy technician career path since the 1990s.

Technician training programs may offer credit or noncredit courses, so the educational requirements for pharmacy technician educators may vary. For credit-based programs, an associate's or bachelor's degree may be required. Often the education requirement is an undergraduate degree or equivalent experience. Individuals who wish to pursue a career in technician education may begin by seeking out opportunities to become involved in the orientation and training of new employees in their practice setting.

Future Roles for Pharmacy Technicians

An article for a popular pharmacy information technology company cited the following potential information technology (IT) roles for pharmacy technicians who have completed education and training:

* Initiating medication reconciliation, including obtaining and documenting patients' medication information for pharmacists' review
* Scheduling patient outpatient clinic drug therapy management visits
* Providing criteria-based screening of medical records to identify patients who may require pharmacist intervention
* Preparing clinical monitoring information (e.g., international normalized ratios) for pharmacist review
* Managing controlled substances systems
* Managing medication assistance programs
* Conducting aspects of quality improvement programs
* Managing pharmacy department information technology systems, including routine database management and billing systems
* Supervising other pharmacy technicians

A 2008 survey conducted by ASHP lists a variety of "novel" roles for the pharmacy technician including the following:

* Launch the dispensing process by entering medication orders into the pharmacy management system to obtain and document medication histories; participate in patient assessment, data collection, and interpretation.
* Keep patient records; review EMRs to identify patients in need of intervention; review patient charts for medication allergies; clarify medication orders.
* Perform benchmarking surveys and put together quality improvement reports.
* Manage vaccination databases, inventory, medication assistance, and quality assurance programs, inventory for controlled substances, information technology, medication disposal, and destruction.
* Supervise and review the work of other technicians.
* Work in a telepharmacy environment and dispense medications remotely under video supervision of a pharmacist.

Starting on the Right Foot and Moving Forward

SUCCESSFULLY ENGAGING JOB SEARCHES, INTERVIEWING, AND CONTINUING YOUR EDUCATION AS A PHARMACY TECHNICIAN

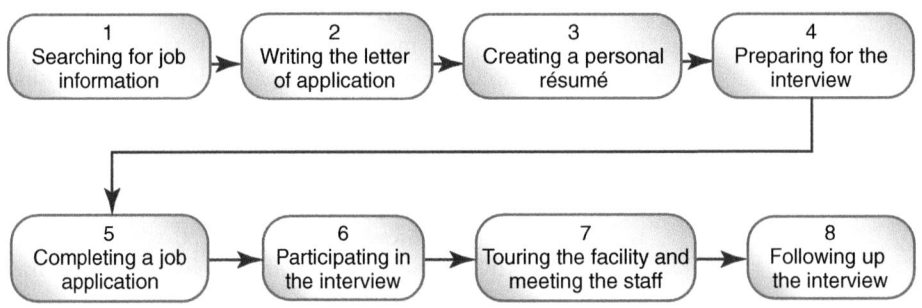

The career planning process. (From Finkbeiner BL, Finkbeiner CA: *Practice management for the dental team,* ed 7, St. Louis, 2011, Mosby.)

At this point in their pharmacy technician training, students will have explored the knowledge, skills, and attitudes that will prepare them for a successful entry-level career as a pharmacy technician. After successfully passing the certification exam, new technicians may begin the process of seeking out new positions by logging on to one of the popular career and job search websites, apply-ing for a few pharmacy technician jobs, then sitting back and waiting for the calls to roll in, right? Not exactly. There are a variety of activities that one should engage in to prepare for the job search and interview process. The first step to selling yourself is to write an appealing advertisement that will convince an employer to want to buy what you're selling. Your *résumé* is your personal/professional advertisement.

Making a Good Impression in Writing: How to Write an Effective Résumé

There are a few subtle differences between a good résumé and a great one. It is a lot like comparing a television commercial that is produced for the Super Bowl to one that is aired during the rest of the year. Super Bowl commercials are designed to be eye-catching, captivating, and with the inten-tion of leaving a lasting impression and becoming one of the commercials that viewers recall when discussing their favorites. The same is true of résumé writing. A résumé should be written in a way that catches the eye of a potential employer, highlights compelling information about that person, and leaves a lasting impression that will cause that employer to *remember* that person and his or her qualifications.

A few basic structural elements must be in place for a résumé to present a professional appearance to an employer. A basic résumé should include the following elements:

- Personal/professional contact information
  - Ensure that your contact information is kept current so that an employer does not have a problem contacting you. Make sure that the contact phone number is correct and the e-mail address is one that you check frequently.
  - Ensure that your e-mail address does not communicate unintended or undesirable messages about you. The e-mail address Johnnyhottubparty2009@hotmail.com will not leave a positive impression. If necessary, create an e-mail address for business-related messages only. John.Smith2009@hotmail.com would be far more appropriate.
  - Change your voicemail message on your cell phone or any other messaging system that a potential employer might hear.
- Objective
  - Some may consider an objective to be similar to a mission statement: it lets an employer know what direction the applicant wishes to go in his or her career and what skills the applicant possesses that would help an organization to achieve its goals.
  - Objectives should be brief, specific, and powerful:
    "Highly motivated pharmacy technician seeking a position in a community pharmacy that will allow me to use my excellent customer service skills"
    "Entry-level pharmacy technician with great listening and speaking skills who is willing to learn a new area of pharmacy practice and contribute positively to a diverse pharmacy team"
    "Entry-level pharmacy technician with a strong customer service background seeking a new role in which to apply knowledge and skills acquired during formal pharmacy technician education"
- Education
  - List educational background in reverse chronological order (most recent first).
  - If still in school (or a pharmacy technician training program), list the projected date of completion/graduation.
  - List high school or General Educational Development (GED) certificate information. If your high school was attended outside the United States, ensure that all necessary information is included:
    For those who attended high school outside of the United States, it may be useful to obtain U.S. equivalency through an educational credentialing agency.
    For around $75, your high school or college degree course work can be evaluated by a profes-sional for the reporting of U.S. equivalency.
    Be sure that if the agency requires original documents, you are aware of the process for return-ing your original documents.

- Experience
  - Experience can come from a paid position, volunteer work, internship/externship experiences, and involvement in student organizations.
  - List only experience that is relevant to the position for which you are applying.
  - Be brief. Describe relevant details related to what you did and how you succeeded in that position using action verbs:

    "Provided exemplary telephone support service in a call center, ensured that customer concerns were resolved by the end of each call"

    "Reduced 30+ overdue accounts by 20% within the first 90 days of my employment with the company"

    "Supervised five employees within the sales division"

    "Applied knowledge of C++ to troubleshoot customer software issues"
- References
  - The statement "References Available Upon Request" may be used; ensure that a reference sheet is prepared and available and that it includes your name and contact information.
  - Always gain the permission of the individuals listed on the reference sheet before citing them, and ensure that their current contact information is provided.
  - References could be past faculty members, co-workers, or supervisors/managers.

The following valuable basic tips may also be followed:

- Try to condense résumé content to one page, unless relevant experience is extensive
- To further emphasize a mission or objective statement, place that information on a cover letter instead; doing so will provide the employer with more detailed information concerning why you wish to gain employment with the organization
- Present past experience within the context of how it would be useful in the position for which you are applying
- Proofread your résumé to ensure the following:
  - There are no grammatical, punctuation, or typographical errors
  - Font type and size are consistent (and select a basic font like Times New Roman or Arial)
  - All action verb tenses are consistent (e.g., "processed laboratory samples," "dispensed medication orders")
- Emphasize important details using capitals, bold type, or italics
- Spend a little extra for quality paper, but stick to white or ivory colors

Once you have formatted your résumé, find a qualified person whose opinion you value to proofread your résumé and provide objective feedback. A second (or third) pair of eyes is always better than one. After preparing a résumé, you can then begin to seek positions for which you may qualify.

TECH NOTE!
Résumé objectives should be brief, specific, and powerful!

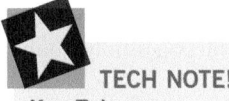

TECH NOTE!
Key Takeaways
- One page
- Error-free
- Basic font
- Intentional action verbs in past tense

ACTIVELY SEEKING PHARMACY POSITIONS

Some organizations require that applications be completed online; other organizations allow them to be filled out in person. Ensure, when job seeking, that you keep with you information needed to complete an application, such as job history information and reference information (Figure 21-1).

Some organizations require all job inquiries to be handled through a human resources (HR) office or through an HR client representative. Find that information out as early as possible, so you will know who to follow up with after submitting an application (Figure 21-2).

Make a note of all jobs for which you have applied and the dates on which you applied so that you can provide that information if an employer asks.

Don't wait for a personal invitation to interview or follow up on a submitted application; follow up if you haven't heard anything after a few days, and inquire as to how long one should reasonably wait before following up. Some hospitals may allow personal inquiries concerning the availability of positions, even when the applications themselves must be submitted through the human resources department.

Don't let the phrase "1-2 years of experience required" scare you away from a position. Even if you don't qualify for that position, there may be other entry-level positions that you do qualify for that were not posted. Also, don't express frustration or irritation if there is a delay in follow-up—and never be rude when communicating over the telephone. Strive to present yourself as open, flexible, and friendly.

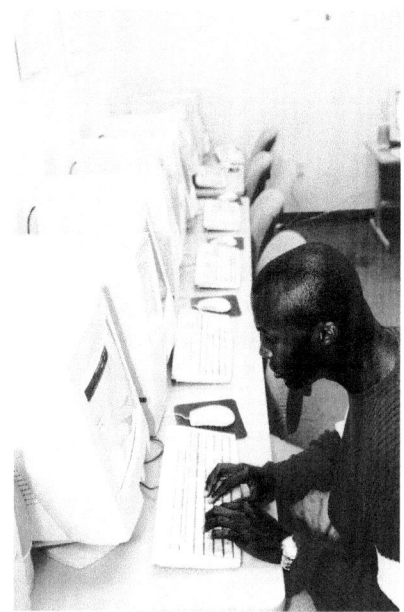

FIGURE 21-1 Student doing an online job search. (From Fordney MT: *Insurance handbook for the medical office,* ed 12, St. Louis, 2012, Saunders.)

EMPLOYMENT APPLICATION
All information listed on this application will be considered and handled as personal and confidential. Please write or print legibly.

AN EQUAL OPPORTUNITY EMPLOYER
This employer provides equal opportunity to all persons without regard to handicap, race, color, religion, sex, age, or national origin.

Name:				Date of Application:
Address:	City:	State:	Zip:	
Home Phone:	Cell Phone:	Social Security Number:		

GENERAL INFORMATION

Position applied for: _____

Available to work: ☐ Full-Time ☐ Part-Time ☐ Temporary

Date available to start work: _____

Are you over 18 yrs. of age? ☐ Yes ☐ No   Will transportation be a problem for you? ☐ Yes ☐ No

If you are not a U.S. Citizen, do you have the right to work in the United States?   ☐ Yes ☐ No

Have you ever been convicted of a felony?   ☐ Yes ☐ No

   (A conviction is not an automatic bar to employment. Each case will be considered on its own merits.)

Does the sight of blood bother you?   ☐ Yes ☐ No

EDUCATION

	Name and address of School	Major/Degree(s)	No. of Years Completed	Did you Graduate?
High School				
Community College				
4 Year Institution				
Vocational				
Other (specify)				

Describe Specialized Training, Apprenticeship, Skills, Seminars, Courses, Extra-Curricular Activities

A

FIGURE 21-2 A, Sample application for employment. (From Finkbeiner BL, Finkbeiner CA: *Practice management for the dental team,* ed 7, St. Louis, 2011, Mosby.)

Continued

SKILLS

Task	Circle One		Task	Circle One	
Keyboarding WPM _____	Yes	No	Pour Models	Yes	No
Bookkeeping	Yes	No	Cavitron	Yes	No
Computer Operations	Yes	No	Cast Onlays	Yes	No
Handling Group Insurance	Yes	No	Plaque Control Instruction	Yes	No
Expose, Process, and Mount X-rays	Yes	No	Oral Evacuator	Yes	No
Panoramic X-Rays	Yes	No	Knowledge of Dental Instruments	Yes	No
Have you used insurance software?	Yes	No	Knowledge of Dental Terms	Yes	No
Other: (Describe if yes)					

EMPLOYMENT RECORD

Beginning with your current employer, please list your work experience over the past ten years. You may include pertinent volunteer activities.

Name of Employer		Start Date	End Date
Address	Phone	Start Salary	End Salary
Job Title	Supervisor	Phone	
Duties			
Reason for Leaving			

Name of Employer		Start Date	End Date
Address	Phone	Start Salary	End Salary
Job Title	Supervisor	Phone	
Duties			
Reason for Leaving			

Name of Employer		Start Date	End Date
Address	Phone	Start Salary	End Salary
Job Title	Supervisor	Phone	
Duties			
Reason for Leaving			

B

FIGURE 21-2 B, Sample application for employment (cont'd).

MAKING A GOOD IMPRESSION: HOW TO ENGAGE IN A SUCCESSFUL TELEPHONE OR LIVE INTERVIEW

A potential employer will have already screened résumés for qualified individuals to whom they wish to extend a telephone or live interview. Often employers prescreen qualified applicants using a telephone interview. It is important to prepare for a telephone interview, because the impression you create may determine whether you are granted a second, live interview. Follow these tips for telephone interviews:

- Check your telephone connection, volume, and speakerphone to ensure that you are able to hear and understand as well as to be heard and understood. It may be useful to verify this information with the interviewer before proceeding with the call.
- Plan ahead and make sure that any roommates, pets, or children present will not create distractions or background noise.
- Be prepared with pen and paper to jot down notes, the name and job title of the interviewer, and other important information.
- Be prepared for silence on the line while the interviewer is taking notes; don't feel the need to fill spaces of silence with embellished responses.
- Speak with a smile in your voice.

REFERENCES

Please provide the name, address, and phone number of at least two non employer/relatives as references.

NAME	ADDRESS	PHONE

EMERGENCY CONTACT

Name	Relationship	
Address	Phone	Alt. Phone

DUTY PERFORMANCE

Are you able to perform the essential duties of the position for which you are applying, either with or without reasonable accommodations? ☐ Yes ☐ No

If yes, please indicate what type(s) of reasonable accommodations are needed:

In the course of making an employment decision, this employer makes it a practice to verify with previous employers information such as dates of employment, description of job duties, attendance records, reason for leaving, etc. If there are any employers you want us to contact, please indicate their names below and reasons why:

_____

_____

_____

_____

I understand that if I am employed and any statement herein is not true, I may be released immediately, I will be paid only through the day of release and this employer may cancel any rights to accrued benefits.

_____   _____
Date   Signature

C

FIGURE 21-2 C, Sample application for employment (cont'd).

- Be aware of verbal distracters that you may use during conversations, such as "uh," "um," and "like." Avoid slang, such as "yeah" or "uh huh."
- Speak clearly and enunciate your words, ensuring that words are pronounced correctly.
- Have questions prepared to ask the employer, but do not ask a question that you should already have the answer to, like "So you're a hospital facility?"
- Contemplate the types of questions that you may be asked, but don't script your responses or answer too quickly; it's okay to ask for time to consider your response.
- Do your homework! Find out information about the organization, its mission, and the services it offers. Find an appropriate moment to share that information during the interview.

Don't talk an employer out of considering you for a second interview by doing any of the following:

- Communicating your negative attributes or using self-effacing statements like "I'm kind of gullible, so I tend to be taken advantage of."
- Projecting arrogance as confidence: "You'll be missing out if you don't consider me for this position" or "I won't require training because I am already qualified for this position."
- Mentioning what you didn't like about your current or last employer: "My last boss didn't really know what he was doing" or "This girl Suzy used to drive me crazy!"
- Immediately asking about the pay.
- Sharing personal information: "I was in the emergency room for 7 hours last night, so pardon me if I sound sleepy."

- Using profanity or sharing inappropriate information or jokes.
- Sharing information that would lead an employer to view you as potentially unreliable or inflexible.

GAINING A LIVE INTERVIEW

The live interview may follow the telephone interview, if there was one. The expression that one "never gets a second chance to make a good first impression" holds very true. Strive to make a positive impression with every person that you come into contact with. A motivational speaker once mentioned a practical example of how a department's administrative assistant was among the most trusted and influential members of the pharmacy team. Learn that person's name, and show the assistant genuine courtesy and respect. Your interviewer is sure to find out if the administrative assistant was not impressed with how you treated him or her, and that could weigh heavily on whether you are offered a position!

There are different types of interviews, and the format used will depend on the pharmacy organization. Interview styles include the following:

- *Board/panel interview.* Meeting with multiple individuals who are likely involved in the hiring decision
- *Onsite interview.* May include touring a facility and speaking with individuals who may be involved in the hiring decision or with whom you may work and with whom it would be useful to make a good impression; during this tour, you may be asked if you are familiar with different pieces of equipment or specifics about a tool's functionality.

Often, the types of questions being presented in an interview will be one or more of the following:

- *Theoretical questions.* Present a hypothetical situation (i.e., "How would you respond if you were asked to stay late on a day when you already had plans?")
- *Leading questions.* Include a clue to the type of response an interviewer is seeking (i.e., "You don't mind a little heavy lifting, do you?")
- *Behavioral questions.* Call for specific examples from past professional or personal experiences.
- *Behavioral interview.* Many employers have moved to a behavior-based interview question style, as past behavior is a good predictor of future behavior or performance. It is important to recognize when you are being asked what you *might do* in a situation versus what you *have done* in the past. Answer properly, depending on how the question is phrased. Whatever the question, be truthful in your response! Don't *overstate* or *understate* your experience. It is possible to communicate when you don't know something while presenting how you might overcome that lack of knowledge. Note the following example: "While I have never been involved in building a schedule, I maintain my own personal schedule and tasks using an electronic calendar and I would be willing to learn how this task is performed."

One successful approach for responding to behavior-based questions is in terms of P-A-R (University of Wisconsin-Eau Claire, 2008):

- Problem: State brief details of the example being given.
- Action: Describe the action that was taken.
- Result: Describe the result or outcome of the action.

Be prepared to describe an occasion in which the outcome was not what you expected or hoped for. Many employers want to know how an applicant will respond when a mistake is made or when a situation becomes unpredictable. Your ability to be adaptable and flexible may be determined based on your responses to those types of situations. Further, an employer wants to know if an applicant can admit to fault and recognize it as an opportunity to learn from a mistake.

Planning ahead is a key to success during the interview process, and it will alleviate a great deal of the anxiety one might feel on the day of an interview. Here are some tips for successful interviewing:

- Drive to your interview location the day before so you will be familiar with traffic, parking, whether parking requires cash, and other details.
- Arrive 15 to 30 minutes early to allow time to find the location.
- Exercise good personal hygiene; keep a mint handy, but avoid chewing gum.
- Dress conservatively and professionally: a suit is best, but business casual is generally fine, so long as shirt and slacks are dry cleaned, pressed, and sharp looking (Figure 21-3).

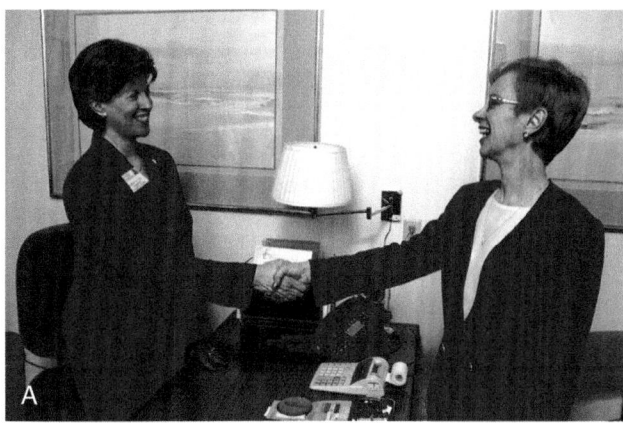

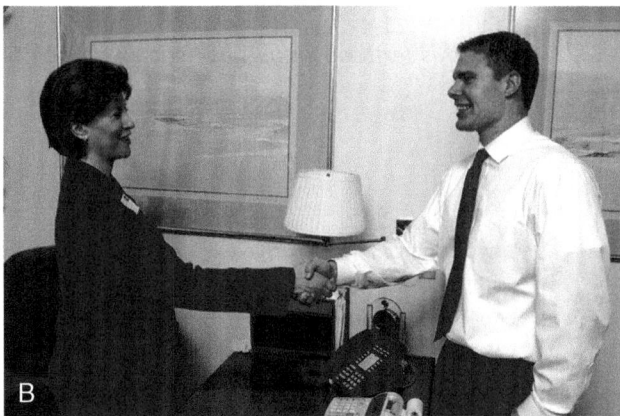

FIGURE 21-3 A, A simple suit is worn for a job interview. **B,** This man wears slacks and a shirt and tie for his interview. (From Sorrentino S: *Mosby's textbook for nursing assistants,* ed 8, St. Louis, 2012, Mosby.)

- For women, skirts should be either slightly below or no more than an inch above the knee; avoid revealing or tight-fitting clothing.
- Artistic self-expression through body art, piercing, and dramatic makeup is fine when you're on your own time; however, prior to an interview it is best to do the following:
  - Conceal visible tattoos when possible.
  - Remove visible facial piercings.
  - Keep jewelry and cosmetics minimal and conservative.
- Avoid strong-smelling perfumes or colognes, and apply a conservative amount.
- Come prepared with multiple copies of your résumé to distribute.
- Have a pen and paper handy for taking notes.
- Know thyself!

Many people are unaware of their own facial expressions or body posture that may send unintended negative messages. Consider the following:

- Sit in front of a mirror and rehearse sample interview responses.
- Practice sitting up straight in your seat.
- Practice speaking slowly and clearly.
- Become aware of distracting facial expressions or gestures (like eye rolling, eyebrow raises, or dramatic hand gestures) that you may wish to avoid during the live interview.
- Practice a soft and genuine smile or friendly expression.

Here are some final tips that may be useful when preparing for an interview:

- Practice a firm and confident handshake, unless your cultural or religious tradition precludes handshaking (and if this is the case, you may choose to share this information with the employer).

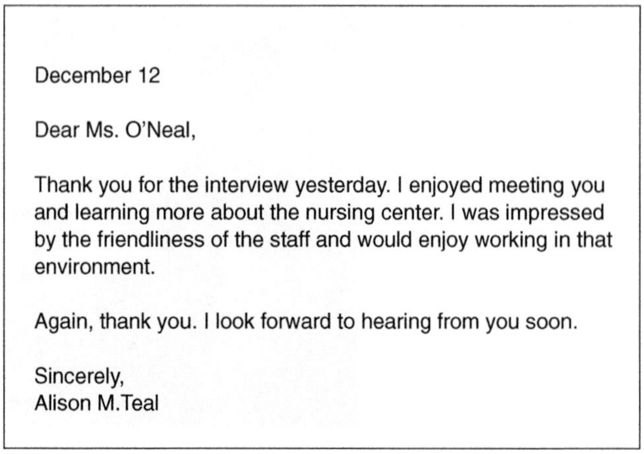

December 12

Dear Ms. O'Neal,

Thank you for the interview yesterday. I enjoyed meeting you and learning more about the nursing center. I was impressed by the friendliness of the staff and would enjoy working in that environment.

Again, thank you. I look forward to hearing from you soon.

Sincerely,
Alison M.Teal

FIGURE 21-4 Sample thank-you note written after a job interview. (From Sorrentino S: *Mosby's textbook for nursing assistants,* ed 8, St. Louis, 2012, Mosby.)

- Eye contact may be driven by cultural norms, although it is important to project a reasonable amount of eye contact during an interview. Try to establish some eye contact with each interviewer when speaking or being spoken to.
- If your mouth tends to get dry when you're nervous, ask if you may bring a bottle of water or a cup of coffee to the interview.
- Practice good posture and a seated position that you will find comfortable during the interview so that you won't fidget or shift in your seat. Never slouch in your seat or lean forward with forearms on your knees.
- Get some sleep the night before an interview—you don't want heavy eyelids when speaking to a potential employer!
- Read between the lines—when formulating responses, consider *why* an employer is asking you the questions being presented.
- Thank your interviewer for his or her time (Figure 21-4).
- Send a thank-you letter, note, or card to each of your interviewers following your interview.
- Be yourself!

Chapter Summary

- As a result of the evolving role of the pharmacist, pharmacy technicians have more career options than ever before.
- Areas of the pharmacy technician practice include telepharmacy technician monitoring, managed care pharmacy, nuclear pharmacy, pharmaceutical sales, marketing and research, and pharmacy technician education.
- Pharmacy benefit management (PBM) companies develop and manage comprehensive and cost-efficient prescription drug benefits for a broad scope of patient populations; the pharmacy technician's role in the PBM setting is primarily to provide information to a broad client base, determine proper the utilization of benefits by patients, and collect and enter clinical data.
- Radiopharmaceuticals are "agents used to diagnose certain medical problems or treat certain diseases [and] may be given by mouth, given by injection, or placed into the eye or into the bladder." Highly specialized training is required for both pharmacists and technicians working in this specialty area of practice.
- Pharmacy technicians possessing a 4-year undergraduate degree can pursue careers in pharmaceutical sales, marketing, and research.

- Pharmacy technicians interested in pursuing a career in technician education should begin by seeking out opportunities to be involved in the orientation and training of new employees in their practice setting.
- A basic résumé includes the following items: personal/professional contact information, education, experience, and references. In addition, some employers require job candidates to complete an application, either online or in person.
- Telephone interviews require the same preparation as live "in person" interviews
- Care should be taken to ensure professional dress, appearance, and body language.

REVIEW QUESTIONS

Multiple Choice

1. Telepharmacy has been in use for at least:
   a. 1 year
   b. 5 years
   c. 10 years
   d. 20 years

2. One of the commonly cited barriers to the implementation of remote monitoring is a lack of:
   a. Pharmacist support
   b. Hospital funding
   c. Room for equipment
   d. Nursing support

3. Job duties for a pharmacy technician in a PBM setting include:
   a. Negotiating contract relationships
   b. Providing plan information to physicians and plan members
   c. Analyzing drug therapies
   d. Offering clinical consultive support

4. According to the Mayo Clinic, nuclear pharmaceuticals may be administered via which of the following routes?
   a. Ear
   b. Cerebrospinal
   c. Eye
   d. Nose

5. Which of the following schools offer specialized training in nuclear pharmacy practice?
   a. Community colleges
   b. University of Arkansas
   c. Purdue University
   d. High schools

6. This specialty area of practice may be available to pharmacy technicians who possess a 4-year undergraduate degree:
   a. Nuclear pharmacy
   b. Pharmacy benefits management
   c. Pharmaceutical sales
   d. Pharmacy technician education

7. During pharmacy technician training, learners should gain foundational knowledge, skills, and _____ that embody the pharmacy technician practice.
   a. Organization
   b. Attitudes
   c. Competence
   d. Proficiency

8. Résumé objectives should be all of the following *except*:
   a. Specific
   b. Powerful
   c. Lengthy
   d. Brief

9. The "A" in the P-A-R approach for answering behavior-based interview questions is an abbreviation for:
   a. Always be punctual
   b. Action taken
   c. Act natural
   d. Avoid the question

10. All of the following interviewing tips may be used *except*:
    a. Bringing a bottle of water to offset dry mouth
    b. Practicing a firm handshake
    c. Asking for a moment to contemplate your answer
    d. Noting what you disliked about a previous employer

TECHNICIAN'S CORNER

1. Explain how remote monitoring is used in the acute care setting.
2. What four key issues do state boards of pharmacy consider when determining whether to allow remote monitoring, in terms of patient safety and how the technology is applied.
3. Describe two to three roles that pharmacists serve in a pharmacy benefits management company.

Bibliography

Bureau of Labor Statistics. (2011). *Occupational Outlook Handbook, 2010-11 Handbook*. Retrieved 10/16/2011, from United States Department of Labor—Bureau of Labor Statistics: http://www.bls.gov/oco/ocos325.htm

Fahrni, J. (2011, March 7). *The Role of the Pharmacy Technician in Pharmacy IT*. Retrieved 10/15/2011, from Talyst: http://talyst.com/2011/blogs/jerry-blogs/the-role-of-the-pharmacy-technician-in-pharmacy-it/

James Madison University. (2011). *How to Write a Resume*. Retrieved 8/16/2011, from http://www.jmu.edu/cap/resumes_cover/write_resume.htm

Mayo Clinic. (2010, November 10). *Radiopharmaceutical*. Retrieved 10/15/2011, from http://www.mayoclinic.com/health/drug-information/DR602307

McFadden, M. (2009, September 9). *New Remote Monitoring Technology Offers Round-the-Clock Care*. Retrieved 9/28/2011, from WNDU.com: http://www.wndu.com/mmm/headlines/58176697.html

Myers, C. (2011). *Opportunities and Challenges Related to Pharmacy Technicians in Supporting Optimal Pharmacy Practice Models in Health Systems*, American Journal of Health-System Pharmacy 68(12):1128-1136.

North Dakota State University (NDSU). (2010, January 15). *Telepharmacy [for Hospitals]*. Retrieved 9/29/2011, from http://www.ndsu.edu/telepharmacy/for_hospitals/

Parker, M. (2011). *What Are the Opportunities Available for Pharmacy Technicians?* Retrieved 10/15/2011, from http://www.ehow.com/list_6762048_opportunities-available-pharmacy-technicians_.html

Pharmaceuticalsaleshelp.com. (2005). *Pharmaceutical Sales Career Information*. Retrieved 10/14/2011, from http://www.pharmaceuticalsaleshelp.com/career.html

Texas State Board of Pharmacy. (2001). *Legislative Changes Affecting Your Practice: 77th Legislative Session.* Newsletter Vol. 25, No.3. Retrieved 9/2011, from Texas State Board of Pharmacy: http://www.tsbp.state. tx.us/Newsletter/Legislative77.htm

University of Arkansas College of Pharmacy—Nuclear Pharmacy. (2000, November). *Nuclear Pharmacy Technician Training Objectives.* Retrieved 10/15/2011, from http://nuclearpharmacy.uams.edu/resources/ Technicians.htm

University of Wisconsin-Eau Claire. (2008). *FAQs about Behavioral Interviews.* Retrieved 8/15/2011, from University of Wisconsin-Eau Claire Career Services: http://www.uwec.edu/career/online_library/ behavioral_int.htm

Young, D. (2006). *Telepharmacy Project Aids North Dakota's Rural Communities, American Journal of Health-System Pharmacy,* 63(19):1776-1780.

22

Identifying Quality Leadership and CQI Process Management in the Pharmacy Practice

Katrina Harper and LiAnne Webster

LEARNING OBJECTIVES

By the end of this chapter, students will be able to competently:

1. Differentiate the characteristics of an effective leader versus a manager.
2. Discuss key attributes that highly effective managers possess.
3. Discuss key opportunities for pharmacy technicians to fulfill management or supervisory roles.
4. Relate each of the steps of the successful change initiative.
5. Describe how medication errors occur as a result of faulty processes.
6. Relate how medication errors may occur throughout the medication order, fill, and dispensing processes and how they may be prevented.
7. Describe each of the steps of the continuous quality improvement (CQI) process, utilizing the methodologies of FOCUS-PDCA.

KEY TERMS

Leadership: Begins with setting a direction and developing a vision for the distant future.

Management: Determines what tasks must be performed and executes them consistently through planning, organization, and coordination.

Introduction

The advancement of quality in the practice of healthcare is paramount to any other goal or objective. Quality patient care optimizes the benefits that patients gain from their medical and pharmaceutical treatment. That increase in quality should lower expenditures by patients, who maintain better control of their wellness and management of disease states. The healthcare team must meet the challenges of providing quality care while seeking opportunities to either justify or lower costs for the services provided.

Pharmacy practice in particular is in a period of profound transition. In addition to providing innovative services and ensuring the effective delivery of the traditional stages of the medication use process, the industry faces the following challenges:

- An aging population
- Public reporting
- Government regulations
- Budget constraints
- Health care reform
- Technological advances

The role of the pharmacist has evolved from primarily dispensing medications to monitoring and managing drug therapy in collaboration with physicians and other providers. According to The Joint Commission of Pharmacy Practitioners' vision for pharmacy by the year 2015, pharmacists will be the health care professionals responsible for providing patient care that ensures optimal medication therapy outcomes.

As a result, pharmacy technicians are beginning to take on some of the technical aspects of the pharmacy practice and are playing an increasingly important role in the delivery of pharmacy services. Pharmacists will need the support of well-qualified, competent pharmacy technicians to ensure they can fulfill their evolving role. The expanding role of the pharmacy technician includes leadership, whether leading a practice, leading a shift, or leading a project.

There is a critical need for increasing quality among the ranks of pharmacy technicians across the United States. Disparities that exist among state boards of pharmacy in the regulation of pharmacy technicians create a quality gap, as there is no nationally recognized practice standard on which a pharmacy technician's performance can be measured. The advancement of the pharmacy technician career path must be leveraged with higher quality standards in light of the increased industry demands for quality patient care.

Recall from the previous chapter the various innovative roles for pharmacy technicians:
- Scheduling outpatient clinic drug therapy management visits
- Screening medical records to identify patients who may require pharmacist intervention
- Preparing clinical monitoring information (e.g., international normalized ratios) for pharmacist review
- Managing controlled substances systems
- Managing medication assistance programs
- Conducting aspects of quality improvement programs
- Managing pharmacy department information technology systems, including routine database management and billing systems
- Supervising other pharmacy technicians

Many of these positions may entail a supervisory or management role within a department of pharmacy, which creates excellent opportunities for advancement within the profession.

Although state boards of pharmacy may not yet have established standards for best practice for technicians, there are certainly standards of practice in existence on which pharmacy technicians may measure their effectiveness and value across the profession. Additionally, the nation's economy has driven many adults away from failing industries or those with a reduced workforce—and those individuals have sought out the stability of the allied health career path. These often seasoned professionals may bring valuable management and leadership skills, along with a fresh perspective on how best to increase quality in the pharmacy technician profession.

This chapter identifies several opportunities for increasing quality in the profession of pharmacy. Key focus areas include the following:
- Describing the characteristics of a quality leader or manager
- Discussing strategies that pharmacy technicians can employ on their way to pursuing leadership roles within their practice settings
- Examining processes involved with *continuous quality improvement* in the health-system pharmacy practice and the unique roles that pharmacy technicians may play
- Discussing how change—an often challenging aspect of continuous quality improvement—must be carefully approached within an organization and how effective leaders can gain the support of employees

Leadership versus Management

When a pharmacy technician considers whether he or she may be suited for positions of leadership in a present or future point of their careers, it is important to take a look at the characteristics that describe each position. The technician can then look introspectively at how those characteristics align with his or her own personal traits and strengths.

WHAT CHARACTERISTICS DESCRIBE A LEADER?

Although leadership and management must go hand in hand, the attributes that describe each role are not the same. Let's begin by examining the characteristics that define a leader in health care, such as a CEO of a hospital or health care organization. On the pharmacy level, that leader may be the director of pharmacy. The role of individuals in leadership is to do the following:
- Set quality standards
- Determine the direction of an organization
- Set the course that will take that organization in the direction that it needs to go.

An organization's mission and vision statements generally outline what leaders envision for the present and future of their organization. Leadership begins with setting a direction and developing a vision for the future. Leadership is strategic and looks to what *could be*. A leader's vision must be clear and effectively communicated to all individuals involved in accomplishing the goal or cause. The emphasis of a leadership team is to inspire and motivate; in this way the team ensures continued commitment to the vision and makes sure obstacles do not get in the way of achieving the set goals.

Although a leader may determine *what* an organization wishes to accomplish, a manager determines *how* the organization and its employees will accomplish its mission. Those in management positions determine what tasks must be performed and execute them consistently through planning, organization, and coordination. The role of management is to ensure things are done right, whereas the role of leadership is to do the right things. One of the most important *right things* that leaders must do is to recruit and surround themselves with highly effective managers who will help the organization to get where it wants to go through the combined efforts of every member of the organization.

WHAT CHARACTERISTICS DESCRIBE AN EFFECTIVE MANAGER?

Managers are generally given titled positions of authority and oversight of a functional area within an organization (such as the central pharmacy or outpatient pharmacy). The manager is also responsible for any employees who work in those functional areas. Some of that authority may be reasonably delegated to area supervisors, depending on their skills and abilities.

A management team must focus on the complexity of tasks involved with accomplishing various jobs and what steps should be taken to avert chaos and maintain order. Among the characteristics of an effective manager are the following:

- Strong communication skills
- Strong organizational skills
- Ability to delegate
- Ability to pair employees with jobs that fit their skills and abilities
- Strong conflict management skills
- Demonstration of strong work ethic and exemplary behavior (leading by example)
- Strong team-building and collaborative skills

These are just a few of the characteristics that an organization (and its employees) would seek in a manager.

DIGGING DEEPER

Aside from the management traits that were previously listed, there are several other characteristics associated with highly effective managers. A web article paraphrased key concepts from Alyssa Dver's "7 Habits of Highly Effective Product Managers" seminar. These concepts are equally applicable to anyone who is in, or wishes to pursue, a management role. They include the following:

- Know your limits. Have command of your expertise while deferring to those who know more than you do about other things.
- Listen first (get information before forming an opinion or making a decision).
- Ask "why," not "what." Doing so can actually help you to understand the situation.
- Be decisive. Although you may not have all of the information you would like to have, you can still make the best decision possible with the information you have at that time. This equates to confidence, which equates to credibility.
- Be responsive. Good managers are attentive, and that means being responsive.
- Communicate frequently.
- Manage passion. Dyer has noted that "Passion motivates you to execute, but passion is not execution. And without execution there is no success."

Think of each of these characteristics in terms of the relationship that exists between pharmacists and pharmacy technicians. Pharmacy technicians who fill supervisory roles must demonstrate these characteristics within the scope of technician practice. Interestingly, these are the types of traits that would be useful to cite in a personal mission statement, but be prepared to explain how these traits characterize your current or past workplace behavior.

TECH NOTE!
Pharmacy technicians interested in supervisory roles should take care to demonstrate that they have leadership qualities within the context of their role as a technician.

Leading Change

According to leadership and change management guru John Kotter, management promotes stability and copes with complexity as leaders press for and cope with change. The practice of pharmacy is in a constant state of change. Managing change is not enough. Change must be led as it is resisted. A leader must be able to guide followers through the change process effectively in order to be successful. Kotter developed an eight-step process that leads to successful change initiatives:

Area of Focus	Step	Lessons from Successes
Set the stage		
	1	Urgency
	2	Coalition
Decide what to do		
	3	Vision
Make it happen		
	4	Sharing vision
	5	Enabling action
	6	Short-term wins
	7	Hold gains
Make it stick		
	8	Anchor culture

STEP 1: URGENCY

The first step in leading change is to create a sense of urgency. A leader must help others see the immediate need for change and the consequences of not acting or moving toward the change initiative. A leader must convince others that standing still or remaining in one's comfort zone is not an acceptable option.

STEP 2: COALITION

The next step is to build a coalition of individuals who support the change initiative. This group of individuals, referred to as a guiding team, helps bring others on board with the new idea. The guiding team should consist of individuals who are influential, credible, and able to effectively communicate the sense of urgency to others.

STEP 3: VISION

The third step is to develop the change vision and strategy. The vision needs to give a clear and concise picture of what the change will look like once implemented to everyone who the change initiative will impact. The vision should also clarify how the future will differ from the past, as well as spark interest and motivation. Once the vision is decided, specific, detailed steps to achieve the vision should be determined.

STEP 4: SHARING VISION

The fourth step is to communicate the vision for buy-in. Every existing communication method, style, and perspective should be used to share the vision and strategy with all stakeholders and agents of change. The message should be delivered multiple times by various members of the guiding team whenever an opportunity presents itself.

STEP 5: ENABLING ACTION

The next step is to empower others to act on the vision. A leader must identify barriers that may hinder change and remove them so that anyone who wants to make the vision a reality can do so.

Key individuals should be released from existing responsibilities so they can concentrate on the new change initiative. It is frustrating for individuals who have accepted and bought into the shared vision of change to be unable to affect it by not having the time, money, resources, or support needed to succeed.

STEP 6: SHORT-TERM WINS

The following step in the "make it happen" phase is to produce short-term wins. Change can be a long process, and the sense of urgency and level of commitment can diminish over time. Successful change leaders actively plan and achieve short-term gains that people will be able to see and celebrate. These little victories prove to individuals that their efforts are not in vain, and long-term success is possible.

STEP 7: HOLD GAINS

The seventh step is to hold gains by not giving up. Once first successes have been achieved, leadership must continue to initiate change, even after the decided strategy has been modified, until the shared vision is a reality. Most change initiatives fail at this stage because victory has been declared too soon. Change leaders should not dismiss the possibility of regression and that individuals may fall back into their comfort zones. It is their role to keep the momentum for change moving until the vision has been achieved.

STEP 8: ANCHOR CULTURE

The eighth and final step for leading change is to make it stick by creating a new culture. The new behavior or process that has resulted from the change initiative must become the norm for the pharmacy. The now-incorporated vision should be hardwired into daily workflow or routines. It should simply be "the way things are done."

Leading Quality and Safety

As stated in Chapter 3, principle 8 of the Code of Ethics for Pharmacy Technicians refers to the core value of quality assurance that each pharmacy technician must possess. Quality is defined as the degree to which a product or service meets or exceeds a customer's requirements and expectations. Quality assurance (QA) refers to the certainty that products and services meet the requirements for quality. QA in the pharmaceutical industry is often associated with manufacturing and research. But the assurance of a high-quality product or service extends beyond the pharmaceutical industry to all facets of the pharmacy practice.

A pharmacy's customers—which may include patients, nurses, prescribers, administration, or shareholders—have various and sometimes conflicting requirements and expectations regarding an acceptable level of quality. These requirements and expectations include value, accuracy, speed, inventory availability, having their health questions answered, having their problems solved, and not being harmed. Of the many requirements and expectations of the customer, pharmacists and pharmacy technicians must ensure that patient safety is always the first priority. The ultimate goal of a pharmacy QA program is to promote medication safety by reducing errors and increasing performance. QA is a progressive process. Pharmacy personnel should continually seek to improve processes and systems. This concept is referred to as continuous quality improvement (CQI).

As their roles and responsibilities increase beyond traditional dispensing support, pharmacy technicians must be aware of the causes of medication errors as well as the ways to prevent them and reduce the risk that errors will occur. Technicians can work with pharmacists to implement process changes that lessen risk and improve patient care. In order to be a leader in identifying quality and safety practices, pharmacy technicians must first understand the significance of medication errors and realize that medication errors are due to system failures.

In 1999, the Institute of Medicine (IOM) issued a report titled "To Err Is Human: Building a Safer Health System." The report revealed that medical errors rank as the eighth leading cause

TECH ALERT!
Because pharmacy technicians are on the front line of most of the medication use processes, they are in the optimal position to provide an extra layer of medication safety, in addition to the layer of safety provided by the pharmacist.

of death, killing more Americans than motor vehicle accidents, breast cancer, or AIDS. The report also estimated that more than half of the medical errors occurring each year are preventable. As many as 98,000 Americans die each year as a result of preventable medical errors. The cost associated with these errors in lost income, disability, and healthcare expense is as much as $29 billion annually.

Many of these medical errors are associated with the use of medications. The IOM estimated that more than 7,000 deaths per year can be attributed to preventable medication errors alone; 700,000 emergency department visits and 120,000 hospitalizations are due to medication errors each year. In addition, preventable medication errors are estimated to increase hospital costs by about $3.5 billion nationwide.

An adverse drug event (ADE) can be defined as any injury resulting from the use of a medication. One potentially preventable ADE is a medication error. Specifically, a medication error is any preventable drug event that may cause or lead to inappropriate medication use or patient harm. A medication error that does not reach the patient is referred to as a near miss.

More than 10 years after the release of the IOM report, medication errors are still a serious health care problem. It is now estimated that 1.5 million Americans are injured or killed each year by medication errors. Currently, 3 billion prescriptions are dispensed annually in the United States; 82% of adults in the United States take at least one medication, and 29% take five or more medications. The percentage of medication use is likely to increase as a result of the aging of the American population, the development of new medications, the discovery of new uses for older medications, and the increased use of medications to prevent disease. Even with the growing percentage of prescriptions dispensed, there is no acceptable percentage of medication errors.

ADEs and medication errors can occur at any point in the medication use process. The medication use process consists of a series of complex events and comprises five steps:

1. Prescribing
2. Transcribing/documentation
3. Dispensing
4. Administration
5. Monitoring

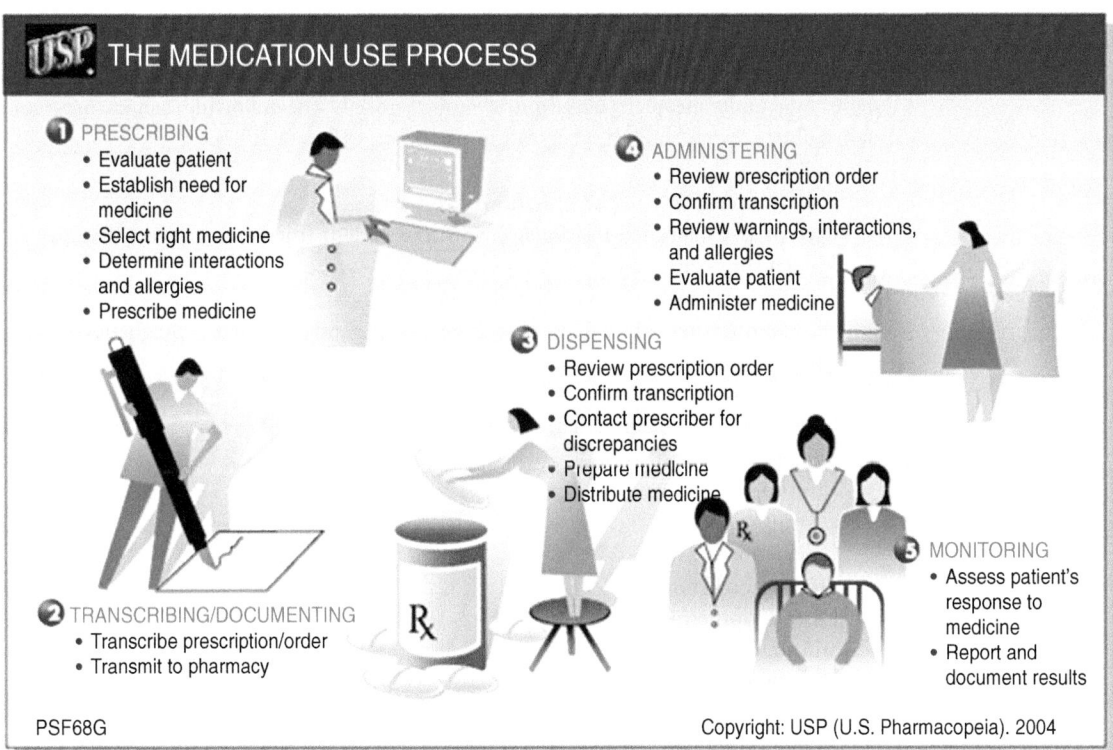

FIGURE 22-1 The medication use process. (Courtesy of USP [U.S. Pharmacopeia], © 2004.)

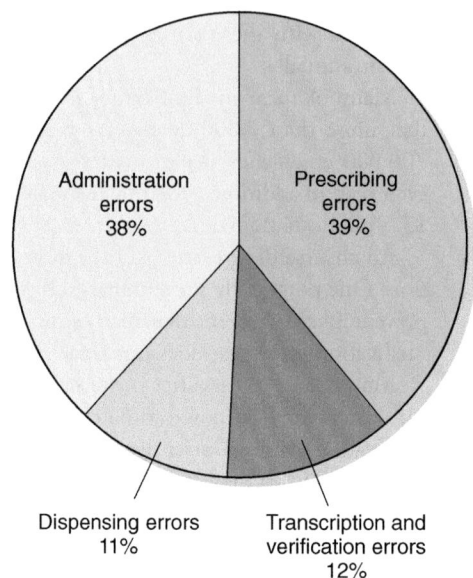

**Percentage of Medication Errors That Occur
at Each Stage of the Medication Use Process**

Administration
errors
38%

Prescribing
errors
39%

Dispensing errors
11%

Transcription and
verification errors
12%

FIGURE 22-2 Graphical representation of when medication errors occur.

"Mistakes are a fact of life. It's the response to the error that counts."
—Nikki Giovanni (American poet, 1943-)

Medication errors are caused by system or process flaws and conditions that lead people to make mistakes or fail to prevent them. Errors are inevitable, yet unacceptable. This notion may lead individuals to hide or cover up errors when they occur, rather than reporting them. A culture of safety must be established to allow individuals to work in an environment where people learn from errors, rather than an environment that blames and punishes the individual who made the mistake. A quality and safety leader should focus on redesigning the system to make it resistant to errors rather than focusing on the individual who made the error. Most medication errors are the result of faulty systems, not faulty people. Causation is multifactorial. The following factors may contribute to system failures throughout the medication use process (Figure 22-2):

1. Prescribing
   - Lack of knowledge of the prescribed drug
   - Lack of an established relationship with the patient (medication reconciliation)
   - Mental slips caused by distractions
   - Calculation errors (overdose, wrong route)
   - Misidentification of a patient (name, age, gender, weight, pregnancy/lactation status, allergies)
2. Transcribing/documentation
   - Inability to read illegible handwritten prescriptions
   - The use of abbreviations
   - Misusing leading and trailing zeros
3. Dispensing
   - Calculation errors
   - Preparation errors
   - Distribution errors
4. Administration
   - Five rights violated
   - Look-alike packaging
   - Failure to double-check
   - Failure to understand what the drug does
   - Unclear medication orders or directions
   - Understaffing

HOW PHARMACY TECHNICIANS CAN ACTIVELY ENGAGE IN QUALITY IMPROVEMENT

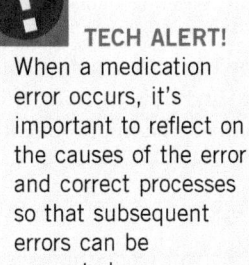

TECH ALERT!
When a medication error occurs, it's important to reflect on the causes of the error and correct processes so that subsequent errors can be prevented.

To lead for quality and safety, pharmacy technicians must know how to prevent or reduce the risk of errors occurring throughout the medication use process. The first step in error prevention is to be knowledgeable and proficient in the area in which you work. It is important for pharmacy technicians to be properly trained and up to date on CE requirements.

Pharmacy technicians should take pride and personal responsibility for the quality of the product or service they deliver. They should follow defined system-based processes, policies, and procedures. They must also inform the pharmacist whenever they have questions, concerns, or feel processes are ineffective or unmanageable. Despite the best individual efforts, medication errors may still occur as a result of system failures. When an error does occur, it is important to focus on improving the work habits that contributed to the error so that the same error will not happen again.

In addition to instituting individual behavioral changes when an error occurs, a systemic review of the factors that led to the error should be examined. Continuous quality improvement (CQI) activities drive significant and measurable improvements by reflecting on what factors contributed to the error, establishing what lessons can be learned, and implementing the lessons learned into practice to reduce the chance of medication error occurring again.

Many process improvement methodologies will achieve CQI results. One method is the use of root cause analysis (RCA) to identify the cause of an error. Another method is conducting a failure mode and effects analysis (FMEA), which proactively looks at risks within processes or systems. The most useful methodology for initiating a CQI project is the FOCUS-PDCA cycle, sometimes called the Deming or Shewhart cycle.

FOCUS

Find an improvement opportunity. Find an area of practice that is currently an issue or needs improvement.

Organize a team that understands the process. The team should consist of people directly involved in the process being improved.

Clarify current knowledge of the process. Collect data regarding the process using data collection tools such as a flowchart of the current procedure, and determine where the variances lie.

Understand the causes of variation in the process. Use a cause-and-effect diagram to determine why the process is not working effectively. If a new process is being implemented, the requirements should be determined.

Select the improvement that needs to take place. The team selects the most appropriate solution, keeping in mind the costs (financial as well as human) and difficulty of implementation.

PDCA

Plan the action aimed at the problem. Study the improvement opportunity, and develop a plan based on what needs to be done. Develop an action plan for how the process will be improved. Also, plan to collect data for monitoring the improvement and the change.

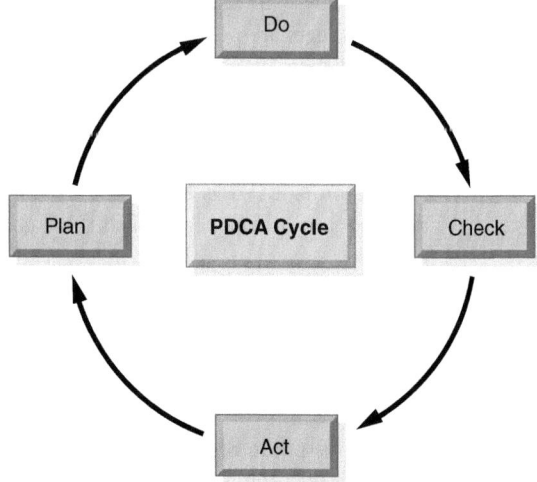

FIGURE 22-3 Plan-Do-Check-Act (PDCA) cycle.

_Do_ execute the plan. Implement the improvement and change, first as a test or pilot on a small scale.

Check the results of the plan to determine whether the plan worked. Evaluate the effect of the improvement and change through data collection and comparison with baseline data or data collected prior to the improvement.

Act to fully implement the plan and continue to improve. If the plan worked, write a policy and standardize the change. If it did not work, go back to the drawing board and try something else while going through the cycle again. Do whatever is necessary to maintain the improvement, such as add education and training, adjust policies, and so on.

Examples of Areas to Monitor for Improvement Opportunities

* Is a date of birth or an identifying piece of information obtained for the patient requesting every new prescription?
* Are complete demographics as well as information on allergies and health conditions obtained for each patient?
* Are patient profiles being accessed and verified using date of birth or some identifying piece of information other than the patient's name?
* Are the prescription data double-checked prior to submitting information and obtaining a label?
* Is the counting technician checking the prescription prior to sending it off for final verification?
* Are expiration dates checked and adjusted if necessary when filling prescriptions?
* Are outdated/expired medications being pulled from inventory?
* Is inventory being put away and rotated properly?
* Is an open-ended question used to verify that the correct patient is receiving the correct prescription?

Leading Yourself to Lead Others

In addition to developing others through teaching and training, a leader must always continue to develop him or herself, particularly in the following areas:
* Organization
* Prioritization
* Time management

A commitment to lifelong learning is one of the traits of a successful leader. Lifelong learning can be accomplished through formal education or courses, on-the-job training, participating in professional organizations, and mentorship.

Because _following_ is a voluntary activity, one does not have to have a title to lead. Sara White, an expert on pharmacy leadership, best illustrates the concept of "titleless leadership" by distinguishing between a "big L" leader versus a "little L" leader. A "big L" leader has a formal management position, such as pharmacy technician supervisor or lead technician. Every pharmacy technician has the ability to be a "little L" leader in his or her practice environment or during the technician's shift. "Little L" leaders are people who, regardless of their job titles, see opportunities to make positive changes and then take action to bring about those changes.

Chapter Summary

* A leader's main task is to identify the organization's goals, whereas a manager determines how the organization will accomplish those goals.
* Characteristics of an effective manager include the following:
  * Strong communication skills
  * Strong organizational skills
  * Ability to delegate
  * Ability to pair employees with jobs that fit their skills and abilities
  * Strong conflict management skills
  * Demonstration of a strong work ethic and exemplary behavior (leading by example)
  * Strong team-building and collaborative skills

- Characteristics of a highly effective manager include the following:
  - Ability to recognize his or her limits
  - Willingness to listening first
  - Tendency to ask "why," not "what"
  - Decisiveness
  - Responsiveness
  - Willingness to communicate frequently
  - Ability to manage passion
- Not only must change be managed, but leadership is required in order for the change process to be effective.
- John Kotter identified eight steps to successful change initiatives: urgency, coalition, vision, sharing vision, enabling action, short-term wins, hold gains, and anchor culture.
- The goal of a pharmacy's quality assurance program is to promote medication safety by reducing errors and increasing performance.
- The process of continuously seeking to improve processes and systems is referred to as continuous quality improvement (CQI).
- Most medical errors are associated with the use of medications; an adverse drug event (ADE) can be defined as any injury resulting from the use of a medication.
- A medication error is any preventable drug event that may cause or lead to inappropriate medication use or patient harm. A medication error that does not reach the patient is referred to as a near miss.
- The medication use process consists of five steps: prescribing, transcribing/documentation, dispensing, administration, monitoring.
- Pharmacy technicians can support quality improvement by adhering to defined system-based processes, policies, and procedures; following up with pharmacists whenever they have inquiries; and assessing and improving work habits/processes if a medication error occurs.

REVIEW QUESTIONS

Multiple Choice

1. An adverse drug event may be considered:
   a. Any injury resulting from the use of a medication
   b. A quality improvement process
   c. A preventable drug event that may cause or lead to inappropriate medication use or patient harm
   d. Unavoidable

2. The behavior of displaying professionalism at all times is a leader's demonstration of:
   a. Relationship building
   b. Leading by example
   c. Displaying authenticity
   d. Aligning people with their vision

3. A pharmacy manager's ability to show technician staff the immediate need to change from nonsterile to sterile gloves for increased infection control would demonstrate this step in the change management process:
   a. Coalition
   b. Urgency
   c. Vision
   d. Sharing vision

4. The steps that a pharmacy management team would take to formulate a picture of how the intravenous (IV) clean room will look and function following a large-scale renovation would demonstrate this step in the change management process:
   a. Vision
   b. Sharing vision
   c. Short-term wins
   d. Enabling action

5. A pharmacy manager's insistence that nursing staff members use the new automated dispensing cabinets instead of inappropriately reverting to an old habit of storing medication in their pockets demonstrates this step in the change management process:
   a. Short-term wins
   b. Enabling action
   c. Holding gains
   d. Anchoring culture

6. The inability to read and correctly decipher poor handwriting on a prescription may generate a medication error at this stage of the medication use process:
   a. Prescribing
   b. Transcribing
   c. Dispensing
   d. Administration

7. An error in the proper preparation of an oral solution by a pharmacy technician would result in a medication error at this stage of the medication use process:
   a. Prescribing
   b. Transcribing
   c. Dispensing
   d. Administration

8. As a means of preventing the occurrence of errors, pharmacy technicians' workplace skills should be evaluated for proficiency at least:
   a. Daily
   b. Weekly
   c. Monthly
   d. Annually

9. When an error does occur, it is important to focus on improving the work habits that contributed to the error so that the same error will not happen again:
   a. Communication
   b. Work habits
   c. Distractions
   d. The work of others

10. This step of the FOCUS quality improvement process involves assembling a team of individuals who are directly involved in the process that needs to be changed:
    a. Find
    b. Organization
    c. Clarify
    d. Understand

TECHNICIAN'S CORNER

1. Why is it important to identify barriers that may hinder the process of change?
2. How would you respond if a manager asked you to serve on a guiding team? What do you perceive your role would be?
3. How might a manager work toward empowering others to act on a vision that involves new change?

Bibliography

Blackburn, J. (2010). *A Technician's Role Optimizing Patient Safety and Minimizing Medication Errors: A Knowledge Based Course for Technicians*. Woodlands, TX: J&D Educational Services, Inc.

Hawn, C. (2007). *7 Habits of Highly Effective Managers*. Retrieved 5/31/2013, from http://gigaom.com/2007/10/18/7-habits-of-highly-effective-managers/

Health Notes. *Quality Assurance: Preventing Medication Errors*. California State Board of Pharmacy. http://pharmacy.ucsf.edu/ce/qa/qa.pdf

Kohn, L.T., Corrigan, J.M., Donaldson, M.S. (1999). *To Err Is Human: Building a Safer Health System.* Washington, DC: National Academy Press.

Kotter, J. (1995, March-April). *Leading Change: Why Transformation Efforts Fail. Harvard Business Review.*

Medication Error Reports, U.S. Food and Drug Administration. http://www.fda.gov/drugs/drugsafety/medicationerrors/ucm080629.htm

Permal-Wallag, M.S. *Safety Culture Chapter.* In *University of Michigan Health System Patient Safety Toolkit.* The Regents of the University of Michigan.

Preventing Medication Errors. Quality Chasm Series. http://www.nap.edu/catalog/11623.html

Quality Assurance Requirements. Oregon Board of Pharmacy. http://www.oregon.gov/ODOT/HWY/OPL/docs/QA/qa_guidebook.pdf?ga=t

USP. (2004). http://www.usp.org/pdf/EN/patientSafety/medicationUseProcess.pdf

Van den Bemt P.M., Egberts, T.C., de Jong-van den Berg, L.T., Brouwers, J.R. (2000). *Drug-Related Problems in Hospitalized Patients, Drug Safety,* 22(4).

White, S.J. (2006). *Leadership: Successful Alchemy, American Journal of Health-System Pharmacy,* 62:1497-1503.

23

Certification Review for Pharmacy Technicians

Michelle D. Remmerden

By the end of this chapter, students will be able to competently:

1. Explain the purpose and requirements for gaining professional credentialing as a pharmacy technician, including licensure, registration, and certification.

2. Describe the structure and content of the Pharmacy Technician Certification Exam, as prepared by the Pharmacy Technician Certification Board (PTCB), and the Institute for the Certification of Pharmacy Technicians' (ICPT) ExCPT exam.

3. Discuss strategies for preparing to perform successfully on a Pharmacy Technician Certification Examination.

4. Gain a better perspective of the structure and content of a certification exam by completing the 100-question practice certification exam provided at the end of the chapter.

KEY TERMS

Certification: A credential awarded to an individual who successfully passes a national certification exam.

Licensure: The process of gaining a license to work in a particular state as a pharmacy technician.

Registration: The process whereby a pharmacy technician is added to the public record on file with a particular state that affirms his or her legal eligibility to work within that job title.

Pharmacy Technician Credentialing: How Do Licensure, Registration, and Certification Differ?

Most states regulate the pharmacy technician practice by requiring some type of prerequisite knowledge or validation of skill to go with some type of work in the field. Some states require pharmacy technicians to be licensed, whereas other states have a registration process. In either case, an individual must provide documentation to prove that he or she has met the requirements to be eligible to work as a pharmacy technician in that particular state. Additionally, prospective pharmacy technicians may pursue national certification by taking a national certification exam. The terminology can be confusing, as one or more of the following titles seem to be used interchangeably:

- Licensed pharmacy technician
- Registered pharmacy technician
- Certified pharmacy technician

There is no single method by which a pharmacy technician can become eligible to work in the United States, as each state sets the requirements according to its own regulations. Some state requirements must be completed prior to working in the field, so it is important that individuals residing in those states prepare ahead of time and become familiar with those regulations. The material that follows provides a broad overview of the differences among licensure, registration, and certification.

LICENSED PHARMACY TECHNICIAN

Licensure is the process of gaining a license to work in a particular state as a pharmacy technician. Each state has a regulating body known as the board of pharmacy. For example, Florida's regulating body is known as the Florida Board of Pharmacy. As students learned in the law chapter of this text, each state board of pharmacy has the authority to write regulations and rules that pertain to all pharmacies within that state. The board of pharmacy is also in charge of issuing licenses for each pharmacy and pharmacist according to the state regulations. Increasingly, states are beginning to require that pharmacy technicians be granted licenses in order to perform the duties of a pharmacy technician.

The licensing process assures employers that each pharmacy technician has completed adequate education prior to his or her initial licensure, and it often provides a mechanism to require continuing education to renew existing licensure. Each state differs in the exact requirements to obtain a license, but, in addition to an application fee, requirements may include the following:

- Proof of a high school diploma or a general education development (GED) certificate
- Completion of a pharmacy technician training program
- Successful passing of a national certification exam

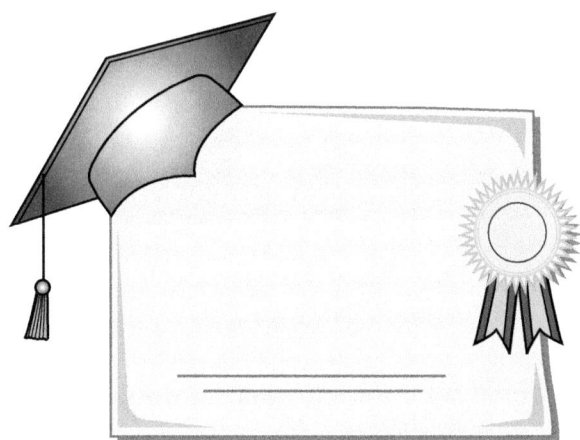

Generally, an online or hard-copy application must be completed, along with an application fee that is submitted to the designated state board of pharmacy. Some states also require the submission of fingerprints as part of the background check process. Following successful completion of the licensure process, a registrant may receive proof of registration via a certificate or wallet card in the mail. Some state boards of pharmacy require that the license certificate be displayed in the pharmacy where an individual is employed.

Individuals with a criminal history related to theft, drug use, or drug distribution may be disallowed from gaining registration. Misdemeanor offenses, such as driving while intoxicated (DWI), driving under the influence (DUI), public intoxication, or indecency, are generally evaluated and investigated on a case-by-case basis by state board compliance officers. Anyone who is unsure as to whether or not he or she is eligible for licensure should review content on the state board's website to gain a better understanding of the types of criminal history that are automatically disqualifying. For someone with a criminal history that includes offenses other than those listed earlier, it is best to simply apply and go through the compliance investigation process. It is also best to provide the state board with as much information as possible concerning the nature of the offense, along with any supporting documentation.

To determine the requirements of individual state boards of pharmacy, check out the board's website or call the office directly. The National Association of Boards of Pharmacy is a professional organization that oversees the state boards of pharmacy. Its website, www.NABP.net, provides a link to each state board of pharmacy's website. If a particular state requires pharmacy technicians to be licensed, the license must be kept current in order for the pharmacy technician to remain eligible to work. Licenses must be periodically renewed (usually every 2 years), and each state establishes a renewal schedule and a renewal fee. Often there is a requirement to complete a certain number of continuing education credits to be eligible for renewal. Continuing education requirements also vary from state to state.

REGISTERED PHARMACY TECHNICIAN

Registration is the process whereby a pharmacy technician is added to the public record on file with a particular state that affirms his or her legal eligibility to work within that job title. Pharmacies generally check on their pharmacist and technician staff registration status to verify eligibility to work, as the pharmacy could face fines for noncompliance. The registration process typically involves fewer requirements than the licensure process, and these requirements vary by state.

To register as a pharmacy technician, in addition to an application fee, an applicant may be required to do the following:

* Show proof of a high school diploma or GED certificate
* Provide proof of satisfactory work experience as a pharmacy technician trainee
* Complete a pharmacy technician training course or program

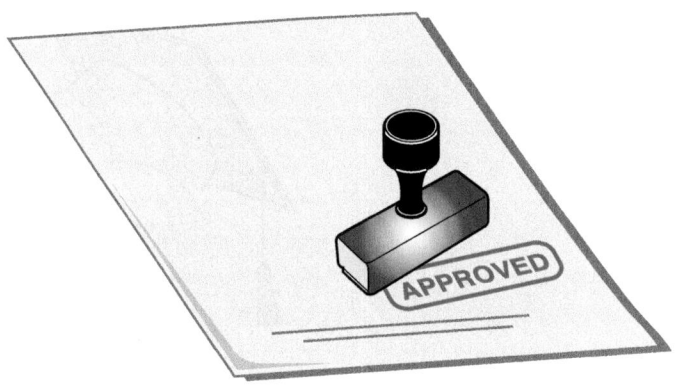

Following the successful completion of the registration process, a registrant may receive proof of registration via a certificate or wallet card in the mail. Some state boards of pharmacy require that the registration certificate be displayed in the pharmacy where an individual is employed.

Some states may also require national certification or accept national certification in lieu of a pharmacy technician training requirement. As with licensure, registration must be kept current and usually is renewed either annually or biannually. Most states require a renewal fee, and often there is a requirement to take a certain number of continuing education credits to be eligible to renew registration. Again, each state has its own rules, so it is up to each individual to gain an understanding of the requirements, not only for initial registration but for renewal as well.

CERTIFIED PHARMACY TECHNICIAN

Certification is a credential awarded to an individual who successfully passes a national certification exam. Typically, individuals attempt the national exam after completing a training course or after gaining experience in the field. In some cases, an employer will require national certification, meaning that employees have passed a national exam. In many states, the licensing or registration processes discussed here will include passing a national exam and becoming a certified pharmacy technician. Even if an employer or state regulations do not require certification, an individual may elect to voluntarily take this exam. The advantages of taking the certification exam include the following:

* Increases an individual's marketability when applying for pharmacy technician positions
* Usually increases entry-level pay for those who are certified versus those who are not

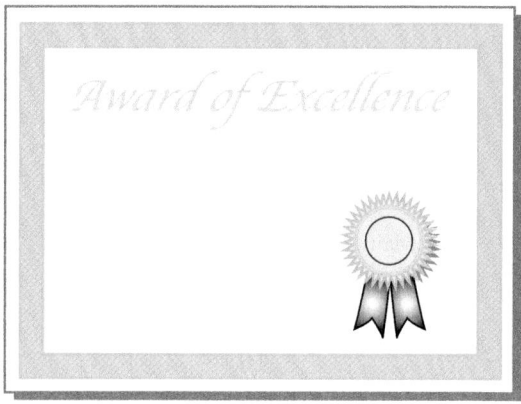

National certification exams are offered by either the Pharmacy Technician Certification Board (PTCB) or the National Institute for the Certification of Pharmacy Technicians, which is now part of the National Health Career Association (NHA). Both organizations offer national certification testing in all 50 states. The exams are known as the PTCE and the ExCPT, respectively. A few states only accept the PTCE for licensing or registration requirements, so it is important to review each state's board of pharmacy requirement. A table and map of the state's certification requirements are on the Pharmacy Technician Certification Board website at www.PTCB.org.

A nationally certified pharmacy technician is one who successfully passes either of the two exams identified earlier. Once pharmacy technicians are certified, they are able to add the credentials "CPhT" to the end of their name. This distinction is made to inform employers and representatives of the industry that you are a certified pharmacy technician. Certification also demonstrates to the public that the individual pharmacy technician has attained the necessary level of knowledge, skill, and experience in the field. Further, certification of pharmacy technicians assists pharmacists and state boards of pharmacy by upholding high quality standards to protect public safety. Thus, becoming a certified pharmacy technician is beneficial to the technician and the pharmacist and advances patient care and safety.

Following the successful passing of the certification examination, a certified pharmacy technician receives proof of certification via a certificate or wallet card in the mail. Some state boards of pharmacy require that the license certificate be displayed in the pharmacy where an individual is employed. Included with the certificate is information related to the scores that the examinee earned in each of the three sections of the designated examination, in addition to the final composite score. Those who do not pass the exam on their first attempt must wait a period of time before another exam attempt. Applicants must reapply and pay the full application fee for each subsequent exam attempt, and the examination may be attempted up to three times (both the PTCE and the ExCPT).

After gaining the certified pharmacy technician credential, there are continuing education requirements to keep certification active. Assuming that the pharmacy technician completes the renewal requirements, retesting is not required. If the pharmacy technician misses the renewal deadline or does not complete continuing education credits by the deadline, then retesting may be required. Pharmacy technicians certified by the Pharmacy Technician Certification Board (PTCB) must complete 20 hours of approved continuing education every 2 years as one of the requirements for certification renewal. The continuing education requirement for ExCPT is also 20 hours every 2 years for renewal. Generally, at least 1 hour of continuing education must be in pharmacy law.

Preparing for the Certification Examination

The PTCE is administered as part of the Pharmacy Technician Certification Board (PTCB; www.PTCB.org), and the ExCPT exam is administered as part of the National Health Career Association (www.nhanow.com). Each testing agency has eligibility requirements to take the exam, so please check out their websites to ensure you are ready and able to sit for the exam. The exams themselves are administered by approved professional testing centers. Applicants generally schedule the date and time to report to the testing center to take the examination.

Both of the exams have similar multiple-choice layouts with four possible answers and a 2-hour time limit; the PTCE currently consists of 90 questions and the ExCPT has 110 questions. For both tests, 10 questions from the total are not scored but evaluated for future exams. These 10 unscored questions are inserted randomly and are not otherwise distinguishable from the scored questions.

The following is an overview of the content areas of the two exams. The makeup of these exams may change, so for a more detailed comparison, please visit the websites of the respective testing bodies.

The exam content for the PTCE covers the following:
1. Assisting the pharmacist in serving patients (66% of exam)
2. Maintaining medication and inventory control systems (22% of exam)
3. Participating in the administration and management of pharmacy practice (12% of exam)

The exam content for the ExCPT covers the following:
1. Regulation and technician duties (25% of exam)
2. Drugs and drug products (23% of exam)
3. The dispensing process (52% of exam)

To successfully gain certification from the PTCE, the applicant must achieve a score of 650 points out of 900 possible points. For the ExCPT exam, the applicant must achieve a score of 390 points out of 500 possible points in order to pass. Both exams are scored immediately and a result is provided to the test taker once the exam is complete. Study materials are available for both exams. However, because the exams are administered by computer, using practice tests on the computer provides the best simulation of the actual test experience and thus provides the best preparation for most people.

Strategies for Success on Certification Examinations

It is important to keep the following points in mind when preparing physically and mentally for the certification examination:
- Don't rush through the test.
- Read each question in its entirety, including possible answers, *before* answering.
- Attempt to strategically pace yourself throughout the exam.
- Maintain breathing.
- Once finished with the exam, check all answers if allowed.
- Remember that calm, rational thinking will reduce the symptoms of test anxiety.
  For critical thinking questions, consider the following:
- Try to determine the answer without looking at the possible choices.
- If your answer is among the options available, it is likely the correct choice.
- Trust your instincts! Generally the first answer selected is the correct one.
  For mathematical questions, use the possible answers to your advantage, or at least to eliminate the incorrect answers:
- If a particular unit of measurement is listed in the answers, this will give you guidance on which direction to head in the problem or maybe what formula to use.
- Read each question carefully to identify what the question is asking and what information is most important. Questions are often loaded with distracters to assess a student's ability to pick out the most important information
- Use scratch paper or wipe boards to note any formulas or units of measurement from memory for easy recall during the exam.
  For questions you are not sure of, skip and come back:
- Other questions may help you answer the questions you skipped; it is best not to consume exam time agonizing over a particular question.
- Do not leave any questions unanswered: a guess has a 25% of being correct, whereas a blank response has a 100% chance of being marked as incorrect!
  Prepare your body before taking an exam:
- Get a good night's sleep.
- Don't overload on sugar or caffeine prior to the exam, as this may negatively impact recall.
- Eat a high-protein breakfast, and drink plenty of water.
- Wear something comfortable and appropriate for the weather—depending on the test center, outer coats or jackets may not be allowed in the testing area.

SHOW WHAT
YOU KNOW:
PRACTICE
CERTIFICATION
EXAM
QUESTIONS

Here are 100 sample questions. These questions are tailored to the PTCE but could also be seen on the ExCPT. They will not be in the exact wording or format of the actual exam, nor will they cover the same content, but they are offered as examples of what you might encounter. The answer key is provided at the end of the practice exam.

1. If a prescription calls for Flagyl 500 mg q8h for 7 days, and 0.25 g tablets are available, how many tablets should be dispensed for the 7 days?
   a. 21
   b. 14
   c. 22
   d. 42

2. Preparing oral medication into single-unit doses from a multiple-dose stock container is known as:
   a. Bulk compounding
   b. Parenteral admixture
   c. Prepackaging
   d. Supplemental

3. Which Drug Enforcement Administration (DEA) form should be used when disposing of expired controlled substances?
   a. DEA Form 41
   b. DEA Form 106
   c. DEA Form 222
   d. DEA Form 221

4. Which U.S. law required pharmacists to provide consulting services to Medicaid patients?
   a. Omnibus Budget Reconciliation Act
   b. Poison Control Act
   c. Occupational Safety and Health Act
   d. Durham-Humphrey Amendment

5. Which reference book would be used to find the average wholesale price (AWP) of a medication?
   a. Orange Book
   b. Red Book
   c. PDR
   d. Facts and Comparisons

6. A patient is to receive a TPN with 2400 ml over 24 hours. How many milliliters per minute will the patient receive?
   a. 100
   b. 6000
   c. 1.67
   d. 40.2

7. In which controlled substance schedule would you find Ritalin?
   a. Schedule II
   b. Schedule III
   c. Schedule IV
   d. Schedule V

8. A 100-ml piggyback is given over 60 minutes every 6 hours. If the first bag was given at 0900, when will the next bag be due?
   a. 1800
   b. 1500
   c. 2100
   d. 1000

9. Which of the following is an antineoplastic medication?
   a. Acyclovir
   b. Neurontin
   c. Cisplatin
   d. Requip

10. How much diluent is needed to prepare 250 ml of Heparin 100 units/ml from a concentrate of Heparin 5000 units/ml?
    a. 5 ml
    b. 225 ml
    c. 25 ml
    d. 245 ml

11. A prescription is received for 30 tablets of Coumadin 5 mg. The pharmacy's cost for 100 tablets of Coumadin 5 mg is $165.75. If the pharmacy charges a dispensing fee of $5 and a markup of 30% of cost, what would be billed to the insurance company after the patient paid a co-pay of $15?
    a. $54.64
    b. $39.73
    c. $69.64
    d. $64.64

12. A 6-year-old child that weighs 55 lbs is to receive Cephalexin. If the child dosing for Cephalexin is 50 mg/kg/day in two equally divided doses and the suspension concentration is 250 mg/5 ml, what amount of suspension would be needed for a dose?
    a. 25 ml
    b. 27.5 ml
    c. 12.5 ml
    d. 5 ml

13. When using a Class A balance:
    a. Can only weigh up to 120 mg
    b. Only has one pan, which is where the powder goes
    c. Left pan: the weights are placed; right pan: the powder is placed
    d. Left pan: the powder is placed; right pan: the weights are placed

14. What is the percentage concentration of a 1-mg/0.2-ml solution?
    a. 500%
    b. 0.5%
    c. 5%
    d. 0.005%

15. If a vancomycin vial is reconstituted to a concentration of 0.1 g/ml, what volume is needed to prepare a dose of 125 mg?
    a. 0.1 ml
    b. 1 ml
    c. 1.25 ml
    d. 125 ml

16. To compound 500 g of a hydrocortisone 2.5% cream, how much hydrocortisone is needed?
    a. 12.5 g
    b. 5 g
    c. 1.25 g
    d. 50 g

17. If the Food and Drug Administration (FDA) reports a shortage of ACE inhibitor agents, which of the following medications could be involved?
    a. Temazepam
    b. Enalapril
    c. Simvastatin
    d. Esomeprazole

18. What is the flow rate of a 1-liter bag of D_5W with 20 mEq of KCl if infused over 24 hours?
    a. 50 ml/hr
    b. 100 ml/hr
    c. 42 ml/hr
    d. 35 ml/hr

19. Which of the following medications is not available as an over-the-counter (OTC) product?
    a. Loratadine
    b. Omeprazole
    c. Ibuprofen
    d. Metformin

20. When preparing a unit dose of medication, all of the following information must be included on the container *except*:
    a. Lot number
    b. Expiration date
    c. Patient's name
    d. Manufacturer's name

21. Medication used to reduce gastric acid production is classified as a(n):
    a. Calcium channel blocker
    b. Benzodiazepine
    c. HMG-CoA reductase inhibitor
    d. Proton pump inhibitor

22. The Material Safety Data Sheets (MSDS) provide:
    a. Information concerning hazardous substances on hand
    b. A collection of monographs
    c. The USP and NF drug standards
    d. Pregnancy codes for medications

23. If a pharmacy technician needs 45 units of insulin, how much insulin is drawn out of a U100 insulin vial?
    a. 22.5 ml
    b. 0.45 ml
    c. 45 ml
    d. 0.225 ml

24. Which FDA recall class includes a product that may cause temporary but reversible adverse effects?
    a. Class I recall
    b. Class II recall
    c. Class III recall
    d. Class IV recall

25. An intravenous (IV) solution containing 25,000 units of heparin in 500 ml of D5W to be infused at a rate of 1,000 units/hr. How many drops per minute should be infused if the drop kit is 20 gtt/ml?
    a. 4 gtt/min
    b. 7 gtt/min
    c. 13 gtt/min
    d. 20 gtt/min

26. A handwritten prescription is received for hydralazine. It is difficult to tell from the handwriting whether the dose is 10 mg or 100 mg. As a pharmacy technician, what should you do?
    a. Ask the patient for clarification
    b. Use the 10-mg tablet to fill the order because it is the smaller dose
    c. Alert the pharmacist to contact the physician for clarification
    d. Assume the prescription refers to a 100-mg tablet because a trailing zero should not be used

27. _____ is an OTC medication that must be recorded in a book before it is sold to a customer.
    a. Acetaminophen
    b. Simethicone
    c. Aspirin
    d. Pseudoephedrine

28. A child who weighs 74 lbs and is 8 years old is prescribed Tylenol. Tylenol elixir comes as a concentration of 160 mg/5 ml. How many milliliters should the child receive for a dose if Clark's rule is used and the average adult dose is 650 mg every 6 hours?
    a. 10 ml
    b. 8 ml
    c. 13.5 ml
    d. 5 ml

29. Which class of medication does acyclovir belong to?
    a. Analgesic
    b. Antibiotic
    c. Antifungal
    d. Antiviral

30. How often should the inventory of controlled substances be noted?
    a. Weekly
    b. Twice a month
    c. Twice a year
    d. Every 2 years

31. In what proportions should a 25% ointment be mixed with white petrolatum (which has no active drug) to produce an 8% ointment?
    a. 17 parts of the 25% ointment and 8 parts white petrolatum
    b. 8 parts of the 25% ointment and 17 parts white petrolatum
    c. 25 parts of the 25% ointment and 17 parts white petrolatum
    d. 17 parts of the 25% ointment and 25 parts white petrolatum

32. Doxycycline is to tetracycline as cephalexin is to _____?
    a. Cephalosporin
    b. Macrolide
    c. Quinolone
    d. Penicillin

33. Which route of administration has the quickest onset of action?
    a. IM
    b. IV
    c. PO
    d. PR

34. An example of a drug with a sublingual dosage form is _____.
    a. Synthroid
    b. Warfarin
    c. Nitroglycerin
    d. Nortriptyline

35. In a DEA number, the first letter for a nurse practitioner or physician's assistant who can prescribe controlled substances would be _____?
    a. A
    b. B
    c. M
    d. X

36. What is the generic name for Augmentin?
    a. Piperacillin-tazobactam
    b. Amoxicillin-clavulanate
    c. Ampicillin-sulbactam
    d. Ticarcillin-clavulanate

37. An insurance company might reject a prescription for any of the following reasons *except*:
    a. One number missing in a National Drug Code (NDC) number
    b. Incorrect member number
    c. Coverage has expired
    d. A compound medication includes a legend drug

38. Which dosage form does not enter the digestive system?
    a. Oral tablet
    b. Suppository
    c. Oral capsule
    d. Enteric coated tablet

39. How many milligrams are in 150 ml of a 1:400 solution?
    a. 375 mg
    b. 0.375 mg
    c. 3.75 mg
    d. 37.5 mg

40. A federal program for individuals older than 65 years of age or individuals with certain diseases is known as:
    a. Medicaid
    b. Medicare
    c. Welfare
    d. Workers' compensation

41. A pharmacy receives an order for 0.5 L of 0.8% sodium chloride IV solution. The stock IV solutions are NS and 1/2NS. What amount of each solution is needed?
    a. 400 ml NS and 100 ml 1/2NS
    b. 100 ml NS and 400 ml 1/2NS
    c. 111 ml NS and 389 ml 1/2NS
    d. 389 ml NS and 111 ml 1/2NS

42. When stocking medication shelving, why is it important to rotate the product?
    a. To give more shelf space
    b. To prevent look-alike products
    c. To ensure medications with shorter expiration dates are used before medications with longer expiration dates
    d. To ensure medications are stocked in the correct spot

43. Amlodipine is what classification of medication?
    a. ACE inhibitor
    b. Beta-blocker
    c. Calcium channel blocker
    d. HMG-CoA reductase inhibitor

44. An intravenous solution is running at 150 mg per hour. The 100-ml IV bag has a concentration of 5 mg per milliliter. If 40 ml remain in the bag, how long will the current bag last?
    a. 80 minutes
    b. 60 minutes
    c. 90 minutes
    d. 30 minutes

45. If 15 g of hydrocortisone is mixed with Aquaphor to prepare a total of 500 g of ointment, what is the percentage strength?
    a. 33.3%
    b. 3%
    c. 30%
    d. 0.03%

46. A 2-g vial has a powder displacement of 0.5 ml. A pharmacy technician adds 9.5 ml to the vial for reconstitution. What will the concentration be after reconstitution?
    a. 2 mg/ml
    b. 20 mg/ml
    c. 200 mg/ml
    d. 2000 mg/ml

47. For which pregnancy rating would a drug be contraindicated for pregnant patients?
    a. A
    b. B
    c. C
    d. X

48. What flow rate should be run to achieve a dose of 0.25 mg/kg/minute for a patient weighing 187 lbs (assuming the IV solution has a concentration of 50 mg/ml)?
    a. 25.5 ml/hr
    b. 127.5 ml/hr
    c. 141.2 ml/hr
    d. 21.25 ml/hr

49. How often should a laminar hood be inspected and certified?
    a. Every 3 months
    b. Every 6 months
    c. Every 12 months
    d. Every 24 months

50. Which vitamin helps in blood clotting?
    a. Vitamin B_1
    b. Vitamin C
    c. Vitamin D
    d. Vitamin K

51. DAW stands for:
    a. Dose as weight
    b. Dispense at will
    c. Determine at window
    d. Dispense as written

52. Insulin is administered by what route?
    a. SC
    b. PO
    c. IM
    d. PR

53. Amoxicillin is to antibiotic as ibuprofen is to a(n):
    a. Diuretic
    b. Steroid
    c. NSAID
    d. Antifungal

54. A task that cannot be completed by a pharmacy technician is:
    a. Taking inventory
    b. Refilling a prescription
    c. Counseling patients
    d. Compounding medications

55. Which of the following medications is a controlled substance Schedule IV?
    a. Ambien
    b. Morphine
    c. Vasotec
    d. Pepcid

56. How many refills are allowed on a controlled substance Schedule IV prescription?
    a. 0
    b. 3
    c. 5
    d. 6

57. What amount of dextrose is delivered to a patient if 250 ml are received of a 2.5% dextrose solution?
    a. 500 mg
    b. 625 mg
    c. 5000 mg
    d. 6250 mg

58. Because of the acidic nature of fruit juices and colas, which type of antibiotic should not be taken with either of these fluids?
    a. Macrolides
    b. Penicillins
    c. Tetracyclines
    d. Sulfas

59. Aspirin is available in the form of 325-mg tablets. If 15 gr of aspirin are ordered for a dose, how many tablets must be dispensed?
    a. 1
    b. 2
    c. 3
    d. 4

60. A 143-lb patient is to receive clindamycin for 4 days. If the dosing is 25 mg/kg/day, how many total grams of clindamycin will the patient receive?
    a. 14.3 g
    b. 6.5 g
    c. 1.43 g
    d. 0.65 g

61. Interpret the sig: i gtt ad tid
    a. One drop in the right ear three times a day
    b. One drop in the left ear three time a day
    c. One drop in both ears three times a day
    d. One drop in the left eye three times a day

62. A pharmacy technician needs to prepare 250 ml of a 1:10 solution. If a 25% stock solution is available, how much of the concentrate is needed?
    a. 50 ml
    b. 100 ml
    c. 150 ml
    d. 200 ml

63. If a partial fill of a controlled substance C-II takes place, the remainder of the prescription must be filled within _____ hours of original fill?
    a. 12
    b. 24
    c. 36
    d. 72

64. Diazepam is a(n):
    a. Steroid
    b. Benzodiazepine
    c. Diuretic
    d. Anti-inflammatory

65. Which of the following needles has the largest diameter?
    a. 10 G
    b. 16 G
    c. 18 G
    d. 20 G

66. To prepare a D5 and 1/2NS 1L IV bag with 40 mEq of KCl, how many milliliters of a KCl vial with a concentration of 2 mEq/ml would be added to the bag?
    a. 2.5 ml
    b. 10 ml
    c. 20 ml
    d. 40 ml

67. A medication has an expiration date of 01/2015 printed on the bottle. When will the medication expire?
    a. 01/01/2015
    b. 01/31/2015
    c. 12/31/2014
    d. 02/01/2015

68. In a 7.5% dextrose solution, how much dextrose is in a 1-L bag?
    a. 7.5 g
    b. 75 g
    c. 750 g
    d. 7500 g

69. How much diluent is added to a 2-g vial to reconstitute to a concentration of 250 mg/ml? (Assume no powder volume.)
    a. 8 ml
    b. 10 ml
    c. 12 ml
    d. 15 ml

70. A prescription for NuvaRing is received. What is the maximum number of refills allowed?
    a. 3
    b. 5
    c. 9
    d. 12

71. A prescription for prednisone is as follows: 60 mg daily and reduce by 10 mg each day until finished. If prednisone 10-mg tablets are available, how many tablets are needed?
    a. 15
    b. 20
    c. 21
    d. 25

72. Which auxiliary label is needed for tetracycline?
    a. Take with food
    b. Avoid dairy products and antacids
    c. Avoid aspirin
    d. May cause drowsiness

73. If a laminar flow hood is turned off, it should not be used until it has been running for at least:
    a. 15 minutes
    b. 30 minutes
    c. 45 minutes
    d. 60 minutes

74. Licensing pharmacies, pharmacists, and pharmacy technicians are overseen by:
    a. ASHP
    b. USP
    c. State boards of pharmacy
    d. American Pharmaceutical Association

75. The Orange Book provides what type of information?
    a. AWP
    b. Pregnancy codes
    c. Investigational drugs
    d. Generic equivalents

76. What would be the last digit of this DEA number: AB620164?
    a. 2
    b. 4
    c. 6
    d. 8

77. HCTZ is an abbreviation for which drug?
    a. Hycodan
    b. Heparin
    c. Hydralazine
    d. Hydrochlorothiazide

78. A prescription is written for TobraDex ophthalmic suspension 2.5 ml. Assuming 15 gtt/ml, what is the day's supply?
    a. 5 days
    b. 9 days
    c. 12 days
    d. 15 days

79. What is the generic name for Cozaar?
    a. Verapamil
    b. Losartan
    c. Amoxicillin
    d. Latanoprost

80. Which auxiliary label is needed for warfarin?
    a. Take with food
    b. Avoid dairy products and antacids
    c. Avoid aspirin
    d. May cause drowsiness

81. If an adult dose is 500 mg, how much should a 55-lb child receive?
    a. 110 mg
    b. 83 mg
    c. 410 mg
    d. 183 mg

82. A medication used to reduce nausea or vomiting is called an:
    a. Antiemetic
    b. Antitussive
    c. Antipyretic
    d. Analgesic

83. Premarin belongs to which drug classification?
    a. Antibiotic
    b. Benzodiazepine
    c. Hormone
    d. Vitamin

84. Which form of medication has solid particles dispersed in liquid?
    a. Elixir
    b. Gel
    c. Lotion
    d. Suspension

85. How many times a day would a patient take a medication if it is prescribed q4h?
    a. 4
    b. 6
    c. 8
    d. 2

86. A 30-year-old patient who weighs 135 lbs has a BSA of $1.64m^2$. The chemotherapeutic medication, Mesna, has dosing of 240 mg/m^2. What dose of Mesna should this patient receive?
    a. 394 mg
    b. 146 mg
    c. 221 mg
    d. 439 mg

87. If a pharmacy technician had to prepare 60 capsules each containing 0.25 g of drug X, how much of drug X needs to be in stock?
    a. 60 g
    b. 15 g
    c. 250 g
    d. 25 g

88. What would 25°C be in °F?
    a. 17°F
    b. 50°F
    c. 107°F
    d. 77°F

89. Which regulatory agency would initiate a Class I recall on a prescription drug?
    a. FDA
    b. DEA
    c. OSHA
    d. TJC

90. According to The Joint Commission, the temperature of a medication refrigerator should be checked:
    a. Daily
    b. Weekly
    c. Biweekly
    d. Monthly

91. What DEA form is used for transferring drugs that have been loaned/borrowed between two pharmacies?
    a. DEA Form 41
    b. DEA Form 106
    c. DEA Form 222
    d. DEA Form 221

92. A maximum of 2 ml may be injected using the following route of administration:
    a. Intradermal
    b. Subcutaneous
    c. Sublingual
    d. Intravenous

93. Medicare Part _____ provides benefits for inpatient hospital stays and hospice care.
    a. A
    b. B
    c. C
    d. D

94. Medicare Part _____ provides benefits for regular preventive care, like visits to a physician's office.
    a. A
    b. B
    c. C
    d. D

95. Medicare Part _____ provides benefits for prescription drug expenses.
    a. A
    b. B
    c. C
    d. D

96. The area on an outpatient prescription where the name, strength, dosage form, and dispense quantity of medication prescribed is indicated is traditionally known as the:
    a. Inscription
    b. Signa
    c. Directions
    d. Superscription

97. A DAW code of _____ indicates that the prescriber does not authorize generic substitutions.
    a. 0
    b. 1
    c. 2
    d. 3

98. A DAW code of _____ indicates that the patient requested the brand name product only.
    a. 0
    b. 1
    c. 2
    d. 3

99. This oral dosage form should be held between the cheek and gum to slowly dissolve:
    a. Sublingual
    b. Intradermal
    c. Buccal
    d. Suboral

100. A maximum of 5 ml may be injected using the following route of administration:
    a. Intradermal
    b. Subcutaneous
    c. Intramuscular
    d. Intravenous

Answer Key for Practice Certification Exam Questions

1. D   2. C   3. A   4. A   5. B   6. C   7. A   8. B   9. C   10. D   11. A   12. C   13. D   14. B
15. C   16. A   17. B   18. C   19. D   20. C   21. D   22. A   23. B   24. B   25. B   26. C   27. D
28. A   29. D   30. D   31. B   32. A   33. B   34. C   35. C   36. B   37. D   38. B   39. A   40. B
41. D   42. C   43. C   44. A   45. B   46. C   47. D   48. A   49. B   50. D   51. D   52. A   53. C
54. C   55. A   56. C   57. D   58. B   59. C   60. B   61. A   62. B   63. D   64. B   65. A   66. C
67. B   68. B   69. A   70. D   71. C   72. B   73. B   74. C   75. D   76. C   77. D   78. B   79. B
80. C   81. D   82. A   83. C   84. D   85. B   86. A   87. B   88. D   89. A   90. A   91. C   92. B
93. A   94. B   95. D   96. A   97. B   98. C   99. C   100. C

Index

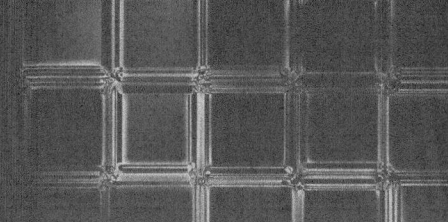

Page numbers followed by "f" indicate figures, "t" indicate tables, and "b" indicate boxes.